Level 5

Diploma in Leadership and Management for Adult Care

SECOND EDITION

The City & Guilds textbook

Tina Tilmouth

HODDER Education

AF621614

The Publishers would like to thank the following for permission to reproduce copyright material.

Text credits

Extracts from the Care Quality Commission's 'Key questions and quality', the Health and Social Care Act 2008 (Regulated Activities) Regulations 2014, reg 18 and NHS England 'What are integrated care systems?' are all used under the Open Government Licence v3.0; extract from Skills for Care and Skills for Health, 'Code of Conduct for Healthcare Support Workers and Adult Social Care Workers in England' (www.skillsforcare.org.uk/resources/documents/Support-for-leaders-and-managers/Managing-people/Code-of-conduct/Code-of-Conduct.pdf) is reproduced with kind permission from Skills for Care; extract from Dignity in Care, 'The 10 Dignity Do's', www.dignityincare.org.uk/About/The_10_Point_Dignity_Challenge/ is reproduced with kind permission from Dignity in Care; the NEWS2 scoring system is reproduced from Royal College of Physicians, the *National Early Warning Score (NEWS) 2: Standardising the assessment of acute-illness severity in the NHS*. Updated report of a working party. London: RCP, 2017.

Photo credits

p. 6 © John Wildgoose/Istock/Getty Images; p. 49 © Care Quality Commission, Enforcement Policy 2015; p. 157 © JPC-PROD/stock.adobe.com; p. 183 © Dorde/stock.adobe.com; p. 208 © PoppyPix/stock.adobe.com; p. 225 © Kali9/E+/Getty Images; p. 228 © Jacob Lund/stock.adobe.com; p. 232 © Jules Selmes/Hodder Education; p. 326 © B. BOISSONNET/BSIP SA/Alamy Stock Photo; p. 341 © Andrzej Tokarski/stock.adobe.com; p. 379 © Nirat Makjantuk/123RF.com; p. 393 © SDI Productions/Getty Images; p. 400 © Syda Productions/stock.adobe.com.

City & Guilds and the City & Guilds logo are trademarks of The City and Guilds of London Institute.

City & Guilds Logo © City & Guilds 2023

Although every effort has been made to ensure that website addresses are correct at time of going to press, Hodder Education cannot be held responsible for the content of any website mentioned in this book. It is sometimes possible to find a relocated web page by typing in the address of the home page for a website in the URL window of your browser.

Hachette UK's policy is to use papers that are natural, renewable and recyclable products and made from wood grown in well-managed forests and other controlled sources. The logging and manufacturing processes are expected to conform to the environmental regulations of the country of origin.

To order, please visit www.hoddereducation.com or contact Customer Service at education@hachette.co.uk / +44 (0)1235 827827.

ISBN: 978 1 3983 7933 6

© Tina Tilmouth 2024

First published in 2016 by
Hodder Education,
An Hachette UK Company
Carmelite House
50 Victoria Embankment
London EC4Y 0DZ

www.hoddereducation.com

The authorised representative in the EEA is Hachette Ireland, 8 Castlecourt Centre, Dublin 15, D15 XTP3, Ireland (email: info@hbgi.ie)

Impression number 10 9 8 7 6 5 4 3

Year 2028 2027 2026 2025

All rights reserved. Apart from any use permitted under UK copyright law, no part of this publication may be reproduced or transmitted in any form or by any means, electronic or mechanical, including photocopying and recording, or held within any information storage and retrieval system, without permission in writing from the publisher or under licence from the Copyright Licensing Agency Limited. Further details of such licences (for reprographic reproduction) may be obtained from the Copyright Licensing Agency Limited, www.cla.co.uk

Cover photo © Jade Maas/peopleimages.com - stock.adobe.com

Illustrations by Aptara, Inc

Typeset in India by Aptara, Inc

Printed and Bound in Great Britain by Bell & Bain Ltd, Glasgow

A catalogue record for this title is available from the British Library.

FSC www.fsc.org
MIX
Paper | Supporting responsible forestry
FSC™ C104740

Schools have a *Licence to Copy* one chapter or 5% for teaching
CLA Copyright Licensing Agency

Contents

How to use this book

This textbook covers all 21 mandatory units for the City & Guilds Level 5 Diploma in Leadership and Management for Adult Care.

Key features of the book

Learning outcomes: find out what you are going to cover in each unit. Learning outcomes and assessment criteria are clearly stated and fully mapped to the specification. Examples given in the topic sections are not intended to be an exhaustive or prescriptive list, but to provide guidance.

Getting started: a short activity or discussion to introduce you to the topic.

Key terms: understand important terms and concepts.

Reflect on it: learn to reflect on your own experiences, skills and practice, and develop the skills necessary to become a reflective practitioner.

Research it: enhance your understanding of topics with research-led activities encouraging you to explore an area in more detail.

Evidence opportunity: test your understanding of the assessment criteria, apply your knowledge and generate evidence.

Case studies: learn about real-life scenarios and think about issues you may face in the workplace.

Reflective exemplars: explore examples of reflective accounts tailored to the content of the unit and understand how you can write your own accounts.

Legislation: summaries of legislation relevant to the study of each unit. Legislation and guidance are frequently updated so it is important to stay up to date with the most recent and applicable versions.

Stretch and challenge: activities to help you to apply your skills in the workplace.

Useful resources and further reading: references to books, websites and other sources for further reading and research.

More information about adult care

You can find more information about this City & Guilds qualification and specification by searching for 'Level 5 Adult Care' or '3096' on the website: www.cityandguilds.com

Note: Those who use adult care services have been referred to as individuals.

Unit 500

Understanding leadership and management in adult care

GLH 30

About this unit

Effective team performance requires the development of a positive and supportive culture in an organisation. Only in this way can you expect staff to be supportive of a shared vision to meet the agreed objectives for an adult care setting. The most important person in your team will be the individual using the service and they need to be central to any teamworking.

This unit will introduce you to the roles of the manager and leader of teams in the adult care sector and the models of management and leadership that are relevant to this type of work. You will be encouraged to examine strategies of leading and managing teams in order to identify your own strengths, responsibilities and learning needs, and to reflect on best practice within the care context.

Your understanding of this unit should help you to develop your skills in leadership and management, your vision for the service you manage, and how to involve others in driving forward a strategy that will be successful for all those you care for and support in your setting.

The unit will help you to develop an understanding of the importance of leadership and management in ensuring the implementation of required policies and procedures, the development of existing and new strategies in service design and delivery, the management of quality outcomes, and ways to support and develop your teams in creating a shared vision for all.

As part of this unit, you will critically evaluate your own effectiveness as leader and manager, be aware of your strengths and areas for further development and learn how to adapt and apply your skill sets to varying needs, situations and circumstances within your role.

You will explore how theories and models of leadership and management practice apply in your practice, and how they can be used to overcome some of the barriers and challenges faced in a leadership and management role in adult care settings.

Learning outcomes

By the end of this unit you will:

1. Understand leadership management theories and styles.
2. Understand how coaching and mentoring can be used to complement leadership style.
3. Understand leadership and management in adult care services/settings.

Getting started

Before you study the unit, think about the following:

- How do leaders and managers differ in their practice?
- What do you consider to be the required qualities of a good leader and how could you justify whether you/others fulfil these qualities?
- What are the challenges to effective leadership and management?

LO1 Understand leadership management theories and styles

AC 1.1 Analyse the differences between leadership and management

Here, you will be required to define the terms leadership and management and analyse how they differ. You will also look at theories and styles of leadership.

The terms 'leadership' and 'management' are often used interchangeably but they are slightly different. Management is concerned with process and developing systems that relate to organisational aims and objectives and communicating those systems across the organisation. Leadership is about the behaviour and personal style of the person leading and their ability to influence others towards goals (Stewart, 1997).

In this section you will gain an understanding about the differences in leadership and management by looking at important terms related to the way in which organisations operate and add value to their purpose.

In trying to understand the differences between a leader and a manager it is useful first to address the vision and purpose of a setting.

Reflect on it

1.1 Identify vision and purpose

What is the purpose of the organisation for which you work? Think about what it does, how it operates and where it is going.

Having identified these things, think about who it was that delivered the vision. Who was it who said, for example, 'we are going to be the best adult care provider in the county?' Was it one person or a group of senior people who made that decision? Perhaps it was a team member? For the organisation to develop that vision to become a reality it will require the skills of both leaders and managers.

As you read through this book you will note that the terms 'leader' and 'manager' are used interchangeably; this is because it is quite hard to determine where one role ends and the other begins.

> *Leadership is more about change, inspiration, setting the purpose and direction, and building the enthusiasm, unity and 'staying-power' for the journey ahead. Management is less about change, and more about stability and making the best use of resources to get things done ... But here is the key point: leadership and management are not separate. And they are not necessarily done by different people. It's not a case of, 'You are either a manager or a leader'. Leadership and management overlap.*

Source: Scouller (2011)

The following headings show some of the areas in which leadership and/or management is required to ensure that a care provision is the best it can be.

Vision/direction

Leaders display an ability to influence and motivate their staff to contribute toward the success of the organisation. They have vision with respect to the mission and purpose of the organisation and this is translated into operational strategy that seeks to influence and inspire others.

Motivation of self and others

A transformational leader will motivate and inspire staff, gaining their loyalty by building confidence and ensuring that they buy into the vision. This is achieved by developing a solid operational strategy.

Operational strategy

Operational strategy involves the development of strategic initiatives and operational and resource plans. Leaders develop these plans by translating the vision into goals and values that inform processes, systems and people. Managers are tasked with delivering these measurable goals and processes.

Cascading the organisation's vision and its shared values is a crucial step to ensure that employees buy into organisational strategy. This is known as organisational alignment and is sometimes referred to as a '**golden thread**'.

KEY TERM

Golden thread: A description of how an organisation's goals, vision and values link together to inform its processes.

Organisation and co-ordination

The smooth running of any organisation is dependent upon the ability of a manager to ensure that all employees perform the work for which an organisation exists. They co-ordinate the processes required to ensure that the leaders' vision, mission and purpose is organised into tasks designed to meet the goals outlined in the operational plans.

Service representation

Working directly with the individuals using the service also provides useful feedback as to how the setting is working. Managers and leaders need to take this part of the work seriously, resolving complaints, answering questions and offering assistance.

Resource planning

Planning resources and staffing are part of the operations of an organisation, and this is largely a manager's responsibility. Drawing up a resource plan will ensure that resources are used in the most effective way, and in adult social care this will mean looking at material and staff resources. It is essential to allocate appropriate resources to provide facilities for individuals using the service. Financial planning and the ability to create and manage budgets is therefore a crucial part of the role of manager. As well as the materials to do the job, you also need to ensure that sufficient and qualified staff are part of your resource planning.

Improvement, innovation and change

Adult social care constantly changes as care services and national strategies evolve. Leaders need to scan the horizon for such changes and plan for them. Strategic decisions in response to a range of changing priorities must be made, as leaders steer organisations though daily challenges.

Such changes may require you to make improvements to the services offered and you can encourage your team to consider how to make processes better. This might be the opportunity to really make a difference to what you offer and to be creative about the way your setting is heading. Innovation is about looking at processes and rethinking them where possible.

Some organisations shy away from innovation as they deem it too risky or because it can lead to conflict with staff, but this might also be the difference between your setting gaining a reputation as 'the best in the county' because of its innovative approach to care or simply being a slightly shinier version of what it was before. Innovation is forward looking and requires leaders to ensure that staff are invested in changes that may initially seem challenging.

Decision making and accountability

Decisions must be made as to how an organisation is going to move forward to embrace change or whether it will simply make the minimum changes required to keep the organisation afloat. Managers may implement the changes, but it will be the leader who is **accountable** for any risks in taking the organisation forward.

KEY TERM

Accountability: Taking responsibility and being liable or answerable for something.

Contingency planning

When taking decisions that involve risk, drawing up a contingency plan allows for an alternative plan of action if needed. Identifying and managing threats to the organisation and taking steps to reduce the impact of incidents will enable you to minimise those risks.

Having a contingency plan in place will help to protect your organisation's reputation if things go wrong, as you can quickly take positive action to reduce the impact of any negative consequences. Day-to-day operations can continue with little or no impact on the individuals using the service.

Conflict resolution

Change in organisations can lead to resistance and conflict. Often, this arises out of misunderstandings and poor communication. The leader must understand this and adapt their communication methods accordingly.

Asking your team to contribute ideas to effect a change in the setting or to give you an update on something may be viewed by some as an opportunity to share their knowledge and skills, but others may interpret this as a problem with their performance.

Dealing with this sort of conflict requires effective communication. You should take time to think about how the staff will receive your message and how they will interpret the language you are using. What may seem a neutral or positive statement may be interpreted negatively by others.

Taking time to communicate clearly and to listen properly will prevent a change opportunity that would be great for your setting from spiralling into a conflict.

Conflict can be positive, however. If a debate ensues about what is changing, enabling your team to provide different points of view can lead to innovative solutions and new ideas. As a manager, it is important to support debate and not to stifle communication. Manage the debate as a positive force and an opportunity to learn.

Managing conflicting values and addressing difficulties

There are two types of conflict that are most common in a work setting:

- those that relate to disagreements on approaches to work
- those that stem from differences in personal values and beliefs.

Badly managed conflict leads to ineffective teamwork. People start to avoid each other, and rifts develop. This inevitably leads to ineffectual or poor care practice for individuals who use the service.

Reflect on it

1.1 Nature versus nurture?

Are leaders born or made? Having studied the requirements of running and managing an organisation, try to identify those things you do in your role as a manager and/or leader.

Evidence opportunity

1.1 Leadership and management skills

List all of the things you deem to be a leadership skill or a management skill. Then, investigate and analyse how they differ.

Leadership

Leadership is a trait that can be developed, and the view that leaders are born not made is fast losing its credibility. The Melbourne Business School's research in this area contends that everyone has leadership qualities that can be brought to the fore to make them a great leader and these are usually aspects of an individual's experience, personality and skills. By being aware of personal blind spots when it comes to managing staff and developing knowledge of what is holding us back, you can start to develop skills and attributes that good leaders possess. There is no single way to be a good leader; it will depend on the people with whom you work and how you interact and lead them. It is about knowing yourself and recognising your own skills and qualities.

Coaching and mentoring

Another role of a leader and manager is that of coaching and mentoring and this is covered later in this unit in learning outcome 2.

AC 1.2 Analyse key theories of leadership and management relevant to own role

In this section, you will be required to analyse theories and models of management and leadership, including the ones covered here.

Urwick's ten principles of management

Lyndall Urwick (1943) compiled a list of ten general principles for being an effective manager. These are detailed below.

- **Objective or the overall purpose of an organisation**: As a manager your objectives will reflect those of the organisation, and you will have to ensure that your team is working to meet them. This requires the team to be invested in what the organisation wants to achieve so your leadership to that end is crucial.
- **Specialisation**: This means one group having one function. Understanding the strengths and weaknesses of each member of staff means you can choose the right person for a situation or task. For example, more senior members of staff may be best to undertake training of newer members of staff.
- **Co-ordination**: This refers to organising the team to facilitate 'unity of effort'. Every effort in a team project needs to be co-ordinated and as a manager you must be able to organise this. Tasks and jobs will be done only if there is a clear co-ordinated plan of action, and all are aware of it.
- **Authority**: There should be a clear line of authority in every organised group. Although you have overall authority within the team, there are times when you may delegate this to a group member in order to get a job done. For example, you may delegate the training of staff to one member of the group who has the authority to book and organise training.
- **Responsibility**: Somebody must be accountable for the actions of subordinates. All team members are accountable for the jobs they do and the actions they take in the course of their duty. As a manager you need to make it clear that this is expected of staff and to explain clearly what that means in practice.
- **Definition**: All roles, jobs and relationships must be clearly defined. As a manager you should ensure that all job descriptions are up to date and clear.
- **Correspondence**: This demands that every position, responsibility and authority correspond with one another. Teamwork demands that every member is aware of what others do. This enables people to know how their role affects the work of others. For example, a care assistant may be responsible for stocking shelves with equipment and ensuring that supplies are available. If this is not carried out, then it has a direct effect on those who need the supplies and equipment and can make their job more difficult. Your managerial role is to see that all members of the team are aware of that effect.
- **Span of control**: No person should supervise more than five or six **line reports** whose work is **interlinked**. As a manager you should ensure that no staff member is overwhelmed by their duties or the number of staff they are responsible for.
- **Balance**: This is the requirement to maintain the units of an organisation in balance. Each part of the organisation can run well only when there is balance. If one team is not functioning well this will have a detrimental effect on others. For example, in residential care staff are often called upon to cover different roles. Shortages of domestic or catering staff may mean that

care assistants are required to undertake these roles alongside other duties.

- **Continuity**: This ensures that reorganisation is a continuous process and provision is made for it. As a manager you should ensure that when things are not working well and continuity in the service is disrupted for whatever reason, there is a contingency plan that can be put into place.

Source: Adapted from Urwick (1952)

KEY TERMS

Line reports: Members of staff who report to you.

Interlinked work: Work that is connected and has similar objectives.

Reflect on it

1.2 Urwick's ten principles

How do Urwick's ten principles fit with your experience of being a manager? Do they still work for you today or are they outdated? Undertake a professional discussion with your assessor covering the following points.

You may recognise some of the principles as being part of your role, so it is useful for you to take a critical look at what you do in each instance. For example, when analysing this theory you might ask why such principles are useful, if they are, and give examples from your own practice to demonstrate your understanding.

How can you demonstrate balance in your own workplace? What about co-ordination and authority? How do you ensure that this is part of the team function and how useful is it?

Write a short piece giving examples of your experience.

Trait theory

While Urwick's ten principles were developed for managers, Gordon Allport's trait theory (Allport and Odbert, 1936) is a leadership model which describes characteristics of good leaders. The idea that 'leaders are born rather than made' asserts that by identifying those characteristics in a person, it is possible to identify who might be an effective leader. On the other hand, behavioural theory suggests that leadership can be learned, and that people may be taught to display the appropriate behaviours. This theory assumes that 'leaders are made, not born. Some theorists argue that by learning to behave in a manner which makes you a 'good' leader, it is possible to become a good leader.

What do you think about trait theory? You might criticise it for being too general and subjective. For example, the belief that a person is born with certain traits and remains the same means that people are either born to leadership or not. If you do not have the traits identified in Allport's theory, this implies you will not be a good leader. Behavioural theory suggests the opposite – that we are able to learn how to lead and can develop the characteristics needed.

Behavioural theory

You will now look at four different behavioural leadership theories that were developed between the 1930s and 1970s:

- Kurt Lewin's leadership styles
- Ohio State University leadership studies
- University of Michigan leadership studies
- Blake and Mouton's managerial grid.

Lewin's leadership styles

In 1939, Kurt Lewin described leadership styles and, although somewhat dated, they remain relevant to team leadership and management today. He identified three very different leadership styles (Lewin et al., 1939). You may be familiar with the terms **authoritarian**, **democratic** and **laissez faire** applied to styles of leadership. The traits of these styles and their advantages and disadvantages are as follows:

Autocratic/authoritarian or 'I want you to ...'

- The leader/manager makes decisions on their own without consulting the team. They expect the team to follow the decision exactly.
- The task is to be accomplished in the least amount of time possible.
- Instructions must be clear and concise.
- Team members may become dissatisfied when they have ideas but are unable to voice them.
- Team members are not consulted on decisions being made. This can make them feel less involved and their commitment to the task is likely to be lukewarm.
- This type of leadership is good in situations requiring immediate or emergency action – for example, in an emergency department or crisis situation when decisions have to be made quickly.

Democratic/participative or 'Let's work together to solve this'

- Involving the team in the decision-making process leads to team members feeling they have ownership of the task.

- This style is democratic and is the most popular style of leadership.
- A drawback is that teams are made up of individuals with vastly different opinions and decision making can therefore be a lengthy process. The leader must be prepared to make the final decision in a collaborative way.

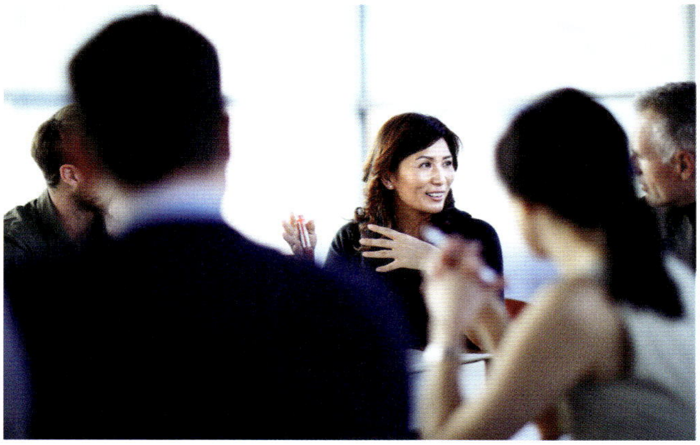

▲ **Figure 1** A collaborative leader values participation from employees

Laissez faire or 'You two take care of the problem while I go'

- Team members are enabled to make their own decisions and get on with tasks.
- This works well when people are capable and motivated to make their own decisions.
- A problem with this style is the tendency for people to go off task, with the result that the outcome is never achieved. It may lead to the team becoming impatient with the amount of time it takes to make a decision.

> **KEY TERMS**
>
> **Authoritarian**: Having total authority and control over decision making; keeping everything under close scrutiny.
>
> **Democratic**: Sharing type of leadership in which employees' participation in the decision making is favoured.
>
> **Laissez faire**: Leadership style that favours leaving things to take their own course, without interference.

Ohio State University leadership studies

Lewin's trait theory was still dominant in the 1940s when researchers at Ohio State University started to look at leadership behaviours and how they affected leadership performance. Two categories emerged:

- Initiating structure are leadership behaviours which aim to create clarity and structure for an organisation. When there are high levels of initiating-structure behaviour, employees have their roles, tasks and expectations clearly defined with little uncertainty about what needs to be done. The leader takes all decisions and punishes poor performance. This type of leadership is results driven.
- Consideration behaviour focuses on relationships and the welfare of people. A high consideration behaviour engenders an ethos of trust and interest in staff and a willingness to create warm relationships within the team. A leader with high consideration behaviour is an active listener who understands the strengths and weaknesses of each team member.

Further research suggested the most effective leaders display high consideration behaviour and a high initiating structure at the same time and that leadership can be learned.

University of Michigan leadership studies

In the 1950s, the University of Michigan leadership studies identified behaviours common to the most effective leaders, which would lead to increased job satisfaction among workers and improved productivity. They found two categories of leadership behaviours: task-oriented and employee-oriented. Although both could deliver excellent performance, the behaviours are mutually exclusive, and a leader cannot display both types of behaviours.

The studies suggested that leaders who are employee-oriented and provide general supervision of workers are more likely to obtain favourable results than leaders who are production-oriented and who opt for direct supervision of workers. However, a criticism of the approach is that the studies did not consider all situations and types of organisations, leaders and employees.

Blake and Mouton managerial grid

The Blake and Mouton managerial grid is a behavioural leadership model developed in the 1960s by Robert Blake and Jane Mouton. The grid is a visual aid enabling leaders to assess which leadership style they use, according to their levels of concern for people versus production.

Five management styles are plotted on a graph, where the y-axis shows the leader's level of Concern for People, and the x-axis shows the leader's Concern for Results.

The management styles are as follows:

- **Impoverished management**: There is little concern for production and little concern for people. This manager only does the minimum required to avoid being fired and this results in a disorganised team that is often unhappy.
- **Country club management**: The manager shows excellent concern for people but low concern for production, so staff are happy but they do not do much work.
- **Produce-or-perish management**: Also known as authority-compliance or authority-obedience,

this type of management is high on production and low on concern for people. This leader gives orders and directs people but does little to care for them, believing that performance is what matters. This style leads to a toxic environment with unhappy people resulting in a high turnover of staff.

- **Middle-of-the-road management**: Also known as organisation management, this shows a balance of concern for people and production. It results in less than maximum output, but better situations for the staff.
- **Team management**: This type of management shows great concern for both people and production and is the most effective leadership style of the Blake and Mouton Managerial Grid Theory. The concern for people results in a great team climate, with committed, engaged and empowered staff.

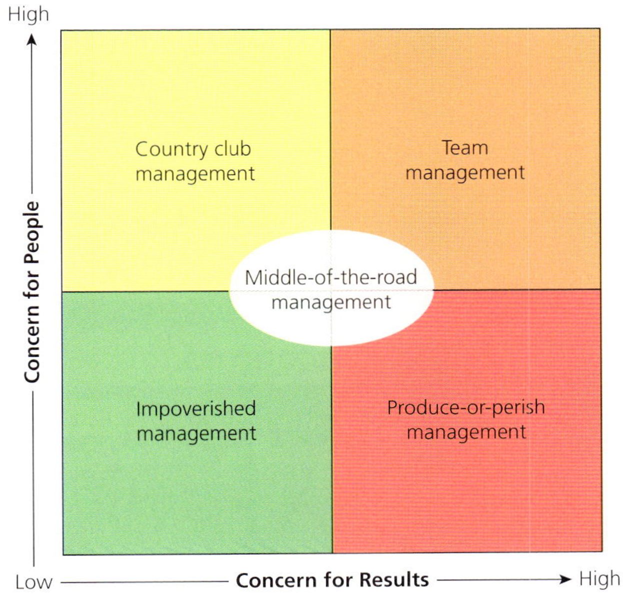

▲ **Figure 2** Blake and Mouton's managerial grid

Goleman's leadership styles and emotional intelligence (EI)

Daniel Goleman (1995) stated that emotional intelligence is:

> *the capacity for recognising our own feelings and those of others for motivating ourselves, for managing emotions well in ourselves as well as others.*
>
> Source: Goleman (1995) p.137

For Goleman, self-awareness is about knowing our own emotions and recognising those feelings as they happen. So, you may feel angry at something somebody has said, but as a manager and leader, showing that anger inappropriately will have a negative effect on relationships.

Social awareness refers to the empathy and concern you have for others' feelings and the acknowledgement that people under threat in an organisation may show aggression and anger. Decisions affecting people's jobs may have to be made and a manager who sees only the task at hand is failing to acknowledge the effect this is having on those at risk and those who have to continue to work in such a climate of change.

Relationship management is the ability to handle relationships competently in order to best deal with conflict, and to develop collaboration in the workforce.

Finally, Goleman refers to motivation, particularly your own motivation, to enable the workforce to meet an organisation's goals.

In a management situation your awareness of the impact of your actions and responses can go a long way towards defusing situations that might be potentially threatening. You may not be feeling very happy or friendly towards the other person but being in a position of authority demands that you have an awareness of the feelings of others. A good manager has a level of **emotional intelligence** (EI).

EI as a theory has been criticised for being unscientific; some writers question how we can accurately measure the traits of 'emotional stability', 'agreeableness', 'extraversion' and 'conscientiousness', which are often referred to in the theory. Self-report personality-based questionnaires can be falsified (were you truly honest the last time you completed a questionnaire in a magazine?) so the measurement is potentially flawed.

KEY TERM

Emotional intelligence: Being aware of and having the ability to control your emotions in order to manage interpersonal relationships empathetically (i.e. thinking about and understanding how others are feeling and seeing things from their point of view).

However, Goleman's research did show that leaders with EI performed better than those who did not have this ability. He also suggested that EI in leaders was more useful than just having technical expertise or a high IQ.

Maslow's hierarchy of needs

Abraham Maslow's (1908–70) work has been influential in many disciplines and you may be aware of his hierarchy of needs theory, which outlined the things that contribute to a person's wellbeing (see Figure 3). According to this theory, we are motivated by unsatisfied needs. For example, our physiological need for food and water, once satisfied, is no longer a motivator and leaves us free to pursue the next level in the hierarchy, that of safety and security, and so on. The theory has been used in social care settings, when managers have recognised the impact that motivation has on workplace success. The biggest and most expensive resource in any organisation is its employees and therefore motivation theory has become a valuable tool for managers.

Criticisms of Maslow's theory (and other theories of motivation) include the lack of empirical research to support its conclusions, the assumption that all employees are alike and will therefore respond in similar ways, and that all situations are alike. Another criticism is the assumption that the lower needs must be satisfied before a person can reach self-actualisation. For example, there are cultures in which large numbers of people live in poverty, but they may still be capable of higher order needs such as love and belongingness. Also, history tells us of many creative people, such as authors and artists, who manage to reach their potential despite living an impoverished life.

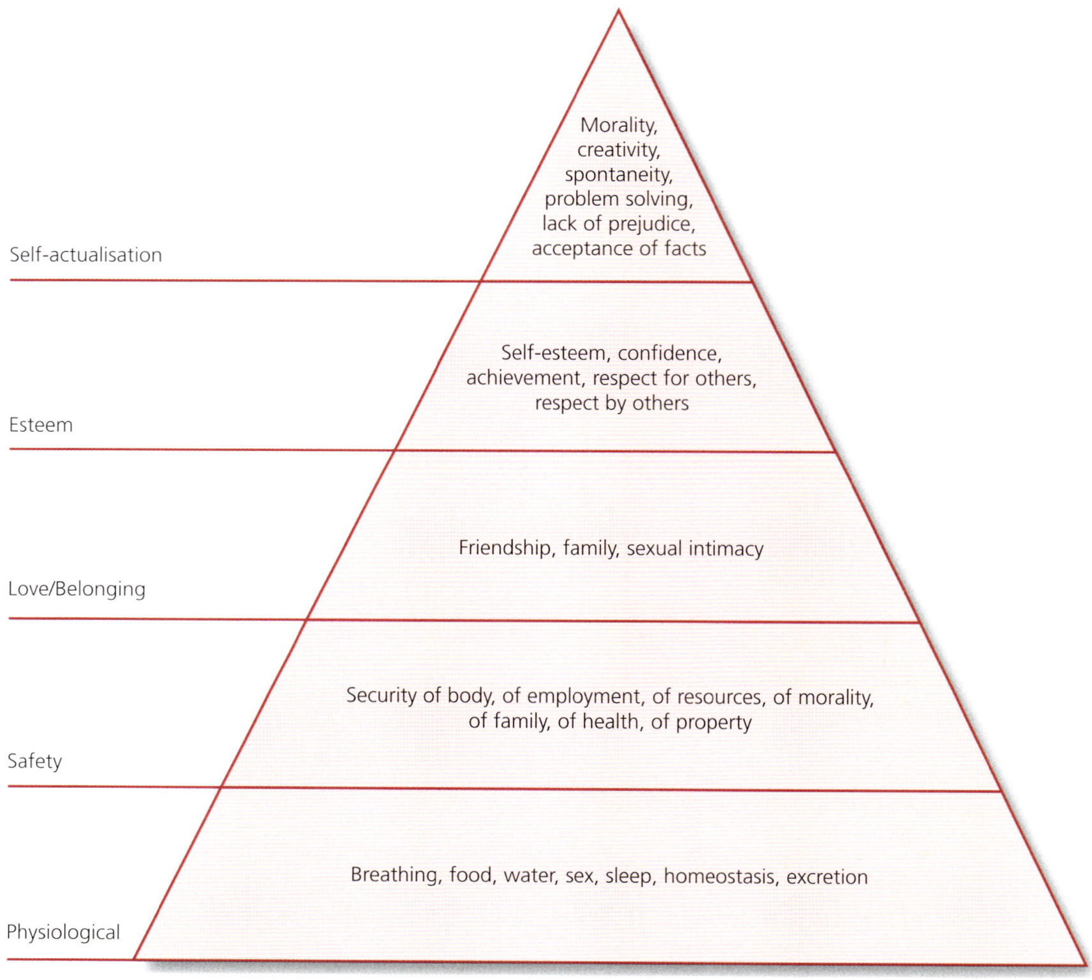

Figure 3 Maslow's hierarchy of needs

Case study

1.1 Managing difficult situations

A member of staff has recently undergone a traumatic separation from her husband. She has three small children and is struggling to make ends meet. She finds it difficult to get to work on time and has been late a number of times recently. You know she does not have family to help her get the children to school.

When you ask to see her to try to resolve some of her issues, she is aggressive and quite rude. This has made you feel angry, particularly as you are trying to come up with a solution. However, fighting anger with anger does not work and you need to consider how you might approach this problem in a different manner.

How might you deal with this situation? Perhaps you might empathise with the staff member's plight and ask her how she can see a way forward. It is likely she has been unable to take time out to note the decline in her work or her lateness. You could suggest a change in hours to help her to get to work on time, or a reduction in her hours of work until she can settle her children into a more favourable routine. Perhaps she might work the same number of hours but at times when the children are at school.

The way you deal with this situation will have an effect on the whole workforce.

What do you think are the main issues in this case study? For example, how would you deal with your anger and your staff member's aggression to resolve the situation? How would emotional intelligence help here?

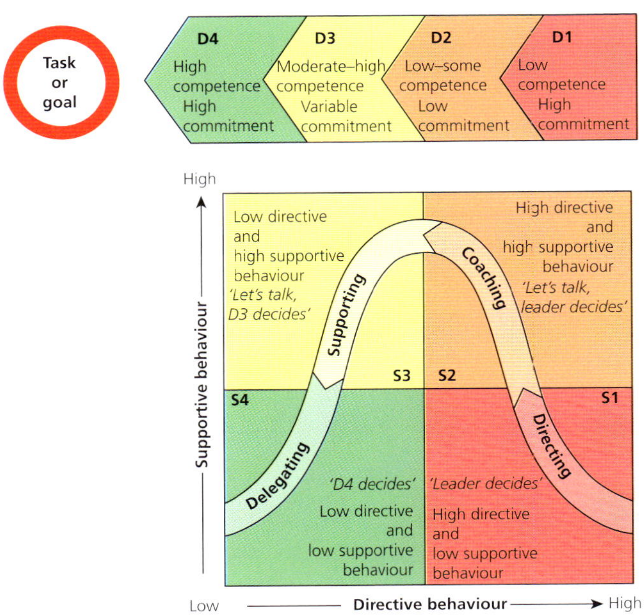

▲ **Figure 4** The organisation's situational self-leadership model

Hersey and Blanchard's Situational leadership theory

Situational leadership theory, devised by Paul Hersey and Ken Blanchard, describes leadership as being led by the situation that is presented to you and adapting the leadership style to that situation. This approach depends upon the leader having the ability to adapt to the task in hand by evaluating the competence and commitment of the workforce to accomplish that task (Northouse, 2018). For example, if during your daily routine an emergency were to arise, situational leadership would require you to adapt to this and you would have to decide at that moment the best course of action. To be a situational leader requires an ability to adjust according to what is happening.

Situational leadership further classifies leadership style into four different behaviours of the leader, which are shown in Figure 4. The leadership behaviours, directing and supporting, can be shown to be high or low.

- The team receiving instructions and carrying them out is the High Directive–Low Supportive function (S1).
- The leader handing over control to the workforce but facilitating their development to help them to achieve the goal is the High Supportive–Low Directive approach (S3).

Research it

1.2 Situational theory

Research Hersey and Blanchard's situational theory. Show how the S2 High Directive–High Supportive style and the S4 Low Directive–Low Supportive style of management of tasks might work in your workplace.

Read more about this on the Leadership-central website (Leadership-central.com, n.d.).

Kouzes and Posner – the leadership challenge

Contingency theories put forward the view that situations lend themselves to different styles of leadership and that the team leader's flexibility to adapt in response to those situations is key (Fiedler, 1967; Martin et al., 2010; McKibbon et al., 2008). Successful outcomes in this respect depend on the leader adopting a style based on several variables, including the job in hand, the qualities of those in the team and the context in which the team is working.

James Kouzes and Barry Posner's (2003) Leadership Challenge model, based on Fred Fiedler's theory, identifies 'Five Practices of Exemplary Leadership':

1. **Modelling the way**: Leaders create incremental objectives so the team can experience win-wins on the way to achieving the larger goal. Standards of excellence are established and the leader models outstanding behaviours.
2. **Inspiring a shared vision**: This enables leaders to create a better future that their teams are also excited about.
3. **Challenging the process**: Innovative ways, experimentation and calculated risk taking become part of the process. This may be uncomfortable as mistakes will happen, but it is part of growth.
4. **Enabling others to act**: Leaders empower their teams and make them feel valued and confident. Building a culture of trust will lead to team cohesion.
5. **Encouraging the heart**: This means celebrating success and recognising the team's input as well as sharing rewards with the team to shows how they are valued.

KEY TERM

Contingency theories: A theory that suggests there is no single best style of leadership; the leader's effectiveness will depend on the situation.

Character traits generally associated with good leaders:

- honest
- inspiring
- forward-looking
- competent
- intelligent
- dominant
- consciousness
- enthusiastic
- sense of humour
- integrity
- courageous
- visionary.

The bottom line is that good leaders and managers are able to generate enthusiasm and commitment in others. They lead by example with consistent values and break down barriers which stand in the way of achievement. Kouzes and Posner (2003, in Tilmouth et al., 2011) argue that a good leader:

- will also inspire a shared vision and enlist the commitment of others
- will promote collaborative working, which builds trust and empowers others
- recognises others' achievements and celebrates accomplishments.

Management by wandering around (MBWA)

In this style of management, the manager sets aside time to walk through their departments to make themselves visible and available to staff. They see the problems staff face and have time to listen to concerns. This is the sort of manager who operates an 'open door' policy. This means that you do not have to make an appointment to see the manager; you simply go to them when you need to.

Reflect on it

1.2 Unpopular decisions

Some decisions may be unpopular and yet as a manager you are asked to ensure that they are followed. How might you do this? What if you believe a decision to be a bad one? How will you motivate staff to undertake the unpopular outcome?

In their book *A Passion for Excellence* (1985), Tom Peters and Nancy Austin stated that as leaders and managers wander about, three things should be going on:

- Managers should be listening to what people are saying.
- They should be using the opportunity to transmit the organisation's values.
- They should be able to give people on-the-spot help.

This theory seems to have much to commend it, but do you have the time to 'wander around'? Some managers may work for care providers that operate outreach services, so staff are employed in individuals' own homes or in the community. It would require a general rethink of how you use your time to facilitate this way of working.

Power and empowerment

Dimensions and sources of power

In most organisations, there will be people who have more power than others simply because they are in a higher position in a hierarchy. This power can be used in a positive way, but often the concept of power suggests negative connotations of abuse and harassment and this kind of thinking can lead us to distrust anybody who is in a position of power. In this way, power can be perceived as influencing or controlling somebody in a negative way.

If you are the manager in a work setting, you are already in a position of power. You may have recruited the people you manage. You have influence and authority over those people.

Reflecting on power

It is useful to consider the power you hold in your position and to reflect on how you use it. For example, do you get a sense that people in your employ are wary of you? Could this be because of the way they perceive you? Do they think you try to control them? Or perhaps you do not exercise your power at all and find that maybe the team take you for granted and often fail to deliver on deadlines?

Defining empowerment

Empowerment is 'a process by which people, organisations and communities gain mastery over their affairs' (Rappaport, 1987) and in order to do this, individuals need to have more control over what they are doing and should be encouraged to work autonomously.

Leadership in this instance is not about control and making decisions on behalf of staff but is more about empowering staff to lead on ideas and innovations to make the workplace more efficient. This approach links in with motivation theories (such as Maslow's theory, see pages 7 and 8) but this is not an easy approach to take.

Essentially, the leader refrains from directing the staff and telling them what to do and how to do it. Rather, they enable the team to do it on their own. They give staff the problem to solve and then enable them to work through solutions without stepping in and giving the answers. Staff should feel more motivated when they work in this way.

Care and control

Empowering staff means relinquishing control of some of your power to some extent in terms of management. Care should be taken to support staff so that they feel safe to carry out the tasks and make decisions, and to seek help if they need it.

Power and influence leadership theory

John French and Bertram Raven's (1959) Power-and-Influence leadership theory shows leaders what type of power is most effective. The theory identifies five types of power:

- Coercive power, the least effective form, is when a leader uses coercion to get employees to do something they do not want to do.
- Reward power is similar to coercive power and is the offer of a reward to undertake the task. Although slightly more palatable, the rewards need to increase over time as the team starts to expect to be rewarded.
- Legitimate power refers to the **obligation** and responsibility a team feels to complete tasks. This common type of power relies on a traditional system of reward and punishment.
- Referent power is reliant on the charismatic quality of the leader who may be hero-worshipped by staff. This becomes a problem if there is a loss of faith in the leader.
- Expert power is the most important form of power. It results from having expertise, ensuring that staff have respect for the leader's seniority. Leaders are seen to be more effective in directing others as they know what needs to be done, offering advice where needed.

Ultimately, by improving your knowledge, experience and expertise in your work, you will gain the respect and loyalty of a motivated team.

KEY TERMS

Empowerment: Giving someone authority.

Obligation: An action or restraint from action that a person is morally or legally bound to owe to (an)other(s).

Reflect on it

1.2 Reflecting on power

Think about the types of power that you may have come across during your work life. Using John French and Bertram Raven's (1959) Power-and-Influence leadership and the five types of power, provide an example of each type from your own experiences. For example, have you ever had to undertake work you were coerced into?

SWOT analysis in leadership and management role

The acronym SWOT stands for strengths, weaknesses, opportunities and threats and involves making lists and using a template to showcase those lists. SWOT analysis is a useful tool to help you to analyse what your setting is doing well, and what areas of the setting are potentially holding you back or might pose a threat to you.

- Strengths are things that your setting does well or that set you apart from your competitors.
- Weaknesses are areas of the organisation that could be improved or practices you should avoid. As the manager, you may have blind spots when it comes to assessing areas of weakness, so it's important to seek **feedback** from others.

KEY TERM

Feedback: An open two-way communication between two or more parties.

- Opportunities are the chances for something positive to happen. They may arise from things happening outside your organisation. They may also be things that will happen in the future, perhaps as a result of a policy or legal change, so being able to anticipate these can make a huge difference to your setting and its ability to compete.

- Threats include negative effects on your setting from the outside. These could include cuts in funding or an increase in spending, or a lack of staff in a decreasing labour market. Anticipating and taking action against threats is crucial to enable you to future proof your organisation.

Strengths	Weaknesses
Motivated staff Expertise Brand reputation	Staff who are nearing retirement Changes to legislation leading to financial downturn
Opportunities	**Threats**
Succession planning and training Promoting staff to senior positions	Further legislation coming online which will affect service Social and economic change affecting staff recruitment

▲ **Figure 5** SWOT analysis

The strengths of SWOT analysis lie in being able to analyse both internal and external factors, as it is easy to see what factors will be within your control and those which might not. Carrying out such an analysis can help you to challenge risks and uncover dangerous blind spots. You may, for example, be aware of the strengths of your setting, but until you record them alongside weaknesses and threats you might not realise how unreliable those strengths are.

Each section in the template asks questions to get you started, such as asking you what you do well (strengths), what might you improve (weaknesses), what opportunities are open to you (opportunities) and what threats might stop you (threats).

Evidence opportunity

1.2 Analysing your role

Describe your own role in the organisation.

Using the theories you have learned, make an analysis of how they might be used in day-to-day practice.

For example, you might address the Situational leadership theory by Paul Hersey and Ken Blanchard and describe a situation that was presented to you and how you adapted your leadership style to that situation.

AC 1.3 Explain how key theories of leadership can be applied in practice in a range of situations in the leadership role

In this section, you will be required to explain how three theories and/or models of management and leadership (which you learned about in AC1.2) apply to adult care practice.

You will need to explain how theories and/or models of management and leadership apply to adult care practice. You should explain in your critical evaluation to what extent you agree with the three management styles you discuss. You will need to conduct further research into your chosen management styles, argue 'for' and 'against' the use of each style in your own workplace and provide evidence of how you have used the theory in the workplace.

Defining what makes a great leader and manager

As you saw in AC1.1, leadership and management are different. According to Stewart (1997), 'Management is essentially about people with responsibility for the work of others and what they actually do operationally, whereas leadership is concerned with the ability to influence others towards a goal.'

A leader inspires others to work towards a shared vision for the future and is able to empower and motivate people. A manager, on the other hand, may simply give out tasks and ensure that the day-to-day operations of the organisation are running smoothly. However, good managers also inspire staff to perform and command respect. They show empathy and consideration for the staff and have good communication skills and discipline.

Figure 6 highlights some of the traits of a good leader, including confidence, good interpersonal skills and charisma.

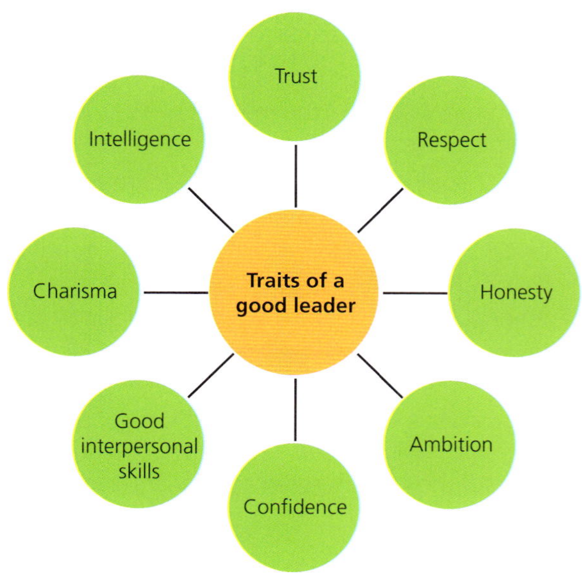

▲ **Figure 6** Some traits of a good leader

Look back at Kouzes and Posner's Leadership Challenge model (pages 9 and 10) which identifies character traits associated with good leaders, especially if you want to use this as one of the theories on which to base your critical evaluation.

Evidence opportunity

1.3 Theories and models of management and leadership

Provide a written account explaining how you apply the theories and models of management and leadership, including the ones covered in AC1.2.

You must consider how these apply to adult care practice.

Explore the evidence for and against each theory.

Your role as a leader and manager

Adair (1983), an influential writer on leadership and management, identified three key roles for leaders:

- Achieving the task.
- Developing team members.
- Maintaining the team.

These may sound obvious, but how often do you become so task orientated that you forget the needs of the team?

Team members need to understand the task and be given the resources to achieve that task if the outcome is to be successful. In this respect, team and individual development is critical to ensure that individuals can perform in the team (Martin et al., 2010).

Identify and understand your own management style(s)

As a manager in a care setting, it is important that you identify and understand your own management style so that you can adjust your style to the different people in your team. Not everyone responds well to a direct approach. Some may wish to use their own initiative and to feed back to you. Others may require gentle handling, so you may need to adjust to this.

Think about the managers you worked for in your first few roles. Reflect on what you liked or disliked about them. Was it purely their friendly nature or were you a little in awe of them? Did they inspire you with confidence or were you a bit scared of them? Did they show an interest in you as a person or were they more task-focused? Your style of leadership will be more effective if you are wise in your choice and adjust to each person.

Adjusting styles

In 2011, the American Management Association collected data on the managerial effectiveness of 622 leaders across hundreds of organisations and highlighted three competencies that spanned all industries. This is reflected in work by Terry (1993) and George (2003) on authentic leadership.

The three competencies are as follows:

- **Building trust and demonstrating personal accountability**: A leader who keeps their promises and honours commitments to staff will be regarded by them as somebody who can be trusted. Far from being weak, the leader/manager who accepts responsibility for their actions and communicates honestly is seen as accountable and trustworthy.
- **Action orientation**: Staff want somebody to act decisively and to suggest a solution in a crisis, so action orientation is about maintaining the momentum and sense of urgency about a project or a piece of work.
- **Flexibility and agility**: Working for somebody who has fixed ideas can be demoralising, so if you are able to adjust to the situation and change your behaviour according to the change in circumstances, you demonstrate that you are open to new ways of doing things.

By being authentic in this way, you develop a sense of trust with staff, who can then be held accountable for their actions. By adjusting the way in which you manage and lead, you can be more effective in your role.

KEY TERM

Action orientation: A type of leadership in which practical action is taken to deal with a problem or situation.

Research it

1.3 Characteristics of a good leader

What do you think are the characteristics of a good leader/manager?

Conduct some primary research and ask your peers and colleagues for their views. Figure 6 on page 12 outlines some of these characteristics. You may be able to think of other characteristics, too.

The following may be helpful for secondary research and will help you to gain a greater understanding of the traits of good leadership and management:

- *Effective Leadership: How to be a successful leader* (2009) by John Adair.
- *Foundation Degree in Health and Social Care* (2011) by Tina Tilmouth, Liz Davies-Ward and Briony Williams.
- 'People development and teamwork', Department of Trade and Industry (n.d.)

Reflect on it

1.3 Your own role

How would you define your own role in the workplace?

How is your role different from those you lead or manage?

Make some notes to support your learning.

You explored Lewin et al.'s (1939) leadership styles in AC1.2 (pages 5 and 6), so you may like to reread this section if you plan to use one of these for your critical evaluation. Allport (1936) also looked at leadership styles and you should revisit the section on trait theory (page 5) if you would like to base your critical evaluation on this.

Adapting management styles to meet requirements of role and with individuals and teams

The social skills needed in different leadership roles vary, and leaders need to adjust their styles at different times to facilitate or help group process (Wheelan, 2005).

At times you may need to be more directive and assertive to address and reduce any anxiety in team members, but this needs to be accomplished in a positive and open way. Supplying the resources needed to get the job done helps the team to accomplish their tasks and feel supported. When the team start to work well and demand to participate more, a good leader will recognise this, and step back rather than risk resentment caused by too much influence from the leader. At times your competence as leader will be questioned and it is important not to take this personally. Ultimately you want the team to take the leadership role on themselves to become more autonomous and responsible.

Whatever qualities you possess or need to develop, you will use these in various ways and adopt certain styles with respect to how you lead and manage. Part of a manager's role is to encourage others to work effectively so whichever style you adopt, you need to be able to rationalise why you chose that way to work. Outcomes will be affected if you fail to recognise the impact your style of leadership is having on the team. In AC1.2, you looked at Goleman's style of leadership which emphasises the role of emotional intelligence in managing people. If you become more attuned to your own emotions and can see how they affect others, you will be in a better position to handle situations which may require empathy and an understanding of the other person's feelings.

An effective team is committed to working towards the same goals and the team members will co-operate with decisions. In well-managed teams, results are produced quickly and economically where there is a free exchange of ideas and information (Tilmouth et al., 2011).

You will have a particular management style that you favour, but the ability to adapt to different situations is good practice. Every individual you manage is unique and you need to treat them as such. Your style of management must adapt to the unique nature of each person in your team, and you should try to draw upon different styles of management to accommodate this.

Positive and negative emotions impact your behaviour and the behaviours of those you lead and manage. An awareness of this and an ability to manage your emotions will lead to more positive outcomes in pressured situations.

Stretch and challenge

1.3 Management styles

Explain how different management styles may influence outcomes of team performance.

Senior colleagues/team managers – roles as managers and others

Your role as manager will also impact others in the wider team and you need to be aware of how your behaviour and the way in which you manage impacts these individuals.

Senior colleagues/team managers

- **Deputy**: A deputy needs to work closely with you and adopt the same values and attitudes towards the organisation as you. There should be a strong link between how you both manage the team and a clear understanding of the tasks or operations you wish them to undertake.
- **Team leaders/supervisors**: It might be that a delegated task for a deputy will be to manage the team leaders and supervisors. If this is the case, then your responsibility will be to ensure that you support the deputy in this role. You may take a step back from the line management of these people, but you should always be aware of what is happening at this level by getting regular updates from your deputy.

Others

- **Company directors**: These people have a financial interest in the organisation and may also make strategic decisions. As a manager it is your responsibility to ensure that they are aware of the day-to-day running of the setting and any related issues.

- **Trustees**: They serve on the board of an institution, charity or local government. They are not normally paid for their role but have control over how the organisation is run. They will need to be aware of the administrative and legal side of the organisation and will want assurance that the setting is operating in compliance with the law and that high-quality care is a top priority.
- **Families of individuals using the service**: They need to be kept up to date with changes to ways of working, and they have a right to know what is happening.
- **Commissioning agencies**: Commissioning services assess needs, and plan, prioritise and purchase care services. They have an important role to play since they set the requirements for the care provision that they are paying for.
- **Regulatory body (CQC)**: The care manager is responsible to them and will be inspected against a set of standards in a regulated service.

Reflect on it

1.3 Adjusting your management style

Take some time to consider how you might adjust your style when talking to a deputy, team leaders/supervisors, directors and trustees, the families of the individuals using the service, commissioning agencies and regulatory bodies.

Evidence opportunity

1.3 How theoretical models are applied to practice

Using the models discussed in AC1.2, explain how theories and/or models of management and leadership apply to adult care practice. For example, if you choose Kouzes and Posner's leadership challenge, you could include examples of how this applies to your own setting. If you choose Daniel Goleman's EI theory, how would you compare it to Kouzes and Posner?

AC 1.4 Analyse the range of different leadership styles

Here, you will be required to analyse different leadership styles and their impact on working culture and service delivery.

Different leadership styles were addressed in AC1.3 of this unit, and it would be a good idea to recap these now.

Inclusive vs exclusive

Inclusive versus exclusive approaches to leadership and management refer to the way in which recruitment to the workforce is managed. You may have come across the term 'talent management', which is about finding the right person for the job by employing individuals who are considered to be particularly valuable to an organisation because of the qualities they possess. You may find it helpful to look at resources provided by the Chartered Institute of Personnel and Development (CIPD, 2022).

Some organisations approach their workforce planning inclusively by investing in the current staff they have and developing them according to the specific needs of the organisation. In this way the whole workforce is developed. In this approach, there is an acknowledgement that talent exists at all levels of the organisation and the focus is on developing existing staff to the needs of the setting. This type of approach is very motivating as staff feel valued and this will impact morale.

An exclusive approach is the recruitment to the workforce of staff from outside the organisation with specific skills and knowledge according to the needs of the organisation at the time.

Open vs closed

A manager who adopts an open style seeks to develop relationships of trust with their staff. These are based upon mutual respect and will have a positive impact on the workforce as they will feel trusted. A disadvantage is that on some occasions there is a need for a more direct approach to get a job done.

A closed style of management is more directive and autocratic. While this is necessary when, for example, somebody must take the lead in an emergency situation, in everyday management this may have a negative impact upon staff morale.

Positive vs negative

A positive manager will take time to support the team and help them to achieve the goals of the organisation. They will be upbeat and highlight the team's strengths and what they are doing well rather than focusing on things that have gone badly. Adopting a positive style will motivate people and they will be inspired to do their best.

A negative manager will focus on failures rather than the achievements of the team and may resort to sanctions if goals are not met. Under a negative regime a team is likely to feel demoralised, where staff are not inspired or may not feel supported to do their best.

Approaches to management

- **Autocratic**: Autocratic leadership occurs when the decision making and power belongs to only one person with little or no input from others. Rather than collaborating with staff the autocratic leader will simply send the message to 'do it'. This dictatorial type of leadership may be unpalatable to some, but it does have its advantages when applied to certain situations. For example, an autocratic leader does not have to wait for a committee to agree a decision but can make the decision today. This style also gives structure to organisations, with clear rules and streamlined communications. In this type of leadership staff know exactly who to talk to for approval and this can lead to greater organisational efficiency.

- **Authoritative**: Authoritative leadership is where the leader is in complete control. They set the goals, determine what needs to happen and oversee all steps to reach those goals, asking for little or no input from team members. Authoritative leaders drive organisations toward common goals, working with the staff by leading and coaching them. Once authoritative leaders show employees how to complete tasks, they let them continue on their own, which encourages innovation and new ideas.
- **Pacesetting**: This type of leadership focuses on the leader setting the pace for the organisation by adopting a 'Do as I do' approach. By observing the pacesetting leader and their speed, performance and quality of work, the team is given an example to follow. Results are what count in the end. This type of leadership style limits staff development as tasks are rarely assigned to an incapable employee and the leader will also take over from an employee who is failing.
- **Democratic**: A democratic leader is one who collaborates with others and invites participation as part of the decision-making process. The democratic manager is open and enables everyone to put forward ideas and discuss options. This leads to increased feelings of involvement, recognition and satisfaction. However, without some control on the part of the manager it can be chaotic and sometimes a consensus is never reached. It may also be time consuming.
- **Coaching**: Coaching leadership includes collaboration, support and guidance, with leaders focusing on guiding their teams through goals and obstacles. This leadership style is very much the opposite of autocratic leadership, which is focused on top-down decision making.
- **Affiliative**: This was put forward by Daniel Goleman as one of his six leadership styles. This leader wants teams to feel connected and work in harmony. Praise ensures that the team is cohesive. A disadvantage is that there may be a tendency to ignore poor performance, as there is a preference for always being upbeat and positive.
- **Laissez faire**: This type of leader gives staff free rein and lets them make their own decisions while they take a back seat.

Reflect on it

1.4 'Positive' and 'negative' managers

What do you think would be the difference between a positive manager and a negative one?

Evidence opportunity

1.4 How different leadership styles can impact working culture and service delivery

Provide a written account analysing different leadership styles and their impact on working culture and service delivery.

You may wish to determine when you might use certain types of leadership. In what situations might you change your leadership/management style? Give examples.

When analysing, make sure that you give two sides to your argument. Look at the advantages and disadvantages of an approach and then say whether it might be a useful approach to use or not.

LO2 Understand how coaching and mentoring can be used to complement leadership style

AC 2.1 Explain the differences between coaching and mentoring

In this section you will define mentoring and coaching and explain the different roles they play in the development of your leadership style.

Coaching and mentoring

Coaching and mentoring are similar in nature, so you should be clear about what they refer to. Both are used to enable individuals to flourish in their work and also their personal lives.

According to Parsloe (1999), successful coaches require knowledge and understanding of process and have at their disposal a variety of styles, skills and techniques. A coach therefore may not have direct experience of a person's formal occupational role but will be able to use a process to help them to make the changes they desire.

Mentoring is a professional relationship and involves following in the footsteps of a more experienced colleague who can pass on their knowledge and experience of a role. They will share advice and offer guidance when needed.

Sometimes on-the-job training to develop new skills and techniques or simply to update staff regarding new policies, practices and procedures is required. The use of coaching as a strategy to advise and support team members and to enhance team performance is now a well-respected part of team development.

Parsloe and Wray (2000) defined coaching as:

> *a process that enables learning and development to occur and thus performance to improve. To be successful, a coach requires a knowledge and understanding of process as well as the variety of styles, skills and techniques that are appropriate to the context in which the coaching takes place.*

AC 2.2 Outline how the use of coaching can complement a leadership style with self and with others

Here, you will outline how coaching is an essential leadership style and how to use coaching to develop yourself and others.

> *Coaching is unlocking a person's potential to maximise their own performance. It is helping them to learn rather than teaching them.*
>
> Source: Whitmore (2002)

Coaches aim to improve performance by focusing on the 'here and now' rather than on the past or future. The key skill is asking the right questions to help the individual work through their own issues. Coaches believe the individual has the answers to their own problems and focuses on helping them to unlock their own potential.

Coaches have a different function to a teacher or a mentor. A major difference is that coaches are not necessarily subject experts whereas teachers are. Mentoring, while similar to coaching, usually focuses on the future, both in terms of career development and broadening an individual's horizons.

Coaching in leadership

Daniel Goleman identified coaching as one of the essential leadership styles. Coaching in leadership is a leadership style that focuses on high performance, encouraging collaboration and empowerment among staff. To use this style a leader requires a good knowledge of their teams including their strengths, weaknesses and motivations.

The 'GROW' model of coaching (Whitmore, 2002) provides a simple and structured model for the coach:

G = Goal setting asks questions to encourage the coachee to clarify what they want and where they want to get to. The coach will encourage the coachee to explore what achievement would look like to them.

R = Reality promotes questions that require reflection now. What is the situation currently? What is stopping you from achieving your goals? What do you need to achieve your goals? What is a realistic timescale? What do you enjoy and why? What are the key risks?

O = Options. This stage of the model encourages the coachee to explore different means of achieving the goal. Questions that might be asked include: What are the different ways that you could achieve your goal? What else could you do? What are the pros and cons of different options? What would happen if ...? Which of the options would bring about the best result?

W = Way forward. Finally, the coach will encourage the coachee to make an action plan. Questions that might be useful include: What are you resolved to do, and by when? What support do you need? What commitment do you have? When should we/you review progress?

Successful coaching is not easy as it is sometimes necessary to ask sensitive questions of the person you are coaching, which can be quite unnerving for them. Coaches who are self-aware can accurately assess the emotional state of the other person and therefore have a good understanding of how and why they may react and respond as they do. It is therefore crucial for a leader using this style to be self-aware.

You can use coaching with all members of staff you come into contact with, for example deputy managers, team leaders/supervisors, administration staff, teams, partnerships and ancillary staff. Members of the permanent team are likely to be better known to the manager and this will make a coaching approach easier, as there is time to build a good rapport and put plans in place and coaching sessions are more likely to be followed up.

Staff from external teams, such as volunteers, advocates, informal carers, apprentices/learners from schools and colleges and agency staff, may still benefit from a coaching type approach but the time they are working in the area will be limited. You also need to consider how much professional development you are required to undertake for these staff or if their development is part of a different organisation's remit.

Self-analysis, self-evaluation and self-reflection

Self-evaluation, reflection and analysis can all be summed up as 'self-awareness'.

According to 'How To Become a Better Leader' (Toegel and Barsoux, 2012), self-awareness was cited as the most important capability for leaders to develop. Other studies also found that successful companies had employees with high levels of self-awareness.

A core component of emotional intelligence, self-awareness is about knowing what your values are, what type of personality you have, and what your needs, habits and emotions are. Knowing how these affect your actions and the actions of others means you will be in a better position to manage your stress and make better decisions.

Being self-aware means you can see the difference between the things you can and cannot control, and this is important.

Reflect on it

2.2 Understanding the extent of your control

In your daily life what are the things around you that you can truly control?

Make a list.

If you reflect on your list, it is likely that you will cross out a few of the items. For example, you may have included your health, journey to work and daily tasks, but can you really control these?

We like to think we have control of our lives but there are a host of things we have no control over. The important point here is that this can cause worry and stress even though nothing we do can change them.

The only thing you can truly control is yourself. You can take care of yourself and look after your health to reduce your risk of illness, but you cannot fully take away that risk. You can make your own decisions and react to others in the way you think best, but ultimately you cannot control much else. Having this knowledge and accepting it is a step to becoming self-aware, but it is only when you fully realise what is out of your control that you can experience the benefits of self-awareness.

This might seem a little negative. Humans like to control things and as a manager you want to be organised and have a smooth-running organisation. The thought of not having much control over this can seem daunting, but becoming self-aware means understanding what is beyond your control. By doing this you are gaining back some power over your life. When you realise that you have no control over whether somebody will turn up for work or not or whether the much-needed delivery of supplies will come through on time, you can then take a step into determining what in those situations you can control. Worrying about staffing or deliveries not arriving are not useful activities but planning for the likelihood they may not happen is.

Case study

2.2 Responding to difficult situations

Jennifer and Taimor both had their rotas scheduled with their team on Friday. The rotas had been planned for months and on Friday both managers were going to be on a day off. A stock delivery was due that day that required checking; this had been planned for and staff were delegated duties to cover.

On Thursday evening, two staff members called in sick. When Taimor got the call, he slammed the phone down. He would now have to cancel his day off. Not only that, but he would also have to reschedule staff to cover. He was very angry and frustrated.

Jennifer received a similar call. She thanked the member of staff for phoning in early and said she hoped they would be well again soon. She reflected on her options. Her day off may be in jeopardy but she now had a few choices as to what she could do. Change to another day off and come in on Friday instead or simply call colleagues to see if they could cover the shift. She was not angry and solved the dilemma calmly.

Both individuals had no control over their staff members illness, but they reacted in very different ways. Taimor expressed anger, frustration and negativity, while Jennifer opted for power and positivity.

Reflect on it

2.2 Responding to difficult situations

How would you have reacted in this situation? Try to be honest and note down how you would respond.

Problem-solving in a leadership role

To be an effective leader you must be able to problem-solve. Problems are often viewed negatively, as things to be avoided and dealt with immediately, and this is true to an extent. However, problem-led leadership is a new way of working where leaders encourage their teams to get involved in not only identifying problems but also using everyone's expertise and input to solve them.

Here are six steps to follow to solve any problem:

1 Identify the problem. This may seem obvious, but it is often the first step to be missed. Define what the problem truly is before you implement a solution. The following questions are useful starting points:
- What is the problem?
- What should we be doing instead?
- What is it we want to achieve?

- How can we achieve this solution quickly and efficiently?

Only then can you form an action plan with your team.

2 Evaluate the problem. What has caused this problem? Get to the root of it. Is there a pattern? Ask questions using what, who, where, when and how to gain a deeper understanding. There is no need to assign blame; you are simply trying to understand all the perspectives around the issue.

3 Get the facts to back up your solution. Stakeholders such as management peers, external supporters, knowledge specialists, commissioning agencies, specialist care providers, trustees or owners' who invest in your organisation will all require facts about the problem and the solution.

4 Communicate to your team. Being clear to your team and stakeholders about how you plan to act on this problem is a measure of good communication. By showing others that you are transparent, you will gain their respect and they will support the solution.

5 Develop and test solutions. With some solutions to work with you can start putting ideas into action. Creating lists with actions, timelines and priorities is useful. You also need to be mindful of cost and time.

6 Improve the solution. If the solution is not right, then mistakes can be evaluated and used to improve the plan for next time. The most important thing is that any plan should be continuously improved upon.

The coaching approach

In adopting a coaching leadership style you may need to elicit help from others who can support the coaching:

- **Management peers**: Your peers may have some experience of coaching and could offer your staff much needed aid. Some larger care providers may have a team of coaches from different disciplines within the organisation who are available to other areas, resulting in a more objective stance to the coaching. You may find it difficult to coach your own staff so this could be a good approach to coaching your own team.
- **External support**: External companies can come into the organisation and coach individuals. This is quite costly but can reap rewards if changes made encourage a more efficient service.
- **Knowledge specialists**: Although more adapted to teaching than coaching, knowledge specialists can give much needed information to staff and are very useful in training situations.

Evidence opportunity

2.2 Coaching session

Provide a brief overview of how coaching could benefit your leadership style and how you could support others to develop. What benefits will you and the service gain by developing a range of coaching opportunities and skills?

AC 2.3 Outline how the use of mentoring can complement a leadership style with self and with others

Here, you will outline the process of mentoring and how it can develop your leadership style and that of others.

NOTE: In this section we recognise that 'others' who are part of the mentoring process include deputy manager(s), team leaders/supervisors, volunteers, advocates, informal carers, apprentices/learners from schools and colleges, agency staff, administration staff, teams, peer to peer, partnerships and the individuals using the service.

While coaching aims to help staff fulfil both their personal and professional potential, the process of mentoring involves an experienced and trusted advisor sharing information on his or her career path and providing guidance, support and role modelling.

Some organisations offer in-house mentoring schemes as part of leadership training. More senior staff are assigned a mentee to provide support to and to give feedback on performance. They act as guides and advisors.

Mentoring offers a different relationship to that of coaching. For example, a coaching relationship might be a short one, particularly if the outcome is achieved, whereas mentoring can take place over a longer period of time, sometimes years. Coaching focuses on performance, but mentoring is about development.

Mentors have more seniority and expertise in a specific area, so the mentee can learn from their experience. A coach is hired in for their expertise in a particular area, related to the coachee's desired improvement.

In determining whether you require a coach or a mentor, you should consider the goals you wish to achieve. Coaches and mentors help in different ways, and you might decide that for your own career development you will opt for both.

Case study

2.3 Coaching or mentoring?

Simon is a member of a re-ablement team and has been identified as having huge potential for developing assessment skills in order to take on a senior role. At work he is keen, knowledgeable, supportive of the other staff and well-liked by the people who use the service. At team meetings, however, he turns into a different person when he is in front of his senior managers. He is nervous and seems to lack concentration. He stumbles over his words and is very quiet as a result.

1. Would you offer Simon coaching or mentoring? Write a paragraph explaining your choice.
2. Identify a suitable mentor to help you with your own development and approach that person for support. How do you want them to help your development? Write down your plan of action to put this into place.

Maybe you opted for coaching for Simon. A coach could help with how he presents himself in meetings, working on his self-esteem and presentation skills. The coach will give Simon the tools he needs to ease his nerves and to work on his focus.

However, for Simon to develop and engage as a manager in the future, he may need more guidance than this and a mentor could help him move into a management position in the next few years. You might decide to mentor Simon yourself or to ask another senior professional to do so.

Professional development within a leadership role

As a leader, you will need to ensure that each staff member has the required training, coaching and mentoring that is appropriate for their particular area of professional development. This may be provided in-house or by an external organisation and should begin from the point of their induction through to managing their performance once they are established in their role.

As part of formal induction

As soon as somebody starts in a new role, professional development should be an important part of the process. Staff will be expected to achieve certain milestones from the point of induction to the end of the probationary period, but this is also a good time for individuals to address their own development needs. They need to see that their ongoing development needs are going to be met and that they are part of an organisation that values this. This is a good time for someone to draw up their own development plan by stating their learning objectives and developing some **SMART** goals. These are goals that are:

- **S**pecific
- **M**easurable
- **A**chievable
- **R**ealistic/relevant
- **T**ime bound.

For more on SMART goals, see Unit 505.

Having a clear plan of action will help staff to organise their learning time more effectively and will boost their motivation and will help you, as their manager, to identify a way of measuring their progress.

KEY TERM

SMART: Targets that are specific, measurable, achievable, realistic/relevant and time bound.

As part of probationary period

If staff identify their goals at the induction stage, this will help you to measure their progress during the probationary period, as you can see if their goals have been met.

As part of performance management

A personal development plan can be used during an appraisal to determine how far an individual has come with respect to their chosen developmental areas.

Think about how you provide performance feedback to your staff and how it is provided to you. Traditionally, feedback has been limited to a yearly appraisal in which staff are formally judged and appraised on their performance over the past year. If bonus payments are involved, then this can be an uncomfortable meeting and may not be particularly productive.

Feedback which is delivered regularly is far more effective, whether it is positive or constructive in nature. If goal setting is a focus at induction and then at periods throughout the year, staff are clear as to what is expected of them.

One key purpose of performance management is to manage the talent in the organisation. Think back to Case study 2.3. Simon was great at his job and could have stayed in the same position for years. Instead, by coaching and mentoring him and investing in his talent, he is likely to feel valued and respected.

Giving and receiving positive and negative feedback

Feedback is an open two-way communication between two or more parties. Feedback to staff should be regular and a daily part of your work as a manager. In formal feedback sessions, the best way to approach this task is to first ask the member of staff how they perceive their performance of a task. By linking the feedback to their professional development, the person will be able to focus more on what they need to change. You can see what they understand about how well they are doing their job and you are also encouraging them to be reflective about their performance.

Sometimes positive feedback is not given, yet genuine positive feedback is motivating for staff. Thanking somebody at the end of the shift for a job well done or acknowledging a person's work during a shift builds respect and ensures that the member of staff feels secure in their work.

How, though, do you approach giving bad news with respect to a person's role or performance? Everyone makes mistakes from time to time, and we all need some guidance on aspects of our work from time to time. Although the content of feedback may be negative, it should be given in a constructive and encouraging manner. You can help the person to solve a problem or to address an aspect of their behaviour and work towards organisational goals, so they develop, grow and improve.

So how do you go about giving constructive feedback? You may have heard of the 'feedback sandwich'. This is a three-step procedure to help provide constructive feedback, consisting of praise, followed by the problem area or criticism, followed by more praise. In this way, the unpalatable news is sandwiched by good news and the blow of receiving it is softened.

Although it has come in for criticism from some writers, it is a good way for new managers and supervisors to help to deliver news that may otherwise be seen as purely negative.

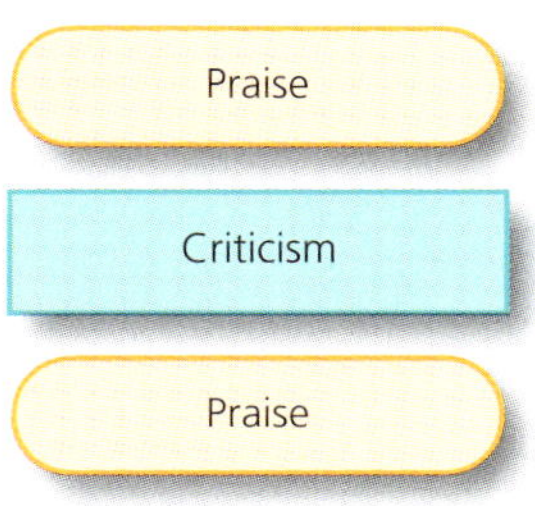

▲ **Figure 7** The praise sandwich

Reflect on it

2.3 Supporting staff

As a manager, how do you undertake responsibility for providing professional supervision for staff to ensure that they are supported in their roles and to enhance their skills and performance?

By focusing on both your own development needs and those of others, including internal and external staff where appropriate, individual performances will improve and the setting as a whole will show an improvement in performance.

Stretch and challenge

2.3 Benefits of mentoring

How do you think that mentoring can complement your leadership style? Outline how you will use mentoring to benefit others.

LO3 Understand leadership and management in adult care services/settings

AC 3.1 Analyse the impact of internal and external drivers on leadership and management in adult care services/settings

You will be required to analyse current national and local **policy drivers** *and how these impact your leadership and management role, including those discussed in this section.*

Earlier in this unit you looked at strategic plans and how these shape your setting. Internal and external policy drivers refer to both UK government policies and the policies stated in the mission and values statements of your setting. They determine how services need to be developed to uphold current standards and meet future targets. They are broad aims, targets or statements that various bodies of government or non-government organisations consider to be desirable to satisfy overall goals. These policies drive the way in which care is delivered and managed in this country.

In this section, you will look at some of the current initiatives you need to be aware of in your leadership and managerial role.

You will now look at some of the internal and external drivers that may impact care services and the way they work and therefore affect the way you lead your setting.

KEY TERM

Policy drivers: Documents, research, laws and information that can lead to change in practice and drive forward new procedures and ways of working.

Wellbeing of self

As the impact of the COVID-19 pandemic was felt across the UK, working in the care sector became a very difficult place to be. Staff were left demoralised and burnt out and this led to large numbers of care staff leaving the profession, the impact of which is still being felt now.

The Skills for Care 'Wellbeing for registered managers: A bite size practical guide' is based on the New Economics Foundation's 'Five ways to wellbeing: Connect … Be active … Take notice … Keep learning … Give …'. Registered managers may find it a useful guide to generate ideas around promoting positive wellbeing. See Skills for Care (n.d. b).

Stress and burn-out have become real issues for adult social care staff, so workforce wellbeing has never been so important. Support for the health and wellbeing of the staff ensures that people with care and support needs and their families can still receive good quality care. The wellbeing guide provides self-assessment activities and guidance by means of support groups, webinars and podcasts. The five ways to wellbeing and suggested activities to meet each one are outlined.

Staff wellbeing is a driver in terms of whether your setting will flourish or fail. If staff are not looked after they will become unsettled. The setting should provide support for mental health issues and adjustments should be made to ensure that staff can continue to work if they are able to.

Research it

3.1 Health and wellbeing

Go to 'The care exchange – Series 2' page on the Skills for Care website (Skills for Care, n.d. a). Here you can access a number of different resources for wellbeing at work, including the managers' guide mentioned above.

How might you integrate these into your own care setting?

Professional confidence

Professional confidence has increasingly become an area for concern. The impact of the COVID-19 pandemic in particular has affected the professional confidence of many care workers. You may find your team are concerned about the level of care they are able to provide and if care has suffered, it is likely that staff morale will be low. Your staff may feel worried so building their confidence is a key driver.

Developing a mentoring system is a good place to start. Encourage staff to work with others to build their confidence in what they do. Self-belief may be an issue that needs to be tackled; many people, particularly women, experience '**imposter syndrome**', where they feel their success is undeserved, which they put down to luck rather than the results of their own efforts or skills.

Praising staff, ticking off every small success and telling them they are good at what they do will develop confidence (and the same applies to telling yourself too!). Staff need to feel valued and invested in, so motivating them is crucial. You may need to adapt your personal style of leadership from a task-oriented style to one of collaboration and care.

KEY TERM

Imposter syndrome: Feelings of doubt that a person might experience about their abilities, which can lead them to feel like a fraud or assume that their success is due to luck rather than talent. People suffering from imposter syndrome often feel that they are underqualified or lacking in ability to do their job properly.

Making changes to existing policy and strategy

As mentioned earlier, organisations are required to develop organisational policies and strategies as these provide guidelines for action for staff. However, circumstances may change. For example, you may have to manage staff shortages or increased care needs. As a result your existing strategy may be unfavourable towards staff and could have a negative effect on them, causing stress.

Policies around the delivery of care changed during the COVID-19 pandemic. These included the requirement for care staff to be vaccinated, relatives being unable to visit their loved ones and a lack of personal protective equipment (PPE), all of which caused many issues for care staff, and some of these changes are likely to become the new normal for care.

These necessary policy changes were sometimes delivered to staff with little or no rationale and this caused stress and dissatisfaction. If a policy or strategy needs to change then staff need to be part of that change for it to be effective.

Reflect on it

3.1 Changes to policy or strategy

What policy or strategy changes have been evident in your care setting recently? How did staff react to the changes and what might you have done to reduce anxiety?

Staffing/recruitment and service delivery

A Unison survey conducted in November 2021 revealed that 31 per cent of care staff reported dangerously low staffing levels that were getting worse and 97 per cent of workers said their care employer was currently experiencing staffing shortages due to burnout, overwork and low pay. Another finding stated that two thirds (67 per cent) of staff were thinking of leaving social care.

It is therefore imperative that you address how your setting recruits and retains its staff. Staff recruitment can impact an organisation both positively and negatively. Finding the right people for the vacant roles with relevant skills and abilities is not just about filling an immediate vacancy but about the impact hiring somebody will have on the long-term success of the organisation.

Having an effective recruitment and selection policy ensures that a transparent and fair recruitment process is in place, clearly outlining your setting's recruitment methods and practices.

Funding/budgets and quality of care delivery

The delivery of quality public services across the UK was severely affected by the COVID-19 pandemic, including services provided by care homes and other provisions. Despite care staff rising to the challenge, the pandemic has had a devastating impact on these.

In March 2022, the government announced significant investment in social care of around £12 billion per year on average across the UK, funded by the introduction of a Health and Social Care Levy and increased rates of dividend tax from April 2022.

In September 2021, the government set out to reform adult social care in England and promised £5.4 billion to fund the reforms between 2022/23 and 2024/25. A reform payment of £3.6 billion was to be used for social care, which included £1.4 billion for local authorities to move towards paying a 'fair cost of care' to providers. The funding was initially planned to come from the new Health and Social Care Levy, but in September 2022 the government announced the levy would be cancelled.

At the time of writing (May 2023) funding for social care remains unchanged with proposed reforms being delayed to October 2025. The Autumn Statement of 2022 announced that the reforms would be delayed for two years, with funding being allocated to local authorities to provide more care packages.

The government now plans to introduce a new £86,000 cap on the amount an individual in England will need spend on their personal care over their lifetime, irrespective of their age or income. The legislative framework for a cap is already provided by the Care Act 2014.

Public health challenges/initiatives

Any new initiative will impact care settings as they seek to make the required changes.

Public Health England strategy

In 2019, Public Health England outlined a strategy focusing on protecting and helping people to live longer and in good health. Addressing the current reliance on the NHS and the care provided by hospitals and GPs, the plan also includes the need for a prosperous economy and addresses the choices we make as individuals and families.

The PHE Strategy 2020 to 2025 aims include:

- keeping people safe
- preventing poor health
- supporting a strong economy.

National Strategy for Autistic Children, Young People and Adults

The National Strategy for Autistic Children, Young People and Adults sets out a vision for what autistic people and their families' lives should be like by 2026. It covers six priority areas:

- improving understanding and acceptance of autism
- improving autistic children and young people's access to education and supporting positive transitions into adulthood
- supporting autistic people into employment
- tackling health and care inequalities for autistic people
- building the right support in the community and supporting people in inpatient care
- improving support within the criminal and youth justice systems.

For more information, see Department for Education and Department for Health and Social Care (2021).

Quality Matters

The Adult Social Care Quality Matters initiative, published in 2017, focuses on care that is person-centred, safe, effective, caring and responsive. The purpose of the initiative is to build on existing partnerships and commitments and set out clear action plans to support the improvement of quality.

The highlight of the initiative is that quality is everybody's business and it sets out a shared commitment to high-quality, person-centred adult social care. The aim to make a difference in care services includes working across the sector with people who use these services and their carers.

For more information, see ADASS et al. (2017).

Care Data Matters

Following the pandemic, it became evident that data on social care was important. New data was collected directly from care providers through a 'capacity tracker system', detailing what was happening in care homes and home care agencies. This enabled the government and local authorities to help those who provided support with the challenges they were having at the time. Recognising that the use of data, digital tools and technology is crucial to supporting care for vulnerable individuals, it was noted that the adult social care sector lags behind healthcare with its use of technology.

It was further noted that the far-reaching reforms of social care to increase the quantity and quality of care available is better achieved through the use of better social care data, with joined-up health and social care records, and more digital technologies and innovation in care.

The People at the Heart of Care plans (see Unit 503) outlined a ten-year vision for adult social care, and published the health and care data strategy 'Data saves lives', making a commitment to improving the collection and sharing of social care data.

See GOV.UK (2023).

Evidence opportunity

3.1 Internal and external drivers

Identify and analyse the impact of internal and external drivers on leadership and management in adult care settings/services. You might refer to internal drivers such as staffing, workload and funding.

External drivers, such as those imposed by law, commissioning agencies, national initiatives and locality-specific issues, all impact leadership and management within your own service/setting. Identify and analyse the impact these have had on how you deliver your service.

Diversification in business models

Catastrophic events, acute situations and changes in the market often mean that organisations fail. Although care services will always be needed, large numbers of staff leaving the profession and changes to ways of working have resulted in some care organisations having to close.

Business diversification is a growth strategy, which means entering into new markets or industries or creating a new product for that new market. There are different types of diversification:

- Horizontal diversification is when new services are developed that complement the core business. For example, you might develop a community-based care service with staff going into people's homes. New technology, skills or a different marketing approach may be required to achieve this.
- Conglomerate diversification is the addition of services that are entirely different from the core business. For example, perhaps you wish to develop a new service within the setting that local people can also access. The risks of entering a new market, particularly if costs are involved, may be high at first so need to be considered carefully.

Deciding how and when to diversify will require:

- detailed market research for the new product or service
- making an assessment of the needs of the individuals using the service
- developing a clear product development strategy and market testing
- identifying the sales, marketing and supply chain operations to manage the changes
- commissioning agency requirements as a lot of care services are commissioned by social workers and monitored by local authority adult care providers.

Being successful will lead to increased sales and revenue and grow your market share while you develop new revenue streams. Conversely, diversification will incur costs and require additional skills, management and operational resources and if these demands exceed the profit gains, it can put your setting at risk.

Self-motivation

A potent driver for your setting is your own self-motivation. A leader who is self-motivated evolves with the setting and improves themselves continuously. This characteristic will inspire those around you and will influence the motivation of your staff.

Motivation helps a person achieve their objectives and encourages them to work hard.

External policy and/or strategy

Legislation, statutory guidance and regulations that underpin adult care need to be followed if organisations are to succeed. Some of the laws your care setting must be aware of and develop policy for are outlined below.

Health and Social Care Act 2008 (Regulated Activities) Regulations 2014

The Health and Social Care Act 2008 (Regulated Activities) Regulations 2014 were introduced following the public inquiry and publication of the Francis Report into care at the Mid Staffordshire NHS Foundation Trust (Francis, 2013) and established new fundamental standards for care. Should care not reach the required standards, provision is made within the guidelines to take enforcement action.

As a result of the Francis Report, there have been changes to the way in which adult social services are led and managed. New practices continue to be introduced including changes to the way in which care is delivered and monitored. In part 5 of the Regulations, section 1 introduces requirements relating to persons carrying out or managing a regulated activity, which state that providers must not appoint a person to an executive director or associate director level post or to a non-executive director post unless they meet the fit and proper person requirements (CQC, 2015). People employed in management roles must show they:

- are of good character
- have the qualifications, competence, skills and experience that are necessary for the position
- can perform the function and tasks for which they are employed
- are not responsible for any serious misconduct or mismanagement (Department of Health, 2014).

Equality Act 2010

The Equality Act 2010 brought together four major EU Equal Treatment Directives and replaced previous anti-discrimination laws, simplifying the law and making it easier to understand. It is an umbrella Act, bringing together legislation that deals with race, disability and gender.

The Act highlights protected characteristics of age, gender reassignment, pregnancy, religion, marriage and civil partnerships and sexual orientation in an attempt to end discrimination. Additionally, it strengthens protection by setting out the different ways in which unlawful treatment may occur. Individuals are now fully protected from discrimination in the workplace and in wider society.

Additionally, the Equality Act clearly identifies that any organisation (including social care settings) that provides goods, facilities, services or functions to the public must ensure that it does so within the requirements of the law. The Act applies to private, statutory and voluntary organisations, no matter what their size. Equality law affects those running an organisation as well as those working within the organisation, such as staff and volunteers.

The Act has enabled protected groups to gain employment and to not be discriminated against. There has also been a positive move to address the gender pay gap and equal pay and fair pay for all are also being addressed.

Care Act 2014

The Care Act 2014 sets out the key responsibilities of local authorities in meeting the needs of individuals who require help and support to promote their wellbeing. Some of these responsibilities include promoting individual wellbeing and the ability to stay as independent as possible, preventing the need for care and support, promoting integrated care and support and the right to an assessment of need for care and support.

Those in need of care and support

The impact of these Acts of Parliament in the adult care sector has led to changes in the way care is delivered and paid for and will also affect how care is managed and led. Leadership and management must change to meet new needs in the care sector. For example, changes to how the **Care Quality Commission (CQC)** carry out inspections in most adult care provision will drive forward change to internal policies and the way in which staff deliver care.

> **KEY TERM**
>
> **Care Quality Commission (CQC)**: The independent regulator and lead inspection and enforcement body for all social care services in England.

Inspection – internal and external

The CQC's Key Lines of Enquiry (KLOEs) were introduced in 2013 and highlight how an adult social care provider will be inspected and judged against five key questions:

- Is it safe?
- Is it effective?
- Is it caring?
- Is it responsive?
- Is it well led?

The KLOEs direct the focus of inspection to make sure there is a consistent and standardised approach to inspection. For managers, it means that there is a more transparent approach to inspection as the five key questions provide clear and concise guidelines as to what is being looked at.

The Care Certificate

Training is a further driver for leadership and management. Any new care worker must be trained and inducted into the role. The Care Certificate was developed by Skills for Care, Health Education England and Skills for Health and provides a set of standards that social care and health workers should cover as part of their training. It links to National Occupational Standards and other qualifications such as the Regulated Qualifications Framework (RQF) for new staff, as well as those already in post who wish to undertake further training. The Care Certificate provides a good basis for staff new to the profession from which they can develop their knowledge and skills.

As a manager you must be aware of what training is on offer for your staff and be clear about what you will require them to do to access training. This is likely to impact your training budget as you put people through new qualifications.

Research it

3.1 Policies and your setting

Look at a national policy relevant to your care setting and identify how this might change the way in which your provision is inspected.

Research it

3.1 Policies and your setting

Download the Care Quality Commission's standards (Care Quality Commission, 2022a) and choose three of the standards. If you are not a regulated service this is still a useful activity as these are fundamental standards.

Say how your organisation is meeting these particular requirements.

How have changes to legislation and/or the CQC standards described above affected your role as a manager and leader? Think in terms of the positive and negative impact upon your setting of these changes. Show the arguments for and against the changes and the impact they have had in your own setting.

Evidence opportunity

3.1 How policies impact leadership and management

Write some notes to enable you to have a professional discussion with your assessor analysing the current national and local policy drivers and how these impact the leadership and management role, including the ones covered in this section. You may need to do some research around the current national and local policy drivers.

There is more information about the difference between management and leadership in AC1.3 (page 12).

AC 3.2 Explain the role of leadership and management skills in adult care services/settings

Here, you will be required to explain why it is important for managers in adult care to have both leadership and management skills.

Is there a difference between a leader and a manager? As you have already seen in AC1.1, many writers have debated this concept. Fayol (1916) identified the functions of a manager as planning, organising, staffing and controlling. Kotter (1990) believed leadership to have a more far-reaching effect, being a role that sought change and movement. Clearly though there is a need for both and ideally a manager should possess both leadership and managerial qualities.

As a manager you will be expected to co-ordinate the staff to ensure that they carry out their tasks well and deal with any underperformance. You will ensure that the daily routines are carried out so that the service functions well and delivers its strategic plan.

However, as a leader you will also ensure that in the course of their work the staff are taken care of. Leaders inspire others to want to do their best and you can do this by ensuring that you always follow through on any promise you have made and assume responsibility for the team. If, as the manager, you are good at inspiring your team then you are also coming close to being a good leader.

Evidence opportunity

3.2 Reasons managers in adult care settings need both leadership and management skills

Explain to your assessor, or provide a short written account, of the role of leadership and management skills in adult social care and why it is important to have both leadership and management skills.

Reflect on it

3.2 Leadership and management skills

Look at the table below and evaluate your own job description against it. Are you a leader or a manager and how might you change to adapt to both roles? Reflect on the reasons why.

Leaders	Managers
Have ideas	Move people to develop those ideas
Inspire people	Co-ordinate people
Create opportunity	React to situations
Create vision	Provide resources to achieve that vision
Have followers	Show people the way

AC 3.3 Describe how to adapt own leadership and management style for different situations

Here, you will describe how leadership models can assist with adapting your leadership style for different situations that you may face.

In AC1.2 you looked at Hersey and Blanchard's Situational leadership model. Paul Hersey and Ken Blanchard disagreed with the notion that there would be a single, best, 'one-size-fits-all' leadership approach that could be used within organisations but contended that leadership styles should be adapted to the context.

This model suggests that successful leaders are adaptive and flexible, considering the individuals in the team first, before focusing on the factors that impact the work environment. They then adapt their style to the situation presented before making a decision on how they will lead.

According to the Situational leadership model, the following are styles of leadership managers can use:

S1: Directing: In this style, leaders emphasise directive behaviour and have low emphasis on supportive behaviour. The primary concern here is to get the job done by giving step-by-step instructions and clearly explaining the consequences of non-performance.

S2: Coaching: This style is highly directive and highly supportive of staff who are willing to do a task but are not able. The leader here adapts their style to increase the confidence and skills of staff so that they can take on more responsibility.

S3: Supporting: This style shows high support but low direction in which the leader may listen, praise and put a high level of trust in the staff to achieve the day-to-day tasks as the competence grows.

S4: Delegating: The final leadership style assumes a low support and a low direction and is a 'hands-off approach'. Staff are able and willing to perform the tasks independently and with great autonomy.

Evidence opportunity

3.3 Leadership styles for managing situations

Consider the following different situations that arise in the course of your work. For each one give an example of how you have adapted your style. You can refer to the Hersey and Blanchard model if this is appropriate.

- ✔ Formality/informality of different working. Here you might consider how a formal situation such as a board meeting or an appraisal requires a different approach to leading than an informal situation such as an event happening on shift.
- ✔ Working under pressure. Give an example of a situation where work was challenging, and you were required to make a decision quickly. What leadership style did you use and why?
- ✔ Management and leadership roles in particular situations. Consider two situations you have been in when a problem has occurred, or a decision has been needed. Which leadership style was appropriate? For example, how did your style differ during an emergency compared to when you have been compiling work rotas?
- ✔ Managing conflict: How did you deal with a difficult conversation or a conflict in the workplace.

Note: Ensure that any sensitive information you share with an assessor or include in a portfolio of evidence is anonymised and remains confidential.

AC 3.4 Describe how to adapt own leadership and management style for internal teams, external teams and partnerships with other professional teams

Here, you will describe how different teams have different requirements from you as a leader and how you adapt your leadership style for their needs.

You will adapt your leadership approach according to the situation you find yourself in. Leadership is about guiding and influencing others, whether they are members of your internal team, external to the organisation or partners. With constant change a part of our everyday lives, the difficulty this brings can prove to be particularly challenging for a leader. To successfully emerge from a period of change you need to work on your leadership skills and change your leadership style to suit the situation. Some useful steps are outlined below.

Recognise the need to change

By being clear about what needs to change and why, you can start to be constructive rather than panicked. Change may be uncomfortable but a leader who can see the bigger picture and work out what the change will lead to will be able to adapt well to the new situation and will help staff to see this too. For your internal team there may be changes to work patterns. For those who are external there may be changes to how they can enter the setting and what they are allowed to do once there.

Lead with purpose and set clear goals

Whoever you are dealing with, your style of leadership must be clear and purposeful. During a period of change or crisis, leaders need to become more involved with the staff.

Planning is essential and a step-by-step plan of how you will carry your team through the challenges is needed.

Communicate clearly and share decision making

Leaders who communicate clearly with their team members and who make sure staff are aware of their role during a period of change will gain their trust and loyalty. Enabling staff to voice ideas and concerns will reduce the risk of misunderstandings.

Delegate

Delegation is a key aspect of leadership, so identifying key team members who share your view and agree with your vision is a crucial task. These team members can then act as role models, encouraging other staff through the change.

Addressing problems and reviewing the plan

No plan is without issues, so you need to be able to predict what issues might arise along the way and have an alternative plan to overcome them. Regularly review your plans and make opportunities to celebrate the wins. This will help boost the team's morale and motivation.

Lead with empathy

Leaders who lack empathy find it difficult to relate to others, whereas empathetic leaders know about the lives of their team members. They listen when they are being spoken to and recognise and celebrate each team member's input. Having empathy means being able to determine how decisions will affect members of a team, so teach yourself to become attuned to how your team are feeling.

> **Evidence opportunity**
>
> **3.4 Describe leadership styles using examples**
>
> Describe how you adapt to varying situations with reference to the Hersey-Blanchard situational leadership model. Use examples from your practice to describe your leadership styles, ensuring confidentiality of sensitive information if it is to be shared with an assessor or included in a portfolio of evidence.

AC 3.5 Evaluate the interaction between the values and culture of an adult care service/settings and own leadership behaviours

In this section, you will be required to evaluate both internal and external factors that impact your leadership and management role and related interactions considering the topics discussed in this section.

Organisational culture and values

The term 'culture' is a complex one but refers to the rules, norms, values or beliefs that are shared by a group. In the context of an organisation, culture is about the professional values and beliefs shared by that group. As a leader, one of your roles is to ensure that staff have clarity about what is expected of them with respect to the values of the organisation.

An effective organisation works towards the same goals and the members will co-operate with the decisions made. Effective teamwork requires all team members to relate well to each other; as a leader you need to recognise the similarities as well as the differences in the individuals who make up your team. Your challenge is to respect those differences in personality and to work with them to ensure that team members do not clash or that the team does not become dysfunctional. Teamwork is not about getting people together and dictating your orders but rather about developing a commitment to the goals by establishing trust and cohesion and recognising everyone's efforts and input.

Staff who work on their own in the community are part of a more remote team but the same applies. They still need to buy into the culture of the organisation and should still follow the rules, norms, values and beliefs of the wider group.

When properly managed and developed, teamwork improves processes and produces results quickly and economically through the free exchange of ideas and information.

Effective governance and partnerships

Governance refers to the system of rules, practices and processes by which an organisation is directed and controlled. It identifies who has power and accountability, and who makes decisions.

Culture plays an important role in the governance of an organisation and defines the way in which things are organised and people relate to each other.

A negative culture in a setting, for example where secrecy, bullying and abuse are common, is likely to also experience bad governance as there is a lack of challenge and dominant people in significant roles.

Good governance structures and mechanisms are essential for effective partnerships. There must be clear lines of responsibility and decision-making structures and systems to ensure that partners, such as health professionals, social workers, advocates and commissioning agencies, are clear about what they have agreed to do and also that internal staff are clear about where roles and responsibilities start and end.

Responsiveness

Good governance requires that organisations try to serve all stakeholders within a reasonable timeframe. Your setting also needs to be responsive to changes coming through with respect to how you care for the individuals using the service.

Person-centred care and safeguarding/ protection

The principles of person-centred care include:

- treating people with dignity, compassion and respect
- offering personalised and co-ordinated care, support and treatment
- supporting people so that they can live an independent and fulfilling life

(The Health Foundation, 2014).

Person-centred care places the individual at the centre of their care, recognising them and not the care professional as the expert in their own care. In this way, the individual, and their family, become equal partners in the planning of their care, ensuring that their needs, goals and outcomes are met. The emphasis becomes one of doing rather than being done to, and enables individuals to be active not only in their own care but also in the design and delivery of services.

These principles should be part of the values and culture of an organisation to ensure that all those involved in the provision of care put the individuals using the service at the forefront of all they do.

An integral part of providing high-quality personalised care is the safeguarding protocols in place to protect individuals' health, wellbeing and human rights. Staff need to understand their role in identifying, recording and reporting concerns and this is covered in more detail in Unit 507.

Duty of candour

Duty of candour demands that every care professional must be open and honest with the people in their care when something goes wrong.

Individuals using the service, advocates, carers and family members must be informed and an apology made. They must then be offered an appropriate remedy or support and an explanation as to the short- and long-term effects of what has happened.

Safety/risk management

As a leader you are responsible for ensuring that anybody who enters your setting is cared for and that risks are minimised. Rigorous risk assessment and management protocols should be part of your culture and governance procedures.

The Management of Health and Safety at Work Regulations 1999 set out what employers are required to do to manage health and safety in their organisation. The Regulations apply to every work activity and place duties on both employers and employees to ensure a safe and healthy workplace. In particular, you must first identify potential hazards that could cause injury or illness in your setting, then identify how serious this risk is and how likely it is somebody could be injured. Action must then be taken to eliminate the hazard and control the risk.

Personal values

Personal values are underlying beliefs that make us who we are and guide our decisions and actions. Such values include compassion, dignity, independence, privacy, communication, protection, respect, courage, inclusion, pride and integrity. Your setting's mission and vision statements will include clearly stated values to which the organisation must align. These will form the culture of your setting.

Leadership values, similarly, are those values that positively influence the ability to lead effectively and to be a 'good leader'. These can be developed over time.

Openness and transparency with others and inclusion of staff and others

An organisation which promotes openness and creativity, encouraging the team members to share information, to innovate and take calculated risks, will provide a positive climate in which to work. By ensuring that all your staff are included in making decisions, you will help them to feel valued and respected. One of your roles as a manager will be to involve organisation partners as well as the families and friends of those using the service in helping to move the organisation forward in a positive way. By encouraging open discussion and ideas, a more transparent and open culture will develop.

Reflect on it

3.5 Conflict and your managerial role

Reflect on the points above and how they have impacted your work as a manager and leader and give examples.

How have you dealt with conflict within the work setting which may have arisen as a result of differing personal and organisational values?

Positive engagement of colleagues and those receiving care and support

Supervision of staff has been introduced into practice to provide professional support and learning to enable them to develop knowledge, skills and competence in their work and additionally to safeguard those receiving care. It is during these sessions that you as a manager can promote the values of the organisation and this in turn will enhance the experience of the individuals using the service and improve quality and safety in the care setting.

Level of experience in management role and related responsibilities

The transition to manager is a challenge because now you are the one in charge and being looked to for advice and guidance. Ultimately, you are responsible for how the team is working.

The following points might help:

- First you need to establish your style and authority by ensuring you understand your own values and priorities in the role. For example, if communication and trust are important to you then make sure staff are aware of this and stick to these values at all times.
- Be a good listener. By listening to others, you learn about them.
- Recognise that change happens slowly and affects staff morale.
- Attribute success to the team and not just to you.

Stretch and challenge

3.5 Interactions between leadership and the values/culture of an organisation

Evaluate how effectively your leadership practice reflects the values and culture of your adult care service/setting. Reflect on how both internal and external factors impact your leadership and management role.

Legislation

Legislation	Key points
Health and Social Care Act 2008 (Regulated Activities) Regulations 2014	Outlines the fundamental standards for care and sets regulations against which some services are inspected.
Equality Act 2010	An umbrella Act bringing together legislation that deals with race, disability and gender. It highlights protected characteristics of age, gender reassignment, pregnancy, religion, marriage and civil partnerships, and sexual orientation in an attempt to end discrimination.
Care Act 2014	Sets out the key responsibilities of local authorities in meeting the needs of individuals who require help and support to promote their wellbeing. Its main aim was to provide integrated care and to introduce the right to an assessment for all.
Care Quality Commission's Key Lines of Enquiry (KLOEs) 2013	Key criteria against which adult social care regulated providers are inspected and judged.

References

Adair, J. (2009) *Effective Leadership: How to be a successful leader*. New York: Pan Macmillan.

ADASS et al. (2017) 'Adult social care: Quality matters'. https://assets.publishing.service.gov.uk/government/uploads/system/uploads/attachment_data/file/795351/Adult_Social_Care_-_Quality_Matters.pdf

Allport, G.W. and Odbert, H.S. (1936) 'Trait-names: A psycho-lexical study', *Psychological Monographs*, 47(211).

Care Quality Commission (2013) *A New Start: Consultation on changes to the way CQC regulates, inspects and monitors care*. London: CQC.

Care Quality Commission (2015) *Regulation Five: Fit and proper persons: Directors. Information for NHS bodies*. Newcastle Upon Tyne: CQC.

Care Quality Commission (2022a) 'The fundamental standards'. www.cqc.org.uk/about-us/fundamental-standards

Chartered Institute of Personnel and Development (2022) 'Talent management'. www.cipd.co.uk/uk/knowledge/factsheets/talent-factsheet/

Department for Education and Department for Health and Social Care (2021) 'The national strategy for autistic children, young people and adults: 2021 to 2026'. www.gov.uk/government/publications/national-strategy-for-autistic-children-young-people-and-adults-2021-to-2026/the-national-strategy-for-autistic-children-young-people-and-adults-2021-to-2026#our-roadmap-for-the-next-5-years

Department of Trade and Industry (n.d.) 'People development and teamwork'. www.businessballs.com/dtiresources/TQM_development_people_teams.pdf

Fayol, H. (1916) *General and Industrial Management*. London: Pitman.

Fiedler, F.E. (1967) *A Theory of Leadership Effectiveness*. New York: McGraw-Hill.

Francis, R. (2013) *Report of the Mid Staffordshire NHS Foundation Trust Public Inquiry*. London: TSO. https://assets.publishing.service.gov.uk/government/uploads/system/uploads/attachment_data/file/279124/0947.pdf

Goleman, D. (1995) *Emotional Intelligence*. New York: Bantam Books.

GOV.UK (2023) 'Care data matters: A roadmap for better data for adult social care'. www.gov.uk/government/publications/care-data-matters-a-roadmap-for-better-data-for-adult-social-care/care-data-matters-a-roadmap-for-better-data-for-adult-social-care

Health Foundation, The (2014) 'Person-centred care made simple'. www.health.org.uk/publications/person-centred-care-made-simple

Kotter, J.P. (1990) *A Force for Change: How leadership differs from management*. New York: Free Press.

Kouzes, J.M. and Posner, B.Z. (2003) *The Leadership Challenge*. San Francisco, CA: Jossey-Bass.

Leadership-Central.com (n.d.) 'Hersey-Blanchard Situational Leadership Theory'. www.leadership-central.com/situational-leadership-theory.html

Lewin, K., Lippit, R. and White, R.K. (1939) 'Patterns of aggressive behavior in experimentally created social climates', *Journal of Social Psychology*, 10: 271–301.

Martin, V., Charlesworth, J. and Henderson, E. (2010) *Managing in Health and Social Care*. Abingdon: Routledge.

McKibbon, J., Walton, A. and Mason, L. (2008) *Leadership and Management in Health and Social Care*. London: Heinemann.

Northouse, P.G. (2018) *Leadership: Theory and practice*. Thousand Oaks, CA: Sage.

Parsloe, E. (1999) *The Manager as Coach and Mentor*. London: Chartered Institute of Personnel & Development.

Parsloe, E. and Wray, M. (2000) *Coaching and Mentoring: Practical methods to improve learning*. London: Kegan Paul.

Peters, T. and Austin, N. (1985) *A Passion for Excellence: The leadership difference*. London: Collins.

Public Health England (2019) PHE 2020–2025. London: Crown Publishing

Rappaport, J. (1987) 'Terms of empowerment/exemplars of prevention: Toward a theory for community psychology', *American Journal of Community Psychology*, 15(2): 121–48.

Scouller, J. (2011) *The Three Levels of Leadership: How to develop your leadership presence, know-how and skill*. US and UK: Management Books.

Skills for Care (n.d. a) 'The Care Exchange: Series 2'. www.skillsforcare.org.uk/Support-for-leaders-and-managers/Support-for-registered-managers/The-care-exchange/The-care-exchange-Series-2.aspx

Skills for Care (n.d. b) 'Wellbeing for registered managers: A bite size practical guide'. www.skillsforcare.org.uk/resources/documents/Support-for-leaders-and-managers/Managing-people/Wellbeing/Wellbeing-for-registered-managers-a-bite-size-practical-guide.pdf

Stewart, R. (1997) *The Reality of Management*. Oxford: Butterworth-Heinemann.

Terry, R.W. (1993) *Authentic Leadership: Courage in action*. Jossey Bass: Wiley and Sons.

Tilmouth, T., Davies-Ward, E. and Williams, B. (2011) *Foundation Degree in Health and Social Care*. London: Hodder Education.

Toegel, G. and Barsoux, J-L. (2012) 'How to become a better leader', *MIT Sloan Management Review*, 53(3): 51-60

Urwick, L.F. (1952) *Notes on the Theory of Organization*. New York: American Management Association.

Wheelan, S.A. (2005) *Creating Effective Teams: A guide for members and leaders*. London: Sage.

Whitmore, J. (2002) *Coaching for Performance: GROWing people, performance and purpose*. London: Nicholas Brealey.

Useful resources and further reading

Bolton, G. and Delderfield, R. (2018) *Reflective Practice: Writing and professional development*. London: Sage Publishing.

Cavazotte, F., Moreno, V. and Hickmann, M. (2012) 'Effects of leader intelligence, personality and emotional intelligence on transformational leadership and managerial performance', *The Leadership Quarterly*, 23(3): 443–55. https://doi.org/10.1016/j.leaqua.2011.10.003

Care Quality Commission (2022b) 'Consultation on changes for more flexible and responsive regulation – consultation document.' https://www.cqc.org.uk/get-involved/consultations/consultation-changes-more-flexible-responsive-regulation-consultation

Care Quality Commission (2022c) 'How we monitor, inspect and regulate adult social care services'. www.cqc.org.uk/guidance-providers/adult-social-care/how-we-monitor-inspect-regulate-adult-social-care-services

Care Quality Commission (2022d) 'Regulations for service providers and managers'. www.cqc.org.uk/guidance-providers/regulations-enforcement/regulations-service-providers-managers

Covey, S.R. (2004) *The 7 Habits of Highly Effective People.* New York: Simon & Schuster.

Department of Health, Skills for Care and Skills for Health (2013) 'Code of Conduct for Healthcare Support Workers and Adult Social Care Workers in England'. www.skillsforcare.org.uk/resources/documents/Support-for-leaders-and-managers/Managing-people/Code-of-conduct/Code-of-Conduct.pdf

Goleman, D. (1999) *Working with Emotional Intelligence.* New York: Bantam Books.

Gopee, N. and Galloway, J. (2017) *Leadership and Management in Health Care.* London: Sage.

Investopedia, 'What are the Michigan Leadership Studies?'. www.investopedia.com/terms/m/michigan-leadership-studies.asp

Lindberg, C. (n.d.) 'The Ohio State Leadership Studies – What is it? Definition? Conclusions?' www.leadershipahoy.com/the-ohio-state-leadership-studies-what-is-it-definition-conclusions/

Maslow, A. (1987) *Motivation and Personality.* New York: Harper & Row.

McClean, S. (2012) *Power and Empowerment in Health and Social Care.* London: City & Guilds.

McGrath, J. and Bates, B. (2017) *The Little Book of Big Management Theories and How to Use Them.* London: Pearson.

Newton. R. (2011) *The Management Book: How to manage your team to deliver outstanding results.* Upper Saddle River, NJ: Prentice Hall/Financial Times.

Owen, J. (2017) *The Mindset of Success: Accelerate your career from good manager to great leader.* London: Kogan Page.

Peters, S. (2012) *The Chimp Paradox: The mind management programme to help you achieve success, confidence and happiness.* London: Vermilion.

Reynolds, M. and Holwell, S. (eds) (2020) *Systems Approaches to Making Change: A practical guide.* London: Springer.

Skills for Care (2013) 'Leadership starts with me'. www.skillsforcare.org.uk/Developing-your-workforce/Care-topics/Leadership-skills/Leadership-starts-with-me.aspx

Skills for Care (2016) 'Manager induction standards'. www.skillsforcare.org.uk/Support-for-leaders-and-managers/Developing-leaders-and-managers/Manager-induction-standards.aspx

Skills for Care (2022) 'Supporting the development of leadership skills'. www.skillsforcare.org.uk/resources/documents/Support-for-leaders-and-managers/Developing-leaders-and-managers/Supporting-the-development-of-leadership-skills/Supporting-the-development-of-leadership-skills-guide.pdf

Skills for Care (2023) 'The state of the adult social care sector and workforce in England'. www.skillsforcare.org.uk/Adult-Social-Care-Workforce-Data/Workforce-intelligence/publications/national-information/The-state-of-the-adult-social-care-sector-and-workforce-in-England.aspx

Unit 501

Governance and regulatory processes in adult care

GLH 30

About this unit

Adult social care governance is the process whereby good outcomes and good service delivery for people who use the service is promoted, and it is the responsibility of every manager, leader and care worker to ensure that social care governance is central to their practice and the service provision. There must be accountability at every level within the organisation to uphold the standards of social care. The intention of the Health and Social Care Act 2008 (Regulated Activities) Regulations 2014 (Regulations 4 to 20A) is to ensure that adult social care providers have systems and processes in place for effective governance. Assurance and auditing systems need to be in place to drive improvement in the quality and safety of the services provided. Risks relating to health and safety and the welfare of the individuals need to be mitigated against and providers need to continually evaluate and improve their governance and auditing practice. Records of individuals using the service and staff should be maintained accurately and securely.

All adult care providers' systems in the UK are required to provide safe and good-quality care and support, improving the experience of those using the service, as well as continually updating practice in the light of evidence from research. The scandal relating to the Mid-Staffordshire Healthcare Trust, for example, highlighted the treatment of individuals and led to an inquiry into failings in the system. Lessons for adult social care can be learned from the Francis Report. The report highlighted the lack of competent governance, and poor working culture along with ineffective management. This led to a blame culture where staff feared for jobs and reprisals if issues were spoken about.

This unit is about the responsibility to deliver safe adult care. As a manager of care services, you are responsible for the safety and wellbeing of the individuals using those services. To do this, performance management systems need to be put into place that not only identify best practice and focus on continuous improvement but also deliver better outcomes for individuals by acting upon new initiatives, legislation and information.

Learning outcomes

By the end of this unit, you will:

1. Understand legislation and statutory guidance that underpins adult care.
2. Understand internal governance arrangements within own organisation.
3. Understand systems and requirements for the regulation of adult care services.
4. Understand the inspection process in adult care.
5. Understand the inspection process in own setting/service.

Getting started

Before you study the unit, think about the following:

- What do the terms 'governance' and 'regulation' mean?
- Do you understand why these are so important for your organisation and for all adult care?
- What are the internal arrangements for governance within your organisation?
- Do you know your role and responsibilities in the inspection process? If your service is not currently regulated or inspected, how could you use current regulations to support service improvement?

LO1 Understand legislation and statutory guidance that underpins adult care

AC 1.1 Outline current legislation and statutory guidance that applies to all aspects of service provision

Here, you will be required to outline the current UK legislation and statutory frameworks that apply to social care providers and **voluntary sector providers***, including the ones discussed in this section.*

This section highlights the main legislation that impacts adult social care provision in the UK, and that applies to **social care providers** in adult social care provision – statutory, private and voluntary.

Legislation must be applied to all practice. Tragic incidents can happen when the legal aspects of care work are either not followed correctly or ignored altogether. Failure to uphold the law will inevitably lead to consequences not only to the individuals using the service but also to staff and the care establishment as a whole.

Health and Social Care Act 2008 (Regulated Activities) Regulations 2014

The **Regulations** were introduced following the Francis Report into care at the Mid Staffordshire NHS Foundation Trust (Francis, 2013) and introduced new fundamental standards for care for England. These included a new 'professional duty of candour' outlining the need for social care professionals to be open and honest when things go wrong and to be honest about reporting adverse incidents or near misses that may have led to harm.

Other standards highlight the needs for treating people with dignity, respect, with their consent and in a safe way by engaging competent and qualified staff of good character. They should also be offered choice, which is central to support in adult social care. For more on these standards see Unit 500.

Should care not reach those standards, provision is made within the guidelines to take enforcement action.

Fit and proper person

Part 3 of Section 1 of the Regulations introduces requirements relating to people carrying out or managing a regulated activity. These are termed the 'fit and proper person requirements' for directors and determine that directors of care are of 'good character' and 'have the qualifications, competence, skills and experience necessary for the relevant position' (DH, 2014).

> **KEY TERMS**
>
> **Social care providers**: Care providers who operate on one or more sites; these settings vary and can range from individuals' homes to specialised care settings to hospitals.
>
> **Voluntary sector providers**: These are part of charitable trusts or groups who simply volunteer services to support social care services.
>
> **Regulation**: A rule or order that is underpinned by law. In care settings, apart from those concerned with health and safety care, regulations with respect to health protection and control of disease are also available.

Equality Act 2010

The Equality Act 2010 brings together legislation that deals with race, disability and gender, replacing and simplifying previous anti-discrimination laws, making them easier to understand. It highlights protected characteristics of age, gender reassignment, pregnancy, religion, marriage and civil partnerships, and sexual orientation in an attempt to end discrimination. It strengthened protection by setting out the different ways in which unlawful treatment may happen to someone. Individuals are now fully protected from discrimination in the workplace and in wider society.

Care Act 2014

The Care Act 2014 sets out the key responsibilities of local authorities in meeting the needs of individuals who require help and support to promote their wellbeing. Some of these responsibilities include promoting individual wellbeing and the ability to stay as independent as possible, preventing the need for care and support, promoting integrated care and support and the right to an assessment of need for care and support.

The Act simplified and improved the existing legislation for care, changing the way in which care was accessed and financed. People requiring care are now able to access care and support from local authorities or other organisations in the community and have more choice about the type of support and care they receive.

Under this legislation, individuals receiving care and support from any regulated provider are covered by the Human Rights Act 1998. Local authorities are responsible for helping individuals to access independent financial advice to help them with care funding.

Health and Care Act 2022

The Health and Care Act 2022 provides an amendment to the Care Act 2014 and will address the proposed cap on personal care spending due from October 2023. The cap is already provided by the Care Act 2014, but the provisions are not currently in force.

In November 2021, the government announced an amendment to the Care Act so that money paid by a local authority towards meeting a person's eligible care needs will not count towards the cap. Although controversial, this change became law in April 2022.

Further legal changes are expected in 2023 with changes to the social care means test for accessing local authority funding support becoming more generous, with an increase in the upper capital limit of the threshold above which somebody is not eligible for local authority support. This will increase from £23,250 to £100,000 and the lower capital limit or the threshold below which somebody does not have to contribute towards their care costs will increase from £14,250 to £20,000. This will be introduced incrementally from 2023 to 2025. The proposed reforms will mean that people will no longer face unlimited or unpredictable care costs.

Care Quality Commission (CQC)

Regulations

Section 23 of the Health and Social Care Act 2008 (HSCA, 2008) instructed the Care Quality Commission to produce guidance to help care providers meet the changes required by the Health and Social Care Act 2008 (Regulated Activities) Regulations 2014. This document replaced CQC's 'Guidance about Compliance: Essential standards of quality and safety' and its 28 outcomes. The Regulations apply to providers and managers registered with the CQC who carry out regulated activities in any sector.

Fundamental standards

The guidance lays down fundamental standards that must be met by registered persons. Care services must never fall below these standards, and every person who uses a care service has the right to expect such high-quality care. These are stated on the CQC's website and include the following:

- **Person-centred care**: Treatment is personalised to meet the individual's needs and preferences.
- **Dignity and respect**: Individuals have equality, privacy and support to help them remain independent and involved in the local community.
- **Consent**: Prior to any care or treatment, the individual (or anybody legally acting on their behalf) gives their consent.
- **Safety**: Risks are evaluated during any care or treatment pathway, ensuring staff are qualified and competent to keep individuals safe.
- **Safeguarding from abuse**: Neglect, degrading treatment, unnecessary or disproportionate restraint or inappropriate limits on freedom are unacceptable.
- **Food and drink**: Anyone receiving care and treatment has enough to eat and drink to keep them in good health.
- **Premises and equipment**: Settings and items used for care services are suitable, secure and looked after properly.
- **Complaints**: Systems should be in place to handle and respond to individuals' complaints, with a thorough investigation and action being taken if problems are identified.
- **Good governance**: Quality and safety of care must be monitored to help the service improve and reduce any risks to health, safety and welfare for individuals.
- **Staffing**: Qualified, competent and experienced staff are in place and receive the support, training and supervision that they need to help them do their job.
- **Fit and proper staff**: Staff can provide the care and treatment appropriate to their role, recruited via efficient recruitment procedures and after relevant checks such as Disclosure and Barring Service (DBS) have been implemented.
- **Duty of candour**: Settings are open and transparent about individuals' care and treatment. If something goes wrong, the setting offers support and an apology.
- **Display of ratings**: The CQC rating is displayed where stakeholders can see it and should also appear on the organisation's website.

Key Lines of Enquiry

CQC's Key Lines of Enquiry (KLOEs) were introduced in 2013 and highlight how a care provider will be inspected and judged against five key questions:

- Is it safe?
- Is it effective?
- Is it caring?
- Is it responsive to people's needs?
- Is it well led?

The KLOEs direct the focus of inspections to ensure that scrutiny is consistent, but a new framework will replace this in 2023. The questions will remain, but the evidence collected will change. See AC4.4 for more on KLOEs.

Mental Capacity Act

The Mental Capacity Act 2005 protects and supports people who do not have the ability or capacity to make decisions for themselves. The Act applies to people aged 16 and over in England and Wales and makes provision in a number of different conditions for those whose capacity is affected.

A person with capacity is able to understand information that is relevant to the decision they want to make and can retain that information long enough to make the decision. They will also be able to weigh up the information they have been given and to communicate their decision by means such as talking, using sign language, or through simple muscle movements such as blinking an eye or squeezing a hand. If a person is deemed to lack capacity, then any decision made must be in their best interests – you will look at how this is enacted later.

The Mental Capacity Act 2005 is amended by the Mental Capacity (Amendment) Act 2019, although at the time of writing, this is not yet in force. See Unit 508, LO1 for more about the Mental Capacity Acts.

Mental Health Act 1983

The 1983 Mental Health Act (MHA) laid down provision for the compulsory detention and treatment of people with mental health problems in England and Wales and focused upon strengthening individuals' rights to review their treatment.

Mental Health Act 2007

The MHA was amended in 2007 and focused on public protection and **risk management**. The amended legislation extends the powers of compulsion and introduces compulsory community treatment orders, making individuals' compliance with treatment a statutory requirement.

The main changes outlined in the 2007 MHA are as follows:

- **Definition of mental disorder**: A single definition replaced categories of disorder found in the 1983 MHA. The definition covers 'any disorder or disability of the mind'. Individuals with learning disabilities are exempt here as they are not suffering from a mental disorder unless the disability is associated with aggressive or irresponsible conduct.
- **Criteria for detention**: For detention to be put into place a relevant health professional must guarantee that medical treatment, including psychological intervention, is available. This is 'the appropriate treatment test' and replaces the former 'treatability test'.
- **Professional roles**: Anyone with experience in supporting people with mental health problems, such as nurses, occupational therapists and psychologists, can now make assessments and referrals as there have been changes to the roles of professionals. The former title 'approved social worker' has been replaced by 'approved mental health professional'.
- **Responsible clinician role**: This replaced the responsible medical officer, and social workers or other clinicians can now fill this role. Recommendations for detentions under Sections 2 and 3 of the 1983 MHA still have to be made by two 'registered medical practitioners'.
- **Nearest relatives**: Individuals can remove their nominated nearest relative if they feel that person is unsuitable. Civil partners have the same status as husband and wife on the list of eligible relatives.
- **Community treatment orders**: Provided people who are discharged from hospital continue the medical treatment they need they can live at home under supervision. This is called the Community Treatment Order (CTO) and replaces the 'supervised discharge' of the 1983 MHA. Failing to comply with the conditions of the CTO may result in the person being recalled to hospital under Section 17E.
- **Mental health review tribunals**: An individual who has been receiving treatment in the community is referred to a Mental Health Review Tribunal (MHRT) to determine whether they can receive a formal discharge.
- **Age-appropriate services**: Anyone under 18 who is admitted to hospital for a mental disorder must be accommodated in a suitable setting for his or her age.
- **Electro-convulsive therapy (ECT)**: This should be given to an individual without their consent only in an emergency. If the individual lacks capacity to consent, the treatment can be given only if it is appropriate and does not conflict with the safeguards set out in the 2005 Mental Capacity Act.
- **Advocacy**: The UK government in England and the Welsh Assembly are responsible for providing an independent mental health advocate to a person who is liable to be detained. An IMHA is an independent advocate, trained in the Mental Health Act 1983 to support people to understand their rights under the Act. They also participate in decisions about their care.

As of June 2023, a new Mental Health Bill is being prepared, but the likely publication date is unknown.

KEY TERM

Risk management: Forecasting potential risks and taking steps to minimise or avoid them altogether. Your policies should identify how you undertake risk assessment in your area and how you intend to manage risks that arise.

Deprivation of Liberty Safeguards and Liberty Protection Safeguards

In 2009, the MHA introduced Deprivation of Liberty Safeguards (DoLS) by amending the 2005 Mental Capacity Act, and the rights of victims were extended by amending the Domestic Violence, Crime and Victims Act 2004.

The Human Rights Act states: 'Everyone has the right to liberty and security of person. No one shall be deprived of his liberty [unless] in accordance with a procedure prescribed in law'.

DoLS were put in place to keep safe from harm those who lacked capacity to make decisions and who could not therefore consent to necessary treatment. It is important that when restrictions are put in place, they are in the individual's best interest.

However, a Law Commission report published in 2017 concluded that DoLS were too technical and reliant on legal jargon, which meant they were not always meaningful for disabled people and their families or carers and they were not always understood by social care practitioners. As a result, new Liberty Protection Safeguards (LPS) have been introduced which will replace DoLS. The LPS is linked to the provisions in the Mental Capacity Act 2005 and is about safeguarding the rights of those who need high levels of care but who do not have the mental capacity to consent to such arrangements for their care. It will be applicable to everyone over the age of 16 and an LPS will need to be authorised in advance by 'the Responsible Body', which now includes local health authorities.

See Unit 207, AC1.1 for more on LPS and also the Social Care Institute for Excellence website.

Safeguarding Vulnerable Groups Act 2006

The Safeguarding Vulnerable Groups Act (SVGA) 2006 was passed to protect children and vulnerable adults from harm, or risk of harm, from people who are deemed unsuitable to work with such groups. As a result of this Act, the Independent Safeguarding Authority was established and merged with the Criminal Records Bureau to become the Disclosure and Barring Service (DBS).

Protection of Freedoms Bill

The Protection of Freedoms Bill amends the SVGA 2006. It abolished registration and monitoring requirements but retained the national barring function.

Health and Safety at Work Act 1974 and associated regulations

You will be familiar with the Health and Safety at Work Act 1974 (HASAWA), which is the main piece of UK health and safety legislation. It places a duty on all employers 'to ensure, so far as is reasonably practicable, the health, safety and welfare at work' of all their employees. Additionally, it requires:

- the safe operation and maintenance of the working environment, plant (equipment) and systems
- maintenance of safe access and egress to the workplace
- safe use, handling and storage of dangerous substances
- adequate training of staff to ensure health and safety
- adequate welfare provisions for staff at work.

Source: Health and Safety Executive (n.d.)

The Management of Health and Safety at Work Regulations 1999 (the Management Regulations) further highlights and details in greater depth what employers are required to do to manage health and safety under the Health and Safety at Work Act. The main requirement is the need to carry out a risk assessment. Employers with five or more employees need to record the significant findings of a risk assessment.

Evidence opportunity

1.1 Legislation and statutory frameworks

Investigate the current UK legislation and statutory frameworks that apply to adult social care workers, including the ones covered in this section. You could provide a written account of your findings for your portfolio.

Depending upon the sector in which you work, you might also look at the frameworks that have been developed to improve care and support for autistic people and people with learning disabilities.

Forming part of the Autism Strategy and developed by autistic people and people with learning disabilities and their families and carers, the frameworks describe the skills, knowledge and behaviours that social care staff should have to inform the development and planning of the current and future provision. (See Skills for Health et al., 2019.)

The SCIE website also provides information about living with dementia and is worth visiting. The section dealing with supporting people with dementia discusses the person's physical living environment (whether at home or in a care home or other provision), decision making and how to use information and communication technology in activities. (SCIE, n.d.)

Research it

1.1 Legislation, policies and procedures

For each piece of legislation, find out its purpose and investigate the related policies and procedures in your setting.

What are your responsibilities with respect to how legislation is implemented in your setting?

AC 1.2 Explain own role, accountability, and responsibility in applying legislation and statutory guidance within own service/setting

Here, you will be required to explain your accountability and role within your organisation's governance structure.

Personal accountability

If you are accountable for something, you are expected to take responsibility for it. In adult care this means you are competent to carry out tasks and procedures while being acutely aware of the safety of those using the service. For example, adult social care workers are expected to undertake annual training on manual handling to protect themselves and the individuals using the service; and there are standards relating to the use of hoists, slide sheets and other manual handling equipment. But what happens in the workplace? Perhaps you do not have the equipment or perhaps staff are simply not using it, thinking it is too time consuming.

Being accountable means you must be able to justify what you are doing and why, and also prove that you are competent to carry out the task in question. Staff must be clear that they will be held accountable for errors, mistakes or problems, so they should be confident to speak up if they are unable or unwilling to do something.

As a manager you are accountable for the whole team too and need to be aware of what your staff are doing and how they are doing it. You are also accountable to the individuals using the service (duty of candour), your line manager and others for what you do.

The individuals using the service are owed a duty of care, which means that staff must deliver person-centred care in a safe and compassionate manner.

Evidence opportunity

1.2 Personal accountability

Provide a written account explaining your accountability and role within your organisation's governance structure.

You might like to consider what you are accountable for and who you are accountable to. For example, what actions and processes are you responsible for and entrusted to complete? Give an example of an area of your work for which you are accountable and discuss the positives and negatives of this situation.

Reflect on it

1.2 What are you accountable for?

What are you accountable for in your role as manager? Who are you accountable to?

Evaluate how your role and accountabilities help you to maintain your organisation's governance structure. Give an example from practice and demonstrate how you are accountable in practice. Show the pros and cons of your role with respect to accountability. For example, how do you ensure that staff are upholding practice policy and how do you deal with those who do not conform?

Your responsibility and accountability also applies to how you adapt and meet legal requirements. There is a strong association between legislation and **policy** on person-centred care and positive outcomes-based procedures and practice. All these laws should be enshrined in the policies and **procedures** you are required to have in your workplace.

Policies set out the arrangements you have for complying with the law and procedures identify the activity surrounding practice needed to implement the policy. As a manager, one of your roles is to ensure that staff are aware of the importance of carrying out practice according to policy. Failure to do so can have major consequences for the individuals using the service, the organisation and the staff.

KEY TERMS

Policy: A plan or principle of action proposed by an organisation, also known as a guideline or code.

Procedures: These state how policies will be carried out or actioned in a setting.

Person-centred care

The principles of person-centred care include showing respect for individuals and treating them with dignity and compassion, offering them choices in the support and care they seek. By offering care that is personalised to the individual and ensuring that all care, support and treatment is co-ordinated, you can help individuals to live an independent and fulfilling life.

It is therefore about making the individual requiring care the central figure in the process. The government publication 'Putting People First: A Shared Vision and Commitment to the Transformation of Adult Social Care' was published in 2007 and outlined its personalisation agenda – the government's vision of enabling individuals to live independently with complete choice and control over their lives.

Personalisation is about enabling individuals to build a system of care and support tailored to meet their needs and designed with their full involvement. It is about ensuring that the individual has their choices taken into account and their culture and ethnicity respected, with care tailored to these factors. Historically, a one-size-fits-all approach to care was in practice and this meant the individual had to fit into and access existing care services, whether they were appropriate or not.

The term 'person-centred care' is now used to describe care which is user focused, promoting independence and autonomy. Collaborative and partnership approaches to care often use the term 'person-centred' to describe their ethos (Innes et al., 2006).

Table 1 outlines some of the legislation, white papers, reports and guidance that affect person-centred care. The legislation from AC1.1 may also be relevant here.

Table 1 Documentation and its relevance to person-centred care

Date	Act/guidance	Purpose and effect
2008	'Valuing People Now'	The government's three-year plan to improve the lives of people with learning disabilities and their families. It covers all aspects of life, including health, housing, getting paid work, personalisation, transition, advocacy, hate crime and relationships.
2009	'Living Well With Dementia: A national dementia strategy'	Strategic framework for making quality improvements to dementia services. It also addresses health inequalities.
2010	The Francis Report	The failings in care at the Mid Staffordshire NHS Foundation Trust between 2005 and 2009 forced the person-centred care agenda back into public awareness. It focused sharply on dignity, compassion and respect.
2010	'A Vision for Adult Social Care: Capable communities and active citizens'	Set out the plans for a new direction for adult social care, putting personalised services and outcomes centre stage, based on six principles, personalisation being one such principle.
2012	Health and Social Care Act	Requires Clinical Commissioning Groups to promote the involvement of every individual.
2014	Care Act	Requires local authorities to involve adults in their assessment, care and support planning and review.
2022	Health and Care Act	Amends the Care Act 2014 and addresses the proposed cap on personal care spending already provided for by the Care Act 2014.

As you can see from the laws and guidance published since 2000, there has been a major revamp of adult social care law in England, all with the intention of seeking to transform care. The Care Act 2014 was a move to a single piece of legislation, so people were clear about their rights.

Evidence opportunity

1.2 Effects of legislation and policy on practice

- ✔ Provide a written account describing the association between legislation and policy on person-centred care and positive outcomes-based procedures and practice. This should include effects on a range of policies relevant to own area of provision. Think about the things that have been discussed in this section.
- ✔ Discuss with your assessor in a professional discussion how your application of legislation and statutory guidance within your own service/setting demonstrates that you are responsible and accountable.

Reflect on it

1.2 Legislation and your setting

Reflect on the ways in which the laws and papers in Table 1 have affected the way in which your setting delivers its care.

List five procedures or policies in your work setting which have developed as a result of legislation.

For example, you might look at how the Mental Capacity Act 2005 has impacted your work and comment on the changes the setting has made.

AC 1.3 Describe the roles, remits and responsibilities in a registered service

Here, you will be required to describe the different roles within your organisation's structure and be aware of the legal responsibilities of particular individuals.

Registered manager

All providers must have a registered manager with the exception of some day care, outreach and multidisciplinary or social work teams. This is a legal requirement under the Health and Social Care Act 2008, as set out in Regulation 7 relating to registered managers. The person undertaking this role must apply for a CQC counter-signed DBS check and demonstrate their fitness to be registered as a manager. This person must:

- be of good character
- be able to properly perform tasks that are intrinsic to their role
- have the necessary qualifications, competence, skills and experience to manage the regulated activity
- have supplied their employers with documents that confirm their suitability.

Source: Adapted from Care Quality Commission (n.d. a)

The registered manager will be expected to take appropriate action to address any shortfalls in practice and to improve the situation. This means your role will be to look to the teams with which you work and ensure that they take responsibility for updating their knowledge and continually improving their practice.

As a registered manager, you are responsible for the level of care your organisation and staff provide. The daily tasks you will be required to perform depend on the setting in which you work but essentially you will oversee the running of the service, managing staff so they can perform their roles safely and to a high standard.

You will also have control of budgets and contracts and will be involved in making strategic decisions about the future and growth of the setting.

Nominated individual

To register as a care organisation you need to nominate an individual to act as the main point of contact with the CQC. This may be the registered manager but is more usually another person in the organisation who can support the manager. In small care homes this may be the owner or manager. They will have overall responsibility for supervising the management of the regulated activity and ensuring the quality of the services. Therefore, they must be a senior person, with authority to speak on behalf of the organisation. The role of this person is to supervise and take responsibility for the management of the service and to show how it provides quality of life for the people who use it.

Fit and proper person

This person has met the criteria to be a registered provider, nominated individual or registered manager in terms of character and qualifications but does not have a specific role. It is a term that is becoming increasingly familiar in the care sector. All employees should be classified as 'fit and proper' persons, who are responsible for the quality and safety of care, and for meeting the fundamental standards.

Evidence opportunity

1.3 Roles and responsibilities

Who are the people in regulated services who carry out the roles described above? How have they been chosen for the role and what qualifications do they have? Describe the roles and responsibilities of these individuals and engage with your assessor in professional discussion.

LO2 Understand internal governance arrangements within own organisation

AC 2.1 Describe internal governance procedures used within own service/setting

Here, you will be required to describe your own organisation's governance procedures and mechanisms. You will be required to describe your own organisation's governance mechanisms to be able to identify how these relate to the identity of the organisation. This will include the topics discussed in this section. You will also consider the inspection process in your work setting. If your service is not currently regulated or inspected, you can think about how you could use current regulations to support service improvement.

The Department of Health and Social Care defines clinical and care governance as the system by which accountability for the quality of social care is monitored and assured. It is about creating an environment in which clinical and social care excellence will flourish with high standards of care. It includes quality assurance and improvement and risk and incident management.

We want adult social care to be safe and of good quality. Good **governance procedures** provide a framework through which this can be assured.

KEY TERM

Governance procedures: Monitoring actions, practices and policies which guide the decisions of organisations and their stakeholders.

Governance processes

Risk management

This is about making sure the risks to the individuals using the service are minimal. You must identify what can go wrong in care and ensure that if something does happen you learn from it and change it for the future. For example, an individual may make what the care worker deems to be an unwise choice. Training for staff in the requirements of the Mental Capacity Act will enable adult care workers to support individuals to make their own informed decisions safely and within the law.

Clinical audit

An audit compares one thing against another to check its quality. For example, you may be required to audit compliance with handwashing in your setting. There are certain standards expected with handwashing and by monitoring performance against such standards you can check efficiency. The audit on handwashing would therefore check and identify if you were not meeting the standards and you can then make changes to practice. Auditing may be a local practice but there are also national audits into which all care organisations supply data.

Education, training and continuing professional development

Your staff are a major resource, so time and money spent in upskilling them and ensuring they have the knowledge to do excellent work are required under the governance principles. This can range from mentoring to formal training courses. All upskilling activities should be recorded.

Your staff need to be aware of their responsibility to update their knowledge and to attend health and safety training and safeguarding on a regular basis. It is your responsibility to ensure that the opportunity to do this is available and that staff are encouraged to take time to attend training courses so that there is no reason for not complying with health, safety and risk management policies and procedures. Failure to comply could mean the staff member would be put at risk of losing their job and there will also be consequences for the organisation.

Evidence-based care and effectiveness

Care should be based upon researched evidence that it is the best practice. The National Institute of Clinical Excellence provides guidelines for practice that care organisations must follow. To go back to the earlier example on hand washing, this activity has been researched and nationally accepted guidelines as to the most effective way in which to carry out the procedure are available.

Behaviour that challenges can be very distressing for people with learning disabilities. It shows that something is not right and that they need help and support. The principles of Positive Behavioural Support (PBS) and other evidence-based approaches ensure that people with learning disabilities have a right to receive support and care based on good and up-to-date evidence.

The British Institute of Learning Disabilities (BILD) sets out a values-led PBS initiative that supports 'human rights and promotes respect, dignity, inclusion and a life without unnecessary restriction'.

The overall aim of PBS is to improve the quality of a person's life and the lives of the people around them. It aims to provide the right support at the right time and uses different methods to gather information to work out what people's behaviour means. The intention is to empower people to use less harmful methods to achieve their needs, instead using approaches that will enhance their lives.

However, it recognises that this approach may require staff training, as well as changes to service structures and cultures.

For more information, see BILD (n.d.).

Inspection

When an inspection is expected the registered manager is responsible for preparing the staff for the event and preparing the paperwork. You can start by reading the CQC guidance about compliance and encourage the individuals using your service to complete 'please tell us your experience' evaluation surveys. Ensure that staff understand the role of the CQC and what happens during an inspection visit, and that they have received training that is appropriate for their role.

There are five key questions that you will need to review to make sure that you are prepared for an inspection.

1. Is the service safe?
2. Is the service effective?
3. Is the service caring?
4. Is the service responsive?
5. Is the service well led?

Research it

2.1 CQC inspection

The CQC provides details of the legislation and guidance required for inspection, which you can access on their website (Care Quality Commission, 2022b)

Familiarise yourself with the guidance and consider how you might start to engage with collection of evidence now.

You can find more information on the five key questions on page 47. News of a pending inspection can sometimes cause unnecessary stress, but if good practice is the norm in your service, you can reduce this anxiety by helping staff to see and appreciate that they are doing the best they can do and that they are supported. Being inspection-ready at all times will reduce the anxiety that might come with unannounced visits.

Individual and carer experience and involvement

Complaints and compliments are a vital link to how others feel about the service, and you should take these on board. It is important to establish close partnerships with families, friends and others who work with the individuals in your care. Governance is about establishing policies and procedures and monitoring processes to ensure that the organisation meets the needs of the people who use it. Efficient monitoring of complaints is a necessary part of the process.

Staffing and staff management

Highly skilled people working to provide quality care need to be supported and motivated. Part of governance is the training and upskilling of staff. Additionally, you need to ensure that staff are motivated to encourage them to stay with the organisation.

Roles and responsibilities within the governance process

As a manager, you are responsible for the safety and wellbeing of the individuals using your service and for ensuring that the components of governance are in place and being worked towards.

As a manager and leader in adult care, your knowledge of the law and how it is translated into practice through policy and implemented by your staff must underpin your practice. Undoubtedly, you will already have a good working knowledge and practice related to the legal aspects of care work, but it is wise to revisit this from time to time. You will need to offer strong induction activities and training for staff. Staff need to understand their roles and responsibilities about health and safety record-keeping and reporting, safeguarding and person-centred practice, and must also be aware of the necessity of complying with policies, procedures and practice. Any breaches must be dealt with effectively and quickly to avoid unsafe practice. By monitoring compliance to the policies and procedures, ensuring that checks/audits take place and risk assessments are updated, you will be practising safely with respect to this part of your management role.

To maintain such high-quality care in your organisation you need to create a performance management system that:

- identifies areas of best practice and focuses on continuous improvement
- delivers better outcomes to individuals
- improves adult care services by acting upon new initiatives and information
- ensures that organisational activities are linked to the overall goals of the organisation.

Performance management is a process where managers and employees work together to plan, monitor and review a team member's work objectives and to review how they contribute to the organisation. It requires the establishment of formal, regular and rigorous systems of data collection to measure the performance of services.

Understanding of the governance process within the organisation

Adult care should be standardised, of good quality and good reputation, and conform to government legislation. Above all, organisations must be accountable for what they do and be transparent so that all involved can see the decisions being made and understand why they are needed. Governance also requires that you work in partnership with other sectors, including the private and voluntary sectors. This requires the individuals using the service and their families, as well as the partners you work with, to participate in the decision-making process.

The World Health Organization publishes information on health system governance, including fact sheets, data and tools and resources (World Health Organization, n.d.)

Additionally, the Skills for Care website provides their GO Online: Inspection toolkit, which provides support for a 'well led service'. It defines good governance and management in adult social care services and provides managers with resources to support them in inspection (Skills for Care, n.d.).

Evidence opportunity

2.1 Governance mechanisms

Provide a written account describing your organisation's governance procedures and mechanisms and reflect on your organisation's governance mechanisms so that you can identify how these relate to the identity of the organisation. Include governance concepts, governance processes, roles and responsibilities within the governance process, and understanding of the governance process within the organisation.

Reflect on it

2.1 Governance mechanisms

Describe your organisation's governance procedures and mechanisms, saying how you evidence:

- risk management
- clinical audit
- education, training and continuing professional development
- evidence-based care and effectiveness
- individual and carer experience and involvement
- staffing and staff management.

Pick three of these aspects and explain how successfully your organisation uses these procedures and mechanisms to ensure positive outcomes. It is a good idea to question why you do certain things and what is good (or otherwise) about what you do. For example, if you undertake a clinical audit of handwashing and find that staff are not complying with the practice, what do you do about this? Ask questions such as: 'Why are staff non-compliant?' 'What else is happening?' 'What might be done to change this?'

What are your roles and responsibilities within these areas of work?

AC 2.2 Explain own role in applying, leading and evaluating own service/setting's governance procedures and agreed ways of working

Here, you will explain your own role in following the governance procedures outlined in AC2.1 and how you apply these to the rest of the organisation.

The difference between procedures and policies lies in the fact that policies are designed to help an organisation meet its objectives and so may grow and change. A **protocol** is a standardised way of doing something and is generally a step-by-step directive to be followed to help accomplish a task. Not following a protocol leads to misunderstandings or miscommunications. For example, you will have an infection control policy in place and this provides care staff with guidance on best practice. A procedure attached to this policy may provide a set of instructions describing the steps on how to control infection. Protocols are more explicit and provide written plans that specifically outline what, when, and how procedures are to be followed in defined situations, for instance should an infection breakout occur, the protocol will be used.

As the registered manager of the setting you must ensure that the **agreed ways of working** and governance procedures are clearly understood and followed by staff. Agreed ways of working are really about the culture of the organisation and the policies and procedures that are laid down in that culture. A culture is the way in which things are done and it will be reflected in the values and attitudes of the staff who work in that organisation. For example, a culture of safety within your organisation will be reflected in everything that you do – if you work in a high-pressure environment, you may be aware that there are in-house counsellors who can be contacted should you require psychological or emotional help to stay safe. Your staff will be educated about safety and your policies and procedures will have the safety of the individuals using the service at the heart of their practice.

Additionally, the stakeholders and those who use the service or are in partnership with you will be aware of your agreed ways of working.

KEY TERMS

Protocol: A set of rules that explains the correct procedure to be followed in a situation.

Agreed ways of working: Procedures and policies that workers in an organisation are required to follow.

Evidence opportunity

2.2 Evaluate your own role

Provide a written account to explain your own role in applying, leading and evaluating the organisation's agreed ways of working, protocols, policies and procedures relating to governance and accountability. Include feedback from those using services, those acting on their behalf and other stakeholders so that you can continually drive improvement.

Your organisation's agreed ways of working, protocols, policies and procedures all relate to governance and accountability and link to quality of care provision. For example, failure of staff to work within a policy or to follow a strict protocol could have a detrimental effect on the service and an individual using the service may suffer as a consequence. This will lead to the service being accountable for errors.

In evaluating your own role, look at the positive and negative effects of the ways of working and how they impact the service. What is good about having such practices in place? Are there any limitations?

Reflect on it

2.2 Agreed ways of working, protocols, policies and procedures

What are your organisation's agreed ways of working, protocols, policies and procedures? Do these reflect a particular culture, for example of safety or person-centred care?

Review how these relate to governance and accountability and to quality of care provision.

LO3 Understand systems and requirements for the regulation of adult care services

AC 3.1 Outline current legislation and statutory guidance underpinning and supporting inspection processes in England

Here, you will be required to outline the key drivers and impacts of legislation for the inspection system, including the topics discussed in this section.

Health and Social Care Act 2008 (Regulated Activities) Regulations 2014 and the Care Act 2014

The HSCA 2008 (Regulated Activities) Regulations 2014 and the Care Act 2014 both set out key responsibilities of local authorities to meet the needs of individuals who require help and support to promote their wellbeing. The HSCA also sets out the Care Quality Commission's (CQC) statutory powers and duties. The CQC is the lead inspection and enforcement body for safety, quality of treatment and care matters involving individuals in receipt of a health or adult social care service from a provider registered with the CQC.

The Health and Safety Executive (HSE)/local authorities are the lead inspection and enforcement bodies for health and safety matters involving individuals who are in receipt of a health or care service from providers not registered with the CQC.

The process recognises that certain bodies may be more appropriate to deal with specific cases. So, for example, the CQC will be called to investigate an incident where an individual is seriously injured or dies after being physically restrained by staff, but the HSE and local authority may be asked to investigate a manual handling injury to an employee.

Both pieces of legislation focus upon quality and standards in care to address some of the catastrophic failings within the care sector (see below) that resulted in neglect and abuse of individuals in a number of settings. As a result of these laws, the inspection framework for care settings has changed.

Recent local/national queries and findings from Safeguarding Adult Reviews

As a manager you are required to have policies and procedures in place to protect the individuals using your service, staff and visitors from breaches of health and safety law. The Francis Report, published in 2013, reported on the Mid Staffordshire NHS Foundation Trust where a major failure in care was uncovered. As a result, an important change was introduced in April 2015, giving new enforcement powers to the CQC with respect to health and safety in the care sector. The main purpose of the group is to monitor, inspect and regulate services to ensure standards of quality and safety are being met. Failure to do so will result in prosecution.

The change ensures that there is effective and co-ordinated regulation of health and safety for the individuals using the service, workers and members of the public, and a shared responsibility between the CQC, the HSE and local authorities to ensure safety.

Other appropriate topical reviews and reports

Examples of findings that have led to reform

In May 2011, a BBC Panorama documentary showed shocking undercover footage of abuse and humiliation carried out by a team of carers at Winterbourne View hospital in South Gloucestershire, which was owned and operated by a private company, Castlebeck. As a result of this programme, a **serious case review** led to 11 employees being charged and the closure of Winterbourne View, as well as criticism of the CQC for its failure to act when complaints had been made. Lessons learned from this serious breach of human rights led to a review of Castlebeck's management structures and they were eventually sold in 2013. In 2016, the CQC launched a new strategy for quality.

In another example, Orchid View was a West Sussex private nursing home registered as a care home with nursing for up to 87 people in the categories of old age and dementia. Opened in November 2009, it closed in October 2011 following revelations of several safeguarding alerts and investigations and possible criminal offences. In October 2013, an inquest found that five people had 'died from natural causes attributed to neglect' and that several other people 'died as a result of natural causes' with 'insufficient evidence before me [the coroner Penelope Schofield] to show that this suboptimal care was directly causative' of their deaths ... This suboptimal care caused distress, poor care and discomfort to residents and the families of people who were not the subject of the Inquest' (WSASB, 2014).

A further example is that of Steven Hoskin, a 39-year-old man with learning disabilities and living alone in Cornwall, who was tortured and murdered in 2007 by people who targeted him because of his learning disabilities. Steven's death has since been described as a disability hate crime and links have been made with the deaths of others with learning disabilities with known support needs. The details of the treatment Steven underwent at the hands of his abusers is very difficult to read and investigations of the safeguarding review showed that he had made numerous calls to a number of agencies, including the police and social care services, to alert them to the danger he was in and revealing how scared he was.

As a result of this awful crime, significant improvements in communication, sharing information and partnership working between the agencies in the area have been made. There has been an improved staff training programme and the police have introduced a 'neighbourhood harm register', ensuring that an alert is raised when repeated calls from the same people with the same problems are received.

Data is now shared with the appropriate agencies who work together to provide a joint response.

KEY TERM

Serious case review: This takes place after a person who should be safeguarded is seriously injured or dies, particularly if abuse or neglect is thought to have been a causative factor. It looks at what can be learned from the situation to help prevent similar incidents in the future. Serious case reviews are now known as Safeguarding Adults Reviews (SARs).

Evidence opportunity

3.1 The inspection system in England

Outline the key drivers and impact of legislation for the inspection system.

Reflect on it

3.1 Impact of legislation

Explain to your assessor the impact of legislation such as the Health and Social Care Act, the Care Act and any other recent local/national queries and findings from Safeguarding Adults Reviews that may have affected the way your service is inspected. In evaluating such cases, ask yourself some questions such as:

- What might have been the cause of the breach of the policy?
- What lessons can your service learn from these incidents?
- How does your service ensure that staff are aware of their duty with respect to adhering to policy?

AC 3.2 Identify types of service provision subject to registration and inspection

Here, you will be required to identify services subject to registration and inspection, covering a range of provision for all adult services, to include service provision in social care.

The CQC is responsible for the inspection and regulation of social and acute care providers including prisons, GPs, health centres, NHS and independent hospitals, care homes and other provisions.

Social care

Social care is a generic term relating to services available from social care providers. It relates to the provision of social work, social support services and personal care, and protects adults at risk or adults with needs arising from illness, disability, old age or poverty. It also includes caring for children in these circumstances.

Evidence opportunity

3.2 Services subject to registration and inspection

Identify the services you are aware of in the sphere of adult social services that require registration and inspection.

You may wish to identify the settings you work in partnership with and try to find out what their CQC ratings are. The ratings should be displayed on their websites.

LO4 Understand the inspection process in adult care

AC 4.1 Explain the purpose of the inspection system

Here, you will explain who carries out inspections and the purpose of inspections.

The Care Quality Commission (CQC) carry out the inspection process within certain care settings. Their purpose is to register health and adult social care service providers and to check, through inspection, that standards are being met, thereby ensuring the safety and quality of care.

The CQC is required to carry out inspections and monitoring visits which are usually announced and require settings to provide evidence in relation to the five key questions (see KLOEs, page 47). This will lead to the award of a rating on a four-point scale. For more on ratings see AC4.5.

AC 4.2 Explain how services are inspected and the role of the regulator

Here, you will understand the implementation of the assessment and inspection framework.

A new single assessment and inspection framework is planned for implementation in 2023, with a change in focus on what matters to people who use social care services and their families. See Care Quality Commission (n.d. b).

The ratings and the five key questions remain but new quality statements focusing on specific topic areas under a key question are to be included. Six new evidence categories are being introduced, which show the types of evidence the CQC use to understand the quality of care being delivered against a quality statement. For more on the five key questions, the quality statements and the evidence categories, see AC4.4.

AC 4.3 Describe different types of inspection

Here, you will describe the different types of inspection and the circumstances in which they will take place.

There are four types of inspection carried out by the CQC, as discussed below.

Comprehensive inspection

Comprehensive inspections are carried out when the CQC believe there is a risk to the safety or wellbeing of the individuals using the service or there has been a significant deterioration in the quality of care. These inspections are in-depth so there will be scrutiny of all care processes and procedures, systems and practice. The inspection team reviews the information they already have about the service, contacting stakeholders and professionals for feedback. An inspection site visit will then take place and conversations will be had with individuals using the service, visitors, staff, volunteers and other professionals to assess the key questions.

Records are reviewed and the premises are inspected for safety. Cleanliness, facilities and equipment are also looked at. After the inspection the setting will be given a rating of either 'Outstanding', 'Good', 'Requires improvement' or 'Inadequate'.

Although comprehensive inspections are usually unannounced, small residential services may receive 48-hours' notice to make sure people are available, while a week's notice may be given to complicated community services where planning is required.

Focused inspection

Focused inspections are usually a response to specific information received or to follow up on findings from a previous inspection. They:

- are normally unannounced
- do not look at all five of the key questions; instead, they concentrate on the well-led key question, (see AC4.4) and any other key questions relevant to the information that triggered the inspection
- are structured according to the reason they are being conducted
- raise any concerns or risks about the setting
- are smaller in scale than a comprehensive inspection but follow the same process and can result in a change to the overall rating of a setting.

Targeted inspection

Targeted inspections have a narrower focus than focused inspections and assess a particular risk, such as whether the requirements imposed by a **warning notice** have been met. It may be triggered if there are real concerns about specific risks to people's safety. Targeted inspections are usually unannounced and will not lead to a change of ratings.

KEY TERM

Warning notice: This is issued when the quality of care falls below what is legally required. A section 29 warning notice for all types of regulated provider is issued in writing when there has been regulation breach. A warning notice will state the relevant regulation that has been breached or the section of the Act or condition that is not being complied with and what further action will be taken and in what timescale if compliance is not met.

Combined inspection

Where providers deliver services across both health and social care sectors, inspection may be conducted in a different way. Each service is inspected by specialist inspectors who report on and rate each type of service in comparable ways.

Reflect on it

4.1, 4.2 and 4.3 Inspection process

What has been your experience of inspection? Think about the purpose it served and the type of experience your setting had.

Research it

4.1, 4.2 and 4.3 Well-led guidance

Download a copy of the Inspection toolkit from the Skills for Care website (Skills for Care, n.d.).

The CQC evaluates services against five key criteria: Safe, Effective, Caring, Responsive and Well-led, and Skills for Care supplies a toolkit that provides care providers with resources to help and support with the CQC expectations.

You might also like to look at and download a copy of NHS Improvement's 'Developmental reviews of leadership and governance using the well-led framework: guidance for NHS trusts and NHS foundation trusts'. Look at section 4 'The well-led framework and descriptions of good practice'. Although this framework may not be directly applicable to your service it provides a useful insight into the KLOEs (NHS Improvement, 2017).

Familiarise yourself with how inspections are carried out in your setting: see Care Quality Commission (2022b).

Evidence opportunity

4.1, 4.2 and 4.3 Prepare for inspection

Prepare a PowerPoint presentation for your assessor that explains the purpose of the inspection system and how services are inspected. Describe also the role of the regulator and the different types of inspection.

AC 4.4 Describe the standards that the inspection process reviews

Here, you will describe the different stages of the inspection process and what is covered at each stage.

Key questions

The CQC will continue to assess against five key questions:

- Is it safe?
- Is it effective?
- Is it caring?
- Is it responsive to people's needs?
- Is it well led?

Each question will be accompanied by several questions that inspection teams consider during inspection.

The well-led framework

The Well-led framework on the Skills for Care website looks at the culture, strategy, values and governance of your service. It details what the CQC will look at to ensure that the organisation continues to improve, and continues to deliver the best care possible.

The CQC will focus their inspection on key lines of enquiry (KLOEs), to answer five key questions: is the service safe, effective, caring, responsive and well led?

Is it safe?

This section investigates the safeguarding and protection from abuse procedures in place and how risk is managed and investigated. It scrutinises the suitability of the staff and staff cover and the way in which medicines are managed. Your infection control protocols are also looked at.

Is it effective?

In determining the effectiveness of the service, how you assess individuals' needs and whether you are delivering evidence-based treatment together with how consent is gained for care and treatment will be investigated. Training plans will also be looked at to determine that your staff's skills and knowledge are up to date. Nutrition, hydration and the support you give to help people to live healthier lives will be looked at, as well as how your staff teams work together and with other services. The premises will be assessed as to how accessible they are for the individuals using the service and visitors.

Is it caring?

A caring service is one where kindness, respect and compassion are evident. Involving people in decisions about their care will be a way of determining how far person-centred practices are being used.
Privacy and dignity are also part of this KLOE.

Is it responsive?

A responsive service is one where person-centred care is at the heart of the care, concerns and complaints are taken seriously, and lessons learned are put into place. There will also be an end-of-life care strategy in place.

Is it well led?

The final KLOE looks at the vision and strategy, governance and management of the service. Partnership working, engagement and involvement are investigated by looking at how staff are actively involved in developing the service and whether they are encouraged to propose new ways of working. Links with the local community are also looked at.

See Skills for Care (n.d.).

CQC quality statements

Quality statements are the commitments that providers should live up to. They are expressed as 'we statements' and show what is needed to deliver high-quality, person-centred care. They directly relate to the CQC regulations and show how services and providers work together to plan and deliver high quality care. Each of the five questions have quality statements applied to help you to plan and collect the evidence required to show you are meeting the requirements. The quality statements for the 'Key question: effective' are shown below.

- **Assessing needs**: We maximise the effectiveness of people's care and treatment by assessing and reviewing their health, care, wellbeing and communication needs with them.
- **Delivering evidence-based care and treatment**: We plan and deliver people's care and treatment with them, including what is important and matters to them. We do this in line with legislation and current evidence-based good practice and standards.
- **How staff, teams and services work together**: We work effectively across teams and services to support people. We make sure they only need to tell their story once by sharing their assessment of needs when they move between different services.
- **Supporting people to live healthier lives**: We support people to manage their health and wellbeing so they can maximise their independence, choice and control. We support them to live healthier lives and where possible, reduce their future needs for care and support.
- **Monitoring and improving outcomes**: We routinely monitor people's care and treatment to continuously improve it. We ensure that outcomes are positive and consistent, and that they meet both clinical expectations and the expectations of people themselves.
- **Consent to care and treatment**: We tell people about their rights around consent and respect these when we deliver person-centred care and treatment.

Source: Care Quality Commission (n.d. b)

Research it

4.4 CQC key questions and quality statements

Go to the CQC website and look at all the key questions and the quality statements arising from them. How do they differ from previous key lines of enquiry? Can you use evidence you have already collected to cover these statements? (Care Quality Commission, n.d. b)

Evidence categories

The evidence categories used to assess each quality statement are referred to as 'required evidence'. The amount of evidence required depends upon the service type, the level of assessment (service, provider, local authority or integrated care system) and whether the assessment is for an existing service or at registration.

People's experience of care services

In this category the CQC are interested in what matters to the people who use the service. The evidence will include individuals' perspective of how good their care is, so feedback will be sought.

Feedback from staff and leaders

Evidence from surveys, interviews , focus groups, self-assessment and compliments systems will be sought from the people who work in a service, and other groups who provide care. These might include commissioners, other local providers or multi-agency bodies.

Feedback from partners

This evidence will be collected in a similar way to the above. Your partners may be GP surgeries, pharmacies, the local hospital or physio services. They may also include charities and local authorities and social workers.

Observation

The quality of care delivery either off-site, on-site, or a combination of both will be observed.

- Off-site observations will include interviews with staff and professionals who work in the service as well as telephone and video interviews with people using services and their families and carers.
- On-site observations or inspections will be spent observing care and the care environment, including equipment and premises, speaking to people using services and staff to gain an understanding of the culture and to see how staff interact with each other.

Processes

This focus is on how effective policies and procedures are. The CQC will look at information from the provider and data sources that measure processes. For example, they will review care records, infection prevention control and any reported incidents/notifications.

Outcomes

Outcomes cover the impact of care processes on the individuals using the service and the CQC will consider outcomes measures in the context of the service. For example, they may look at the number of complaints received in the service and how these are acted upon and what lessons are learned.

AC 4.5 Explain how the ratings system is used

Here, you will explain the ratings system and the implications of the different grades.

The CQC will rate or grade each of the five key questions and will give an overall rating of either outstanding, good, requires improvement or inadequate.

Outstanding means that the service is performing exceptionally well, while good means the service is performing well and meeting expectations. If a service requires improvement this shows that the service must improve as it is not performing well enough according to standards.

An inadequate service is performing badly and actions against the person or organisation are put into place. An inadequate service is likely to be closed down until radical changes are made.

Evidence opportunity

4.5 Inspection grades and boundaries

Explain to your assessor in a professional discussion or provide a written account that describes and differentiates between the different grades available at inspection and evaluate the implications of each grade for a service. Try to use an example from your own service to show the differences between the grade boundaries. For example, if in your last inspection you received a good for leadership and management, how are you improving your practice to ensure that you receive outstanding next time?

Research it

4.5 Grading system and implications

Locate your last inspection report and look at the grading for each of the five key questions. Evaluate the implications of the grades for the services you offer.

As a manager, how will you address each rating to ensure that an improvement is made for the next inspection?

Compare the grades to those of a similar setting or service in your area. Explain the implications for your service when comparing the grades.

AC 4.6 Explain when and how enforcement action may be used

Here, you will explain the different types of enforcement actions that may occur and when they will be put into place.

If the individuals using a service are at risk of harm, the inspection team will put in place enforcement action to protect them. Enforcement action will also be taken if services are unregistered or registered persons or managers breach the conditions of registration by failing to follow the relevant sections of the Health and Social Care Act 2008, the Care Quality Commission (Registration) Regulations 2009 and the Health and Social Care Act 2008 (Regulated Activities) Regulations 2014.

The action or enforcement taken is proportionate to the risk or the seriousness of the legal breach but takes into account the impact action will have on the individuals using the service.

Enforcement policy

The CQC has an enforcement policy and inspectors follow a decision tree, in which steps are clearly covered to decide which action is needed (Figure 8).

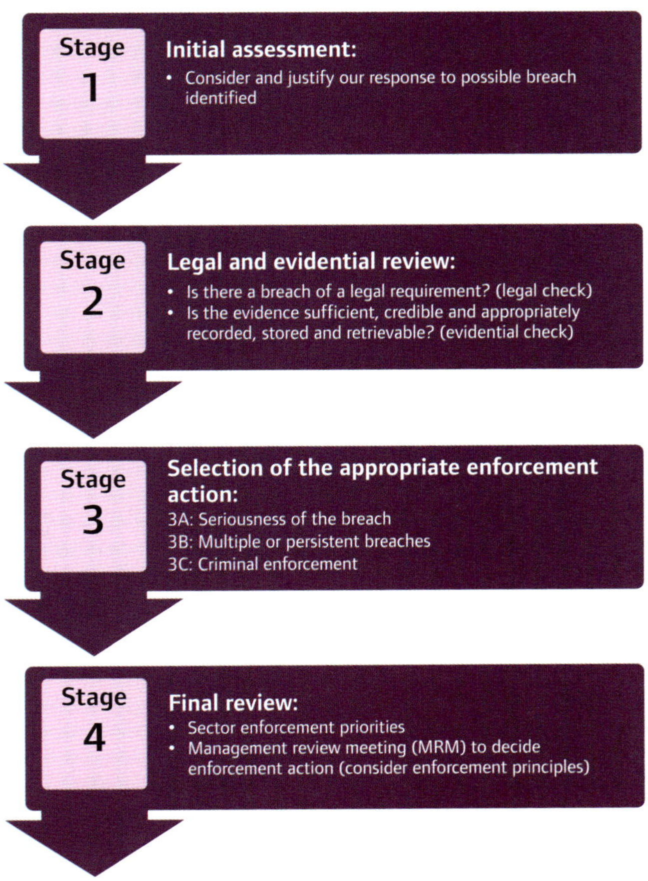

▲ **Figure 8** CQC enforcement decision tree

Possible actions required

If individuals are not at immediate risk of harm but the provider is not meeting a legal requirement, the CQC will require a report or plan to show how the setting will rectify the situation. This is called a 'requirement notice'.

It is up to the service to undertake the actions to meet the legal requirement and to inform CQC when this is done.

If a service is repeatedly rated as 'requiring improvement', an 'improvement action plan' will need to be provided explaining what actions the service intends to take to achieve a better overall rating.

Enforcement action

Two types of enforcement action can be taken. These are:

- enforcement action to protect people, or
- criminal enforcement action if the service fails to meet prosecutable fundamental standards.

If the care provided by a service harms people or puts people at risk of harm, the CQC take enforcement action and employ the enforcement policy (see Care Quality Commission, 2015).

This sets out the principles and approaches that will be followed when using enforcement powers under the Health and Social Care Act 2008, as amended by the Care Act 2014.

Evidence opportunity

4.6 Explain when and how enforcement action may be used

What is your understanding about enforcements? Write a short piece explaining when an enforcement action may be employed and how it might be used.

AC 4.7 Describe the ways information is collected about the service and used to inform inspection activities

Here, you will be required to describe how the regulators prepare for an inspection, the role of the inspection team and the sources of information used for inspection of adult care services, to include the topics discussed here.

At the start of an inspection, the inspection team will contact the senior staff and set up a meeting at which they will introduce the team and explain what they intend to do. In some care sectors, they will expect to see a presentation where the care provider gives its own view of its performance.

The team will then gather views and information from staff, the individuals using the service, their families and carers. This may include face-to-face discussions, emails or surveys.

The team collects evidence towards the quality statements by observing care, looking at care/support plans, checking policies and how they are working, and looking at where the care is given.

At the end of the inspection, a feedback meeting is held with senior staff and the findings are summarised. Any issues that have been highlighted are discussed and subsequent actions are planned. These findings are then published in a report, quality assured, and a grading of the service is given according to the grading detailed on page 48 of this unit.

- **Local information**: inspectors will be informed about the setting and the location within the community by looking at local information. They may also look at complaints and gather information from staff, carers and people who use services.
- **Information collected before the inspection and information from people who use services, their families and carers, staff and other professionals**: the CQC will collect information from the service provider and from any records they already have. They will also look at local and national data.
- **The inspection**: includes observing care and looking at records and documents and for adult social care they will also look at local information and any data they have collected from people who use services, their families, carers, staff and other professionals.
- **Reports that are quality assured, graded and published**: at the end of an inspection, a report is produced with ratings shown. This provides an overall judgement of the quality of care on each of the five key questions. Quality assurance panels are set up to look at samples of inspection reports to check consistency.

Evidence opportunity

4.7 Inspection process and information required

Prepare a written account describing how regulators prepare for an inspection, the role of the inspection team and the sources of information used for inspection of adult care services, to include the areas covered in the bullets.

LO5 Understand the inspection process in own setting/service

AC 5.1 Describe how the requirements of regulations are met within own service

Here, you will gain a better understanding of the inspection standards to assess your own setting.

At this point a good exercise will be to determine how your own setting meets the requirements of regulations. A review of the CQC's five key questions and the quality statements required for inspection is an excellent place to start and you might collect evidence under each of the following headings.

Is the service safe?

Inspectors will want to check that people are being protected from abuse and harm and that risks are carefully monitored.

Evidence for this can be provided by looking at safeguarding notifications, for example complaints, concerns and incidents. Inspectors may also approach staff and the individuals using the service to ask questions about how safe they feel. Observations of care in the service can also provide detail about how staff approach people and how they interact and deal with difficult situations.

Is the service effective?

An effective service is one in which people's care, treatment and support achieve good outcomes. This can be assessed by looking at evaluation forms and feedback from the individuals using the service and their families. By talking to staff and stakeholders, the inspection team can gain evidence of training and support. The inspector may also want to be present at handover when staff discuss the care of individuals to determine their level of knowledge about the service and those using it.

Is the service caring?

A caring service is one that treats people with compassion, dignity, respect and kindness. The inspectors may need to access care/support plans and files and to see what others say about the care they have received. Communication is also looked at and evidence of systems in use shows whether staff are communicating with individuals effectively and with kindness.

Is the service responsive?

A responsive service is organised and meets people's needs in a well-structured manner. Observation of care will quickly show whether a task-orientated approach is used or whether person-centred care is truly practised. The inspection teams again may wish to view satisfaction surveys of individuals using the service and staff training records.

Is the service well led?

A service that is well led will show that it is open and fair and delivers high-quality person-centred and innovative care. Staff will be well-trained, and morale is likely to be good. The general atmosphere of the service will immediately show how well you as a manager have performed to engage staff to ensure that they deliver care that is excellent. Inspectors will look at how staff interact with each other and how this affects the care they provide. Unhappy staff are unlikely to be motivated to do a good job and this will be reflected in how they approach the care.

The inspection team may also wish to access team meeting minutes and staff training and supervision records.

Evidence opportunity

5.1 Describe how the requirements of regulations are met within own service

Using the five key questions, prepare evidence folders for each of the questions and provide evidence for each folder. Describe to your staff or assessor how your service meets the requirements for inspection.

AC 5.2 Explain who needs to be aware of, and involved in, the inspection process

Here, you will be required to explain who the different people and organisations are that need to be informed of any pending inspection and the importance of ensuring a culture of inspection readiness.

In this section you need to identify who will undertake key roles in an inspection and what will be expected of others in the organisation and the team.

As the registered manager you will take a lead role in ensuring paperwork is easy to access and up to date and have a list of people to contact if any of the nominated people are unavailable at short notice. If you are fortunate to have a nominated person in place, then you can support this individual in their preparations as they will take the lead.

Inspection can sometimes cause anxiety but if good practice is the norm for your setting, you can support staff by showing appreciation for what they are already doing.

How to prepare for an inspection

Read the CQC guidance about compliance and encourage the individuals using your service to complete the 'please tell us your experience' evaluation surveys. Ensure that staff understand the role of the CQC and what happens during an inspection visit, and that they have received training that is appropriate for their role.

There is useful information on the CQC website in the section 'How we monitor, inspect and regulate adult social care services' (Care Quality Commission, 2023).

Evidence opportunity

5.2 How to prepare for an inspection

Identify the key people within your setting and any stakeholders outside the setting who will need to be informed about a pending inspection and explain how you will undertake this. You should include organisations that need to be informed of any pending inspection. Explain to your assessor the importance of ensuring a culture of inspection readiness, i.e. working in a setting that is ready for inspection at all times.

AC 5.3 Explain the range and types of evidence which can be used to demonstrate the setting/service is meeting requirements

Here, you will explain different types of evidence that the organisation can use to show that the setting/service is meeting requirements of regulation processes.

If you are to deliver adult care that is safe, fair and of high quality you must ensure that information systems within your organisation are sound and that the records you keep are safe.

Your own setting will have custody of many forms of information about the individuals using the service, the staff and the organisation itself, as well as the stakeholders and the partners you work with. For example, you will have records of satisfaction surveys and reports of how you have managed complaints and concerns.

Written communication from individuals and families can also provide information about the service and its delivery. Your staff supervision, appraisal and training records are also key pieces of information which show how well you meet statutory standards. Care records and meeting minutes provide valuable evidence of how well care aims are achieved. To integrate this information, you will need to train staff in how to use it. Additionally, you will have policies which detail how you work with others to deliver care, meet health and safety regulations, and manage information within the system.

If your care setting wishes to continue to provide care, it must be accountable for its practices and must be able to show evidence of the care it is providing.

The quality of the information stored can be assessed by looking at the source of the material gained and its reliability. Surveys of individuals using the service, for example, in which only five people completed the questionnaire are not a good source of information to recommend a change in service delivery.

Reflect on it

5.3 Types of information required for regulation processes

Speak to your assessor and explain the different types of information that the organisation is required to keep. Then reflect on the quality of the information stored.

Reflect on it

5.3 KLOEs and information

Look again at the CQC's KLOEs about services:

- Are they safe?
- Are they effective?
- Are they caring?
- Are they responsive to people's needs?
- Are they well led?

Under each question, list the information you can supply to support your organisation in answering these questions. For example, under 'Are they safe?', you may supply accident records, your health and safety policy, confidentiality policy, safeguarding and maintenance records.

AC 5.4 Describe ways to address the outcome and impact of an inspection of own service/setting

Here, you will be required to describe the ways to address the outcome and impact of an inspection.

Responding to areas of concern

Any areas that require improvement need to be addressed urgently. You and your team will need to develop an action plan to address them and make improvements.

Acknowledging areas of good practice

This is the positive outcome of inspection and clearly staff, the individuals using the service and the stakeholders should celebrate areas of good practice. This should be part of your website and promotional materials.

Developing an action plan

An action plan to address areas of concern and the improvements to be made should be developed immediately as there will be a follow-up on any action by a focused inspection.

Follow-up focused inspections

The inspectors will return to check that action plans have been completed and that areas of concern have been addressed.

Evidence opportunity

5.4 Respond to recommendations

Look at the last inspection report for your setting. Write a short report to describe the recommendations and say how you met those. What changes did you implement and how did you acknowledge good practice?

AC 5.5 Explain how outcomes of inspection can be used to drive setting/service improvements

Here, you will explain how the results of an inspection can improve the service in your own setting.

Since 2015, the CQC, Health and Safety Executive and local authorities in England have worked together to ensure that 'there is effective, co-ordinated and comprehensive regulation of health and safety for service users, workers and members of the public visiting these premises. It is one of the measures taken by Government to close the "regulatory gap" identified by the Francis Report into failings at the Mid Staffordshire NHS Foundation Trust' (CQC, HSE and Local Government Association, 2015).

The memorandum outlines the responsibility of each of the parties involved. The CQC is the lead inspector and enforcement body for the safety and quality of treatment and care involving individuals in receipt of a health or adult social care service from a provider registered with the CQC.

The outcome of your inspection may be a cause for celebration if you receive a rating of outstanding. However, you will still need to avoid complacency to ensure that you keep this rating.

If action is required, this should be addressed by meeting with staff and individuals using the service to clearly determine the ways forward, addressing not only the shortfalls but also the overall improvement of the service. It should be viewed as an opportunity to develop the service.

In June 2018, the CQC published a resource about adult social care called 'Driving improvement'. This provides useful research into adult care and shows how nine adult social care services achieved a significant improvement on their rating. These services were approached and asked to discuss the actions they had taken to help them learn and improve.

Key themes were identified, including their initial reactions of shock or surprise to the inspection report and how the report helped the provider to reflect and then address standards that might have been slipping. Leadership and the importance of a good leader who engages with staff, the individuals using the service and their families were also noted. Those leaders who were open to suggestions and willing to take tough decisions were valued. Also noted was that failing settings had closed cultures in which staff were afraid to speak out or did not feel valued or listened to.

You may find it useful to read this document and to identify areas in it that might be useful for development in your own setting. For example, there are case studies to support better pressure area care and one in which a significant improvement to an individual's mobility and weight loss was addressed.

Research it

5.5 Driving improvement

Share the CQC report 'Driving improvement' (Care Quality Commission, 2018) with your staff and ask for their comments and suggestions about what you can do to improve the care you provide.

Survey the individuals using your service and ask them to comment on the inspection report. What might they suggest as a good developmental change for the service?

Evidence opportunity

5.5 Improvements to service following inspection

Following on from the 5.5 Research it activity, make a list of the improvements your service has experienced as a result of the last inspection report. Explain the most significant change you made.

How might you turn a good rating into an outstanding rating? You may find it helpful to draw on the case studies in the 'Driving improvement' report referred to above.

In a non-regulated service, undertake your own mini inspection and use your findings to improve the care service.

Legislation

Legislation	Key points
Health and Care Act 2022	This Act introduced new legislation to make it easier for health and adult social care organisations to deliver joined-up, integrated care for people who rely on different services.
Health and Social Care Act 2008 (Regulated Activities) Regulations 2014	Outlines the fundamental standards for care.
Equality Act 2010	An umbrella Act bringing together legislation that deals with race, disability and gender. It highlights protected characteristics of age, gender reassignment, pregnancy, religion, marriage and civil partnerships, and sexual orientation in an attempt to end discrimination.
Care Act 2014	Sets out the key responsibilities of local authorities in meeting the needs of individuals who require help and support to promote their wellbeing. Its main aim was to provide integrated care and to introduce the right to an assessment for all.
Mental Capacity Act 2005	This act informs individuals about what they can do to plan and ensure that someone else can make decisions for them if they ever lack capacity to do so for themselves.
Health and Social Care Act 2008 (HSCA 2008)	The Health and Social Care Act 2008 requires providers of 'regulated activities' in England to register with the Care Quality Commission (CQC). They must also comply with the requirements and standards set out in regulations made under that Act.
Health and Social Care Act 2012	This Act introduced the role of the Care Quality Commission. Safeguarding and protection of individuals are specifically mentioned in these laws to address concerns about abuse. The Act aims to safeguard people who use care services from suffering any form of abuse or improper treatment while receiving care and treatment. To meet the requirements under this Act providers must demonstrate zero tolerance of abuse, unlawful discrimination and restraint.
Mental Health Acts 1983 (amended 2007)	The Mental Health Act 1983, amended by the Mental Health Act 2007, is designed to give health professionals powers to detain, assess and treat people with mental disorders in the interests of their health and safety or for public safety. The legislation also provides safeguards for individuals to ensure that they are not inappropriately treated under the provisions of the Act.
Health and Safety at Work Act 1974	This Act is the primary piece of legislation governing workplace health and safety in the UK. It defines the general duties of employees and employers, owners, managers and maintainers of work premises (etc.) for maintaining health and safety within the workplace.

References

BILD (n.d.) 'Vision and values'. www.bild.org.uk/vision-values

Care Quality Commission (2015) 'Enforcement policy'. www.cqc.org.uk/sites/default/files/20150209_enforcement_policy_V1-1.pdf

Care Quality Commission (2018) 'Driving improvement: Case studies from nine adult social care services' www.cqc.org.uk/publications/evaluation/driving-improvement-case-studies-nine-adult-social-care-services

Care Quality Commission (n.d. a) 'Guidance for providers'. www.cqc.org.uk/guidance

Care Quality Commission (n.d. b) 'How we will regulate'. www.cqc.org.uk/about-us/how-we-will-regulate

Care Quality Commission, Health and Safety Executive and Local Government Association (2015), 'Memorandum of Understanding between the Care Quality Commission, the Health and Safety, Executive and local authorities in England'. https://care2improveblog.files.wordpress.com/2015/01/cqc-mou__between_cqc_hse_las_in_england_final-feb-15.pdf

Department of Health (2001) *Valuing People: A new strategy for learning disability for the 21st century; planning with people; towards person-centred approaches – accessible guide*. London: HMSO.

Department of Health (2007) *Putting People First: A shared vision and commitment to the transformation of adult social care*. London: HMSO.

Department of Health (2008) *The Wanless Report: Securing good health for the whole population*. London: HMSO.

Department of Health (2014) *The Health and Social Care Act 2008 (Regulated Activities) Regulations 2014*. London: TSO.

Francis, R. (2013) *Report of the Mid Staffordshire NHS Foundation Trust Public Inquiry*. London: TSO. https://assets.publishing.service.gov.uk/government/uploads/system/uploads/attachment_data/file/279124/0947.pdf

Health and Safety Executive (n.d.) 'How to trace legislation'. www.hse.gov.uk/legislation/trace.htm

HM Government (2009) *Shaping the Future of Care Together*. Green Paper.

Innes, A., Macpherson, S. and McCabe, I. (2006) *Promoting Person-Centred Care at the Front Line*. York: Joseph Rowntree Foundation/SCIE.

NHS Improvement (2017) 'Developmental reviews of leadership and governance using the well-led framework: Guidance for NHS trusts and NHS foundation trusts', 4. The well-led framework and descriptions of good practice. www.england.nhs.uk/wp-content/uploads/2020/08/Well-led_guidance_June_2017.pdf.

Skills for Care (n.d.) 'Good and outstanding care (GO): Inspection toolkit'. www.skillsforcare.org.uk/Support-for-leaders-and-managers/Good-and-outstanding-care/inspect/Inspection-toolkit.aspx

Skills for Health, Health Education England, NHS England (2019) 'Core capabilities framework for supporting people with a learning disability'. www.skillsforhealth.org.uk/wp-content/uploads/2020/11/Learning-Disability-Framework-Oct-2019.pdf

SCIE (n.d.) 'Living with dementia'. www.scie.org.uk/dementia/living-with-dementia/

West Sussex Adult Safeguarding Board (WSASB) (2014) 'Orchid View Serious Case Review'. www.westsussex.gov.uk/media/5168/orchid-view-scr-final-report.pdf

Useful resources and further reading

Cameron, A., Lart, R., Bostock, L. and Coomber, C. (2012) 'Factors that promote and hinder joint and integrated working between health and social care services,' *Research Briefing 41*, SCIE.

Care Quality Commission (2022a) 'Guidance for providers: About this guidance'. www.cqc.org.uk/guidance-providers/regulations-enforcement/about-guidance

Care Quality Commission (2022b) 'Guidance for providers: Legislation'. www.cqc.org.uk/guidance-providers/regulations-enforcement/legislation

Care Quality Commission (2022c) 'How we inspect services: Adult social care services.' www.cqc.org.uk/guidance-providers/adult-social-care/how-we-inspect-services-adult-social-care-services

Care Quality Commission (2022d) 'State of care'. www.cqc.org.uk/publications/major-report/state-care

Care Quality Commission (2023) 'How we monitor, inspect and regulate adult social care services'. www.cqc.org.uk/guidance-providers/adult-social-care/how-we-monitor-inspect-regulate-adult-social-care-services

Department of Health (2014) *Hard Truths: The journey to putting patients first. Volume One of the Government Response to the Mid Staffordshire NHS Foundation Trust Public Inquiry*, 2 volumes. London: TSO.

Health Foundation, The (2016) 'Person-centred care made simple: What everyone should know about person-centred care'. www.health.org.uk/sites/health/files/PersonCentredCareMadeSimple.pdf

NHS Employers (2022) 'People performance management toolkit'. www.nhsemployers.org/case-studies-and-resources/2018/04/people-performance-management-toolkit

NHS England (n.d.) 'Clinical audit'. www.england.nhs.uk/ourwork/qual-clin-lead/clinaudit

Renz, D. and Eddy, W. (1996) 'Organisations, ethics and healthcare: Building an ethics infrastructure for a new era', *Bioethics Forum*, 12(2): 29–39.

Social Care Institute for Excellence website: www.scie.org.uk

Wanless, D. (2002) *Securing Our Future Health: Taking a long-term view*. London: HM Treasury.

World Health Organization (n.d.) 'Health system governance'. www.who.int/health-topics/health-systems-governance#tab=tab_1

Unit 502

Decision making in leadership and management within adult care

GLH 20

About this unit

In your role as manager or supervisor, you will make decisions daily on various issues relating to staff, budgets, the setting and the people who use care services. Decision making is, therefore, a key part of adult care work and management and will be a key part of your role, so it is important that you understand how to make decisions effectively that consider the best interests of those that will be affected by them.

In this unit, you will understand what it means to make choices, identify the decisions that need to be made and gather the information that is needed to inform effective and positive decisions in your role. You will gain a better understanding of what it means to make thoughtful decisions by carefully organising the information you have and considering alternatives. You will explore models and methods of decision making and understand how you can apply these to your own management practice. You will understand how you can use and analyse qualitative and/or quantitative data to inform your decision making and how you can justify decisions. You will also learn how to evaluate your own management of the range of situations in which decisions are required and to reflect on and critically evaluate your skills in decision making and recommendations to enhance your future practice.

Learning outcomes

By the end of this unit, you will:

1 Understand effective decision making.

2 Be able to demonstrate effective decision making within a leadership and management role.

Getting started

Before you study the unit, think about the following:

- What safeguards are in place for the decisions managers make? In other words, what in law protects you when you make decisions on behalf of others? When do you think it is right to make a decision based on intuition?
- What are the potential challenges to decision making when working with difficult situations and if there are disagreements? Have you experienced these?
- How does legislation impact decision-making processes?

LO1 Understand effective decision making

AC 1.1 Describe different types of decisions required in own role

Here, with examples from your own practice, you will be required to describe:

- *the meaning of effective decision making at senior management level*
- *what constitutes an effective management decision*
- *the effects of not making timely decisions in management*
- *the impact that making a management decision has on others, e.g. for colleagues, teams, others*
- *the impact that not making a management decision has on others, e.g. colleagues, teams, others*
- *the relationship between decision making and accountability.*

Effective decision making at senior management level and what constitutes an effective management decision

What decisions have you made today? What to have for breakfast? What to wear? How to get to work? You had to go through a process to make those decisions. In your role as manager you will be making decisions daily. Some of those may be life changing for somebody, so you need to be aware of the impact of the decisions you are making.

Reflect on it

1.1 The decisions you make

What decisions do you make on a daily basis in your management role? Make a list of some you have made today and then say how you feel about this as part of your management role. What are the pros and cons of making a list of the decisions you have made? What are the pros and cons of reflecting on how these decisions are part of the management role?

Types of decisions

There are a number of different types of decisions that you will need to make in a leadership role:

- Strategic decisions are long-term complex decisions, usually made by the senior leaders. These are part of the mission statement for an organisation, which forms part of the strategic plan.
- Tactical decisions are medium-term decisions and are less complex, focusing on a change at team level. For example, you might decide to undertake a project to make a change in the service delivery.
- Operational decisions are those you make on a daily basis. They relate to processes you might undertake regularly, such as ordering stock or scheduling staff shifts.

Peter Drucker (2015) highlighted seven elements of decision making.

1 Determining whether a decision is necessary

This sounds simple but if a decision does not need to be made then a lot of time and resources may be wasted. It is important then that you are able to distinguish between necessary and unnecessary decisions.

2 Classify the problem

As a manager, you will face a variety of issues. Some will be of a general nature, which can be answered with reference to policy and procedure. For example, if somebody asks for a decision about annual leave you might direct them to the organisation's policy. Occasionally, though, an event may occur that cannot be answered in this manner, such as an emergency situation. When this happens, a decision must be made. Drucker refers to these events as 'unique' problems requiring a unique solution but makes the point that these are rare occurrences and should be carefully examined and defined.

3 Define the problem

Sometimes you may look at a problem and jump to a conclusion. This is dangerous. For example, you may be presented with an issue by a colleague who is making an assumption that the problem lies with an individual using the service, but in reality it is how the staff dealt with the individual that was the real issue.

Sometimes what the problem appears to be is not what it really is. So, how can you make an effective decision here? Drucker suggests asking questions to define the problem:

- What is this all about and what is going on? Here you will need to think about the situation as it is happening and the people or resources surrounding the situation. For example, you may be faced with an emergency and need to make a decision quickly. You will need to evaluate in that moment what you are seeing happening.
- What is key to this situation? In this case, you want to know what the priority is in this situation.

4 Decide on what is right

The next step is to form the decision. It is here that you need to decide who in the wider organisation might be affected. You will start to think about what others may think about your decision or how the finance team might view it, for example. Perhaps a compromise is needed.

Making a decision implies that there are alternatives that may need to be considered, but those alternatives should be ones that fit with the goals and values of the organisation and any compromise also needs to reflect those values.

5 Get others to buy into the decision

This is when you form the decision and start to 'sell' it to the organisation. For example, a new way of working is not always received well. In this case, you will need to explain to staff why the change is necessary and good for the organisation. Staff need to understand that the decision has been made with the wider organisation's objectives in mind and therefore has meaning and purpose.

6 Build action into the decision and make it happen

If this is missing, then the decision simply remains an idea. You now need others to do something to move the action forward and this requires more than just a memo informing staff of a change. You will need to identify the following:

- Who needs to know of this decision?
- What action has to be taken and who is to take it?
- What do they have to do?

As the decision maker, you must be assured that the staff who are involved in making it happen are not only capable of doing so but are aware of how they will show that they have accomplished the action. They will be impacted by the decision and therefore you should be aware of how that decision may affect them. Almost any decision may involve some conflict or dissatisfaction and you need to be ready to justify your decision.

7 Test the decision against actual results

Finally, the results of a decision that has been made may be seen in the future – you may not see the results immediately, but monitoring and reporting should be built into the decision to provide evidence of its progress.

Source: Adapted from Drucker (2015)

Effective management decisions

A good decision is one where the choice made has been considered against other alternatives. In making a good decision you will be aware of the positives and negatives of the options you have and think about the outcome by weighing up the options. For example, you may have two members of staff who need to attend a training course but there is only one place left. Your decision will depend on the information you have about the members of staff and perhaps who might benefit from it more or who can wait until the next course is available. You may make the decision based on the need of the organisation and send the most experienced member of staff who will be able to cascade their learning to the rest of the team. The decision, then, will be based upon several factors but will require information gathering to make it a good one.

Impact of management decision making on others

In the case of the staff training example above, the decision you make will impact at least one member of staff; that is, the one who will not at this time attend the training. This can be negative and will require careful handling, but a well-reasoned and informed choice will ensure that staff understand why you made the decision. You need to justify what you have decided.

Sometimes, not making a decision can also have an impact on others because the decision may be taken out of your hands and made for you. If this happens it may not lead to the best result for your team. Ignoring the need to make a decision will not make it go away, it will simply make somebody take the decision for you.

Effects of not making timely decisions

It is tempting sometimes to leave a decision alone and to simply not make one. We all procrastinate from time to time. Perhaps you hope the problem will go away or that if you leave it long enough it will magically get better. However, putting off a decision may result in somebody else making the decision for you and that may not be palatable. Your team may start to lose confidence in you if they are waiting for a decision to be made and you are seen to be 'dragging your feet'. The impact may be that you have a team of very demotivated staff who feel you are unable to lead them.

Relationship between decision making and accountability

Being 'accountable' means taking responsibility for your actions. It is the same in making decisions. Any decision you make in the course of your work must be accompanied by the knowledge that you are liable for what you have done. Therefore, a good decision-making process will ensure that you can stand by the decisions you make and can justify why you made them. Sometimes, though, you may make a bad decision and you must take responsibility for this too. In such cases, you need to look back at the process you went through and the choices you made to determine what went wrong.

Purposes of decision making

As a leader and manager, you are making decisions for many different reasons and purposes daily. Some require a negotiable, collaborative approach with members of the team, while others are made independently or on behalf of somebody in your team or in your care.

Decision making is a primary function of management, the purpose of which is to drive the organisation forward and to ensure that goals are achieved. It involves the process of deciding what is important in a situation and acting upon it.

Stretch and challenge

1.1 Effective decision making

With examples from your practice, describe:

- the meaning of effective decision making at senior management level
- what constitutes an effective management decision
- the effects of not making timely decisions in management
- the impact that making a management decision has on others, for example colleagues, teams, others
- the impact that not making a management decision has on others, for example colleagues, teams, others
- the relationship between decision making and accountability.

1. Provide evidence of a decision you have made at work and show the process you went through and how effective it has been.
2. How have you measured its effectiveness and impact on staff and service providers? What would be the consequences of not making this decision?
3. How did you justify the decision you made and who were you accountable to in making the decision?

Make sure that you record your thoughts. You could provide a reflective piece.

Making management decisions

Making management decisions supports the organisation's strategic plan and objectives, including those that are sometimes difficult to make. Occasionally, a decision may be unpopular among staff but, as manager, you should ensure that you can supply a rationale for why the decision has been made and how it will help the organisation to move forward.

Managers making independent decisions without consultation – negotiable vs non-negotiable

As a manager, you will have certain rules that are simply non-negotiable. For example, some settings have protected mealtimes, where every activity except eating and helping individuals with their food stops until the meal is finished. Traffic through the area is discouraged and other tasks are postponed until the meal is completed. As a manager, you may have developed this rule to ensure that the individuals using the service are well nourished, and this may be a value you hold and will not waver from.

You may also have rules that are negotiable, or you may be prepared to undertake discussion on. For example, you may be prepared to discuss the off-duty rota and negotiate shift changes among the staff.

Managers making collaborative team decisions

Although often a time-consuming exercise, with clearly defined goals, good communication and the right people in the group, collaborative team decisions are generally more acceptable to employees than those made in a 'top-down' manner. Collaboration on a problem helps the team to accept the outcome of the decision more readily than if a decision is made without their input. Although it is easier for a manager to present a decision to a team, it may not be accepted, and staff may be reluctant to 'buy in' to that decision. By involving staff in the process of making the decision, you may find that the time it takes is well spent and produces a better outcome in the long run.

Managers having to make decisions on behalf of others

Sometimes, you need to make a decision that may have an effect on the team and is made on their behalf. Errors in doing so can have consequences so you must have good decision-making processes in place to ensure that you are clear about what you are doing and why you are doing it. When managers make decisions on behalf of staff, it is important to define the problem clearly to have a good understanding of it. Only then can you determine alternate solutions to the problem, weigh the pros and cons of each decision, and then opt for one you feel is beneficial to all. You need to be aware that your choice will result in change at some level and may not be a popular one, so you should be able to justify the choice made, such as a change to the time staff start and end a shift.

Reflect on it

1.1 Negotiable and non-negotiable decisions

What are your non-negotiable and negotiable rules, or the negotiable and non-negotiable decisions you make? Which would you be prepared to change?

Evidence opportunity

1.1 Purpose of decision making

Describe the purpose of all the decisions you make daily, including:

- ✔ making management decisions
- ✔ managers having to make independent decisions without consultation – negotiable vs non-negotiable
- ✔ managers making collaborative team decisions
- ✔ managers having to make decisions on behalf of others.

Provide a written account.

AC 1.2 Evaluate how data, information and intelligence inform evidence-based decisions to improve quality

Here, you will be required to critically evaluate sources of support and information available. These will include local, regional, national and professional networks.

Evidence-based decision making is reliant on the collection of quality data and facts to inform the decision. It ensures that decisions are made on the evidence available and not just gut instincts and opinion. Gathering information from research, reports and data collected from surveys in the setting is only useful if it is the best possible information for the task in hand. Your evaluation must therefore determine that you are using reliable sources for your data collection and that accurate information is being considered.

Local and regional

Information and support can be gained from a number of different sources locally, and nationwide through various support groups and networks.

Your local integrated health board (ICB) is the clinically-led statutory NHS body responsible for the planning and commissioning of care services in local areas, and will be able to provide information and guidance on care issues. ICBs replaced Clinical Commissioning Groups (CCGs) in July 2022. They work closely with the local authority, safeguarding boards, providers and groups representing the individuals using the service. These groups are made up of individuals, their carers and/or their families who have an interest in adult social care services and wish to provide additional help or advice to the statutory services.

National

There are a number of websites and organisations where you can access information and support for your care sector. The Department of Health and Social Care (DHSC) oversees social care nationally and provide information on the latest legislation and policies regarding all aspects of social care.

The DHSC then delegate responsibility to regional and local health authorities and the CQC, which is the main social care regulator. The government has given the CQC responsibility for inspecting and regulating social care in England and for compiling reports for providers of social care.

UK-wide, the following societies and organisations also offer information and support:

- UK Online – provides government information and services
- Government Carer Information
- Skills for Care
- Skills for Health
- Age UK
- Alzheimer's Society
- Bettercaring – helps care professionals and consumers find care homes in the UK
- Careaware – a public information and advisory service specialising in issues relating to long-term care
- Care Directions – an internet guide to care and the rights of older people
- Centre for Policy on Ageing – an independent organisation promoting social policies that enable older people to achieve their full potential in later life
- Action on Elder Abuse – aims to prevent the abuse of older people
- Help the Aged – provides practical support to help older people to lead independent lives, especially those who are frail, isolated and poor
- Carers Trust
- Carers UK – offers advice on benefits and services available to carers
- National Autistic Society – has been helping autistic people since 1962 by running specialist schools, campaigning for improved rights and encouraging more autism-friendly practice in society
- Mencap – supports people with learning disabilities, and their families and carers
- Mind – provides advice and support for anyone experiencing mental health problems, and raises awareness of mental health issues.

Reflect on it

1.2 Sources of information and support

How does the data and information available to you inform the evidence-based decisions you make to improve quality? Give an example to demonstrate this.

Research it

1.2 Support in local areas

Make a list of the local areas of support that are available to help improve the service you give. This might include for example, your local ICB or a branch of Age UK.

AC 1.3 Explain the importance of reviewing and evaluating decisions to improve quality

Here, you will explain how to ensure that your review of your setting leads to quality decision making.

Improving quality in care settings is about ensuring the care you give is safe and effective and centred upon the individual. It also means ensuring that the teams closest to the problems affecting care quality are given the time, skills and resources they need to solve them.

Let's review the steps in making a quality decision. The processes will vary for different people, but here is a popular one:

1. State and explain what the problem is in order to make it clear. First, think about the purpose of the decision and the timing of it. Why does it need to be made and when? Is it an urgent one or can it be left until you have more facts? If it is about failing quality, then the decision needs to be made quickly
2. Examine, analyse and look carefully at the problem. Remember, the problem you see may not be the actual problem, so don't assume you know what it is until you have investigated it. For example, staff morale seems low, and the care being given is unsatisfactory. You believe it is to do with pay cuts, but in fact, the staff are fed up with the poor communication in the team.
3. What might be the limiting factors that stop you from making a decision? It might be you procrastinating, for example.
4. Is there anyone else that might influence the decision you want to make? Who else needs to know? Who drove the last decision you made? It might be people in the team who resist the change you want to make.
5. Identify potential alternatives and other means to solve the problem if you are unable to agree on a decision. Start by looking at the formal process and determine who or what might be involved in agreeing the decision.
6. Analyse the alternatives. Look closely at what you have and decide if the alternatives are feasible. Are they viable, or justifiable? Can everyone agree on the alternatives?
7. Choose the best alternative. Think about whether this is the best way forward. Does it effectively respond to the issue at hand?
8. Whatever decision has been agreed on, you must now implement it and justify its purpose. Make an action plan showing the way forward and make sure deadlines and dates for completion are in place. It is useful to consider whether deadline dates are realistic and achievable.
9. Put into place a system to measure and evaluate the decision. What are the markers you will set? How will you know that the decision has been implemented effectively and successfully?

An effective decision maker is somebody who is thoughtful about the process, the purpose and the timing of a decision. Keeping lines of communication open and being prepared to discuss the reason for the decision are imperative. The timing of a decision may also be important. If you try to introduce too many changes at once, your team may reject the decision and morale will be low. Remember, you are accountable for the decisions you make.

Research it

1.2 and **1.3** The decision-making process

What data, information and intelligence inform the evidence-based decisions to improve quality that you make?

Research the various processes others in your setting use to make decisions or look at ones discussed online.

Makes notes detailing your findings.

Stretch and challenge

1.3 Evaluating decision making

Managers are required to set objectives, organise tasks, motivate and develop staff, communicate and establish targets. All of these tasks require you to make decisions. Ensuring that the decisions you make benefit your team and the organisation means that you need to evaluate how effective they are. You may need to ask your colleagues, stakeholders or the individuals using the service for input and feedback, both positive and negative, about decisions you have made.

Explain your management of the range, purposes and situations for which decisions are required in your service. Draw conclusions in respect of your decision-making practice. Make sure you cover at least five of the headings/topics discussed in this section. Provide a written account.

When formulating your explanation, think about the strengths and weaknesses of the decision-making process.

AC 1.4 Analyse how values and priorities influence decision making processes in relation to self and others

Here, you will analyse how your values and priorities affect decision making.

The 6Cs (Skills for Care, n.d. b) articulate the values of care, compassion, competence, communication, courage and commitment and were developed to underpin quality social care. As the integration between social care continues, a set of common values across all settings is a way to increase consistency within care work.

The values or beliefs you hold impact all areas of your life, including decision making. When you make a decision that honours your values, you feel satisfied and fulfilled. Decisions that conflict with your values can cause discontent and dissatisfaction. This is why it is important that your own values fit with the organisation's values.

For example, you may value honesty and openness, but your senior leaders have told you that you must not tell staff that changes are being made that may result in redundancy for some. This would be a most uncomfortable situation to be in and might cause you stress and discontent in your role.

AC 1.5 Explain how to enable others to contribute to the decision making

Here, you will explain how you can encourage others to be involved in the decision-making process.

The success of your organisation is dependent upon the staff that you employ and how they conduct themselves in the setting. Every day they will be required to think and act quickly in various situations and to make decisions. As a leader you should support your staff to make decisions without having to come to you each time they need to do so. Having clearly defined values in the setting is a step towards this. Values affect behaviour and if they are fully understood and practiced in the setting this will aid decision making.

You can help staff become more confident in their work by showing them how you make decisions and encouraging this behaviour in them. Once your staff understand how they should be doing things, you can encourage them to become more autonomous in their decision making, which will in turn lead to increased confidence, both yours and theirs. When situations arise you can be sure that they will make the right decisions.

Reflect on it

1.4 and 1.5 Analyse and reflect on decision-making processes

Remind yourself of the values of your organisation and reflect on how these affect the decisions you make. How do you ensure that your staff are able to make decisions? What have you put in place to give them the autonomy to make decisions when a situation demands?

LO2 Be able to demonstrate effective decision making within a leadership and management role

AC 2.1 Establish when decisions need to be made within own role

Here, you will be required to establish the reasons, purpose and benefits of why managers:

- *make decisions about strategy, policies and procedures in adult care practice that might and might not involve others*
- *make decisions for those in receipt of care and support those who might struggle with making management decisions in respect of the above.*

Strategy, policies and procedures in adult care practice are in place to ensure that the organisation functions well. Sometimes you will need to make decisions that involve others in the process or that others will simply have to accept. Decisions made on behalf of those in your care, however, need to be shared.

As the manager, it is important that you keep others 'in the loop' with regard to your decisions and inform them about these to help them understand why decisions have been made. It may be that you need to comply with legislation or regulations to address the day-to-day running of the organisation. The rationale behind the decision is important. You will be expected to make decisions on various issues, perhaps to do with staffing issues and deciding you need emergency cover in an employee's absence, for example, or broader decisions with regard to strategy. It may be that an unpopular change to work practice may be ill received; however, as mentioned, if you inform staff as to why it needs to be made, they can then start to understand.

Decisions also need to be made for and with the individuals in your care. When their needs change, decisions must be made about how their care will be delivered in the future. Research has shown that people who have been actively involved in their own care, treatment and support have improved outcomes which help them to stay well and manage their own conditions in a more productive way.

The CQC's publication 'Better care in my hands' (Care Quality Commission, 2016) highlights how enabling people to have more control of their own care leads to better outcomes. It undertakes a literature review of a growing body of knowledge that demonstrates how people benefit from being involved in making decisions about their care and how that care can be delivered to meet their needs.

Make decisions about strategy, policies and procedures in adult care practice that might and might not involve others

Strategies and policies provide guidelines for decision making and are different from rules or procedures. Policies enable discretion and judgement to be exercised within certain limits whereas rules must simply be followed. For example, 'No Smoking' is a command with no room for negotiation or discretion. We simply follow that command. A policy, on the other hand, is a guide that establishes certain boundaries in which we can exercise judgement. The purpose of policies, which are formulated by managers, is to ensure that decisions made will meet the organisation's objectives and these will be part of the organisation's strategy. Some policies may be generated at team level and will be more applicable to your specific department.

Make decisions for those in receipt of care and support

People with mental capacity can make decisions about their own health and care. However, occasionally this may be compromised, and it falls to care professionals to make decisions on their behalf and this must be assessed carefully. As far as possible, a person in your care should be helped to make their own decisions, but if deemed to lack capacity the decision made on their behalf must be in the person's best interest and according to the law must be the least restrictive option (MCA, 2005).

A person-centred approach

The systems you have in place to ensure that the personalisation agenda is met in your setting need to show regard for the views and needs of the individuals using the service. Your systems must hold the individual at the centre of the decision making if this is to work. Care or support planning is a good example of a system that is in place to ensure that care is individualised. The development of these systems puts the individual at the centre of the process.

Decision making about the day-to-day running of the adult care setting and the general state of repair and decorations should not only be left to the staff but should include those using the service as well. Many care establishments now run a weekly or monthly meeting in which such things can be discussed.

You should also refer to Unit 509 Leading and managing partnerships in adult care.

Why managers might struggle with making management decisions in respect of the above

It is difficult to make a decision on somebody else's behalf, particularly when there may be a moral or ethical principle involved. For example, without **advance directives** in place, individuals may be subject to treatment that could be considered very invasive and of little benefit. In such cases, you would need to ask close relatives to make the decision on behalf of the individual, but difficulty arises if you are not in full agreement with their choice. From a management point of view, you might need to take advice from health professionals and may even have to involve the courts in such cases (MCA, 2005).

KEY TERM

Advance directive: Also known as a living will, this is a legal document that specifies what actions should be taken for a person if they cannot make decisions for themselves because of illness or incapacity.

A person who has a profound learning disability may also struggle to make decisions and might not understand information they are being given, or have the capacity to retain that information. Someone lacking capacity because of a disability or illness might also be unable to communicate their decision. Whilst a person with a profound learning disability may not be able to make major decisions, this does not mean that they cannot decide what to eat or what to wear each day.

For more major decisions social care workers may need to refer to the Mental Capacity Act 2005, which outlines the criteria for assessing a person's mental capacity.

Evidence opportunity

2.1 Reasons why you might need to make decisions

Explain the reasons, purpose and benefits of why you as a manager:

- ✔ make decisions about strategy, policies and procedures in adult care practice that might and might not involve others
- ✔ make decisions for those in receipt of care and support
- ✔ might struggle with making management decisions in respect of the above.

What might be difficult about the whole process of shared decision making? Think of a time when you have had to make a decision and think about these questions in relation to your experience. Provide examples from the workplace.

When collecting examples, you need to ensure that confidentiality is maintained and any material from the individuals using your service is anonymised.

Management decision making

As a manager, you will be required to make decisions on a range of issues and in a range of situations. The following headings outline your areas of responsibility as manager of a setting.

Quality management and improvement and the role of evidence-based decisions

An evidence-based decision is made by critically thinking about the information or facts you have that either support or contradict what it is you are making a decision about. Research is at the heart of this type of management and in developing and improving the quality of your service you should focus upon the way in which you use quality assurance processes to achieve consistent results.

Estates management

This is about managing the day-to-day operations within the setting. In a care setting you may also be managing the domestic, catering and laundry staff and services, which means ensuring that all these services are able to fulfil their roles and that they meet the needs of those using the service. In this area of work you will be making decisions about how the budget is spent on laundry facilities and other resources.

It is also possible that you will have to update premises and buy furniture or decorate areas, so you will be making decisions as to how to fund such large capital expenditure.

Financial planning

As a manager, you will have a budget and as such are responsible for managing how that money is spent. The way in which you financially plan will feed into all other areas of your role. Without finances you cannot, of course, pay for staff or services, so a plan needs to be put into action, and you will be responsible for financial decisions. Go to Unit 503 for more information on financial resources and responsibility.

Care/support planning and partnership working

Although the team will be responsible for the individual care/support plans of those using the service, you will need to have an overall understanding of how the care is being delivered on a daily basis and you may be required to make decisions when changes are needed. While you may not be involved in individual plans, your role will be to co-ordinate the care in the adult care setting.

Care/support plans that are negotiated well and include partners from other services mean that individuals can live lives that are meaningful despite having serious physical or mental health issues. Any activity that helps with a person's wellbeing will be an important part of their care. In working with partners, you are able to offer more services to achieve this. For example, you may work closely with a team of physiotherapists or counsellors and have a partnership deal with them. Their expertise can add to the quality of the care/support planning that you offer.

Policy and procedures

As a manager, you need to ensure that staff are working within the policies of the organisation and you may also be the person who ensures that the policies and procedures remain up to date and relevant. You may, of course, decide to delegate this role but ultimately you have responsibility for ensuring that all staff are aware of their roles with respect to the policies.

Staffing – recruitment

In recruitment, decisions must be made as to what staff are needed, what roles they must undertake and how you will recruit the team. You need to be clear about the type of person you want to fulfil a particular role in the organisation, and you will have some responsibility in a small organisation for drawing up a job description and person specification.

In larger organisations, your role will be to work with the HR team on this, but you will still need to make decisions about the staff needs in your area.

Environmental factors

All organisations are subject to changes in their internal and external environments. The internal environment may refer to staffing and the way the setting works to meet the needs and mission of the organisation. It might also include other resources in its vicinity that are needed for it to function effectively. As a manager, you will have control over this and will also be responsible for it. It will be in the scope of your role to be able to make decisions to effect change and to ensure the smooth and effective running of your setting. The external environment is less pliable and for staff working in a community or domiciliary setting there will be factors that you will not be able to control, but safe working is the key here. Also included are your organisation's competitors, economic conditions, policies and procedures that are determined by legislation, and changes to legislation itself. As environmental factors that are external to the organisation are not in your control in the same way that internal environmental factors are, you will need to ensure that you keep up to date with any changes that will require action to ensure the smooth running of the organisation.

Safety and security and risk assessments

Managing safety and security within your organisation requires decisions about the risks you need to manage and control in the setting. This means you must think about potential hazards that exist and that may cause harm to people and undertake risk assessments to identify the steps to prevent such harm.

Advocacy issues, deprivation of liberty issues and best interest issues

Advocacy, Deprivation of Liberty Safeguards (DoLS) and Best Interests issues provide legal safeguards for the people in your care in either a hospital or an adult care setting. These safeguards are part of the Mental Capacity Act, so as the manager of the setting you must be aware of the implications of this Act for those people using your service and for staff. You may be required to make assessments and decisions about the best interests of individuals, which are often needed towards end of life and when mental capacity is at risk.

Health and safety issues and safeguarding issues

Any health and safety decision you make must be in line with the law and also the policy of your organisation; the same applies to safeguarding. As a manager, you will be required to ensure that safeguarding policies for individuals in your care are followed and that any issues are quickly dealt with for the safety of the individual, the staff and the organisation.

You can appreciate that the range of your decision making as a manager is vast and perhaps you are starting to evaluate just what is essential to your role and what might be delegated or shelved. The 'Reflect on it' activity will help you to identify the decisions that need to be made for you to evaluate the range (are you a designated decision maker or can you seek feedback from others to support your decisions?), purpose (what are the reasons for the decisions you make and who do they affect?) and situation in which you manage.

> **Reflect on it**
>
> **2.1 Your role**
>
> Think about what your role entails and what decisions you are required to make. Write a reflective account about the responsibility of this role and how you manage that responsibility. Think about the range, purpose and situations you come across in your role.

AC 2.2 Gather data, information and intelligence to inform decision making

Here, you will explain different methods of gathering data and which are most relevant to your setting.

Use digital technology to research data and information relevant to adult care service

By conducting online searches, you can gain valuable insights into how others in the care system work. You can also access government documents, care standards and guidelines as well as media reports that can give useful information to help you to make an informed decision. Always make sure the sites you access are reliable and credible. You may need to conduct thorough research to ascertain the reliability and validity of the research and opinions you find online.

The URL at the end of the website address can give you a good idea about the source of the document. For example, if the site ends with .edu then it is an educational setting.

.gov is a government website and is useful for reports and legal documents; and .org refers to an organisation, so you need to be aware of possible bias, particularly if the organisation sponsors political parties or large companies with an agenda to promote a product. For example, you may find useful articles about pain management but need to be mindful of the sponsor who may be marketing a specific type of dressing and using the research data to support their product.

You can also access online journals and magazines for more insights into the issue you are researching and use these to help you to form an opinion and make decisions on the basis of information that has been researched.

National reports and regulatory findings

Reports about health and adult social care can often be found on government websites or the NHS, CQC, Skills for Care or Health Foundation websites. These also comment upon findings that are linked to regulations and guidelines and are good sources of factual data.

Company/internal formal report

Other organisations similar to your own may provide useful information about how they have overcome issues and problems, while reading company reports can help decision making. You do not have to restrict yourself to care settings though. Sometimes, ideas from different sectors – for example, education, manufacturing and customer service – can supply useful information and be adapted to adult care.

Media reporting

Media reports often shed light on issues in adult care. We have all seen investigative journalism reporting upon the lack of adult social care staff and the poor pay structures. We are also aware of the shortcomings and failings in adult care that have been investigated and have led to national inquiries and changes to the law and practice. While the issues these reports highlight may not be an issue in your setting, they could help to inform your decision making. Such journalism may at times be biased so you need to bear this in mind. Remember to check that the information is from a reliable and valid source before using it to make an informed decision.

Validity

This refers to whether a study measures or examines what it claims to. A researcher who is trying to measure people's attitudes towards autism, for example, needs to construct a tool that they know is measuring that specific attitude. In this way, the results can be accurately applied and interpreted for a test to be valid.

Reliability

Reliability refers to the extent to which an experiment, test or other measuring procedure gives the same results in repeated experiments. Other researchers must be able to perform exactly the same experiment under the same conditions and generate the same results in order to reinforce the findings. This is called replicating findings.

Complaints

Your own complaints system can be a valuable source of information in making decisions or justifying something. There may be an area of practice that is constantly complained about and evidence to support a change may be useful here. You will need to carefully explore the issue(s) being complained about, weighing up the positives and negatives, perhaps by having a discussion with the complainant, and determine whether it is a reasonable complaint or simply a subjective point of view. If something can be done about it, then you can start to gather other information to help the situation.

Quality/service provision surveys undertaken which have been completed by others

Surveys are useful if you want to learn what a larger sample of people think, and you need to keep the costs of research down. Surveys tend to have a different way of questioning than interviews and are most useful for gathering data through a wide variety of methods such as email, post or face-to-face interviews to provide useful statistical data. The disadvantage of using this type of method is that poorly written questions can limit the types of responses you get and may also affect reliability and validity of the study if the questions are biased in any way. There may also be a low response rate and of course the answers are subjective. Types of surveys include interview, postal, telephone, internet or online surveys.

Reflect on it

2.2 Validity and reliability

Think about validity and reliability and then write a short piece to show your understanding.

Qualitative and quantitative data to inform management decision making

Informing your decisions will require you to produce evidence in the form of factual data. You will already have this sort of data in the form of surveys or evaluation forms, appraisals and audits. Data that is **quantitative** in nature will focus on answering questions such as 'how many' and 'how often' and is likely to be presented in terms of numbers and statistics. The methods include surveys, experiments and statistical data.

KEY TERM

Quantitative data: Data that is numerical in nature. It will answer questions such as 'how much' or 'how many'.

You might also use **qualitative** methods to gain information, particularly if your decision means you need to gain a greater understanding and depth about what is happening in a particular circumstance.

As a manager, it is important to use all forms of data and information to help you make sound decisions. Whether it is quantitative or qualitative in nature, you also need to ensure that it is both reliable and valid.

> **KEY TERM**
>
> **Qualitative data**: Collected through interviews and observations, this type of information is descriptive and will try to find a meaning in certain phenomena.

Quantitative research

If your research is focusing on questions such as 'how many' and 'how often', then you are likely to present your data in terms of numbers and statistics and it will, therefore, be quantitative in nature.

Originally developed to study natural phenomena, this was the method of choice of natural scientists but is now widely used in education and care. The methods include surveys, experiments and statistical data.

Strengths of the quantitative approach

- Subject to rigorous controls and checks throughout the process.
- An objective approach to data collection is favoured, and therefore the results are often thought to be more accurate.
- Large numbers of participants (samples) are used in this type of research; therefore a large amount of information can be obtained.
- The findings can be generalised to the wider population.
- Studies can be replicated or repeated, and therefore the results obtained can be more readily compared with similar studies.
- In this type of work it is also possible to reduce personal bias, simply because researchers are able to keep their 'distance' from participating subjects.
- This type of research is well controlled and the methods and instruments used, such as questionnaires, are standardised.

Weaknesses of the quantitative approach

- Some of the methods involve the use of laboratory conditions, and this is not entirely appropriate when studying human subjects.
- The validity of the study is questionable.
- The way in which questionnaires or survey methods are written may not elicit responses that are useful or real.
- Misunderstanding about the questions can occur.
- The relationship between what somebody says and actually does cannot always be truly tested.
- We all have our own unique experiences and this can certainly change how we behave. In other words, we may all bring a different way to behave to an experiment, which is not useful for quantitative research.
- Gathering primary data can result in data unreliability.

Qualitative research

Qualitative research methods were developed in the social sciences when it was felt that the study of social and cultural phenomena required a different means of enquiry.

This approach seeks to gain insight into people's lives. People's attitudes, behaviours and value systems are the areas of interest for the qualitative researcher, who wants to seek out the 'why' of a particular topic. Rather than simply trying to describe a certain phenomenon, this approach attempts to gain greater understanding and depth about what is happening in a particular situation.

Using the phenomenological approach, as posited by sociologists in an attempt to study the experience of the subjects and how they interpret their world, the researcher becomes an interpreter and attempts to reveal concealed meaning. The four major qualitative approaches are ethnography, phenomenology, field research and grounded theory.

Strengths of the qualitative approach

- Produces some very in-depth work and rich data about phenomena which are impossible to collect from sets of statistics.
- Enables the researcher to look far more closely at the meanings within behaviour and to understand what is happening in settings, and to question participants' responses to certain issues.
- Enables the study of people in their own settings where there are naturally occurring events that provide rich data for study.
- Enables collection of information in areas where there has been little knowledge in existence in the past and where sensitive issues are being studied.
- Enables the researcher to get close to the material under study and to gain in-depth data which can later be subjected to quantitative research.

Weakness of the qualitative approach

- It can be very time consuming to conduct this type of research to gain a valid response.
- Collecting and analysing the material, which is often unstructured in nature, can also be time consuming.
- Finding themes in reams of notes can, at the very least, be a little daunting and trying to find meaning in the materials can also take time.
- The sample size is usually quite small, with just a few participants taking part.
- Some critics are concerned that the type of study lacks rigour since variables cannot be controlled.
- Results produced cannot be readily generalised to the population as a whole.
- This type of research lends itself to small-scale study and therefore data obtained, while rich, is too small to allow valid conclusions.

Table 2 compares the two types of research.

▼ **Table 2** Comparison of quantitative and qualitative research

Quantitative	Qualitative
Quantitative analysis is more objective.	Qualitative data is generally thought to be more subjective.
Has little human bias attached to it.	As it is dependent on people's opinions and assumptions, there are biases present.
Lack of bias because the data collected relies on the comparison of numbers according to mathematical tests.	Bias is thought to occur because the researcher interprets people's statements or other communication, and this might be influenced by the way the researcher sees the world or approaches the work.

Stretch and challenge

2.2 Using factual data, recommendations, suggestions and ideas to inform decision making

1. Evaluate how you use and analyse qualitative and/or quantitative data to inform your management decision making sourced from the areas discussed in this section. Collect evidence of this and show your assessor the data you have gathered. You may wish to include an example of a recent decision you had to make in the workplace and show what qualitative and/or quantitative data informed that decision.
2. Evaluate the sources by saying what the strength of the source was and what limited its use for you. What was good about the information, and what was missing perhaps? Was it relevant or biased in some way? Highlight the sources you used and justify your choice.

AC 2.3 Identify potential solutions used to inform a decision in own role

AC 2.4 Evaluate potential solutions to draw conclusions

Here, you will identify and evaluate different solutions to problems that arise in your role as manager.

Problem solving to reach a potential solution to a problem requires a decision to be made. Some people make decisions based upon feelings and what they call 'gut instinct' whereas others approach the problem in a systematic and rational way. An effective way to inform decisions is to use both rational and creative approaches and to take a step-by-step approach.

There are several steps to ensure that a good decision is made and the first is to identify the problem. This may sound a little confusing since you know what the problem is surely? However, although you may think you know what the problem is, when you start to discuss the situation and to ask questions you may find that you are looking at the wrong issue. Try asking yourself the following questions:

- What have I (or others) observed about this issue?
- What information do I need to address it ?
- What have I tried already to address this problem?

The next step is to look at the alternatives available to you. You may feel step one has already created the answer for you, but now you need to think about possible alternatives.

When you have generated a few ideas, they will need to be assessed as to how effective they might be. Consider each one and look at how it will impact the setting or stakeholders and staff. What costs might be incurred? Is the solution ethical and legal?

Once these steps are complete, the decision can be made. One decision of course is not to make a decision at all, and whilst this may be valid and the right decision at the time, it might also lead to the problem continuing and escalating.

Next, you should implement your chosen decision and this will require a plan to be made as to how the problem will be tackled.

Finally, you need to evaluate the outcome and results. The outcomes may offer some useful advice about the actual decision-making process, and whether the choice made was in fact the right one. The next time a similar decision is needed you will learn from the process and the information gained.

Evidence opportunity

2.3 and 2.4 Review available information and make valid decisions/ justify your decisions

Identify a problem in your setting and follow the problem solving process shown on the previous page. Provide a written account explaining and reflecting on how the decision was made and implemented. You should also include an explanation justifying your decision in order to gain support from internal and external stakeholders. Provide an evaluation of the conclusion you have come to.

AC 2.5 Involve individuals and others in the decision-making process and implementation of the result of decision

Here, you will need to evaluate situations in which others may need to be engaged in decision making, including the topics we cover in this section.

Internal and external stakeholders

Partnerships, both internal and external, are key in any organisation, and form a big part of your work life. These might be with internal staff/adult care workers who are involved in the organisation on a daily basis, and external stakeholders who also have an interest in the running of the organisation. External stakeholders include medical care workers, resource suppliers, advocates and families of individuals receiving care, and commissioning agencies who are involved in the setting of care standards, checks and decision making. The agencies plan and review the services that are needed in the local area to ensure that they are available and appropriate. As a manager, the decisions that you make will affect the different stakeholders, but these stakeholders will also influence the decisions and decision-making process. It may be that these stakeholders are affected by the decisions that are made on a day-to-day basis, or it may be that they have a financial stake.

You will find that projects that you are working on for your setting, as well as policies and procedures, are often carried out across multidisciplinary boundaries, in other words, alongside other disciplines, organisations and professionals. For example, it may be that internal stakeholders are involved in a new strategy in the setting, or in the local health and wellbeing strategy, and may be responsible for organising and planning the project, arranging meetings, sourcing the resources and the funding needed. They may be involved in developing, organising and managing the project. External stakeholders such as the individuals using the service, their families/carers and the local community may also want to contribute their views and guidance. It is important to choose stakeholders who can make valuable contributions that will enhance the overall project and the outcomes.

Making decisions with stakeholders in mind must have the support of relevant information and data (such as that discussed in AC2.2) if support is to be gained from them. By undertaking a thorough search for evidence to support your topic you can present stakeholders with relevant information and justify the decisions you have made. It is important that stakeholders can see and understand the rationale for your decisions as they need to be fully informed in order to give their support. Without this they may fail to understand the importance of the reasons for the decision you have made, and this might compromise care.

Team meetings

A meeting is an opportunity to communicate with the whole team present and can be a useful vehicle through which to encourage staff to discuss the overall aims of the team, communicate ideas with the shared vision in mind and engage the team in the decision-making process.

Meetings enable team members to get to know each other, to discuss issues and make action points. The success of a meeting can depend on the way it is chaired, and this is an important role for the manager to learn.

As the chair leading the meeting, you need to ensure that you encourage participation from the entire group using open questions and occasionally directing your attention to one person in particular. In this way, you are enabling everybody in the team to express what they know and to demonstrate their skills, which may be useful for achieving the whole team's outcomes. It is very important to come away from the meeting with some action points or objectives, if appropriate.

When a planning activity is required the team meeting can be a useful vehicle for this. If all team members understand the background to the project and its relevance to the organisation, they will be more focused on the changes needed and be motivated to ensure a successful outcome.

At the meeting there can be a collaborative approach to the collection of data and timescales can be set that are clear and achievable. With the project broken down into manageable tasks and assigned to team members for completion, the planning process can reach a successful conclusion in a timely manner. You will need to ensure that timescales are achievable and that the team are aware of the need to meet deadlines, otherwise the project may falter.

One of the best ways to get staff involved in planning is to provide time during the regular team meeting for them to communicate their opinions or ideas. Team meetings often become mere information-giving sessions, without an opportunity for the exchange of ideas. If this is the case, then the valuable skills and knowledge of the staff will not be accessed. Team members can learn a great deal from each other through a mentoring process, and the expertise each one possesses as a result of their experience and training can then be used as a valuable resource for planning.

Staff supervision and appraisals

During a staff one-to-one or supervision, you can engage with staff to share decisions about particular areas of their work, such as how they engage with other members of staff or how well they perform in their tasks with the individuals using the service. Performance appraisal meetings enable staff to be involved in decisions about their career and professional development. This is also an opportunity to deal with any negative behaviour or poor performance.

Care assessments and reviews and carer/advocate and/or family meetings

Decisions are required in all aspects of care, and it should not simply be the remit of the manager to make the final decision. During meetings with carers/advocates and families in the care assessment process you need to encourage them to make their own decisions in order to have ownership of the final product. For example, it is easy to put in place a care/support plan for somebody that you have decided is the best course of action. You may have made a decision that the person will engage in activities in the setting and leave a meeting believing that this was a shared decision. Unfortunately, the person may agree at the time that this is the best decision but then not comply with it. Decisions that have been made on a person's behalf and without their engagement are not likely to sit well with them and yet we may be guilty of doing this in our own care practice.

Skills for Care 'Working with families, friends and carers' (Skills for Care, 2016) is a framework for adult social care providers and identifies good practice guidelines about what adult social care employers and their staff need to know and do to work effectively with people's families, friends and carers.

Four sections are covered, including how to establish positive relationships with families, friends and carers, recognising the importance of family relationships and your role, maintaining appropriate communication and offering support to people who need care and support to maintain and manage family relationships.

The document *Making Shared Decision-making a Reality: No decision about me, without me* (Coulter and Collins, 2011) sets out the government's plan to make shared decision making the norm in the NHS.

It highlights a process in which clinicians and individuals work together to select appropriate care packages based upon clinical evidence and the individual's informed preferences. The rationale for this is the 'compelling research evidence that suggests that patients who are active participants in managing their health and health care have better outcomes than patients who are passive recipients of care'.

Partnership working

For others in the care process, such as stakeholders, partners, families and carers, shared decision making reduces the variation in practice across services and duplication. There are many situations in which others will need to be engaged in decision making. In meetings with stakeholders and others such as families or carers, you can support each other in decisions that need to be made and provide clarity about what needs to be done for the care package to be delivered. As a manager, your role will be to ensure that the care provided by all partners is seamless and does not overlap any part of the service. Repetition of care is a wasted resource and by analysing the care process you can identify any potential issues which may arise and determine a way forward.

Lessons learned from providing support and encouragement to others

You make decisions on a daily basis in your role as manager, but it is also important to ensure that you empower others to take their own decisions. For example, it is easy for staff to come to you with a problem and for you to make a decision for them. This increases your workload enormously and does not encourage or empower staff to take decisions for themselves. Encouraging them to act in an autonomous way, making decisions based upon their own professional judgement, and supporting them in this, will help you to take a step back.

You can do this by listening to what the member of staff is saying and asking them what they feel they ought to do and what the consequences might be. Ask them if there is an alternative course of action and how this might work. If they get into the habit of engaging with this sort of decision-making process, they will start to build this into their daily routine.

Reflect on it

2.5 Engaging others in the decision-making process

Think about a decision you made for somebody else. How well was it received and what happened? What have you learned as a result of this? How can you involve others and support them to engage in the decision-making process?

Reflect on it

2.5 Providing support to engage others in the decision-making process

What situations are you involved in which may need to engage others in decision making, including the areas/topics discussed in this section? Discuss this with your assessor, giving examples for each situation and say what decision was reached for each one.

What lessons did you learn from providing support and encouragement to others in the various situations?

AC 2.6 Evaluate the decision and decision-making process used

Here, you will need to evaluate your own strengths and weaknesses in the management decision-making process.

As a manager, you make decisions on a daily basis, some of which may not always be palatable. For example, you may need to have a difficult conversation with a member of staff and decide to leave that off the urgent list in the hope that they will rectify their actions before you talk to them. This, of course, may not be the best action to take. As you have learned, decisions can be based on intuitive processes – gut instincts – and you can also gather information for analysis before you make a decision. You will need to reflect on your approach, how you make decisions and think about the strengths and weaknesses of your style. Do you always act on intuition and is it always the right choice? What is good about that approach and how can it sometimes go wrong? Do you prefer to get all the facts before you make your move, but does this sometimes hinder the process? As a manager, you should continually reflect not only on your decision making and decision-making process but generally on your practice to identify areas where you could develop further and therefore ensure that you are able to be as effective as possible in doing so.

Reflective exemplar

Today I worked with a member of the team and my own manager to select a candidate for a support worker for a person with autism. Together we drew up a shortlist of candidates and invited two for interview. One candidate had one year's experience in this type of work setting and the other was new to care work entirely. We appointed the one with more experience after much discussion. Although I was involved in the decision-making process, I was not sure that we were making the right decision.

I had a gut feeling that this was not really the right choice but allowed myself to listen to the other two members of the panel and agreed to appoint the experienced member of staff despite them not really having the correct skills for the job we offered.

I now wonder what it was that led me to this outcome. I realised that gut instinct and feelings were not a useful or factual argument to put forward and therefore did not feel I could argue my point well enough. In future I need to pinpoint exactly what my reasons for rejecting a candidate are and why. I must learn to justify my judgements in a more meaningful manner.

Reflect on it

2.6 Reflect on your decision-making practices and areas for further development

Evaluate your own strengths and weaknesses in the management decision-making process. Discuss this with your assessor.

Include any recommendations to enhance your future practice.

Case study

LO1 and LO2 Effective decision making

You have received notification that your budget is to be cut by 20 per cent from the next calendar month. You are already struggling with under-staffing and are now at risk of losing more staff. One of the rooms in the adult care setting requires redecorating and you are in the process of obtaining quotes and are about to employ a local firm to do the job.

1. What will you do?
2. How can you ensure that the service delivered to individuals remains safe and efficient?
3. What action plans can you put into place?
4. How will you ensure that your decisions are effective and positive?

Legislation

Legislation	Key points
Mental Capacity Act 2005	This act informs individuals about what they can do to plan and ensure that someone else can make decisions for them if they ever lack capacity to do so for themselves.

References

Care Quality Commission (2016) 'Better care in my hands: A review of how people are involved in their care'. www.cqc.org.uk/sites/default/files/20160519_Better_care_in_my_hands_FINAL.pdf

Coulter, A. and Collins, A. (2011) *Making Shared Decision-making a Reality: No decision about me without me*. London: King's Fund. www.kingsfund.org.uk/sites/default/files/Making-shared-decision-making-a-reality-paper-Angela-Coulter-Alf-Collins-July-2011_0.pdf

Drucker, P.F. (2015) 'The elements of effective decision making'. https://rlaexp.com/studio/biz/conceptual_resources/authors/peter_drucker/28-the-elements-of-effective-decision-making.pdf

NHS England (2017) *Next Steps on the NHS Five Year Forward View*. London: TSO.

Skills for Care (n.d. a) 'The care certificate: Work in a person-centred way. What you need to know, Standard 5'. www.skillsforcare.org.uk/resources/documents/Developing-your-workforce/Care-Certificate/Care-Certificate-Standards/Standard-5.pdf

Skills for Care (n.d. b) 'Working with families, friends and carers: A framework for adult social care employers'. www.skillsforcare.org.uk/resources/documents/Developing-your-workforce/Care-topics/Working-with-families/Working-with-families-friends-and-carers-A-framework-for-adult-social-care-employers.pdf

Useful resources and further reading

Adair, J. (2009) *Effective Leadership: How to be a successful leader*. London: Pan Books.

Age UK (2018) 'Deprivation of liberty safeguards'. www.ageuk.org.uk/globalassets/age-uk/documents/factsheets/fs62_deprivation_of_liberty_safeguards_fcs.pdf

Cohen, D. (2015) 'What is professional judgment?' www.collegeofdietitians.org/resources/professional-practice/what-is-professional-judgment-(2015).aspx

Hansson, S.O. (1994) 'Decision theory: A brief introduction'. http://people.kth.se/~soh/decisiontheory.pdf

Kapur, N., Parand, A., Soukup, T., Reader, T. and Sevdalis, N. (2016) 'Aviation and healthcare: A comparative review with implications for patient safety', *JRSM Open*. https://doi.org/10.1177/2054270415616548

Mental Capacity Act 2005 www.legislation.gov.uk/ukpga/2005/9/contents

Merriam Webster Dictionary (2015) 'Definition of professional'. www.merriam-webster.com/dictionary/professional

Unit 503

Understanding business and resource management for adult care

GLH 40

About this unit

In an adult care setting, 'resources' include the finances, staff and materials at your disposal to deliver good care. However, effectively managing resources can be tricky to master and there are concerns that a lack of such resources is causing problems in care work today. Careful and effective management of resources is therefore essential in order to run a successful care setting and, as a manager, you will play a key role in ensuring this.

A business is defined as an organisation that engaged in commercial, industrial or professional activities. They can be for-profit or non-profit organisations and range from limited liability companies to sole proprietorships and partnerships.

Mismanagement or not managing resources effectively can result in budget overspend, lack of resources for people using care services and even the closure of the organisation. In this unit you will understand the principles of effective resource management and effective human resource management. You will be required to demonstrate your ability to manage resources within your care setting.

Learning outcomes

By the end of this unit, you will:

1. Understand the principles of effective resource management within adult care.
2. Understand principles of effective human resource management.
3. Understand market provision in adult care.
4. Understand integrated approaches in health and social care.

Getting started

Before you study the unit, think about the following:

- What resources are available in your workplace?
- How can you as a manager learn to trust staff enough to delegate or assign tasks?
- What do you think effective resource management is?
- As a manager, what are you accountable for?

LO1 Understand the principles of effective resource management within adult care

AC 1.1 Explain the meaning of the term 'resource management' in adult care

Here, you will explain what resource management is with reference to your setting.

Resource management refers to the things needed to deliver adult social care, such as people, time, money, facilities, equipment and information. Implementing and managing resources efficiently affects staff as well as the individuals using the service. When resources are managed well, adult care is maximised and staff satisfaction is increased.

AC 1.2 and AC 1.3 Analyse and describe the impact of national and local strategies and priorities on resource planning and management in relation to financial, physical and human resources

Here, you will be required to analyse and describe the impact of different strategies and priorities on resource planning and management, including financial, physical and human resources.

A number of national strategies have addressed financial, physical and human resources in the care system.

In 2021 the government set out long overdue reforms for adult social care. This white paper, 'People at the heart of care', set out a ten-year vision to transform support and care in England with person-centred care as a key theme.

The reforms describe a range of policies for the sector and those who use care and support to implement over the next three years. These include finances to support:

- a range of new supported housing options
- greater adoption of technology for widespread digitisation across social care
- finance to train the social care workforce
- increases in the upper limit of the disabilities facilities grant for home adaptations such as stairlifts, wet rooms and home technologies, as well as a new practical support service to make minor repairs and changes in people's homes
- changes to the services provided to support unpaid carers
- a new national website to explain the upcoming changes
- an increase in the support offer across adult social care to improve the delivery of care and support services
- assistance for local authorities to better plan and develop the support and care options available.

Source: Department of Health and Social Care (2022c)

National strategy for adult care settings

The Care Act 2014 sets out the law for market development in adult social care. It details the duties and responsibilities for the Department of Health and Social Care, CQC and local authorities to promote efficient and effective adult care and support.

For adult social care it is the local authority that is responsible for services provided to people in their homes and residential care services. The Health and Social Care Committee report 'Social care: funding and workforce' (UK Parliament, 2020) made the case for more sustained investment in social care, citing the toll the COVID-19 pandemic has had on the sector. Highlighting the funding problems in social care, including funding shortfalls and the impact on pay levels, the threat to the sustainability of the care market was apparent. The report called for an immediate funding increase to avoid the risk of market collapse caused by providers withdrawing from offering services to council-funded individuals and focusing exclusively on the self-pay market. The crisis in social care funding has been brought into sharp focus by the COVID-19 pandemic, and the government has been urged to respond as a matter of urgency.

The 'Government Response to the Health and Social Care Committee report on Adult Social Care: Funding and Workforce' (GOV.UK, 2021a) was an inquiry into the funding and workforce for social care with recommendations and the government's official response to the Health and Social Care Committee report referred to above. The government responded by pledging to provide substantial funding to support the social care sector through the pandemic and beyond. Local authorities would receive £4.6 billion through un-ringfenced grants, and an estimated additional £3 billion of support for COVID-19 pressures in financial years 21–22 to local government.

The report also contains a commitment to social care workers and an intention to develop a wellbeing package of emotional, psychological and practical resources for the social care workforce. The government stated that they would continue to commission and fund a range of training opportunities to help recruit people into the sector, and to support staff that want to progress to management and leadership roles.

Since 2022, and with the inception of the Health and Care Act 2022, further changes have occurred. In July 2022, the government published 'Guidance on the preparation of integrated care strategies' (Department of Health and Social Care, 2022b). Work had been undertaken to increase integration through health and wellbeing boards, and the Better Care Fund framework 2022 was set up to ensure that health, social care and housing services were working together to help older people and those with complex needs and disabilities to enable them to live at home for longer.

The passing of the Health and Care Act 2022 recognised the Integrated Care Systems (ICSs) and empowered them to govern NHS finances at a local level.

Local strategy

Local strategies for care set out the strategic priorities for the development and delivery of care in local areas, bringing together social care organisations with the ICSs, health and wellbeing boards (HWBs), general practitioners (GPs) and local councils. In this way, the financial, physical and human resources in a local setting can be looked at in a holistic way to ascertain the most efficient way in which to resource the care for a diverse population of people. Not all areas are the same and some locations in the country will have different care needs according to their population demographic. For example, an area where there is a large elderly population will require different care services, which may need to be resourced. Financial, physical and human resources are clearly identified in the local strategic plan, which should identify the action needed to address deficits.

Research it

1.1, 1.2 and 1.3 National strategy

Take a look at the following reports:

- the government response to the Health and Social Care Committee report on Adult Social Care: Funding and Workforce (GOV.UK, 2021a)
- 'Guidance on the preparation of integrated care strategies' (Department of Health and Social Care, 2022b)
- 'People at the heart of care: Adult social care reform' (Department of Health and Social Care, 2022c).

Choose two of the reports and write a short piece to show how each report has influenced your own organisation with respect to resource planning in relation to:

- financial resources
- physical resources
- human resources.

Organisational strategy

The local strategy and the groups involved (such as the STPs, ICSs, HWBs, GPs and the local council) will allocate finance to organisations within their area that have responsibility for delivering care within the budget. The organisational strategy will be outlined in a strategic plan but will support the national and local priorities for care.

Budgets and financial resources

Effective organisations need organisation plans and as a manager you may have been asked to prepare such a document. However, some managers in social care will have no involvement in preparing organisation plans as this is something the owner or director of the organisation will undertake. The Department of Health and Social Care requires all care establishments to have organisation and financial plans in place for external inspection.

You may have been asked to present financial accounts to the Care Quality Commission or the commissioning agency to demonstrate that individuals' fees are being used in an effective way towards their care and that you are providing the best value in your service delivery (again, this is something that not all managers are involved in). To do this, you need to know how to set budgets and monitor the expenditure of your own organisation. This expenditure is likely to be in relation to supplies, staffing, equipment and overhead expenses.

A budget refers to the allocation of finances for specific purposes and will form part of your action plan for the future. If you are part of a large organisation, you will be allocated a small part of the overall financial income and will be expected to audit the expenditure you undertake and to keep within the limits of your budget for a specific length of time, usually known as the financial year. If, however, you work within a small care home or other provision and are in total control of all income and outgoings, then you need to ensure that the budget is carefully allocated to different areas and to avoid overspending.

Budgeting is a continuous process and to manage the process effectively requires the ability to see beyond the barriers of the yearly divisions and to project future trends for the setting. In preparing a budget, the expected income for the year needs to be predicted, along with the predicted expenditure for the year.

Whichever way you choose to set your budget, variations may occur, for instance, the cost of services may be far more expensive than it was last year, and you need to be aware of the potential to overspend. Accuracy is key to managing finances effectively.

You may also need to undertake a cost–benefit analysis, which is weighing the effectiveness of the resources and services you wish to purchase against alternatives. For example, you may have decided that the setting needs to be updated and decorated and new furniture purchased. However, if the washing machine breaks down and a new one is needed, you might have to change your plans or at least reassess the needs with respect to the decorative update. Planning, therefore, needs to be on both a long-term and a short-term basis.

The flowchart in Figure 9 may be helpful in the planning process.

Access the aims and objectives of the organisation

↓

Access last year's income and expenditure

↓

Prepare a statement for the team as to the spending plans for the coming year

↓

Supervise and monitor the control of the budget
Ascertain who is responsible for what

↓

Evaluate your performance against the aims and objectives

▲ **Figure 9** The planning process

Regular reviews and monitoring of budgets

Regularly reviewing and monitoring the budget is essential as the amount you spend throughout the year is likely to vary. The cost of fuel and travel for domiciliary staff must be considered here and, in the winter, the expense of heating and lighting is likely to be higher than during the summer months, so seasonal fluctuations need to be considered. Such planning is called budgetary profiling and if you do not take this into account, you are likely to have cash flow problems, which can be stressful. Your staff may not understand how the budget is set and why they are sometimes unable to purchase certain items or undertake activities with individuals.

It is important to ensure that the team is aware of how the budget functions. You will need to discuss changes with your team and clarify the costs of any changes. For example, some staff may not understand why they are now being asked to finance their own training when in the past these costs have been met by the organisation. Clear discussions in an open and transparent manner can help to clarify this for them.

Physical resources

The physical resources of any adult social care service, care home or other provision refer to the land and buildings as well as the care and administration equipment owned by the organisation.

At national, local and organisational levels these resources need to be managed and maintained to keep the care system safe and efficient. You may be responsible for maintaining a residential care setting or part of one. You will have a budget that will require careful balancing to reduce the financial pressures on an already depleted social care service.

As a manager, you will be responsible for the maintenance of equipment, monitoring its use and ensuring that equipment and premises remain fit for purpose.

Human resources

Human resources are by far the biggest resource in the care service today. In 2022, Skills for Care published a report entitled 'The workforce employed by adult services departments in England'. This shows that in 2021 there were 115,100 jobs in local authorities in England held by 111,100 people, which was an increase of 0.8 per cent from 2020. Vacancies have risen to the highest rate since 2012–13, increasing by 52 per cent in 2021/22 to 165,000 vacant posts, with the decrease in filled posts due to recruitment and retention difficulties (Skills for Care, 2022a).

Evidence opportunity

1.2 and 1.3 Reviewing effectiveness of approaches to resource management

Write an account describing and analysing the impact of different strategies on resource planning in your setting in relation to:

- ✔ financial resources
- ✔ physical resources
- ✔ human resources.

How did you ensure that staff were kept aware of how they can contribute to the financial stability of the organisation? Would you make any changes in the next year and if so, why?

For adult care the vacancy issue is a problem. According to figures published by Skills for Care in October 2022, the number of vacant posts in adult social care increased by 52 per cent during the period 2021–22, which meant there were 165,000 vacant posts. Furthermore, it is suggested that there will be a need for an extra 480,000 people working in social care by 2035 to meet demand (Skills for Care, 2022a). This urgently requires a solution, particularly as there will be further losses to the workforce as people retire.

Developing a workforce plan

One of your key responsibilities at a more local level will be to ensure that you have addressed your staffing needs and developed a **workforce plan**. Additionally, as staff are a major resource, you must ensure that you retain the staff you have and develop them to meet the needs of future developments in adult social care.

As a manager, you will be aware of the need to determine what skills each staff member has and to ensure that during a span of duty you have the right people in place for the care that needs to be given. You also need to develop trust in the team so that you can be confident that delegated tasks will be undertaken. Developing trust is dependent upon certain behaviours, such as listening to your staff, seeking input from them in decision making, recognising good work, praising them and enabling them to develop. When there is trust in a team, staff will feel secure and empowered to undertake delegated tasks.

In developing your workforce development plan, you will need to:

- analyse your current workforce and identify the skills mix required in your setting to deliver the type of service you provide
- ensure that staff receive any training that is required to meet the needs of the individuals using the service.

KEY TERM

Workforce planning: Allocating staff with the necessary skills to a task when they are needed in order to deliver organisational objectives.

Workforce planning is not only about your current provision, though. You need to be aware that future changes to the type or number of individuals coming to your setting will need to be considered so that your plan can highlight any gaps that need to be filled.

In developing your plan, it is useful to consider the stages outlined by the Social Care Institute for Excellence (SCIE). See SCIE (2006) for further information.

Audit of current provision – where the organisation is now

You need to have up-to-date records of all staff working in your setting, with details of working hours, training undertaken, retirement ages and turnover. You should also consider the diversity of your staff to see whether the workforce matches that of the individuals using your service. If not, you may wish to plan for future campaigns to bring in more diverse staff.

The context of your service – the current trends and changes

In this section of the plan you should make reference to the trends in the setting, whether it is expanding or otherwise, the changing needs of the individuals using the service, new regulations or national and local initiatives that may change the service delivery.

Forecasting – or what will you need in the future

This refers to the gaps in the service that you have identified in stages one and two. You may have realised that with the growth of the older population in your area, not only will you need more staff, but you may also need to recruit qualified nurses if individuals using the service have chronic conditions requiring nursing care.

Planning – action plan

Three areas are necessary in this part of your plan:

- Recruitment and succession planning (i.e. replacing staff who leave or retire).
- Career development plans for staff and retention plans.
- Changes to remuneration packages, pay increases or benefits to staff.

Implementation – putting it into practice

In this stage, the plan needs to be integrated into the strategic plan of the organisation and should then be reviewed in line with it.

Workforce development helps to identify current trends and forecast future workforce structures to meet service delivery requirements. The care system is concerned with productivity and outcomes, and with changing structures in social care, workforce development planning is critical to maintaining a good service and achieving positive outcomes for people.

Skills for Care also offers advice and guidance on developing your workforce. Go to the Skills for Care home page and click on 'Developing your workforce'.

Strategic planning

Your organisation's strategic plan or vision will identify a corporate strategy and highlight the way in which the setting is run and how resources are allocated.

The first part of the strategic plan should identify a mission statement, which outlines the direction in which the setting wishes to go. There will then be short-term, long-term and operational plans:

- **Short-term plans** cover the day-to-day operation of the organisation and have specific timeframes in place. These can then be measured by conducting research to check whether deadlines have been met and plans fulfilled. A simple checklist or survey can be carried out to assess this.
- **Long-term plans** link to finances, such as how profitable the setting is and how it can survive in the long term. They are linked to the overall strategic planning process and operational planning.
- **Operational plans** detail the specific objectives and milestones for an organisation and consider the budgetary, physical and human resources needed for the success of the organisation.

The strategic plan in your organisation will have been put together with reference to national organisational strategies and priorities on resource planning and management, and with consideration of government-led spending reviews and plans.

Reflect on it

1.2 and 1.3 Resources and your setting

Think about how your own service has changed with respect to the resources at its disposal. Why do you think this change has come about? If you are new to the setting, and are unaware of how the organisation has changed, you could ask a colleague. How has the organisation evolved?

AC 1.4 Explain the importance of accurate forecasting for resource requirements including contingency planning, crisis management and day-to-day requirements/resources

Here, you will be required to explain the role of forecasting in resource management. This must include reference to maintaining accuracy, validity and reliability.

It is easy to come to work every day and take for granted that your shift will run smoothly and you will have access to stock you need, food for the people in receipt of services and a full team of staff for the care required that day. This requires accurate and reliable planning. As a manager, you will be responsible for the duty rota and must ensure that agreed care is provided. This means that you need to have knowledge of the staffing resources available to you and the needs of the people in receipt of services on each shift. Different service areas, such as residential, domiciliary and outreach care, will have different staffing needs, for example according to the type of people in receipt of services being cared for.

It is important too that you plan for unlikely events, known as contingency planning.

Contingency planning

A contingency plan or 'plan B' is an action plan designed to help an organisation respond to a significant event or a future situation that may or may not happen. It is a bit like managing a risk. Some care homes or other provisions, having listened to increasing stories in the media about the possibility of a pandemic, may have devised a contingency plan which outlined what should be done in the event of such a national emergency. Building projects often feature contingency plans; this usually refers to a pot of money that has been set aside in case something happens that had not been accounted for in the original budget. A contingency plan is a backup plan or an alternative action if expected results fail to come about.

Crisis management

Similar to a contingency plan, crisis management is a plan to minimise the damage a crisis would cause and is a process that is put into practice before a crisis happens. Crisis management practices are engaged before, during and after a crisis. A major incident plan is a good example of crisis management. Pre-crisis planning is undertaken to determine the best way to respond when a crisis occurs and to then identify risks and find ways to reduce them. Risk management is therefore part of crisis management, but crisis management covers incident response.

Although it seems counterintuitive, a crisis can be planned for. For example, early warning signals can be monitored. It might be that power cuts may happen in your area or even staff shortages may be problematic from time to time. Changes to the weather can also have a major effect on service, so these all need to be planned for.

It is useful to identify a 'crisis manager' to direct the organisation's response so that if a major incident occurs staff can be ready to undertake other roles that have been previously assigned under the terms of the incident response plan. The crisis manager is also the communication link to the public and must ensure that any health or safety risk is identified and passed on to the media as soon as possible.

Evaluating what has happened following a crisis will determine whether the plan was useful or requires changing.

Day-to-day requirements/resources

Resource management is the way in which you manage the organisation's physical, financial and human resources every day and you will need to do this in the most efficient way possible. These resources include stock and equipment, your budget and the staff at your disposal.

SCIE gives a definition of resource management as the practice of:

'balancing competing priorities for resources while still delivering good outcomes for people who use services, e.g. resourcing personal budgets and support for disabled adults and children, safeguarding services for adults and children, preventative strategies to promote well-being, and workforce costs.'

Source: Social Care Institute for Excellence (2018)

Forecasting

The strategic plan for the whole organisation will forecast how the service is expected to function in the year ahead. It will set out the budgets available and how these will be spent in order for the service to be sustainable in the short term and how it will grow and develop in the long term. If you are part of a large organisation, part of the budget will be devolved to your section of the service, and you will be expected to manage it by predicting demand and supply of your own service in an accurate and valid way. In a small organisation you may have the whole budget to oversee.

In using the funds, you may feel (and your staff will probably agree) that you require many more staff to accomplish a quality service. If, however, you spend money on more staff earlier in the year, by the end of the year you may have a redundancy situation because you no longer have the budget to pay them. However, if you work in a smaller organisation, such as a care or nursing home, you will have a smaller budget but will be responsible for setting a budget for all the resources in the setting.

It is important to forecast in a quantitative and qualitative manner and you may find you are referring to the forecasts on a weekly basis. Staffing will be your biggest budgetary spend so your forecast will show 'how many' and 'when' you need those staff as well as what the desired personal qualities and role-related qualifications are to fulfil those needs.

Forecasting is an important part of resource management. It means thinking ahead to build a clear picture of what future expenses are likely to be, and how the setting might allocate the money that is available. For example, you may look at equipment to see what needs to be replaced or repaired, or staffing needs, and then budget accordingly. Human resources forecasting involves looking at the staff that you need in the coming months and years based upon growth of the organisation or changes to roles within the team.

Accuracy

Forecasting must be done in an accurate manner, and this requires a critical analysis of the needs of the organisation. This can be done by looking at how the setting met targets in the previous year and what plans there are for the future. You may assume that the future is going to be like the past and simply plan according to last year's data. But this would not produce an accurate result. If, for example, your service is changing or growing then you may need to accurately plan for more staff, more equipment and more financial support to meet this need. Your forecast will be based upon last year's budget, with adjustments due to inflation and costs to cover new services. If the service is to remain the same, you will still need to forecast for inflation.

Validity and reliability

The data you collect to forecast your future resource needs must be valid, which means it must be based upon data that is correct and reliable. Reliability simply means that it is precise and sound. For example, a reliable forecast is one that takes into account expenditure from the previous year, cash flow for the next year, and an accurate analysis of the staff needed to ensure that a quality service is delivered. Forecasting does involve some subjective judgement because you are looking at uncertainty in the future. You cannot know for certain what might happen, so your prediction may fall short of the actual outcome. This might be because the demand for your service changes, inflation may rise more than you had anticipated, meaning cutbacks are inevitable, and there may also be changes in legislation which impact how your service is run. All these are factors that can result in different outcomes to the ones that had been planned.

Evidence opportunity

1.4 Importance of accurate forecasting

Provide a written account explaining the role of forecasting in resource management in your setting. You must refer to maintaining accuracy, validity and reliability. You might also like to use your own strategic/service plan and analyse how you undertook the role of forecasting in resource management. Ensure that you refer to how you maintained the following:

- ✔ Accuracy: How accurate are you likely to be with your planning? For example, will there be major changes to your service or will it remain the same?
- ✔ Validity: What sort of data are you going to use, and do you consider it to be valid?
- ✔ Reliability: How reliable was your planning last year?

Look at the crisis management or major incident plan for your setting. Is it fit for purpose? Make changes if necessary and discuss the plan with staff. What responsibilities will they have?

AC 1.5 Explain the value of using assets and resources outside traditional services and in the community

Here, you will be required to explain the use of alternative resources and assets. This could include volunteers and voluntary services, alternative non-traditional therapies, community and educational resources.

Partnership working

Partnership working developed because it was recognised that it was impossible for one care provider to provide all of the care for an individual and a seamless care provision. To that end, there are valuable resources that can be accessed in the community via voluntary groups, alternative therapies and education and in other parts of the service area.

Working in this way is now integral to the way local authorities have developed community strategies, with a huge number of people all delivering services in different areas and locations. Joint working is paramount if individuals are to receive the best service.

Working with other organisations

You may already be working with other agencies within the wider multidisciplinary team such as advocacy agencies or care teams. An advantage of working closely with organisations is that they may be able to offer advice on specific issues. They may also have access to equipment which your service does not have and could share this resource with you. A disadvantage of purely relying on other organisations is that some may be affected by lack of funding, which may make it difficult for the sector to fund their work.

In developing links with other services you can improve the experience and outcomes of people who use services as you can then access other resources in terms of staff expertise, advice and even shared physical resources. It might also be possible to access technological services that your own service may lack. For example, shared technology such as computer software or training may be available to you.

Volunteers, voluntary services and non-traditional therapies

Voluntary and other non-traditional or alternative therapy services and organisations make a great contribution to the health service and, as such, are part of the resources you may call upon to enrich your own service. They may be able to deliver preventative services that reduce the need for people to see their GP or go to hospital. For example, day care centres and lunch groups may help isolated individuals to meet up with others. Your care setting may also receive volunteers and other services that enhance the wellbeing of the individuals using your service, but alternatively it could be that your setting provides a day care service for others in the community. New initiatives of care homes or other provisions working closely with their local primary schools encourage a reciprocal arrangement for individuals using an adult care service and young people to enjoy the benefits of each other's company.

The Department of Health (DoH) launched the Voluntary Sector Strategic Partner Programme in April 2009 to improve communication between the department and voluntary social care organisations. It was set up to enable the voluntary sector organisations to work in equal partnership with the DHSC, NHS and social care for the benefit of the sector and has aimed to improve health and wellbeing outcomes.

Community and educational resources

Other agencies within the wider multidisciplinary team include social groups, community exercise or walking groups, befriending services and counselling, advocacy agencies or other adult social care teams, and these may all be available to help your own service. These partnerships need to be part of resource planning and forecasting decisions. For example, if the service you work with is under threat of closure, you need to make plans for the deficit this will create in the service you offer.

The use of these services may well enrich the quality of your own service, but you need to justify their use and inclusion in your care offer. As the manager you must, therefore, evaluate their effectiveness in supplying value for money and provide evidence of what they offer to the individuals using your service. An analysis of the strengths and limitations of the service they offer will provide valid and reliable evidence to include in your resource planning.

Evidence opportunity

1.5 Value of using assets and resources outside traditional services

Explain the use of alternative resources and assets. This could include, for example:

- ✔ volunteers and voluntary services
- ✔ alternative non-traditional therapies
- ✔ community and educational resources.

Think about what voluntary, alternative non-traditional therapies, community and educational resources services your service links or partners with and evaluate how these are useful to the individuals using your service. Consider the strengths and the weaknesses of the alternative resources and assets and make arguments for and against their use.

AC 1.6 Evaluate the place of technology as a resource in service delivery and service management

Here, you will be required to evaluate the use of different technologies within your service provision, including your use of digital technology and use by people in receipt of services, team members and other stakeholders.

Role of technology as a resource in service delivery and management

We use digital technology in our day-to-day lives and the same apps, gadgets and technologies can also be used to support how we care for people.

In adult social care and, more specifically, for those people with learning disabilities, the use of assistive technology means personalised technology for individuals with disabilities that enables them to perform functions that might otherwise prove difficult. This technology can make huge differences to people's independence and helps them to gain more control over their lives.

Augmentative and alternative communication (AAC) can be used to support and enhance communication for people with autism, regardless of speech ability. The technologies range from automatic medicine dispensers and big button remote controls to internet connectivity, artificial intelligence, wearable health trackers and smart homes.

Alice Ainsworth, in her blog 'How can digital technologies support care?' (2023), shows how adult care reform groups are supporting the digital transformation of the adult social care sector. Devices such as mobile phones and tablets can be used to help individuals remain in contact with families and loved ones and can also be used to set medication and hydration reminders. Apps have been developed using touchscreen and eye-gaze technologies, which give individuals different ways to communicate and greater control over how they are supported. Digital solutions can also be used to support reminiscence, which can be a useful technique for supporting individuals with learning disabilities or those living with dementia.

The Department of Health and Social Care announced a technology fund in 2023 to help care providers to adopt technologies that address local priorities (DHSC and Whately, 2023).

Use of digital technology in the setting

For care professionals such as yourself, team members and your stakeholders, technology has improved the quality of the service you can offer, increasing the efficiency of the way in which you do things. For example, you are now able to access online up-to-date lifesaving information wherever an individual is, which means you and your team members are able to link into algorithms for care such as resuscitation and sepsis guidelines, thus reducing the waiting time for life-saving care if you are required and trained to do so as part of your role. You can also access NICE's British National Formulary (BNF) online and software such as MEDUSA, which gives information on injectable medicines, again, if this is part of your role as an adult care worker.

You will need to ensure that your staff understand how digital technologies can help them to work efficiently, and how these resources can be used for professional development. There may be training that you can discuss with them and arrange.

Skills for Care (Skills for Care, n.d. e) highlight the use of technology in adult social care, showing how such use is improving care and support.

Artificial intelligence, a currently new but developing area, already uses a limited number of robots to assist in care. Physical assistance robots (PAR) perform discrete tasks such as lifting and carrying to support people who need such support. Cognitive assistance robots (CARs) support users to perform cognitive tasks and can help people with dementia, Alzheimer's disease and other cognitive impairments. 'Chatbots' or computer programmes can conduct conversation via audio or text.

Socially assistive robotics (SARs) help people with the activities of daily living through non-contact assistance and companion robots are associated with improving the overall wellbeing of their users (Skills for Care, n.d. b).

Surveillance technology, such as CCTV, cameras and microphones, is also considered by the CQC as being useful in keeping people safe, provided it is used in ways that protect people's privacy and human rights.

Digital security

You and your staff will also need to be aware of the importance of security of systems and files that are stored digitally, and so they will need to be aware of how they can ensure that information remains secure. You will need to ensure that you have robust systems in place to protect the setting's systems and data that is stored electronically. This is likely to include ensuring your computer systems are firewall protected, that passwords are used and that information is backed up externally or, for example, online in the cloud. Protecting individuals in your setting when it comes to technology will also be one of your responsibilities. As a manager in an adult care setting, you need to make sure that information about the dangers of being online is readily available, and that your staff are trained in and have an understanding of this, so they are able to confidently advise those they provide care for. This might mean being aware of issues such as cyber-bullying, online data protection, online fraud and identity theft, as well as safety issues around meeting or befriending people online. There are many online training courses which you can access to help you learn about staying safe online. You may even run a training course about this for your staff or offer guidance through leaflets and posters on notice boards.

For more information, see NHS Digital (2021).

Research it

1.6 Skills for Care

Visit the Skills for Care website and access the information highlighting the use of technology in adult social care (Skills for Care, n.d. e).

Make notes on your findings. Think about how you can keep up to date with the latest digital developments and offers, and how this can help you in your role as manager.

Impact of technology on your service

Technology is having a huge impact upon the way services are now delivered in adult social care and in the management of services. Software is available to help you conduct staff reviews and appraisals, for example, in a more efficient manner, and online ordering and next-day delivery are becoming standard.

Mobile phones, apps, computers, social media and electronic health records are all now available. These systems are available for your personal use and for the individuals using your service. They enable you to communicate with team members and stakeholders from any location.

The advantages of this are clear. It is quicker, paperless and you can respond to care needs more efficiently. The disadvantages occur when the technology fails to work or breaches arise in the system, which puts confidential data at risk of being lost or shared.

Electronic care plans/risk assessment

The Fundamental Standards of the Health and Social Care Act 2008 (Regulated Activities) Regulations 2014 state that it is an individual's right to have care provision that is tailored to their needs and preferences. This forms part of the CQC inspection as they will check to see that care/support plans have been agreed with the individual.

The care/support plan is a tool with which you and your team ensure that the individual is supported in a way that enhances their quality of life. The individual must be involved in their care/support planning.

Until recently, care/support plans were paper based, and these could often be quite lengthy. However, electronic care/support plans are becoming more common and their logical layout is easier to update. Care must be taken to ensure that such plans remain person-centred.

All care/support plans should start with how much the person can do for themselves. Those areas where the person needs support should reflect the person's needs and wishes in how their care will be provided. Some plans, including electronic ones, tend to split Activities of Daily Living (ADL) into sections so it is easier to describe the areas that staff need to support.

When risks are identified, care/support plans need to contain clear instructions for staff about the level of that risk and the measures to be taken to mitigate the risk or be closely linked to a risk assessment policy.

Electronic medication administration record system

An electronic medication administration record system (eMAR) contains details of medication type, dosage, strength and frequency. Alerts are sent to carers to ensure that individuals receive the correct medication on time and carers receive specific detailed instructions on what medications need to be administered and when.

Electronic rota systems

Originally a paper document, the work rota lists the staff who need to work during a shift and the dates and times at which they are scheduled to do. The use of electronic rotas simplifies and speeds up this process. A number of software packages such as Findmyshift are available.

Video calling

Most computers and smart phones are equipped with video call apps. There are several providers available for download including Microsoft Teams, Google Meet and Zoom. These are an excellent way to meet with stakeholders and other services as they reduce the need for travel outside the office to attend meetings, thereby saving you time during the working day.

Portals/hubs

Adult Care Portals are set up by local authorities to provide a secure space for individuals to have more control over their care and support. They can complete and submit social forms online and get in touch with the people who work with them.

Individuals must register to open a portal account.

NHS login is a portal service providing a way for individuals registered at a GP practice to access multiple digital social care services with a single login. For example, individuals can access the NHS App or online consultation platform eConsult.

NHS Patient hub is a secure online portal providing information relating to care at the click of a button. It enables individuals to access digital appointment notifications, reminders and more, making the booking process fully automated.

Mind have an online peer support community called Side by Side where people can talk about their mental health and connect with others. It provides a safe place to listen, share and be heard.

Evidence opportunity

1.6 Role of technology as a resource in service delivery and management

Evaluate the use of different technologies within your own service provision, including the following:

- ✔ **Own use**: How useful do you find technology? What apps are you signed up to and how do they help you take control of your own health? How do you use technology in your setting? What are the advantages and disadvantages?
- ✔ **People in receipt of services**: Conduct a small survey of the people using the service and ask them if they use any of the apps or self-help programmes available online. What are their views on the strengths or limitations of such programmes?
- ✔ **Team members**: How does your team use online resources for treatments and information? Which would you say are the most used sites for you and your staff and why are they useful?
- ✔ **Other stakeholders**: Talk to the stakeholders in your organisation and ask them how technology has changed the way in which they work. Find out what the pros and cons are for them.

Provide a written account to evidence this.

AC 1.7 Describe the meaning of sustainability in resource management in adult care

Here, you will be required to describe the use of sustainable resources within adult services, with particular reference to own service provision.

You will be familiar with the term sustainability as this is a much-used term in adult social care. But what exactly does it mean?

Sustainability is about making savings where possible and reducing waste. Sustainable care ensures that the care and support delivered does not harm the environment and provides a positive social impact. It must be affordable now and in the future.

However, with the ever-changing demands upon the social care system, such as increasing population numbers and the needs of an ageing population, the delivery of a sustainable adult care service is a challenge.

Climate change has been identified as one of the biggest global health threats of the twenty-first century. The effects of climate change for people with disabilities are far worse. In the UK, we already experience climate change in the form of increased incidences of severe weather, such as heatwaves and flooding. For those with disabilities, these events have more far-reaching effects.

Heat waves are associated with an increase in mortality, particularly in the over-75 age group. The widespread floods in 2007 showed how self-reported symptoms of mental disorders, distress and PTSD were significantly greater for those who were unable to access essential services.

In 2019, the United Nations Human Rights Council adopted a resolution that urged governments to adopt a disability-inclusive approach to address climate change. The disproportionate effects felt by those with disability include health impacts, as severe heat or cold may make them more susceptible to other health problems due to existing conditions. Also, many may be at particular risk of neglect or abandonment during natural disasters, such as local flooding, which are happening more frequently. Wheelchair users may find that access issues prevent them from being able to escape from harm and those with disabilities where communication and understanding is limited may not have access to adequate resources, information and services to enable them to adapt to the effects of climate change.

For social care, an immediate threat is the increasing demand from an ageing population and, together with cuts to local authority funding places, this increases pressure on adult social care services. Subsequently, with shortfalls in social care places, people are forced to remain in hospital despite them having no acute medical need.

Sustainability within your setting

An internet search for ways to improve sustainability or to set a green plan for your setting will provide you with information on how your setting can become more sustainable. This might include very simple actions such as fitting low energy light bulbs, turning off lights in rooms not in use, using energy efficient appliances and turning off computers not in use. You might also consider where the food you serve comes from and could reduce your carbon footprint by buying locally, thereby sustaining the local economy at the same time.

Research it

1.7 Sustainable models of care

SCIE defines sustainability as the 'balance of positive social, economic and environmental outcomes' and says that taking a sustainable development approach to social care, although difficult, will reap benefits.

Their website has a number of case studies that show how local authorities have planned initiatives such as encouraging walking and cycling instead of driving.

For an example of this approach, the Go Low initiative led by Wiltshire Mental Health Partnership NHS Trust with support from Bristol City Council aimed to reduce the amount of petrol used by community health teams. The purchase of low-emission cars and electric bikes for the team to use improved air quality and therefore health. A side benefit was also noted for the people using the services. Staff were in the habit of offering them lifts in their cars. But travelling to home visits by bike meant this was no longer an option. This promoted a message of independence and some people using the services also started cycling.

Go to the SCIE website and access the case studies (SCIE, 2010).

What small difference might you make to the delivery of care that shows you are taking a sustainable approach?

Stretch and challenge

1.7 Sustainability and resource management

Analyse the use of sustainable resources within adult care services and within your own setting. Are there ways in which you could ensure that you use more sustainable resources? How will you ensure this as a manager?

You could evidence this with a reflective account or discuss this with your assessor.

AC 1.8 Explain roles, responsibilities and accountabilities for resource management within an adult care setting/service

Here, you will be required to explain your role and responsibilities regarding resources management in your service with reference to how potential improvements are implemented.

As a care manager, your role will vary according to your setting, but you are required to ensure that the management of financial, physical and human resources are dealt with efficiently.

You may manage budgets and perhaps report to a financial committee to justify your spending. Even if you do not need to report to a committee, you will need to monitor expenditure and costs. When budget planning you need to:

- plan your income for the year
- plan your expenditure for the year
- review the spend at given points in the year
- keep records of costs.

Physical resources will require you to maintain quality standards in the setting and ensure that health and safety is complied with regarding use of equipment and the fabric of the building and furniture. In managing the physical resources, you need to:

- allocate finances to ensure that you can update and renew equipment, furniture and decoration if needed
- draw up a resource plan at the start of the year to determine what you need in terms of equipment, materials, furniture or other items
- monitor the use of physical resources to determine wastage and stock.

For staffing and human resources, your role is to recruit, train and supervise staff to deliver quality care. This goes beyond these three areas however, as it includes more nuanced responsibilities such as ensuring the wellbeing of your staff, looking at workloads and opportunities for development within staff roles and the setting.

Managing human resources also involves ensuring that your budget allows for additional training, should it be required, so that you can invest in current staff.

Responsibilities and accountability

As a manager in an adult care setting, you are responsible for ensuring that the financial, physical and human resources for your department meet the national standards of care and also the organisation's strategic and operational plans. This means you are responsible for the failure or success of the operations within your organisation. It is your responsibility to see that the quality of the care setting is not compromised due to potential shortfalls in funding and staffing. Should this happen, you will need to be aware of how you can improve the situation. For example, if staffing becomes problematic at times, you may be required to look carefully at workloads and employ agency staff as a short-term measure. If staffing issues are unresolved, then you will be responsible for escalating concerns to higher management and putting together a case for additional staff.

Being accountable means you are answerable for the success or failure of something. If you are held accountable for something, then you will be expected to explain why you acted in a certain way and why that action failed or succeeded.

If you are accountable for the financial, physical and human resources within your setting then you could be asked to justify, for example, overspending on budgets or failure to train staff to required standards. Having control of your budget and an understanding about how you might save on the use of physical resources may enable you to make improvements to the current provision. By undertaking a resource planning exercise at the start of the year, you will be able to see where improvements to staffing, physical resources and finances can be made at certain points in the year. For example, you may wish to allocate funds to train a member of staff to undertake mandatory training for all staff, which means you save on employing external companies that offer the same training at elevated costs.

> **Evidence opportunity**
>
> **1.8 Roles, responsibilities and accountabilities**
>
> What is your role and responsibility with respect to resource management in your own service?
>
> How do you address concerns and implement potential improvements?
>
> Provide a written account explaining this.

AC 1.9 Evaluate the importance of business continuity in respect of planning and processes available

Here, you will evaluate the impact of change on your setting and across the sector.

Review of the sector on a regular basis

Changes in the sector must result in an improvement in the lives of the people using the services, so you need to ensure that any organisational strategic planning takes into account current sustainability issues as well as demographic and technological changes. It is important to keep up to date with government changes and reviews in order to address issues in the sector. Skills for Care published a report in 2021 addressing the impact of the COVID-19 pandemic on the care sector and identifying changes to impact care positively (Swift and Teicke, 2021). Their considerations for future planning include:

- the need to recruit another 520,000 people to work in social care by 2035
- some thought on how to provide social care differently.

Evidence opportunity

1.9 Strategic planning

Go to the Skills for Care website and read about their plans for 2021–2025 (Skills for Care, 2021a).

Look at the four main areas for development:

- ✔ Increasing workforce capacity
- ✔ Supporting workforce capabilities
- ✔ Supporting culture and diversity
- ✔ Improving the social care system

How do they fit into your own strategic plan?

Review of the customer base

In your development and planning you must constantly look at who your actual users are. Demographic changes in your area may require you to plan differently. For example, the income level in the area in which your care setting is located will indicate the sort of services you might be able to provide and at what cost.

You also need to consider the age range of your target market to ensure that you offer services that fit their needs. You might wish to conduct a lifestyle survey to support your planning to determine whether the services you wish to offer would be attractive to the local population and whether or not the service is needed. For example, if your care setting is located in a remote rural area, it may not be the best place to offer a service that people cannot readily access, even if it is a crucial one.

Organisation risk assessment

An organisation risk assessment involves five steps:

1. Identify the hazards that could negatively influence the setting. For example, you might consider further COVID-19 pandemic lockdowns, cyber-attacks or failure to recruit staff.
2. Determine what, or who, could be harmed if the risk occurred and which organisation assets would be negatively influenced.
3. Conduct a risk analysis and develop control measures to minimise or eliminate the risk.
4. Record your findings and make these documents easily accessible. The records should include details of hazards, the risk of such a hazard occurring and plans in place to reduce the risk of the hazard occurring.
5. Review and update the risk assessment regularly.

SWOT analysis

Conducting a SWOT analysis may help you identify threats and unexpected events. You can read more on how to undertake a SWOT analysis in Unit 500 AC1.2.

Exercise programme

In AC1.4 you looked at the development of a crisis management plan, sometimes known as a major incident plan. It is essential to know that your plan will work in the event of a major incident, so you need to undertake a training exercise to ensure that everyone knows what is expected of them and understands how the plan should work. For example, you are required to undertake annual fire evacuation exercises to ensure that all staff and individuals can be safely removed from the building in an emergency.

As part of organisation continuity, you must regularly review your SWOT analysis, risk assessments and major incident plan to ensure that they continue to meet your setting's needs.

Evidence opportunity

1.9 SWOT analysis

Undertake a SWOT analysis to identify the strengths and weaknesses in your setting. What opportunities do you have to ensure organisation continuity?

Evaluate the changes in the setting that the SWOT has raised and how this has had positive and negative effects on the service.

LO2 Understand principles of effective human resource management

AC 2.1 Explain legislation, policy and practices underpinning safe and fair recruitment

Here, you will explain the legal aspects and local policy impacts on recruiting for your setting.

Equality legislation

The Equality Act 2010 brought together four major EU Equal Treatment Directives and replaced previous anti-discrimination laws, simplifying the law and making it easier to understand. It is an umbrella act bringing together legislation that deals with race, disability and gender.

The Act highlights protected characteristics of age, gender reassignment, pregnancy, religion, disability, race, marriage and civil partnerships, and sexual orientation in an attempt to end discrimination. Additionally, it strengthens protection by setting out the different ways in which unlawful treatment may occur.

Equality in the workplace means equal job opportunities and fairness for employees and job applicants. The impact of this legislation has been to enable protected groups to gain employment and to not be discriminated against. Discrimination means treating somebody unfairly, especially on the grounds of their race, sex, age or disability.

There has also been a positive move to address the gender pay gap, and equal pay and fair pay for all are also addressed in the Equality Act 2010.

Pensions and Working Time legislation

As a result of the Pensions Act 2008, workplace pensions have become 'opt-out' rather than 'opt-in'. This means most employees are automatically enrolled into a pension provided by their employer. The law also requires employers to pay into their employees' pension schemes.

The Pension Schemes Act 2021 introduced new duties for those involved in running pension schemes and gives new powers to the Pensions Regulator to protect pension scheme members and the Pension Protection Fund.

Working hours in the UK are governed by the Working Time Regulations 1998, which limit the working week to an average of 48 hours (although there is an opt-out). The working day should average eight hours. This legislation also states that workers and employees have the right to paid leave and specified rest breaks.

Regulatory body

The Employment Agency Standards Inspectorate (EAS) enforces certain regulations and can investigate if an employer is refusing to pay what a person is owed for work carried out.

The Conduct of Employment Agencies and Employment Business Regulations 2003 are a set of minimum standards that must be adhered to when placing a work-seeker into a role in the UK. As an employer you need to be aware of these. More details can be found in a guide published by the Employment Agency Standards Inspectorate (HM Government, 2020).

Disclosure and barring service checks

The Disclosure and Barring Service (DBS) helps employers make safer decisions regarding recruitment and prevents unsuitable people from working with vulnerable groups, including children. It acts as a central access point for criminal records checks for all those applying to work with children and young people.

Confirming identity and seeking references

Identity fraud in the UK grows year on year. When recruiting staff you must ensure that the person you are offering the job to is who they say they are. In June 2022, the government published guidance entitled 'How to prove and verify someone's identity' (Cabinet Office, 2023).

After a job is offered, you may wish to check references for the potential new employee to ensure that they have not given misleading statements about their character and experience. You should not seek references before an interview as you may be influenced by them, which could result in unfair discrimination. Unconscious bias and prejudgement might lead you to read a reference and, in so doing, favour somebody who has a similar background to you or who shares the same interests and beliefs.

The most common form of reference is a written reference. A basic reference will provide a short summary of the person's employment such as their job title and the dates they were employed. A more detailed reference might include information about skills and experience, strengths and weaknesses and how often the person had time off.

One way to speed up the process of getting a written reference is to provide a template; this will ensure that you receive the details that are most important for your setting. You could also ask for a telephone reference, but this may be inconvenient to organise, and you will need to ask the right questions to elicit the information you need.

Evidence opportunity

2.1 Seeking references

Consider your applicant process and explain how legislation and subsequent policy has affected the way in which you practice in this area.

How has equality legislation affected the process of seeking references and monitoring applications?

Will you need to make changes to the process you currently use? If yes, how will you ensure that it is a fair and non-discriminatory process?

AC 2.2 Describe potential challenges for safe and fair recruitment

Here, you will describe the challenges in recruitment and investigate the ways in which you can recruit fairly and safely.

The challenges for safe and fair recruitment start with the recruitment and retention challenge in the care sector. According to Skills for Care annual report 'The state of the adult social care sector and workforce in England' published in October 2022, the number of vacant posts increased by 52 per cent during 2021–22 – the highest on record (Skills for Care, 2022b). This could lead to the recruitment of staff who are unsuitable for roles simply because there is a need to fill vacancies.

In an effort to address this challenge and to help with more innovative recruitment schemes Skills for Care has produced a guide entitled 'Safe and fair recruitment: A guide to employing people with convictions in social care' to help social care employers understand their legal rights and responsibilities when carrying out criminal record checks (Skills for Care, 2020). It aims to build confidence when looking at potential applicants, particularly those who may have had a criminal record or have been subject to allegations which might normally disbar them from working in care roles. The guide highlights how to carry out effective risk assessments on such applicants so that employers can make more informed decisions about their suitability for the role.

Research it

2.2 Criminal record checks

Download 'Safe and fair recruitment: A guide to employing people with convictions in social care' from Skills for Care (2020). Read section 5 'Criminal record checks'. Check your own practice against the information given in the guide.

AC 2.3 Evaluate approaches which improve recruitment and retention of staff in adult care

Here, you will be required to evaluate a range of approaches for retention and recruitment of staff. This includes formal training routes, local recruitment drives and social media.

Recruiting people with the right values and behaviours

Values are the guiding principles by which we live our lives, and they develop from our upbringing and the social contexts we find ourselves in.

Measuring and assessing those values can be difficult though. We may not have a clear idea about our own values so self-reporting is not a useful way to determine these and we may not act on our values.

It is crucial that you develop your workforce to ensure that you attract the right staff and, more importantly, retain them. The recruitment process can be costly so if you find that there is a high staff turnover in your setting, you will need to find out why staff are not staying. It may be that you are recruiting staff who do not share the same values as you or the setting.

For an employer, having staff who believe in the same values means they are working towards the same goals. Individuals using the service will then have a consistent experience at your setting.

Designing a values-based recruitment approach will help to recruit staff who measure up to the organisation values. By determining what 'good' looks like in the role and what behaviours you want to see, you will develop a good analysis of the job role.

By working through each of the setting's values and identifying behaviours for each, your recruitment process can then measure and assess candidates for those behaviours. Asking questions that determine why the candidate behaved in a certain way will give a lot of information about the values that underpin the behaviour. For example, a care worker may talk about the importance of communication care work. By asking them 'why' that is important rather than 'how they did it', you are more likely to understand their value system. It is also common practice now to involve individuals using the service in the recruitment process to identify what sort of care workers they would be happy to have in the setting.

Understanding the local area to inform organisation planning

Recruitment plans make the recruitment process smooth and help employers to ensure that they are recruiting staff with the qualifications and skills needed to do the job.

A recruitment plan is a strategy for hiring new staff and follows a number of steps. Spending time setting up a recruitment plan will mean you will not miss any strategic steps in the recruitment process. For example, when you identify that a new vacancy exists it is good to understand exactly what the role requires before you start to source potential candidates through job adverts. The next stages require a screening of the application forms to prepare a shortlist prior to interview and eventually making a job offer. Devising your recruitment plan means coming up with a strategy around these core steps that will improve recruitment. By covering each step above in a methodical manner you will be able to source the right person for the role.

A workforce plan differs from a recruitment plan in that it helps you to assess your current and future staff requirements, but also looks at the local area and what it has to offer. Workforce planning encourages settings to conduct regular assessments of their staff to ensure that their workforce is future proofed against changes that may happen as a result of external forces. By assessing skills gaps, training and development needs, the effectiveness of your workforce is assured.

To help inform your decisions you might access the Adult Social Care Workforce Data Set (ASC-WDS), an online data collection service that gathers information about the adult social care workforce in England. Doing so will help you identify local labour market information and how your turnover compares to other providers.

Research it

2.3 ASC-WDS

Create an ASC-WDS account. This will help you to manage staff training needs and give you access to the Workforce Development Fund. (See Skills for Care, n.d. a.)

Innovative strategies to attract candidates in the local community

With so many jobs vacant in the care sector, innovative messages to candidates could inspire them to come to your settings. You can be more innovative in your marketing by using your values to attract people. Find out why people love to work for you and use that in your recruitment adverts. How do you stand out from other places to work? What is your unique selling point? Maybe you value work–family balance and can offer shifts that are family friendly. What can you offer in terms of benefits? If the salary offered is a standard one and cannot be more competitive then you may need to think about additional leverage to get people to work for you.

The most dynamic organisations offer additional benefits to their staff. Could you offer flexible working hours or options to buy shares in the company? Could there be child care facilities at reduced rates or a bike-to-work scheme or a gym subscription? Be creative in what you might offer staff who come to work for you.

You could develop a referral system to recruit staff. This involves incentivising current staff to refer a candidate to you in return for a financial reward. You then stand to gain a member of staff who already has the values you require and the process of hiring them could be reduced in time and cost.

One useful method of recruitment is through a recruitment drive where people are invited to an open day. Using local newspapers and social media such as Facebook, Twitter and emails, such events and vacancies can be quickly advertised to a great number of potential recruits.

Some organisations advertise one-day events with a promise of a potential job at the end of that day. This works when there are many posts on offer and can be a useful way of getting staff into the organisation. During the day, the applicants are interviewed and given an initial induction to the organisation which outlines its values and attitudes and what it is looking for in staff members. Applicants can undertake any tests that may need to be completed, have paperwork and certificates checked and are then given a conditional offer of a role at the end of the day. For the candidates, such a day will highlight to them very quickly whether they would feel comfortable working in the organisation and they can then decide for themselves whether to accept the role.

Reflect on it

2.3 Innovative strategies to attract staff

Think about how your setting currently attracts staff. Is there a different way you might try?

What alternative benefits might you be able to offer new staff?

Offering a supportive induction

An attractive induction package where staff can get support to step into the role quickly, together with a clear route to career progression and an offer of training, is a useful device for recruitment and retention.

The offer to fund staff to undertake training, such as the Care Certificate, Level 2, 3, 4 and 5 Diploma qualifications, or, for more qualified staff, foundation degrees or management training will be a good starting point for candidates.

Training enables staff to enhance and develop their skill set by gaining new skills, offering them opportunities to grow in their role, as well as to develop their career. As a manager, you will need to ensure that there are such opportunities for your staff, so that they remain motivated and driven in their roles, and also to meet legal requirements.

Staff recruitment advertising

Social media

Social media can be an efficient way to advertise for staff. By asking people to share advertisements on social media, you can contact thousands of potential candidates. Social media is also a good way to engage employees and make them feel that they are part of a team, as you can share information that they may not always be aware of. Some teams set up closed Facebook groups where messages and posts can only be seen by the team. In that way, social events, requests for information and news can be shared. Email is another way to reach many potential candidates quickly.

Job advertisements, recruitment agencies and job centres

These are also useful for recruiting staff. Local job centres serve the local community and recruitment agencies may be able to widen your search for staff outside the local area.

Analysing and overcoming factors that impact recruitment and retention

In an adult care setting, a 2018 survey showed a shortfall of social care workers, with seven in ten people commenting that a care career is undervalued by society and more than two in ten believing that care work is not valued by the government (Anchor, 2018).

Suggestions for recruiting and retaining staff include a public awareness campaign to raise the profile of social care work and a call for the government to demonstrate how it values social care work.

Both internal factors – such as budget, size of organisation, whether it plans to expand and grow and the recruitment policy – and external factors affect recruitment, although external factors, which we discuss below, are more difficult to control. However, as mentioned in the example of the 'golden handshake', external factors can have positive outcomes.

Location may be an issue, requiring people to travel a greater distance to get to work. There may also be fewer people in the area to choose from or perhaps your organisation has a poor reputation in the area (deserved or not), which will put people off applying. You may also be in an area where there are a number of competitors who are also recruiting from perhaps a diminished workforce in the area. Overcoming such factors can be difficult.

As a manager, you face a number of challenges in recruitment and the external factors affecting your service need to be addressed. For example, if your recruitment package offered the opportunity for further training, then you need to deliver on this, even if budgetary demands sometimes make this a challenge. You must be clear on your offer to potential staff and a compromise may be needed.

Research it

2.3 Factors affecting recruitment and retention of staff

What are the factors that impact recruitment and retention in your own area? How easy it is for you to recruit to your setting?

Reflect on it

2.3 Your own role

What was it that attracted you to your current job role and why have you stayed?

Make a list of some of the reasons that made you apply to your organisation.

AC 2.4 Explain processes in own setting/service

Here, you will explain how the values of your setting are reflected in the recruitment process.

Values-based recruitment

In AC2.3 you looked at recruiting people with the right values and behaviours and how value-based recruitment is a good way to engage with this. Look back at this section if you need to remind yourself before attempting the following activity.

Reflect on it

2.4 Values-based recruitment

Think about the formal values framework for your setting as outlined in the mission, vision and values statement(s).

What roles are you are recruiting for and how are the values relevant to that role?

What values do your high performing staff display and what are their guiding principles? How do they put them into action? Explore their behaviour and find out what principles were behind the decisions they made. For example, you might ask your staff why they felt it was important to help an individual put on her makeup every morning. They might believe that it is about dignity and respect and from there you can start to identify the underlying values beneath the behaviour.

Selection and induction

For more on the selection and induction processes, see AC2.5 below.

Managing staff absence

Managing staff absence needs to be fair and non-discriminatory and should involve supporting employees with health problems to stay in or return to work.

Sickness absence is inevitable and developing policies and procedures to deal with sickness absence is a positive move. Standards of attendance should be clearly set out and employees can be provided with information on any terms and conditions relating to incapacity for work.

For long-term sickness you can seek further information about the employee's absence and obtain a medical report if appropriate.

Employers should investigate the nature, extent and likely duration of an employee's illness. For absences of a week or less you might ask for a self-certification form, while for absences of more than seven days, you should ask for a Statement of Fitness for Work ('fit note').

Maintaining contact with an employee may include emails, telephone calls and meetings. It is important, however, not to be overbearing or intrusive in this contact.

Return-to-work interviews are effective tools for managing short-term sickness and should always take place as they provide line managers with an opportunity to chat with staff about any underlying issues which might be causing the absence.

AC 2.5 Explain own role in setting/service for recruitment, selection and induction

Here, you will be required to explain the recruitment, selection and induction processes within your own service provision.

Recruiting and retaining staff

While an increase in salary may be a factor in applying for a role, that might not be the only reason people apply for the roles and jobs they do. Perhaps it is the reputation of the setting for its fair dealings with people or the fact that it also offers **continuing professional development (CPD)** opportunities (opportunities to develop) or a career progression route. When you applied for your own role, for example, you might have been impressed with the way in which the setting delivered the care or maybe it was the atmosphere of the place or the values and ethos declared in the mission statement.

KEY TERM

Continuing professional development (CPD): The planned process of improving and increasing capabilities of staff. It is an ongoing process and includes training and education activities to ensure that staff remain fit to practise.

The staff you wish to recruit will also have a number of reasons for applying for a new role. The recruitment and selection process, therefore, must be one that attracts candidates with the appropriate skills, values and attitudes for the role you wish them to do. They need to be able to fit well into the team and its culture and to deliver the sort of care that gives the best quality to those who use the service.

At the same time, you need to think about how you will retain staff once they are recruited. An unhappy person will leave the job very quickly or be demotivated and therefore unlikely to perform to the best of their ability, so you need to ensure that you have a retention strategy in place. Methods of keeping staff happy could include the following:

- Formal training routes and career development.
- Good terms and conditions so that potential new staff are likely to want to work for you rather than a competitor.
- Benefits such as family-friendly hours or maybe crèche facilities for staff with children.
- A benefits scheme may make your organisation a more attractive place to work.

The selection process

When you have a post to fill, the outcome you want is to find the right person for the job. That person must not only have the skills to do the job but must be committed to the team and the organisation and share the same values and attitudes.

The selection process is your opportunity to collect evidence about the candidate and to identify their strengths and weaknesses. This process is helped by having documents in place such as a job description, which shows the key tasks and responsibilities of the job, and a person specification, which sets out the characteristics needed for the role, clearly described in terms of competencies that can be measured.

At the point of interview, it is most important that all candidates are offered the same opportunities to present themselves. A consistent approach to interview must be followed, with pre-determined questions that clearly enable candidates to give information about themselves. This will enable the interview panel to assess an individual's strengths and potential weaknesses.

Skills for Care documents and guidance

You may find it useful to refer to the Skills for Care blog, 'What is values-based recruitment?' (Skills for Care, 2021b). This document mentions recruiting people for their values and behaviours to ensure that the right people are attracted to a setting. People who are committed to high-quality care and who have strong values are more likely to be retained in the workplace.

The Skills for Care website provides a wealth of information regarding recruitment and retention of staff, including reports, toolkits, case studies and free online workshops, as well as a resources library to help you deal with some of the most common issues regarding recruitment and retention. See Skills for Care (n.d. d).

Induction

Induction is the opportunity for new staff to become familiar with their new role and working environment. Every organisation should invest in a well-considered induction programme, which should not be just a tick-box exercise of reading policies and signing to say they have done so. It should provide information that new staff need and should be conducted in a way that does not overwhelm them.

Each care worker starting in a new role can be enrolled on the Care Certificate or a tailored training course more applicable to the setting. Employers must provide an induction programme to introduce and meet the essential standards set out by the Care Quality Commission. The Care Certificate has been developed jointly by Skills for Care, Health Education England and Skills for Health. This course provides training that focuses on the specific skills, knowledge and behaviours expected of those working in the social care sector.

The whole induction process can involve orientation to the site on which they are to work, introductions to the team and maybe external partners, and information about relevant policies. This might be covered in a day or over a period of time. The member of staff may be required to complete paperwork that specifies what they have learned, and this provides you as their manager with an audit trail.

If you are a manager in a small organisation, you might be responsible for setting up the recruitment process from start to finish and might, therefore, wish to delegate some tasks to team members. In a larger organisation, you may well work alongside the HR team.

Research it

2.5 Care Certificate

Go to the Skills for Care website (Skills for Care, n.d. c) and look at the information about the Care Certificate.

How might you be able to use these suggestions to enhance your current recruitment strategies?

Evidence opportunity

2.5 Recruitment, selection and induction processes

Explain to your assessor your role in recruitment, selection and induction processes within your own service provision. You might like to:

- ✔ explain the approaches for retention and recruitment of staff in your organisation and identify areas that might present a challenge to the process. What are the strengths and weaknesses of this approach?
- ✔ explain how the recruitment, selection and induction processes within your own service provision might be changed. Highlight the effective or positive parts of the process and the parts you believe require change and why.

AC 2.6 Explain the importance of ensuring employment practices are free from discrimination and harassment

Here, you will be required to explain the importance of ensuring all employment practices are free from discrimination and harassment in line with current legislation, and own policies and procedures.

The issue of workplace **discrimination** and **harassment** is a topic that has been highlighted in the media in recent years, with issues surrounding equal pay also being discussed. Discrimination on the basis of race and religion has also been a prominent issue. As a manager, you will need to ensure that your setting provides an environment that promotes inclusion and diversity, where discrimination and harassment are not acceptable, and everyone understands the importance of respecting each other. You should ensure that policies and procedures are in place and that everyone is aware of them, and be prepared to deal with any instances of discrimination and harassment if they do occur.

KEY TERMS

Discrimination: Treating people unfairly or unlawfully because they have a disability, or are of a different race, gender or age, for example.

Harassment: Unwanted behaviour towards another person that is designed to intimidate or degrade.

The recruitment and selection process must be a fair one and you are legally responsible for ensuring that no unlawful discrimination on the grounds of sex, age, race, disability, sexual orientation, religion or belief occurs. You must also be careful not to use language that might offend or humiliate somebody as this might be construed as harassment. This also applies to employment practices more generally, as staff must be able to perform their roles without fear of discrimination and harassment, be offered equal opportunities and be judged based on their performance rather than on characteristics such as their race and religion.

Equality of opportunity is a major part of the recruitment and selection process. It is, therefore, acceptable for you to advertise for applications from those groups that are under-represented in the organisation as well as those that are not. For example, your workforce may be underrepresented in people with protected characteristics (such as those of a different race or religion) and if you are trying to address this you may choose a candidate who has a protected characteristic over one who does not.

The laws that apply to recruitment and selection are as follows.

Equality Act 2010

The Equality Act outlines what is needed to make the workplace a fair environment. It offers protection to individuals regardless of age, disability, gender, gender reassignment, race, religion or belief, sexual orientation, marriage and civil partnership and pregnancy and maternity. The Equality and Human Rights Commission (EHRC) offers guidance for employers regarding changes to recruitment, in particular in relation to questions about health and disability, and you might wish to look at these to remind yourself of this.

The Equality Act 2010 calls for people to be treated with dignity, which cannot happen where harassment and discrimination occurs.

Employment Rights Act 1996

The Employment Rights Act (ERA) 1996 updated the Contracts of Employment Act 1963, the Redundancy Payments Act 1965, the Employment Protection Act 1975 and the Wages Act 1986.

This Act addresses issues such as dismissal, unfair dismissal, parental leave, redundancy, the rights of employees and the right to request flexible working time. Additionally, the Act deals with employees' rights to a contract, suspension, the notice period that needs to be given when leaving and employer insolvency issues.

Own policies and procedures

Your organisation will have its own policies and procedures for ensuring fairness during the recruitment and selection process. As the manager, you are duty bound to ensure that all employment practices are free from discrimination and harassment.

Your policies may include recruitment and selection, bullying and harassment, anti-discrimination, equality, code of conduct, dignity and respect, whistle blowing and Disclosure and Barring Service (DBS), all of which cover the need for staff to be clear about how they should work in an anti-discriminatory manner.

Staff need to be aware of how they should conduct themselves in the workplace and how they should report any infringements with respect to harassment or discrimination. Treating people with dignity and respect should be a major part of your team values.

Below is a list of other acts that may be covered in your own documentation.

- Rehabilitation of Offenders Act 1974
- Equality Act 2010
- Data Protection Act 2018
- National Minimum Wage Act 1998
- Employment Relations Act 1999
- Agency Workers Regulations 2010
- Safeguarding Vulnerable Groups Act 2006
- Immigration, Asylum and Nationality Act 2006
- Health and Safety at Work Act 1974
- Working Time Regulations (1998) and The Working Time (Amendment) Regulations 2007
- Part-Time Workers (Prevention of Less Favourable Treatment) Regulations 2000
- Flexible Working Regulations 2014
- Health and Social Care Act 2008

Research it

2.6 Employment law

Employment law changes rapidly and often. To keep abreast of these changes, go to the Chartered Institute of Personnel and Development (CIPD) website (see CIPD, n.d.).

Changing care and support needs of individuals

Providing every individual with person-centred care, whatever that might entail, should be every care giver's goal and discrimination due to changes in treatment or support must not be tolerated.

Section 1 of the Care Act 2014 says, 'The general duty of a local authority, in exercising a function under this Part in the case of an individual, is to promote that individual's wellbeing.' Promoting wellbeing means actively seeking improvements when carrying out care and support for individuals.

Everyone's needs are different and specific to them. They will also change over time, so care providers must consider how to meet each person's specific needs rather than simply considering what service they will fit into. They need to recognise that discrimination might occur as seen in the following case study.

Case study

You have observed a member of staff criticising co-workers, and occasionally shaming and insulting them. Sometimes the language is sexist, racist or homophobic, but is referred to as 'banter'. This is clearly a case of bullying behaviour. How will you make clear to the worker that this is unacceptable, in order to ensure that the workplace is free of harassment and discrimination?

Increases/decreases in demand for support services

As demand for services increases there is a potential for **unconscious bias** to occur and for services to be apportioned in potentially discriminatory ways. We may stereotype people unfairly without being aware we are doing so. Such bias may be based on our past experiences and affect how we think. For example, age discrimination is based on a belief that older employees are not going to be as competent as younger employees and may arise out of the belief that age is related to work ability or skill.

KEY TERM

Unconscious bias: Holding unfavourable or unreasonable beliefs and views about other people that are outside our conscious awareness and control.

The Equality Act 2010 prohibits unlawful discrimination in the provision of services on the grounds of 'protected characteristics' (see AC2.1). Under the Health and Social Care Act 2012, adult care settings are required to reduce inequalities between individuals with respect to their ability to access support services.

The local authority has a duty to ensure that organisations must comply with equalities law with respect to the diverse needs of the individuals they serve. They must minimise disadvantage and ensure that under-represented groups are included in decision making and are supported.

Holiday/festive periods

Holidays and festive periods are open to discriminatory practices by employers. Employers need to be aware that not all staff celebrate Christmas, and some staff may wish to celebrate different religious festivals.

Indirect discrimination would occur if one employee is paid overtime for working at Christmas, a traditional religious holiday, but another employee was not paid extra for working during their own religious holiday.

Claims of discrimination are uncommon but a sensible approach to holiday planning and days off at festive times and being reasonable to staff will ensure safe practice.

Sickness

For information on staff sickness, refer to the section on staff absence in AC2.4 of this unit.

> **Research it**
>
> **2.6 Discrimination in the workplace**
>
> Conduct some research online around discrimination in the workplace.
>
> How can you make sure that such discrimination is not an issue in your workplace? Discuss this with a colleague and provide a written account of your discussion.

> **Evidence opportunity**
>
> **2.6 Employment practices that are free from discrimination and harassment**
>
> Provide a written account explaining the importance of ensuring all employment practices are free from discrimination and harassment in line with current legislation, including the legislation covered above. How do you ensure this through your setting's policies and procedures?
>
> You might show copies of your policies to your assessor.

AC 2.7 Describe how to identify the numbers and patterns of staffing required to provide a person-centred, outcomes-based service

Here, you will be required to describe processes that are used in your own setting to ensure effective staffing numbers and patterns and how these ensure that the services are providing person-centred, outcomes-focused care; this includes continuity of care and support, importance of flexibility, varying skills sets, identification of and adaptation to changes, use and management of agency workers.

Impacts of funding

The media constantly remind us about how funding deficits have affected the social care system.

In social care, a funding crisis persists. According to NHS Digital (2022b), local authorities spent £22 billion on adult social care in 2021–22, which was an increase of £0.7 billion from 2020. The findings of the 2021–22 report also show that £16.6 billion or (75.4%) of the total expenditure went on long-term support. Additionally, there were almost 2 million requests for adult social care support from nearly 1.4 million new individuals received by local authorities in 2021–22, which represents an equivalent of 5,420 requests per day in England, up by 170 requests per day on the previous year. Although the number of people receiving long-term care has decreased to 818,000, this continues a downward trend which has been mainly driven by a decrease in those aged 65 and over, as well as the continued impact of the COVID-19 pandemic.

To manage these deficits in funding, local authorities reduce spending by targeting staffing costs, reducing services, cutting back on environmental and regulatory services such as waste disposal, and introducing efficiency measures.

Decisions about which services and treatments will be provided (known as 'rationing') are largely made by the local authorities but may also be made at a national level by local commissioners and providers, and by individual clinicians. Some decisions are made because of law or policy, but others may be based on individual judgements and a range of factors including national policy initiatives, clinical guidelines, local priorities and needs, what has been provided in the past, individual clinical judgements and conversations with the people using the services.

Your role as a manager is to effectively manage the impacts that funding can have and maintain an effective workforce with a variety of skills to ensure that the services provided are person-centred and outcome focused. Staff need to be clear about the importance of continuity of care and support.

Continuity of care and support

You will need to use the budget available to ensure that person-centred and **outcomes-focused care** is not disrupted. This can be managed by looking at the staff you need, the staff you have, and how flexible you are in delivering the current services you have.

Varying skill sets and importance of flexibility

A skill set is a particular group of skills or abilities to perform a role. A qualified nurse in your employment will offer different skills to an adult care assistant and the administration staff will also have a different set of skills to perform their tasks.

The recruitment process and the need for person specifications to show the skills required for a role was discussed in AC2.2. For example, if a position requires somebody with excellent computer or communication skills, then the person specification needs to highlight these as part of the required skill set. Of course, a person who can be flexible and shows willingness to develop skills beyond those required in their role will improve their chance of employment.

Identification of and adaptation to changes

As job roles evolve, staff need to adapt to the changes that become evident. An individual may come into your care with complex needs that require a different approach. The individual's care and support needs may have changed either because they have developed independence and therefore require a reduced support package, or conversely they may need additional support due to a change in their complex needs. Staff training, therefore, becomes important and there may be funding issues around this. As the manager, you must identify the changes that are needed to sustain the service and determine the means to adapt to the change.

Use and management of agency workers

The use of agency staff is a huge expense but a necessary one. To control your budget and to ensure that the skill mix is sufficient for each shift, you may have to employ agency workers. It is useful to develop a good relationship with the agency staff who fit the team profile well and who are valued by other staff in the team. For example, you may require nursing staff and therefore need to contact agencies to fill the shortfall in your team on a temporary basis. Agency staff will still require managing and you need to be very clear about what they can and cannot do in the workplace. An agency will supply you with a clear idea about the roles the staff can undertake and the competency level of each individual. You should provide a short induction to orientate the member of staff to the work setting.

KEY TERM

Outcomes-focused care: An outcomes-based approach is similar to person-centred care in that people should be at the centre of their own care and support planning. By identifying what is important to their lives, and ensuring that the person's independence and quality of life is maximised, everyone involved in the support works together, actively listening to the person without judgement. This differs from the task-based approach, which concentrated on meeting task targets. This was previously common but is gradually being replaced.

Research it

2.7 The King's Fund

In August 2022, The King's Fund published a paper, 'Building capacity and capability for improvement in adult social care', which looks at how local authorities are improving the quality of adult social care (The King's Fund, 2022). With the government intention to increase funding for improvement activities to reform adult social care and plans to introduce a new Care Quality Commission (CQC) assurance framework to assess local authority performance in delivering all their adult social care functions, this is a most timely report.

Download the report and look at the four actions identified in section 3:

1. Prioritising areas for improvement.
2. Exploring and understanding these areas for improvement.
3. Implementing change – testing and embedding solutions.
4. Demonstrating (measuring) impact.

Make notes on how your own setting can make some of the changes, for example:

- What changes will you prioritise?
- Why is this an area for improvement for you?
- How will you make the change?
- How will you know if you are successful?

Evidence opportunity

2.7 Processes to identify the numbers and patterns of staffing required

Provide a written account describing the processes used in your setting to ensure effective staffing numbers and patterns and how these ensure that the services provide a person-centred, outcome-focused care. You could, for example, consider:

- ✔ impacts of funding
- ✔ continuity of care and support
- ✔ importance of flexibility
- ✔ varying skill sets
- ✔ identification of and adaptation to changes
- ✔ use and management of agency workers.

AC 2.8 Analyse factors that could influence staffing requirements and patterns

Here, you will analyse the factors that will affect staffing requirements and availability.

A number of factors that are external to the setting can affect staffing levels. As previously mentioned, the use of technology in care work has increased and your setting may now require staff to have technology training. If there is a shortage of candidates with these skills, then staffing numbers will be impacted.

Care career pathways require education and qualifications to prepare for work in the field. You may offer training programmes for unqualified staff, but you will also require trained care workers. If the number of people pursuing work in the care sector decreases, the talent pool from which you can select staff from shrinks.

Government regulations may also impact an organisation's staffing process, because laws regarding recruitment, compensation, working hours, health insurance and qualifications are sometimes difficult to navigate, while failure to uphold the law may result in fines.

Evidence opportunity

2.8 Influence of job market on staffing patterns

How might your own staffing patterns be influenced by factors affecting the job market? How can you future proof your own setting?

Write a short report analysing the potential issues that may arise.

AC 2.9 Explain how to manage staffing patterns and adjust them to meet changing circumstances

Here, you will explain how to manage staffing patterns and how to adjust them to meet changing circumstances.

There are a range of circumstances where staffing patterns will need to be adjusted and these are outlined here.

Short-, medium- and long-term, and emergency cover

Staffing for care delivery in any setting may be subject to short-, medium- and long-term changes. In the short term, you may need to cover staff who are attending a day-release course which will mean cover for one day each week. Staff sickness and maternity leave may result in medium- and long-term changes that must be covered, although this type of cover can usually be planned for in advance. Occasionally an emergency may occur, and this might be when agency cover is the only option available. You will need to think about the following aspects.

Type and number of staff required

Your role as manager is to ensure that circumstances such as those described above are planned for with the correct number of staff and the correct skill set. You may have established that each shift requires a qualified nurse to oversee medications. If one of your qualified staff is to be absent for a long time, then you will need to look at the number of staff that have such skills to determine how this might be covered.

According to the Health and Social Care Act 2008 (Regulated Activities) Regulations 2014 and the Care Standards, employers are required to provide sufficient numbers of suitably qualified, competent, skilled and experienced staff to meet the needs of the people using the service at all times. Your staff must be supported and provided with training, professional development and supervision.

When planning staffing, you should remind yourself of the CQC's Key Lines of Enquiry (KLOEs) regarding the standards required for a care provider (see Unit 500, AC3.1).

Impact on other resources such as training and equipment

Staff absences for any length of time may require you to address the training and equipment budget. A budget that has not planned for contingencies, such as staff absence, may mean cuts to training for staff and this is short sighted. Your responsibility is to ensure that staff absence does not mean training needs are cancelled so plans must reflect this.

Managing staffing requests for changes to established working patterns

Managers who are flexible and open to different ways of working will get the best out of their staff. Your shifts may be eight hours in length, but some staff may be open to working 12-hour shifts in order to get more days off. Staff with children may wish to work within school hours only. If you can accommodate such requests, you will have a workforce who not only are happier but whose motivation will improve.

Staffing levels

Regulation 18 of the Health and Social Care Act 2008 (Regulated Activities) Regulations 2014 states:

> *... providers must provide sufficient numbers of suitably qualified, competent, skilled and experienced staff to meet the needs of the people using the service at all times ... Staff must receive the support, training, professional development, supervision and appraisals for them to carry out their role and responsibilities. They should be supported to obtain further qualifications and provide evidence, where required, to the appropriate regular to show that they meet the professional standards needed to continue to practise.*

Source: Health and Social Care Act 2008 (Regulated Activities) Regulations 2014: Regulation 18

The Regulation does not, however, indicate what safe staffing levels are or should be. Staffing levels need to be determined based on the needs of the individuals using the service, taking into account the nature of the premises and staff training requirements. You need also to look at the skills of the staff.

Evidence opportunity

2.9 Manage and adjust staffing patterns

Explain to your assessor how you manage staffing patterns and adjust them to meet changing circumstances. Remember to consider the range of circumstances where staffing patterns will need to be adjusted:

- ✔ short term
- ✔ medium term
- ✔ long term
- ✔ emergency cover
- ✔ type of staff and number of staff required
- ✔ impact on other resources such as training and equipment
- ✔ managing staffing requests for changes to established working patterns.

Reflect on the methods you have used to overcome funding cuts, skill mix issues and supply of staff to roles. You can do this by first describing what you did and then commenting upon the effects of your actions. What went well and what needs to change?

Reflective exemplar

I have just compiled my first report which shows my resource planning forecast for the coming year and details the financial, physical and human resources. Not an easy task! I understand the principles of effective resource management and managed to collect the data from last year's report which has helped me to forecast what I will need in terms of staffing and physical resources next year, but the financial part is a little more tricky, particularly as my manager has informed me that my budget is not likely to exceed that which I had this year. This has concerned me greatly as I know we are in need of new furniture for the communal areas and if we spend on this, then it is likely that we will have to make some cuts in another area. I am worried that we may have to lose a member of staff to cover this. Although I have learned a great deal in undertaking this exercise, I now realise that it has opened up a whole new area of potential conflict. But it has also focused my mind on what I need to do next and that is to prepare an argument for an increase in funding to ensure that all staff are safe, that redundancies are not an option and to inform staff that we will need to make some budget cuts elsewhere. I intend to ask them to help me to decide what is best to do.

AC 2.10 Evaluate workforce succession and contingency planning in own adult care setting/service

Here, you will prepare a contingency plan for adverse circumstances and plan for future events where team members may leave the setting.

A contingency plan (covered previously in AC1.4) considers all possible future events or circumstances that may affect the organisation adversely. A succession plan is created for when some staff are planning to leave the setting, for example because they are retiring.

If you are lucky, you will know in advance that an experienced and able team member is going to leave because they have notified you of their intention to retire. However, somebody who leaves as a result of a sudden decision may be a cause for concern in terms of ensuring the required level of skills in a team.

Consider all the key staff roles on your team. Think about each role in turn and what effect it would have on the team if that individual was no longer working in the setting. What would be the impact of the vacant position on the setting and how would that affect operations?

You might be able to choose from other team members who could potentially step into a vacant position and so you should consider which employees would be the strongest candidates should the need arise. There may be an obvious choice for a role, but other promising staff may display the skills necessary for a higher position, regardless of their current position.

Your next step would be to notify those members of staff that you feel might potentially be able to step up to a future vacant role and to put in place professional development to help them develop the skills required. You could enable this newly trained person to step into the role to provide cover for annual leave and sickness to enable them to get used to the demands of this new role.

Once you have identified potential successors for critical roles in your organisation from your existing pool of employees, you can then recruit to fill their roles.

Reflect on it

2.10 Preparing potential successors

If you decide to move to another job or retire, which employee could step into your shoes? How could you help that person prepare for the transition?

AC 2.11 Describe performance management systems and relevance to own setting/service and role

Here, you will describe your own performance management system and identify changes that you might make to the system.

Performance management will help your setting to achieve its aims and objectives by monitoring and improving the performance of the staff.

Using agreed targets and objectives or **key performance indicators (KPIs)** will enable line managers to measure and review performance. This will clearly indicate whether the staff and the activities they undertake contribute to the achievement of organisation goals.

For example, you may want a member of staff to undertake a training course by a certain date and this will be measured by the completion of the course.

KPIs express what you want your staff to achieve and when and help to assess and manage employee performance.

If current levels of performance are insufficient, the introduction of KPIs can help employees to become more productive and develop their skills. The setting can help by improving its processes and procedures. An effective performance management system requires reviews to be conducted with the setting's overall strategic plan in mind to ensure the achievement of the goals that have been set.

Performance management best practices involve:

- understanding current practice and being able to clearly identify intended practice
- agreeing targets to meet organisational goals
- measuring and monitoring changes made, improvements and progress towards goals
- reviewing progress, renewing goals and moving forward.

KEY TERM

Key performance indicator (KPI): A way to measure performance over time for a specific objective or target. KPIs state what must be achieved and when and can be used to assess and manage performance.

Evidence opportunity

2.11 Performance management

Describe the performance management system you use in your own setting and write a short piece on its effectiveness. How is your performance managed? If you were in charge of managing your performance, how might you implement some changes to improve this?

AC 2.12 Describe conduct, discipline and grievance procedures, and relevance to own setting/service and own role

Here, you will describe your setting's disciplinary and grievance procedures and how they are used.

Addressing conduct and performance issues with individuals

In order to be constructive about performance issues, there must be a valid set of measures that can support your judgement. Having a good performance management system in place will give you the confidence to show that an individual's performance is not up to standard. You can then set up a performance review where you meet the member of staff to address the situation and help them improve their performance. Be aware that the employee is likely to feel under threat at such an interview, so you need to approach this with care. Finding out what is causing the poor performance is a useful starting point in this meeting, and a copy of the employee's job description will be needed here. By looking again at the standard of work expected from the employee, you may be able to identify what the problem is and can then work towards remedying this.

Some reasons for poor performance are that the employee is unclear about their role, job description or what it is they are trying to achieve. They may feel they lack training or are having some personal issues that are causing them concern. It may simply be that the employee is not suited to care work. By discussing the reason in a calm and clear way, the employee's poor performance may be relatively easy to resolve.

Discipline and grievance procedures and the impact of a performance management system

The impact of an effective performance management system is successful achievement of organisational goals and strategies and a healthy and reliable workforce. It helps to motivate and retain staff members and is useful in identifying top performers among staff, but also those who are struggling or simply not doing what they should be. One of the ways you can do this as a manager is to identify KPIs (see AC2.11).

With respect to disciplinary procedures, policies to support the staff need to be put into place, as well as a process for raising grievances at work. An approach that deals sensitively with conflict is a more humane approach to performance. If a member of staff is struggling with their work, then their competency and capability to do the job may be in question. In this instance, it is best not to go down the disciplinary route. The best course of action is to determine what the staff member needs to be able to function more efficiently; this may then reveal that further training will resolve the situation.

Feedback provided to staff and performance data collected will help you to see how well your organisation is achieving its objectives. For example, if you are aiming to achieve an 'outstanding' CQC grading and you have members of staff who underperform, the feedback you receive might lead you to re-evaluate staff members' roles and provide additional training. In doing so, the next review meeting may well show a marked increase in performance that clearly meets the objectives of the organisation.

Steps in a disciplinary procedure

Your disciplinary procedure should include the following steps:

- A letter to the member of staff setting out the reason or reasons why disciplinary action is being taken.
- A meeting to discuss the issue.
- A disciplinary decision or the outcome of the hearing which might be no action being taken, a verbal or written warning, a final warning, demotion or dismissal.
- A chance to appeal this decision.

For more information on disciplinary procedures, take a look at 'Disciplinary procedures and action against you at work' on the GOV.UK website (GOV.UK, n.d. a).

Reflect on it

2.12 Your organisation's disciplinary and grievance procedures

Obtain a copy of your organisation's disciplinary and grievance procedures and summarise the main points.

Identify the strengths and the weaknesses of the policies and provide a reflective account. You may like to consider the following when writing your account:

- Why do you need to have these policies in place?
- How do they protect the workforce and the employer?
- How have these policies been used in your workplace and what have the outcomes been?
- How have the policies been measured in the past? Are they linked to KPIs?

Evidence opportunity

2.12 Discipline and grievance policies

Describe the policies in your setting that cover conduct discipline and grievance. Provide evidence to show how staff are informed of these policies and how they are used.

LO3 Understand market provision in adult care

AC 3.1 Explain how adult care services are commissioned, procured and funded

In this section you will explain the ways in which services are commissioned and procured and ways in which they are funded at a national and local level.

Care services are commissioned, procured and funded in response to changes in government policy and economic and social context, including demography. There is now a greater emphasis on outcome-based joint commissioning and the involvement of the individual using the service.

Commissioning

Local authorities are responsible for social care and public health functions as well as other services for local people and organisations, while place-based partnerships lead on the design and delivery of integrated services. Local authorities are responsible for commissioning publicly funded social care services, which include services provided in residential care services and to people in their own homes.

Local authorities are also responsible for commissioning public health services, including sexual health services, health visitors, school nursing and addiction services.

Procurement

In 2021, the Department of Health and Social Care published its white paper, 'People at the Heart of Care: adult social care reform' (GOV.UK, 2022b). As part of these plans, the government set a cap for personal care of £86,000 (although this may change), as well as specific guidance on housing, technology and new models of care. This white paper sets out a ten-year vision for adult social care and provides information on funded proposals for the next three years. In particular, the section *'Providing the right care in the right place at the right time'* outlines measures to encourage local authorities to set out a strategic vision for housing-related care and support for older adults and disabled adults of working age, with the promise to invest at least £300 million over the next three years. Further changes include investing £150 million of additional funding over the next three years to drive digitisation across the sector and launching a £30 million Innovative Models of Care Programme to support local systems to build the culture and capability to embed innovative models of care.

Funding

Individuals using care services have to contribute to the cost of care. The amount they pay depends on the level of need and the amount of assets they currently have. Local councils are required to carry out a care needs assessment as well as a financial means test when assessing people for care:

- The assessment of needs helps to decide the level of care required and whether the person can stay at home with additional care or needs to enter residential care.
- The financial means test looks at the person's income, savings and property assets to determine how much the contribution towards the cost of care and support will be.

> **Evidence opportunity**
>
> **3.1 Funding of adult care services**
>
> Look at the local authority website for your area to see how they commission services. Undertake a professional discussion with your assessor and explain how the services have been commissioned, procured and funded.

AC 3.2 Analyse how current drivers are shaping market provision in adult care and funding mechanisms

Here, you will analyse factors and drivers that could influence growth and change in service delivery, and evaluate the impact that areas discussed in this section might have in respect of supporting an entrepreneurial and innovation culture within your service and related delivery.

Political drivers, regulation, local government initiatives and influence of the media

Political drivers are related to government policy, regulations and initiatives that affect change. New legislation or regulatory changes can have a major impact upon the way in which your organisation develops. A failure to heed such drivers may result in a failure of the actual setting or organisation.

The 2021 publication of the government's 'People at the heart of care: Adult social care reform' white paper sets out a ten-year vision for care and support in England and is based around three key objectives:

- That people have choice, control and support to live independent lives.
- They can access outstanding quality and tailored care and support.
- People find adult social care fair and accessible.

The measures set out in a further publication, the 2021 'Build back better: Our plan for health and social care', included a reform of the way that adult social care is funded and highlighted the proposals for a cap on care costs and more generous financial means-tested thresholds. It also called for the ability for self-funders to ask their council to arrange their care and to move to a fair rate of care in respect of councils' fees to providers. A new

Health and Social Care Levy to fund the changes was also announced.

One of the key drivers in recent years has been the need to improve quality provision in adult social care, with revelations of unacceptable treatment of individuals using care services. The media was a key driver for demanding change when it published reports of demeaning and cruel treatment of individuals with learning disabilities at Winterbourne View private hospital, and the abuse and neglect of people in The Morleigh Group of care homes in Cornwall. These tragic events have resulted in government inquiries being set up and reviews published to effect change within the sector. Some of these reviews are as follows:

- Cornwall and Isles of Scilly Safeguarding Adults Board: Safeguarding Adults Review (2019) The Morleigh Group of care homes
- 'Winterbourne View – time for change: Transforming the commissioning of services for people with learning disabilities and/or autism' (2014)
- 'The Cavendish Review: An independent review into healthcare assistants and support workers in the NHS and social care settings' (2013).

As a result of these reviews, new drivers to improve quality and transparency have been introduced.

As a manager, these factors, political drivers, regulations and local government initiatives all have an influence and impact upon service delivery, including the policies that govern your setting and the procedures you follow. The way in which you respond to this can be innovative and entrepreneurial if you develop a culture of empowerment and trust within your teams. By enabling workers to take ownership of decisions and developing cultures of trust and openness, employees are more likely to try to develop new ways of working that can lead to innovation and an entrepreneurial spirit.

Research it

3.2 Quality improvement in care

SCIE offers a free 'Quality improvement in health and social care' e-learning course.

This resource supports managers and staff working in adult social care with information about quality improvement and the associated tools that can be used within social care organisations.

Find out more about the resource and consider undertaking this free training. Discuss with your assessor how you could use some of the quality improvement tools in your setting.

Internal directorates, access to resources – human, physical

Internal directorates, mainly seen in large organisations, are responsible for the development of internal policies that match the political drivers.

For example, your team in the setting may be likened to an internal directorate and, as the manager, you are responsible for the way the budget is used, how the stock is ordered and monitored and how you staff the team. Actions you take in the way you manage the team must be justified at board level.

A team that is part of a larger organisation benefits from having access to resources from elsewhere in the setting and this can influence the way in which the service delivery is improved and quality raised. For example, a staff member seconded from a different area might bring new skills and ideas to the team, impacting the culture within the team. New ideas and innovation may come from sharing physical resources and applying them to the way in which the team works, changing service delivery.

Gaps in related services and funding and health inequalities

There is often a disparity between services offered in some parts of the country and this disparity leads to gaps in the market, which need to be addressed.

A number of factors impact social care. As the population changes, changing patterns affect complex care and health needs and also increase financial pressures. There is a move to include more community-based practices that breakdown traditional barriers and to address widening health inequalities.

Health inequalities have been an issue for many years and tackling them is a huge social issue. It is now well recognised that the place that a person is born and grows up in, as well as their place of residence as an adult, have a significant impact on their life chances and health. Other factors such as quality of education and subsequent jobs also impact health and wellbeing. These are referred to as 'wider determinants of health' and are often linked. For example, an unemployed person is more likely to live in poor quality housing, have less access to open spaces to exercise in and be less able to afford good quality food. This can lead to poor health.

Some groups in society are more likely to experience poorer health than the general population, including people living in areas of high deprivation, Black, Asian and minority ethnic communities and those from **inclusion health groups**. The reasons cited for this include:

- the availability of services in their local area and service opening times
- lack of access to transport or childcare

- poor levels of English language (spoken and written)
- poor literacy and numeracy skills
- previous experience of hardship
- misinformation
- fear.

KEY TERM

Inclusion health groups: People who are socially excluded and who often have overlapping risk factors, such as poverty, violence and complex trauma. They include people who experience homelessness, drug and alcohol dependence, vulnerable migrants, Gypsy, Roma and Traveller communities, sex workers, people in contact with the justice system and victims of modern slavery.

People who live in the poorest areas of the country are more likely to die on average seven years earlier than those who live in more affluent areas. This gap may be due to lack of services being offered in certain areas or due to other factors such as poor lifestyle choices or lack of education.

The CQC publication 'Our equality objectives 2021–2025' aims to ensure that everyone can access good quality care and equal access, experiences and outcomes from social care services. The CQC recognises the impact the COVID-19 pandemic has had on magnifying and exposing longstanding inequalities in social care. It does not set priorities for reducing inequalities itself and instead aims to work closely with other organisations to help reduce inequalities. Their five equality objectives are:

- Equality objective 1: Amplifying the voices of people most likely to have a poorer experience of care or have difficulty accessing care
- Equality objective 2: Using data to understand and respond to equality risks
- Equality objective 3: Working with others to improve equality of access, experience and outcomes
- Equality objective 4: Using our independent voice to reduce inequalities
- Equality objective 5: Our inclusive future: delivering on our diversity and inclusion strategy for our workforce

Source: Care Quality Commission (2022)

The National Healthcare Inequalities Improvement Programme was set up in January 2021 by NHS England to work with its other programmes and policies, as well as partners, people using the services and communities, to improve healthcare inequalities for those at greatest risk.

Stretch and challenge

3.2 Social care and health inequalities

Although not updated for ten years, SCIE offers useful information about inequality in social care arenas in the article 'Social care and health inequalities' (SCIE, 2013). Social workers and social care workers play key roles in reducing health inequalities and improving social outcomes in the communities in which they work.

Six key themes were identified in the Marmot Review (2010) as being significant to the task of reducing health inequalities. Two refer to children and how a good start in life will significantly help them, but for adults four themes are useful to look at. Fair employment, healthy standards of living, sustainable places and communities and ill health prevention are all ways to reduce the inequalities in care and support.

Make notes on the four themes applicable to adult social care and show how these might affect your service.

Financial constraints

Change and improvement for any service inevitably involves a need for more money, and financial constraints can be a key driver of change. With the drive for new and innovative models of care, such as the implementation of preventative services, the demographic challenge of an ageing population and increasing numbers of people with long-term conditions and disabilities, adult social care needs financial change.

As a manager in a care service, where funds are often scarce, innovative and entrepreneurial ways of working may be the way forward. By encouraging your staff to undertake innovative care to improve quality of care and the outcomes of those using the service, you will be helping to reduce variations in care and developing the entrepreneurial spirit in the adult care setting.

Research it

3.2 Innovation

Do some online research around innovation and adult care settings. Think about how you might encourage and motivate your staff to engage with this activity.

Reflect on it

3.2 Growth and change in your organisation

Identify the factors and drivers that influence growth and change in your own service delivery and provide a written account of them. What impact have these had on your organisation with respect to developing an entrepreneurial and innovative culture within your service? You could begin by thinking about the main issues of each driver and then show how each driver is related to your area of work and what impact it will have.

Analyse the impact the factors and drivers discussed above might have in respect of supporting an entrepreneurial and innovative culture within the service and related delivery. You could think about the effects these factors have on innovation and their strengths and weaknesses, for example.

AC 3.3 Explain how own setting/service meets the needs of the local population and the wider market of adult care

Here, you will explain how your setting is meeting the needs of the local population, and identify the role of your setting in the adult care market.

How your service relates to the wider market and is able to meet potential demand

Adult social care is part of a system of public services and forms of support which include:

- health services, such as GP, counselling, district nursing and care homes or other provisions
- housing, such as supported housing, warden schemes and assisted living
- welfare and benefits, such as advocacy, care and professional support, Citizens Advice
- leisure and wellbeing, such as sports facilities, libraries, education and transport.

As manager of such a service your challenge is to ensure that all parts of the system are working together and that you are accessing wider services for the benefit of the people to whom you provide a care service. For example, with better medical management of long-term conditions a person may be able to stay independent for longer and not have to rely on additional care or support. The adult care sector continues to request more money to support the growth it is experiencing. However, this money cannot always be forthcoming so smarter ways of working and innovation are necessary. Challenges with respect to the demand for additional services from an increasing older population might be envisaged in future and you therefore need to be aware of how your service will continue to supply services. If you work in a large residential organisation you may be required to increase the number of beds offered, with subsequent effect on resources and staffing. Alternatively, you may look at ways of supplying care in an individual's home, therefore changing the way in which your service currently works.

Research it

3.3 Local demographics

Visit the Office for National Statistics' local statistics website (ONS, 2023) and access the demographic statistics for your local area. How does your service meet the needs of the local population and the wider market of adult care?

AC 3.4 Explain how own setting/service will need to evolve to meet future demand for care services

Here, you will explain and compare the wider market in respect of similar care service provision, with consideration of the areas discussed in this section.

National care services (their role and market position) and local services (public, private, not-for-profit and charitable sector and market position)

There is growing pressure on the national social care systems in our country to change to meet the challenges they face now and in the future.

Local public and private care organisations must consider how they can deliver care that meets the needs of an ageing and neurodiverse population with complex health needs. Community services are urged to improve, and GP services are also undergoing major change to make stronger ties with the community services. The impact upon the NHS inevitably puts pressure on the adult social care system. With hospital beds in demand, the need to discharge individuals earlier means stretching the adult care system even more.

The government policy paper 'Build Back Better: Our Plan for Health and Social Care' (GOV.UK, 2021b) recognised the pressures created by the COVID-19 pandemic as well as highlighting how it made chronic problems in the care system worse.

The policy paper also confirms that challenges in adult social care have been exacerbated by the COVID-19 pandemic. Funding for care is a problem and people are required to fund their own care and face losing their life savings. The policy paper promises new investment in the NHS and social care, the aim of which is to bring health and the social care systems more closely together so that people can make more informed choices as to where they receive the care they need. The report states that from October 2023, care costs are to be capped so no person starting adult social care will have to pay more than £86,000 for personal care over their lifetime (although this may change).

The charity and voluntary sector, or the 'not-for-profit sector', describes a range of organisations that are neither public nor private sector. It includes voluntary and community organisations, registered charities associations, self-help and community groups, social enterprises and co-operatives.

One government aim is to increase the connection with the voluntary sector and local government to help keep people connected with their own community. Better care can be given if all services work together and share resources.

Managing a care setting means that you need to think about local groups and charities that might add value to the service you provide. For example, you need to consider how local charities and associations may be of benefit to the individuals using your service and how they might be encouraged to work alongside you in supplying care. They might, for example, offer group support services or additional advice on dementia care that your setting may not necessarily offer. You will need to be aware and stay up to date on additional services that are available and how they may benefit your setting and those individuals receiving care, as well as staff, who may also benefit from the knowledge and advice these services offer.

You should also consider innovative ways in which care can be offered and the policy paper supports this. The policy paper shows that better training for staff can enhance staff retention, and being a less risk averse leader may increase levels of innovation. In addition, improving internet connectivity and digital skills would build on digital capacity and would facilitate innovation. It also points out how collaboration between organisations and financial stability boosts innovation.

Outreach working and personal assistance is also a growth area and these services are usually for people who live on their own, wanting to remain independent, yet requiring tailored support. These might be people with milder levels of autism or learning disability.

Developing an innovative culture that supports change and growth

An innovative culture involves the workers in planning and embraces their ideas and views. Their creative thinking about solutions to problems and change is encouraged and, more importantly, they are given the time to develop new ways of working. It is important that in your role as manager you support and encourage innovation, change, redevelopment and growth of the organisation and foster and promote such a culture. This means creating forums where staff feel empowered to contribute ideas and shape ways of working. This could perhaps be through meetings, and suggestion and ideas boxes or even competitions. This in turn will ensure a collaborative workplace culture, staff who are happier in their roles, and higher retention rates. Again, such innovation can help to drive forward more efficient ways of working and improved practice in adult care.

Encourage and exploit entrepreneurship and innovation in others and maintain a culture that supports growth and change

As the population of those aged over 85 grows, and more people with learning disabilities access social care, there is a need for more care provision, yet research has indicated that individuals view the prospect of moving into a care organisation as 'a last resort' and one to be avoided. If there were ever a time for an innovative solution to care for older adults, it is now.

Clearly, the structure of existing care organisations and roles needs to change in order to create a culture based on putting the individual first and changing the way in which care is delivered. As a manager in a traditional type of care setting, one of your roles will be to consider ways in which change can be achieved to respond to the future vision of adult care. See the sections on innovation and entrepreneurship for how you can positively encourage and exploit entrepreneurship and innovation to benefit the care service and maintain a culture that supports growth and change.

Maher et al. (2009) discuss and show how organisations might encourage a more entrepreneurial spirit and maintain the culture of change.

- **Risk taking**: Staff should feel free to try out new ideas. Risk taking encourages the leaders in innovative organisations to demonstrate that they are more 'interested in learning from failure than in punishing it'.
- **Resources**: Create a climate where staff can act autonomously and with authority to move forward on innovative ideas. They should feel empowered and have resources at their disposal to help them to create change.

- **Goals**: These need to be linked to the strategic priorities of the organisation.
- **Rewards for innovation**: It is important to recognise innovative behaviour.
- **Relationships**: Looks closely at how we interact as teams and how innovative ideas are formed over time and through such interactions. The development of an environment where staff are encouraged to be exposed to a wide range of people from a variety of backgrounds provides growth for innovation.
- **Broad-based knowledge**: Refers to any information that can generate new ideas, wherever it is from. The act of filtering or rejecting the knowledge without consideration is seen as damaging to innovation.
- **Tools**: Refers to how leaders can build capability and capacity in staff to ensure that creative thinking becomes a valued and deliberate structure. Within Maher et al.'s document there are tips for developing this sort of training.

Sustainability

Sustainability in adult social care is becoming an increasingly important area that you may wish to research. Care professionals are being asked to deliver more sustainable care and reduce the harmful environmental and social impact of their ways of working. The Sustainability in Quality Improvement framework (SusQI) is an attempt to improve care which has been developed by the Centre for Sustainable Healthcare (CSH) with partners including the Royal College of Physicians. SusQI introduces the concept of sustainable quality improvement, which means delivering the best possible outcomes with minimum financial and environmental costs, while still adding positive social value. For more information, see SusQI (n.d.).

NHS England and Public Health England's publication 'Sustainable, resilient, healthy people and places: A sustainable development strategy for the NHS, public health and social care system' develops an approach to sustainability that embraces the entire social care system. Contributions were sought from local government, public health, social care, professional bodies and NHS colleagues to support all communities to lead healthy lives.

This strategy proposes the vision that a sustainable system reducing carbon emissions, minimising waste and pollution, building resilience to climate change and nurturing community strengths will lead to a healthier population. Organisations can ensure that they contribute by having a sustainable development plan, by measuring and reporting on their progress, by evaluating their approach and by engaging with staff, the people using the services and the public.

Research it

3.4 Sustainable development strategy

Read 'Sustainable, resilient, healthy people and places: A sustainable development strategy for the NHS, public health and social care system' (Sustainable Development Unit, 2014).

Explain how your own setting/service will need to evolve to meet future demand for care services.

Research it

3.4 National Audit Office 2021

You may find it useful to look at the report published by the National Audit Office, 'The adult social care market in England' (National Audit Office, 2021).

The report concludes that high-quality care is critical to the wellbeing of vulnerable adults in society but that with levels of unpaid care remaining high, too many adults have unmet needs, suggesting there will be a growing need for care. Look at the recommendations on pages 12 and 13 of the report and compare what your own setting is doing to meet these.

Reflect on it

3.4 Working within the wider market

How does your own service relate to the wider market for adult care and what do you see as the major challenges to your own setting's sustainability within this?

Evidence opportunity

3.4 Wider markets and potential demands

What do you think the wider market in adult care means to your service provision and what are the future demands with respect to your own service? Provide a written account.

LO4 Understand integrated approaches in health and social care

AC 4.1 Explain what is meant by an integrated health and social care system

Here, you will explain the different aspects of an integrated care system and identify your setting's role within this system.

Integrated care systems (ICSs) are partnerships of organisations that plan and deliver joined up health and care services. The aim of ICSs is to reduce repetition and overlap of services and provide better outcomes for the individuals using the services. By maintaining independence and enabling people to live in their own homes for longer, quality of life is improved. The ICS includes the following:

- **An integrated care partnership (ICP)**: This is a statutory committee between the NHS integrated care board and all upper-tier local authorities. The ICP produces an integrated care strategy on how to meet the health and wellbeing needs of the population in the ICS area. The ICP is a network of care service providers.
- **Integrated care board (ICB)**: This is responsible for planning the health and care needs of the local population and managing the NHS budget. The ICB also provides health and care services in the ICS area.
- **Local authorities**: These provide social care and public health services as well as other services for local people and organisations.
- **Place-based partnerships**: Responsible for designing and delivering the integrated services in their localities and neighbourhoods. They are a partnership between the NHS, councils, community and voluntary organisations, local residents, people who use services, their carers and representatives and other community partners that have a role in the health and wellbeing of the population.

Source: Adapted from NHS England (n.d.)

Integrated care partnerships are in a much better position to provide care that may have previously been unavailable in an area. When joined-up care is offered from a number of partners in a wider area, more services are available.

Evidence opportunity

4.1 Integrated care

What is your understanding of the term 'integrated care system'? Discuss with your assessor the various aspects that are applicable to your setting.

AC 4.2 Analyse the rationale for integrated approaches to service provision

Here, you will analyse the reasoning behind integrated approaches for both the individual and the population as a whole.

Providing person-centred support

Sometimes an individual's care may be provided by several different care professionals across a number of different providers. This can result in a fragmented experience and people can find it difficult to access the services they require. Integrated care can reduce repetition and gaps in the service, reduce confusion as to who is doing what and when, and prevent people being 'lost in the system'. Individuals benefit from person-centred care that is co-ordinated. Integrated care brings together all the different elements of care that an individual needs.

Changing patterns of population needs

The King's Fund published a report in 2022 on 'healthy life' expectancy, which refers to the number of years a person can expect to live in 'full health', taking into account years lived in less than full health/poor health due to disease and/or injury. The report stated that in 2018–20 an English male could expect to live 79.4 years, with an average *healthy* life expectancy of only 63.1 years (i.e. 20 per cent of those years would be in 'not good' health. An English female could expect to live 83.1 years, of which 19.3 years (23 per cent) would have been spent in 'not good' health (Raleigh, 2022).

There remains a socio-economic health gap, with those living in more affluent areas having significantly longer life expectancy than people in deprived areas. The gap in healthy life expectancy between most- and least-deprived areas is even greater, with those living in the most deprived areas spending nearly a third of their lives in poor health.

As discussed in AC4.1, integrated care partnerships are intended to close gaps in care inequalities and begin to address the socio-economic divide.

Prevention and early intervention strategies

In recent years, there have been media articles about the need for early assessment with respect to memory loss and signs of stroke in individuals. NICE recommends that early assessment should take place to enable planning for the future or, if treatment is to be given, to enable its institution at an early stage. In the case of stroke, the quicker the condition is assessed, the sooner the individual can access treatment and the greater the possibility of full recovery. In these cases, then, early assessment is crucial to enable a better outcome for the individual.

In all other cases of need, the assessment process should be initiated immediately or as soon as the care requirements of the individual change. Early assessment enables the care/support plan to be implemented with speed and to meet the needs of the individual as they arise.

When the assessment takes place, the individual needs to be the central figure in the negotiation, and this is recognised in legislation as being the optimum process for care/support planning. Others in the process, including other care workers, family members and advocates, should be clear about their roles and know how to record and report on the process.

Any delay that occurs in the assessment process will mean that risk and needs increase. This could lead to care not being given and the individual suffering as a result. The Care Act 2014 clearly states the obligations of the local authority to ensure that individuals and carers have access to care services, together with an assessment of their circumstances, needs and risks, and early identification of needs and support.

Recognising and recording individuals' current and emerging health and care needs

During a care assessment, the individual's care needs are determined, together with the level and type of care and support required to meet those needs. This is a fundamental role of the care worker and a manager. You also need to ensure that the relatives of the individual are involved in care/support planning processes and assessments if this is appropriate. The care/support plan is a continuous process and does not stop when it has been written. The people involved continue to evaluate and act within the plan to help the individual to achieve the best quality care.

Understanding the importance of early identification and assessment

Importance of early identification

The health and circumstances of an individual can change at any time, and it is good practice to ensure that there are systems in place that can identify these changes early so that treatment and care can be given to accommodate this. For example, a person with a learning disability may have developed their independence skills and require a change to their support plan to reflect this.

Conversely, a person who develops a chest infection or a urinary tract infection can quickly deteriorate and may be at risk of sepsis, which is a life-threatening condition. Using a system by which staff can easily check the current health status will enable them to escalate their concerns more quickly.

One such system is the National Early Warning Score (NEWS)2, developed by the Royal College of Physicians to help hospital staff recognise symptoms of deterioration (Royal College of Physicians, 2017). Widely used in acute settings, it is a scoring system which looks at basic physiological measures such as respiratory rate, oxygen saturations, temperature, systolic blood pressure, pulse rate and level of consciousness. A further review of NEWS2 is expected in 2023.

Role of the manager

As a manager, your role is to ensure that all staff are reporting and documenting changes to the health, wellbeing and expressed needs of the individuals they care for. One way of achieving this is to spend time with individuals and observe the care practices of your colleagues.

> **Research it**
>
> **4.2 Early identification**
>
> What early warning system is available for your staff?
>
> How are they required to document such changes?

Understanding the importance of early assessment

The Social Care Institute for Excellence (2003) states:

> *Although assessment has been recognised as a core skill in social work and should underpin all social work interventions, there is no singular theory or understanding as to what the purpose of assessment is and what the process should entail.*

With no one theory to support it, the process of assessment then becomes a huge subject and one that could differ with each service in a partnership group. This is why, when working with partners, you should bring together people who know the individuals using the service well and who can contribute to the care positively. These people may be from other services but may also include family, friends and advocates.

When this type of working is not done well, it can lead to fragmentation of an individual's care, with many differing approaches to assessing their needs being used at the same time. It becomes imperative, then, to determine how you as a care provider will assess the individual and simplify the process.

Care/support planning

The care/support planning process is a good place to start. In any assessment of an individual's needs, the 'basic helping cycle' shown in Figure 10, as suggested by Taylor and Devine (1993), is useful.

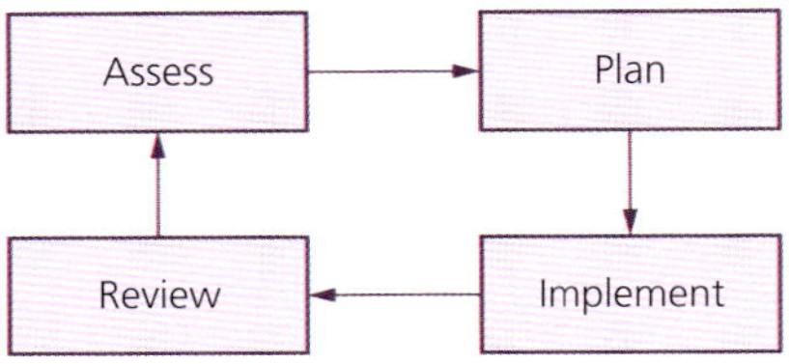

Figure 10 The basic care cycle (based on Taylor and Devine, 1993)

In this cycle, the individual and the care professional work together to assess the needs, resources and potential risks for the individual. In doing this, you are responding to the needs of the individual and are also working in conjunction with policy to ensure, for example, that you are providing individualised care and maintaining independence. The care to meet those needs is then planned and put into action at the third stage and finally evaluated or 'reviewed', starting the cycle again.

In 2006, Thompson described what he called the 'ASIRT' model of care/support planning:

AS – Assessment phase, which is the start of the process and the first part of an action plan leading onto the …

I – Intervention stage when aims and objectives for the intervention are selected

R – Review when the evaluation of what has happened takes place, before finally

T – Termination, when the intervention is no longer needed and can be stopped.

Your role as a manager

As a care professional and manager, your duty is to provide safe care and to ensure that your staff are equally competent. Staff may therefore need to undertake further training on how to carry out assessments or may require assistance to do so and your role as manager is to support them in this. Job descriptions which clearly outline roles in the position for which staff are employed are invaluable in ensuring boundaries are not breached.

As a manager, you are responsible for ensuring that the individuals in your care remain safe at all times and this requires you to put in place systems and processes which enable early identification and assessment of an individual's needs. Staff need to be well-trained to use such systems confidently and they will need to feel supported. You also need to ensure that all methods and systems in use relate ultimately to person-centred care and outcomes.

Moving to more community-based practices

The Care Quality Commission's 2018 report 'Beyond barriers: How older people move between health and social care in England' found that individuals experienced the best care when organisations worked together to overcome the 'fragmentation of the health and social care system' and where there is good evidence of co-ordinated personalised care (CQC, 2018).

Truly integrated care requires change in how performance is measured and how funding is approached. A shared approach to measuring how the whole system meets the needs of people using social care services together with sustainable funding reform, supported by long-term investment, supports collaboration rather than imposes limits. This has already been addressed in government promises to increase funds for adult social care. There is now a move away from efforts to measure the performance of individual organisations working separately, which has previously been a barrier to integrated care.

Planning the workforce and regulating services is seen as a way forward. Integrated care requires a workforce that can move between health and social care, so workforce planning needs to look at the skills and career paths that enable people to work flexibly across the system as services evolve to meet the population's changing needs.

With several organisations working together, the supply of community-based approaches to care improvement could be offered, which would provide an infrastructure for efficient knowledge-sharing and methods of influencing behaviours. Community-based services help people to live independently by offering care, support and treatment for people with learning disabilities, acute or chronic conditions, mental health needs or substance misuse problems.

Reflect on it

4.2 Integrated care partnerships

Consider who your specific care partners are in your local ICP. How has the introduction of the ICP changed or influenced the care you now deliver?

AC 4.3 Evaluate local and national initiatives to better integrate health and social care systems and services

Here, you will evaluate the different approaches to integrating health and social care systems and how these initiatives may apply to your own setting.

Primary care networks

Population growth and people living longer means many more people living with long-term health conditions such as diabetes, heart disease or mental health issues. Access to services may be needed more regularly and to meet this challenge GP practices form primary care networks (PCNs) with various community support groups, mental health services, pharmacies, hospital and voluntary services in their local areas.

PCNs enable greater provision of personalised and co-ordinated care for people, close to their home. In November 2022, there were 1250 PCNs across England, based on lists of GP-registered individuals and serving communities of 30,000 to 50,000 people. Although small enough to provide person-centred care, they achieve impact and economies of scale because of their contact with others in their PCN (NHS England, 2018).

Enhanced Health in Care Homes framework and the Ageing Well programme

The Enhanced Health in Care Homes (EHCH) framework is a new model of care that 'moves away from traditional reactive models towards proactive care that is centred on the needs of individual residents, their families and care home staff' (NHS England and NHS Improvement, 2020).

The NHS Long Term Plan published in 2019 states that between 2020 and 2024, EHCH will be rolled out across England as part of the Ageing Well programme, as part of the NHS goal to strengthen support for people who live and work in and around care homes or other provisions. An Urgent Community Response will now be available to people living in care homes, as well as the appointment of a chief advisor on care home nursing and extra support for nurses that work in care homes or other provisions.

Improvements to information sharing between the NHS and care homes are also part of the NHS Long Term Plan with secure email between the NHS and care homes now available in all care homes or other provisions.

The good practice model described in the EHCH framework is aimed at ensuring those living in care homes or other provisions can obtain both enhanced primary care and specialist services, while continuing to maintain their independence as far as possible by reducing, delaying or preventing the need for additional social care services.

The EHCH framework means that care home staff will now be part of an integrated team that includes primary, community, mental health and specialist care, as well as social care services and the voluntary sector. This will mean that care home staff will no longer work in isolation from other care sectors.

Budgets and incentives align so that all parts of the system work together to improve people's health and wellbeing.

The EHCH model will ensure that the commissioning of social care services is done in a co-ordinated way, and that commissioners and providers working in social care will fully understand the role of the social care provider market.

Source: Adapted from NHS England and NHS Improvement (2020)

Other initiatives include Integrated care systems (see AC4.2) and Sustainability and transformation partnerships (see AC1.5).

Additionally, the Transforming Care programme (ADASS et al., 2017) highlighted three aims for people with learning disabilities: to improve both quality of care and quality of life for people with a learning disability and/or autism, and to enhance community capacity in order to reduce inappropriate hospital admissions and the lengths of hospital stays. The 2015 ADASS report, 'Supporting people with a learning disability and/or autism who display behaviour that challenges, including those with a mental health condition: Service model for commissioners of health and social care services' (ADASS et al., 2015) is a response to the investigation into abuse at Winterbourne View and other similar hospitals. The commitment to transform care and support for people with a learning disability and/or autism who display behaviour that challenges focuses on building up community capacity for care packages to be delivered and introduces a service model for all social care commissioners. It includes learning disability commissioners, mental health commissioners, Continuing Health Care (CHC) commissioners, public health and children's commissioners.

Recognising that local areas are different and that local populations have different needs, each local area is encouraged to draw up its own model for how services should look in the future. Based on an agreed service model, the document provides clarity on 'what good looks like' for health, social care and housing services for people with a learning disability and/or autism.

Research it

4.3 Framework for enhanced health in care homes

Look at 'The framework for enhanced health in care homes' (NHS England and NHS Improvement, 2020) or the Transforming Care programme (ADASS et al., 2017) and make notes on the framework. How might this change the way you deliver care in your setting?

AC 4.4 Explain the impact of more integrated systems and processes on working practices and relationships

Here, you will review the role of integrated systems on care settings and explain the impact of the additional requirements on your setting.

Discharge arrangements

Discharge planning ensures that an individual can transition from the hospital to another medical facility or to their home safely and without their care being disrupted.

In elective care, planning can commence before admission and a screening tool, risk assessment or care pathway should be followed. In emergency or unscheduled care, advance planning is not possible so robust systems to gather information on individuals must be in place. The type of care required should be identified as simple or complex.

Integrated assessment, care/support planning and multi-disciplinary working arrangements

Integrated assessment is an interdisciplinary approach to needs assessment and requires information from a range of healthcare disciplines.

Integrated care is planned and co-ordinated by people who work together to understand the individual and their carer(s) and deliver services to achieve the best outcomes for that individual. (See AC4.2 and 4.3 for more on this.)

A referral to a social worker will start the assessment process for adult social care. This is the point at which an assessment might start. As care needs become more complex, it is likely that an individual may come into contact with a number of different care professionals, so an integrated care/support plan reduces the need for several plans to be put into place.

A social care assessment is carried out by local authority-financed adult care services to find out what help and support is needed to ensure that the individual is supported in their home or residential care setting. A social worker or occupational therapist will carry out the assessment and will ascertain how the individual is managing everyday tasks like washing, dressing and cooking. They will also address mobility needs and discuss changes to the environment, such as the installation of grab rails or other alterations to the home. This may be a separate assessment of home needs.

A single assessment plan should capture all the information required to meet the information needs of a range of health professionals. The introduction of such plans will require changes to working practices and this might require more cross-teamworking than you and your team have been used to in the past. It will mean new practices, including multidisciplinary teams being put into place, as well as reviewing policies and the way communication works between the team. The individual using the service is the key person in this process and should be prioritised at all times.

Data governance

The data protection law outlined by the General Data Protection Regulation (GDPR) and the UK Data Protection Act 2018 has been a problem in the sharing of data. Any consent given by individuals to share their personal data is based on control and choice by those individuals around how their personal data is used. Individuals must be in complete control and have the right to request that their data be erased if they choose. In many care situations, the sharing of personal data for purposes such as protecting public health, ensuring high quality in care standards and scientific research are all recognised as legitimate reasons for using and sharing personal data without the need for consent.

At the time of writing (May 2023), the Data Protection and Digital Information (No. 2) Bill is making its way through Parliament and will regulate the processing of information relating to living individuals. The Bill makes provision for services that use information to ascertain and verify facts about individuals but also addresses who can access personal data and organisation data. There are also provisions about privacy and electronic communications and information standards for social care. This will clarify what type of organisations the wider care system includes, for what purposes personal data can be shared and where it should be anonymised.

Legislation

Legislation	Key points
Equality Act 2010	An umbrella Act bringing together legislation that deals with race, disability and gender. It highlights protected characteristics of age, gender reassignment, pregnancy, religion, marriage and civil partnerships, and sexual orientation in an attempt to end discrimination.
Care Act 2014	Sets out the key responsibilities of local authorities in meeting the needs of individuals who require help and support to promote their wellbeing. Its main aim was to provide integrated care and to introduce the right to an assessment for all.
Fundamental Standards of the Health and Social Care Act 2008 (Regulated Activities) Regulations 2014	This act states that it is an individual's right to have care and treatment that is tailored to their needs and preferences. When carrying out an inspection, the CQC will check to see that care/support plans have been agreed with the individual.
Pensions Act 2008	Workplace pensions have become 'opt-out' rather than 'opt-in'. This means most employees are automatically enrolled into a pension provided by their employer. This law also requires employers to pay into their employees' pension schemes.
The Pension Schemes Act 2021	Introduced new duties for those involved in running pension schemes and gives new powers to the Pensions Regulator to protect pension scheme members and the Pension Protection Fund.
Working Time Regulations 1998	Working hours in the UK are governed by this Act, which limits the working week to an average of 48 hours (although there is an opt-out). The working day should average eight hours. This legislation also states that workers and employees have the right to paid leave and specified rest breaks.
Conduct of Employment Agencies and Employment Business Regulations 2003	This law delivers a set of minimum standards that must be adhered to when placing a work-seeker into a role in the UK. As an employer you need to be aware of these. More details can be found in 'Record keeping for employment agencies and businesses' published by the Employment Agency Standards Inspectorate (GOV.UK, n.d. b).
Employment Rights Act 1996	The Employment Rights Act (ERA) 1996 updated the Contracts of Employment Act 1963, the Redundancy Payments Act 1965, the Employment Protection Act 1975 and the Wages Act 1986. This Act addresses issues such as dismissal, unfair dismissal, parental leave, redundancy, the rights of employees and the right to request flexible working time. Additionally, it deals with employees' rights to a contract, suspension, the notice period that needs to be given when leaving and employer insolvency issues.
Rehabilitation of Offenders Act 1974	This Act describes the rehabilitation of offenders who have not been reconvicted of any serious offence for periods of years, and to penalise the unauthorised disclosure of their previous convictions.
Data Protection Act 2018	This Act controls how personal information is used by organisations, businesses and the government and is the UK's implementation of the General Data Protection Regulation (GDPR). Everyone responsible for using personal data must follow strict rules called 'data protection principles'.
National Minimum Wage Act 1998	This Act sets out the minimum amount of pay a worker is entitled to per hour and this is based on a worker's age. There is also a specific rate for apprentices. It is a legal requirement for employers to pay workers the national minimum wage .
Employment Relations Act 1999	This Act outlines details on employment rights in work. It applies to employees in various sectors.
Agency Workers Regulations 2010	These Regulations entitle agency workers to the same or no less favourable treatment for basic employment and working conditions, if they complete a qualifying period of 12 weeks in a particular job.
Safeguarding Vulnerable Groups Act 2006	This Act helps to avoid harm, or risk of harm, by preventing people who are deemed unsuitable to work with children and vulnerable adults from gaining access to them through their work. The Independent Safeguarding Authority was established as a result of this Act.

Legislation	Key points
Immigration, Asylum and Nationality Act 2006	This Act makes provision about immigration, asylum and nationality.
Health and Safety at Work Act 1974	The Act defines the general duties of everyone from employers and employees to owners, managers and maintainers of work premises (etc.) for maintaining health and safety within most workplaces.
Flexible Working Regulations 2014	This Act outlines changes to the flexible working arrangements so that any employee meeting the minimum service eligibility criteria can request flexible working arrangements.
Part-Time Workers (Prevention of Less Favourable Treatment) Regulations 2000	The Regulations make it unlawful for part-time workers to be treated less favourably than full-time workers which means they have the same rights and entitlements as full time staff.
Health and Social Care Act 2008	This Act requires all providers of 'regulated activities' in England to register with the Care Quality Commission, and to comply with the requirements and fundamental standards set out in regulations made under that Act.

References

Age UK (n.d.) 'Paying for homecare'. www.ageuk.org.uk/information-advice/care/paying-for-care/paying-for-homecare/

Ainsworth, A. (2023) 'How can digital technologies support care?'. Blog: Social care. https://socialcare.blog.gov.uk/2023/05/25/how-can-digital-technologies-support-care/

Anchor (2018) 'Social care sector unites to warn of an impending workforce crisis and raise the perception of care'. www.anchor.org.uk/media/social-care-sector-unites-warn-impending-workforce-crisis-and-raise-perception-care

Association of Directors of Adult Social Services, Local Government Association, NHS England (2015) 'Supporting people with a learning disability and/or autism who display behaviour that challenges, including those with a mental health condition'. www.england.nhs.uk/wp-content/uploads/2015/10/service-model-291015.pdf

Association of Directors of Adult Social Services, Local Government Association, NHS England (2017) 'Transforming care: Model service specifications'. www.england.nhs.uk/wp-content/uploads/2017/02/model-service-spec-2017.pdf

Cabinet Office (2023) 'Guidance: How to prove and verify someone's identity'. www.gov.uk/government/publications/identity-proofing-and-verification-of-an-individual/how-to-prove-and-verify-someones-identity

Care Quality Commission (2018) 'Beyond barriers: How older people move between health and care in England'. www.cqc.org.uk/publications/themed-work/beyond-barriers-how-older-people-move-between-health-care-england

Care Quality Commission (2022) 'Our equality objectives 2021–2025'. www.cqc.org.uk/about-us/our-strategy-plans/our-equality-objectives-2021-2025

Chartered Institute of Personnel and Development (n.d.) 'Employment law dates at a glance'. www.hr-inform.co.uk/employment_law/forthcoming-legislation

Cornwall and Isles of Scilly (CIOS) Safeguarding Adults Board (2019) 'Safeguarding adults review: The Morleigh Group: Final report'. https://ciossafeguarding.org.uk/assets/2/the_morleigh_group_sar_final_report.pdf

Department of Health and Social Care (2022a) Policy paper, 'Data saves lives: Reshaping health and social care with data'. www.gov.uk/government/publications/data-saves-lives-reshaping-health-and-social-care-with-data/data-saves-lives-reshaping-health-and-social-care-with-data

Department of Health and Social Care (2022b) Statutory guidance 'Guidance on the preparation of integrated care strategies'. www.gov.uk/government/publications/guidance-on-the-preparation-of-integrated-care-strategies/

Department of Health and Social Care (2022c) Policy paper 'People at the heart of care: Adult social care reform policy paper'. www.gov.uk/government/publications/people-at-the-heart-of-care-adult-social-care-reform-white-paper/people-at-the-heart-of-care-adult-social-care-reform

Department of Health and Social Care and Helen Whately MP (2023) 'Over £3 million to transform technology in adult social care'. www.gov.uk/government/news/over-3-million-to-transform-technology-in-adult-social-care

GOV.UK (2020) Press release 'Chief nurse for adult social care to provide clinical leadership during winter'. www.gov.uk/government/news/chief-nurse-for-adult-social-care-to-provide-clinical-leadership-during-winter

GOV.UK (2021a) Policy paper 'Social care funding and workforce report: Government response'. www.gov.uk/government/publications/social-care-funding-and-workforce-report-government-response

GOV.UK (2021b) Policy paper 'Build back better: Our plan for health and social care'. www.gov.uk/government/publications/build-back-better-our-plan-for-health-and-social-care

GOV.UK (n.d. a) 'Disciplinary procedures and action against you at work'. www.gov.uk/disciplinary-procedures-and-action-at-work/how-disciplinary-procedures-work

GOV.UK (n.d. b) 'Record keeping for employment agencies and businesses'. www.gov.uk/record-keeping-for-employment-agencies-and-businesses

Health Foundation, The (2021) 'Quality improvement made simple: What everyone should know about health care quality improvement'. www.health.org.uk/publications/quality-improvement-made-simple

HM Government (2020) 'Employment Agency Standards Inspectorate: A brief guide for agencies'. https://assets.publishing.service.gov.uk/government/uploads/system/uploads/attachment_data/file/936515/eas-brief-guide-for-agencies.pdf

King's Fund, The (2022) 'Building capacity and capability for improvement in adult social care'. www.kingsfund.org.uk/publications/building-capacity-capability-improvement-adult-social-care

National Audit Office (2021) 'Report – value for money: The adult social care market in England'. www.nao.org.uk/reports/adult-social-care-markets/

NHS Digital (2021) 'Transforming health and care through technology'. https://digital.nhs.uk/about-nhs-digital/corporate-information-and-documents/transforming-health-and-care-through-technology

NHS Digital (2022a) 'NHS workforce statistics – June 2022'. https://digital.nhs.uk/data-and-information/publications/statistical/nhs-workforce-statistics/june-2022#

NHS Digital (2022b) 'Latest key statistics on adult social care include council spending in 2012–22: Statistical press release'. https://digital.nhs.uk/news/2022/adult-social-care-stats-2021-22

NHS Digital (2022c) 'NHS Outcomes Framework indicators – March 2022 release'. https://digital.nhs.uk/data-and-information/publications/statistical/nhs-outcomes-framework/march-2022

NHS England (2018) 'Primary care networks'. www.england.nhs.uk/primary-care/primary-care-networks/

NHS England (2019) 'NHS Mental Health Implementation Plan 2019/20 – 2023/24'. www.longtermplan.nhs.uk/wp-content/uploads/2019/07/nhs-mental-health-implementation-plan-2019-20-2023-24.pdf

NHS England (2020) 'Delivering a "net zero" National Health Service'. www.england.nhs.uk/greenernhs/wp-content/uploads/sites/51/2022/07/B1728-delivering-a-net-zero-nhs-july-2022.pdf

NHS England (n.d.) 'What are integrated care systems?'. www.england.nhs.uk/integratedcare/what-is-integrated-care/

NHS England and NHS Improvement (2020) 'The framework for Enhanced Health in Care Homes, Version 3'. www.england.nhs.uk/long-read/providing-proactive-care-for-people-living-in-care-homes-enhanced-health-in-care-homes-framework/

NHS England and NHS Improvement (2022) 'Commissioning for Quality and Innovation (CQUIN): 2022/23: Guidance'. www.england.nhs.uk/wp-content/uploads/2022/01/B1477-i-cquin-22-23-march-2022.pdf

NHS England News (2018) 'Dramatic annual surge in online GP services as patients sign up for convenience'. www.england.nhs.uk/2018/03/dramatic-annual-surge-in-online-gp-services-as-patients-sign-up-for-convenience/

NHS Improvement (2021) 'Consolidated NHS provider accounts 2019/20'. www.england.nhs.uk/wp-content/uploads/2021/01/consolidated-nhs-provider-accounts-19-20.pdf

NHS Improvement (2022) 'Monitor Annual Report and Accounts 2020/21: Health and high quality are for all now and for future generations'. Crown Copyright London. https://assets.publishing.service.gov.uk/government/uploads/system/uploads/attachment_data/file/1052210/monitor-annual-report-2020-to-2021-web.pdf

Office for National Statistics (2023) 'Get labour market and population data for areas within the UK'. www.ons.gov.uk/help/localstatistics

Raleigh, V. (2022) 'What is happening to life expectancy in England?', London: The King's Fund. www.kingsfund.org.uk/publications/whats-happening-life-expectancy-england

Royal College of Nursing (2010) *Guidance on Safe Nurse Staffing Levels in the UK*. London: Royal College of Nursing.

Royal College of Physicians (2017) 'National Early Warning Score (NEWS) 2: Standardising the assessment of acute-illness severity in the NHS. Updated report of a working party'. London: Royal College of Physicians. www.rcplondon.ac.uk/projects/outputs/national-early-warning-score-news-2

Skills for Care (2020) 'Safe and fair recruitment: A guide to employing people with convictions in social care'. www.skillsforcare.org.uk/resources/documents/Recruitment-support/Application-and-selection-process/Safe-and-fair-recruitment-guide.pdf

Skills for Care (2021a) 'Our strategy: Explore our plans for 2021–2025'. www.skillsforcare.org.uk/About-us/Our-strategy/Our-strategy.aspx

Skills for Care (2021b) 'What is values-based recruitment?'. www.skillsforcare.org.uk/News-and-events/blogs/What-is-values-based-recruitment

Skills for Care (2022a) 'The workforce employed by adult services departments in England'. www.skillsforcare.org.uk/Adult-Social-Care-Workforce-Data/Workforce-intelligence/publications/national-information/The-workforce-employed-by-adult-services-departments-in-England.aspx

Skills for Care (2022b) 'The state of the adult social care sector and workforce in England'. www.skillsforcare.org.uk/Adult-Social-Care-Workforce-Data/Workforce-intelligence/publications/national-information/The-state-of-the-adult-social-care-sector-and-workforce-in-England.aspx

Skills for Care (n.d. a) 'Adult social care workforce data'. www.skillsforcare.org.uk/adult-social-care-workforce-data/adult-social-care-workforce-data.aspx

Skills for Care (n.d. b) 'Artificial intelligence and robotics in social care: What could the future look like?'. www.skillsforcare.org.uk/resources/documents/Support-for-leaders-and-managers/Managing-a-service/Digital/Robotics-and-the-types-of-Artificial-Intelligence.pdf

Skills for Care (n.d. c) 'Care certificate'. www.skillsforcare.org.uk/Developing-your-workforce/Care-Certificate/Care-Certificate.aspx

Skills for Care (n.d. d) 'Recruitment support'. www.skillsforcare.org.uk/Recruitment-support/Recruitment-support.aspx

Skills for Care (n.d. e) 'Using technology in social care'. www.skillsforcare.org.uk/Support-for-leaders-and-managers/Managing-a-service/Digital-technology-and-social-care/Using-technology-in-social-care.aspx

Social Care Institute for Excellence (2003) *Summary Knowledge Review 1: Learning and teaching assessment skills in social work education*. London: SCIE.

Social Care Institute for Excellence (2010) 'Sustainable social care programme'. www.scie.org.uk/adults/sustainablesocialcare/what.asp

Social Care Institute for Excellence (2013) 'Social care and health inequalities'. www.scie.org.uk/workforce/socialcareandhealthinequalities/

Social Care Institute for Excellence (2018) 'Resource management'. www.scie.org.uk/workforce/peoplemanagement/staffmanagement/resourcemanage/

SusQI (n.d.) 'What is SusQI?'. www.susqi.org/the-susqi-education-project

Sustainable Development Unit (2014) 'Sustainable, resilient, healthy people and places'. www.england.nhs.uk/greenernhs/wp-content/uploads/sites/51/2021/02/Sustainable-Development-Strategy-2014-2019.pdf

Swift, J. and Teicke, J. (2021) 'Evidence review and sector consultation to inform Skills for Care strategy: Final sector report, February'. London: Skills for Care. www.skillsforcare.org.uk/resources/documents/Adult-social-care-workforce-data/Evidence-review-and-consultation-analysis.pdf

UK Parliament (2022) 'Social care: Funding and workforce', Health and Social Care Committee. https://committees.parliament.uk/work/136/social-care-funding-and-workforce/

Useful resources and further reading

Berwick Report (2013) 'A promise to learn – a commitment to act: Improving the safety of patients in England', National Advisory Group on the Safety of Patients in England: https://assets.publishing.service.gov.uk/government/uploads/system/uploads/attachment_data/file/226703/Berwick_Report.pdf

Bubb, S (2014) 'Winterbourne View – time for change: Transforming the commissioning of services for people with learning disabilities and/or autism'. www.england.nhs.uk/wp-content/uploads/2014/11/transforming-commissioning-services.pdf

Cavendish, C. (2013) 'The Cavendish Review: An independent review into healthcare assistants and support workers in the NHS and social care settings'. https://assets.publishing.service.gov.uk/government/uploads/system/uploads/attachment_data/file/236212/Cavendish_Review.pdf

Department of Health (2012) 'Transforming care: A national response to Winterbourne View Hospital'. https://assets.publishing.service.gov.uk/government/uploads/system/uploads/attachment_data/file/213215/final-report.pdf

Department of Health (2018) *Health Inequalities Annual Report 2018*. London: TSO.

Durbin, J. (2022) 'The staffing crisis – regulations must still be met', Ridouts. www.ridout-law.com/the-staffing-crisis-regulations-must-still-be-met/

Francis, R (2013) *Report of the Mid Staffordshire NHS Foundation Trust Public Inquiry*. London: TSO. www.gov.uk/government/publications/report-of-the-mid-staffordshire-nhs-foundation-trust-public-inquiry

Hartley, J. (2013) *The New Driving Force for Improvement across the NHS in England: How NHS IQ intends to support excellence in elective care*. London: NHS IQ.

Medway NHS Foundation Trust (2013) 'The Keogh Review'. https://democracy.kent.gov.uk/documents/s41983/Medway%20NHS%20Foundation%20Trust%20The%20Keogh%20Review.pdf

National Voices (2017) *Person-centred Care in 2017*. London: National Voices.

Nuffield Trust (2013) *The Francis Public Inquiry Report: A response*. Policy response. www.nuffieldtrust.org.uk/files/2017-01/francis-public-inquiry-report-web-final.pdf

Social Care Institute for Excellence (2006) 'Leadership and management'. www.scie.org.uk/workforce/peoplemanagement/leadership/

Unit 504

Team leadership in adult care

GLH 25

About this unit

Effective team leadership requires that strategies of leading and managing teams are positive and supportive. By examining your own strengths, responsibilities and learning needs as a leader, you can support your staff to drive forward an organisational strategy that will be successful for all those you care for and support in your setting.

By reflecting on best practice within the care context and understanding the roles of the manager and leader of teams in the adult care sector, you will be able to develop your skills in leadership and management and gain an understanding of the models of management and leadership which are relevant to this type of work.

This unit will help you to consider your own effectiveness as a leader and manager, be aware of your strengths and areas for further development and learn how to support the wellbeing and resilience of team members.

Underpinned by theories and models of leadership and management practice, you will explore how these apply in your practice.

Learning outcomes

By the end of this unit, you will:

1 Be able to provide leadership for a team.
2 Be able to manage teamwork.
3 Be able to support the wellbeing and resilience of team members.

Getting started

Before you study this unit, think about the following:

In order to provide effective adult social care it is essential to work in partnership with others, either in the same team or across a range of different agencies and disciplines within the care sector. The most important person in your team will be the individual using the service and they must be central in any teamworking.

You will be involved in several different teams in your work setting and this unit will help you to work more effectively in those teams. It will introduce you to models of leadership relevant to the care sector as well as showing how teams move through different stages and cycles. You will be encouraged to examine strategies of teamworking and leadership in order to identify your own strengths, responsibilities, learning needs and to reflect on best practice within the care context. A range of practical skills and suggestions relevant to teamworking will be discussed. Teamworking means taking responsibility for your own work as well as respecting the contributions of all your colleagues and good communication is essential to effective teamworking.

LO1 Be able to provide leadership for a team

AC 1.1 Adapt leadership styles to respond to different stages and cycles within the team's development

Here, you will be required to show that you can adapt relevant leadership and management styles.

A team is a group of people who work together. Wheelan (2005) acknowledges that from the beginning of human history, people have utilised work groups to generate new ideas, get things done and nurture individuals. For a group of people to become a team, they need to be co-ordinated and to be able to communicate and collaborate effectively. Pearson and Spencer (1997) suggest that teams are formed because of a belief that having people work on shared goals interdependently will lead to synergy; the aggregate of each individual's performance will be exceeded by the work group's performance.

For example, social workers, support workers and occupational therapists may work together. This is called a **multi-disciplinary team (MDT)**.

> **KEY TERM**
>
> **Multidisciplinary team (MDT)**: One in which care professionals from a range of disciplines and organisations work together to deliver streamlined care to individuals.

A wealth of leadership styles and models are expressed in literature, suggesting that teams go through various stages and cycles as they develop and grow. The following models could provide frameworks for discussions in your setting about team development and their impact on your leadership style.

Tuckman's theory

Tuckman's theory (1965) describes the changes a team will go through as it develops. This is relevant to teamworking because it demonstrates a process which people go through when forming a team.

Tuckman suggested a mnemonic for common stages of group development. He said that groups go through stages of Forming, Storming, Norming and Performing. Tuckman later added a fifth stage called Mourning or Adjourning.

Forming

This stage is most likely to happen if a team is new, although it may also happen if several new people arrive at the same time. The members of the team are new to each other, and they may be unsure of each other and of the purpose of the team. They may be positive and polite, but others will be anxious.

Their first responsibility is to become a team. Individual team members will look to the leader for direction and support. Being too directive at this stage may result in team members only responding to the instructions given and not forming together as a team. This will slow down the process of achieving team cohesion.

Storming

This occurs as team members become more familiar with each other. As the team leader, you may feel challenged at this stage. This is the time when people start to push the boundaries established in the forming stage. Personality clashes and differences of opinion may occur, and the atmosphere of the group may start to feel uncomfortable. Many teams fail at this point as storming often starts when there is a conflict between team members' natural working styles, making team members feel frustrated.

Norming

The norming stage feels more harmonious and less superficial than the forming stage as it is during this time that the team begins to find some mutual direction and consensus. Creative ideas which may have emerged in the storming stage are focused upon and team members want to move away from the storming stage. The team start to resolve their differences and begin to appreciate others' strengths. There is also a new-found respect for your authority as a leader. This stage can feel complacent but if the storming stage has occured, the team can feel positive and intimate.

Performing

The team starts to get on with the work that needs to be done and apply themselves to the tasks to be completed. They may take on new activities and feel safe to take on different roles because they know each other quite well.

Mourning/adjourning

This stage occurs when a team comes to an end. This may happen when members of the team leave or new members join. If you're about to leave your team it is likely that you'll go through a stage of mourning. You will look back and review events from the past and you will look forward with excitement and fear to future challenges. It is natural at this stage to experience negative feelings for the team as a way of coping and feeling better about leaving them.

Group development and change

All groups develop and change and Preston-Shoot (2007) states that groups may be at different stages for different tasks. He says that the duration of any stage relates more to the groups' history, their function and the personalities within them.

Schiller (2003) agrees with Tuckman's theory and has identified five stages that a team goes through:

1. **Pre-affiliation**: Team members get to know each other and find positive ways of relating.
2. **Mutuality**: Team members learn more about each other and develop greater respect for the other members.
3. **Challenge**: Team members feel comfortable enough with each other and challenge the opinions of other team members without fear of rejection.
4. **Change**: This stage is about action and achieving the task.
5. **Termination**: This is the end of the team.

You may have noticed that the main difference between Tuckman and Schiller's theories lies with the interpretation of the Storming (Tuckman) or Challenge (Schiller) stage. Tuckman argues that teams only start to perform after storming has occurred and team members only get to know each other during the storming process. Schiller's model, however, states that team members only argue and challenge each other *after* they have got to know each other enough to avoid rejection.

Adair's Action-centred leadership model

Rather than believing that leadership is an innate quality, Adair supported the view that leadership is a transferable skill that can be learned.

Adair's Action-centred leadership model consists of three core management responsibilities:

- Achieving the task.
- Managing the team.
- Managing the individual.

This model adapts well to a care setting. It is simple to use and relates to task completion and team building. If you choose to use it, you need to think about the aspects of performance necessary for success in the setting.

Adair also set out the core functions of leadership:

- **Planning**: Information seeking and defining tasks and aims.
- **Initiating**: Task allocation and setting standards.
- **Controlling**: Maintaining standards and ensuring progress.
- **Supporting**: Staff and their contributions and encouraging a team spirit.
- **Informing**: Clarifying tasks and plans and seeking and receiving feedback.
- **Evaluating**: Ideas, performance and enabling self-assessment

The Action-centred leadership model is part of an integrated approach to managing and leading, with a strong emphasis on applying these principles through training.

Hersey and Blanchard's Situational leadership theory

Hersey and Blanchard's Situational leadership theory (also known as the Life cycle theory of leadership) suggests that leadership style is affected by the circumstances that leaders find themselves in and that their ability to lead depends upon certain situational factors. It is only by understanding and adapting to these factors that leaders can influence their surroundings and followers more successfully than if they ignore the factors. For more on the theory, see Unit 500 AC1.1.

Much of Hersey and Blanchard's research focuses on the characteristics of followers in determining appropriate leadership behaviours. They found that leaders modified their leadership style as their followers changed in their ability (task readiness) and willingness (psychological readiness) to perform the task, showing that a leader's relationship with followers is likely to go through different stages as their abilities and willingness change over time.

This led to the four leadership styles of supporting, coaching, directing and delegation to deal with these different stages. For more on the leadership styles, see Unit 500 AC3.3.

Tannenbaum-Schmidt Leadership continuum model

The Tannenbaum-Schmidt Leadership continuum model was developed by Robert Tannenbaum and Warren H. Schmidt in 1958, but it still often used today (Tannenbaum and Schmidt, 1973).

This model puts forward the view that the relationship between the authority of the leader and the freedom of the team is an important consideration and functions between two extremes on a continuum. At one end of the continuum, leaders adopt an authoritarian approach by instructing employees without involving them, while at the other end of the continuum, leaders enable the team to develop freely by using their own knowledge, experience and creativity.

The authoritarian style and the more laid-back approach are two extremes that are unlikely to be applied all the time. Instead, most leaders will adopt a leadership style somewhere in the middle of the continuum using part of each style in different situations. This requires that the manager chooses the most effective leadership style for each situation, which, like the situational leadership model, means their leadership style will vary because different situations need a different evaluation.

The success of a setting is dependent on every staff member as well as the leadership of the manager. It also means that if a staff member makes a mistake that affects the setting, the manager will be held to account as the task was carried out under the manager's instruction.

The Tannenbaum-Schmidt Leadership continuum model identifies the following leadership styles:

1. **Manager makes a decision and announces it**: The manager directly instructs the team without involving them in any discussion. The leader views the problem to be solved as an individual problem to be solved by the team using the solution identified by the manager. This leadership style might be appropriate if a deadline needs to be met or if training is required, but it can create frustration for the team.
2. **Manager sells decision**: This type of leadership style is more persuasive. The manager will still make the decision but will explain it to the team as it is important for them to understand why the decision has been made. The manager will outline the reasons for the decision and its potential positive effects for the team. The manager must receive recognition for the decision that has been made, because this improves their relationship with their team.
3. **Manager presents ideas and invites questions**: The manager gives the team the opportunity to put forward their opinions before the manager makes a decision. As well as receiving input that may be useful when considering a decision, this leadership style also gives the manager the chance to identify which team members have the skills and knowledge to take on more responsibilities.
4. **Manager presents tentative decision subject to change**: This style supports active involvement of the staff in decision making. The manager may have made their decision but offers the team the opportunity to present their reasons why a different decision could be made. This means that all problems are shared group problems rather than solely the manager's problem, and staff feel valued if they feel they can influence a decision.
5. **Manager presents problem, gets suggestions, makes decision**: This is a more team-centred approach as the manager actively involves all staff before a decision is made. The manager presents the problem and requests suggestions to solve it. The difference to the previous style is that the problem is discussed with the group before the leader makes a final decision. This type of leadership requires employees that are skilled and knowledgeable to enable them to be part of the decision-making process.
6. **Manager defines limits, ask group to make decision**: In this style, the manager will outline the problem for the staff, who are then required to come up with a solution. This gives the staff autonomy in their decision, although it is important that the manager sets boundaries for the decision as they will ultimately be responsible for the decision that is taken. This type of leadership can be used with skilled and experienced teams.
7. **Manager permits subordinates to function within limits defined by superior**: This is an extreme type of leadership where the team is given total freedom to make decisions themselves, rather than involving the manager. However, as managers remain responsible for the setting, the team must also consider potential risks in the decisions they make to try to avoid potential problems occurring. This type of leadership mostly occurs in highly experienced and skilled teams working in the top management levels of organisations.

The Tannenbaum-Schmidt Leadership continuum model leadership styles shows that the amount of freedom given to staff to make decisions relates to the level of education and competence of members of the team.

No matter what level of involvement teams have in decision making, managers remain responsible for the setting activities under their control. Managers must also remember that they are still responsible for risks, even when tasks are delegated, so should decide how much involvement they want in working with their teams to achieve the organisation outcomes.

The leadership and management style you adopt can be changed according to the situation that presents itself or the individual you are dealing with. For example, some members of the team may require a more hands-on leadership style or one in which you are more authoritarian. In other situations, you may want to delegate tasks and leave the team to make their own decisions. Your ability to adapt and change will enhance the development of the team.

Stretch and challenge

1.1 Project planning using Adair's Action-centred leadership model

Think for a moment about a project you wish to undertake in your setting. For example, you may need to review policies and procedures, or perhaps you have vacancies to be filled. Using Adair's Action-centred leadership model, plan your project.

Reflect on it

1.1 Adapt leadership and management styles to reflect different situations and stages

Explain to your assessor and show them how you adapt relevant leadership and management styles. How do you adapt leadership and management styles to reflect different situations and stages in a care team's development?

Reflect on it

1.1 Your preferred style of leadership

Say which is your preferred style of leadership and management and provide an example of a time when you have had to adapt this. Reflect on how successful this was and why.

AC 1.2 Establish trust and accountability within the team

Here, you will be required to show you can build positive relationships within the team(s) with consideration of the topics discussed here.

Active listening skills

Developing trust in any relationship is about respect and being transparent and honest in what you are thinking and doing. You can demonstrate you are a trustworthy manager by being consistent and the sort of person who can be relied upon. Communication and listening are at the heart of this.

Think of a time when you know that you were not being listened to and heard.

- What was going on at that time?
- How did it affect the interaction?
- What do you think was going on for the person you were trying to communicate with at that time?

KEY TERM

Active listening: A way of listening and responding to improve understanding. It involves skill in questioning, clarifying, summarising, reflecting, paying attention to body language, offering encouraging verbal cues and refraining from judgement.

Active listening shows that your staff and the individuals using your service have been heard and the ways in which you can do this is are outlined below.

Team cultures

In addition to improving the way you communicate, you can address the sort of culture you wish to develop in the team as this will have a powerful and persuasive influence over the behaviour and practices of the people within that team (Mullins, 2010).

The wider organisation in which you work is complicated and complex interactions occur between individuals. The complexity and interdependency of relationships support an environment in which conflicts of interest and power differentials can be abused if appropriate policies, practices and guards are not in place to counteract this. This will affect your team and its culture. The way in which you approach the leadership and management of the team will impact the way it works. Where this is a positive, value-based influence it can be very useful to the manager in spreading good practice. As a manager, you might use your position to encourage staff to adopt anti-discriminatory and non-judgemental attitudes in their work by challenging discrimination that may come to your notice.

Team values and values-based culture

A values-based culture is one in which the goal is to work by a common set of values that guides behaviours. The 6Cs (care, compassion, competence, communication, courage and commitment) are the collection of qualities and values that all people working in care are expected to demonstrate in their personal behaviour, their beliefs, and the way in which they interact with others at all stages of delivering care and treatment. Culture is developed and built by the values, beliefs and attitudes that people bring to it; these are often deeply ingrained and are acquired through learning and our upbringing. We are encouraged to believe that certain attitudes and behaviours are acceptable. It is only when these values, beliefs and attitudes are challenged, by either new information or different experiences, that they may be seen to be flawed. Even when individuals' views can be shown to be discriminatory, deeply held beliefs may be resistant to change and this is termed prejudice.

A prejudice is an attitude or belief that is based on a faulty and inflexible generalisation/belief which can lead to negative emotions and discriminatory actions. Prejudice does not necessarily cause someone to discriminate unfairly, but examining such beliefs and values and questioning them is a first step in recognising and tackling prejudice.

To eliminate prejudice requires you to redefine beliefs and attitudes in the light of new information and then to change your behaviour in the light of that information. Furthermore, you need to challenge others who articulate similar prejudices. None of this is easy to do, particularly the latter; however, challenging others can have a significant impact on breaking down discrimination and prejudice. Often prejudice is not just an individual issue but represents views that might be more widely held within a group or specific context. When a strong, widespread belief is apparent, challenging it is difficult and individuals who try to do so may fear ridicule, victimisation or reprisals if they stand up against the prevailing beliefs and practices. In an organisation or team, it is important that everyone is aware that prejudice and discriminatory practice cannot be tolerated. Individuals who become aware of such practice must be supported and protected to speak out and not to feel excluded because of it. Creating a culture of discussion and tolerance is important in developing an open-minded community and in preventing abusive practice.

The first step in supporting others to challenge discrimination and exclusion is to accept that they exist and to acknowledge that discrimination is a significant factor in inhibiting equality.

Prejudice can lead to unacceptable behaviours, including harassment, bullying and victimisation, as well as poor standards and abuse of power over others. Harassment, bullying and victimisation are all behaviours that individuals are protected against under the Equality Act 2010; it is important to remember that it is not just individuals and groups that can be prejudiced and discriminatory (adapted from Tilmouth and Quallington, 2016).

Team diversity, roles and responsibilities

We are all products of our culture, experiences and education and, as such, our teams are likely to comprise a diverse mix of people. While discrimination and exclusion may not be intentional, they may come about because of the belief that everyone experiences life in the same way.

As managers it is necessary to communicate to staff that everyone must respect the diverse nature of the team and the differences in the experience, skills and knowledge that people bring to the mix. You should develop a culture of zero tolerance for negative behaviour if the values people have are different to your own. One of the ways in which this might be done is to promote policies that set out expectations of behaviour to others and that remind staff of disciplinary sanctions should they breach the policy. Another may be to look at the roles of each member of the team and to clearly set out the responsibilities they have.

Team activities – internal and external

Regular team activities will help to develop trust within the team. One useful way would be to get staff involved in planning by providing time during the regular team meeting for the team to express their views and to communicate their opinions or ideas. Often team meetings become a mere information-giving session and this does not provide an adequate venue for the exchange of ideas. If this is the case, then the valuable expertise, skills and knowledge of the staff will not be accessed. Using a mentoring process, team members can learn a great deal from each other and the expertise each one possesses through their experience and training can be used as a valuable resource for planning. Other team activities such as learning from peers may also be an influential way to ensure that a cohesive team is developed.

Individual and team accountability, and feedback on team performance and achievement

Good management demands that you hold people **accountable** for what they do or don't do and the way in which you do this can make or break the relationship.

> **KEY TERM**
>
> **Accountable**: Taking responsibility and being liable or answerable for something.

When goals are not met due to something an employee has failed to do, then it is appropriate for them to be held accountable for this failure. However, if you are trying to hold employees accountable for things that are out of their control, this is unreasonable, and you will lose the trust you have with the staff.

To be a good manager, you need to undertake the following:

- **Be consistent**: The key ingredient is consistency, and your staff will expect to be called to account if goals are not met or jobs are not done. The way in which you do this is also important and it is much better to deal with an individual in a firm but kind way in private about a performance error than to berate or criticise them in public for a misdemeanour or mistake. Additionally, it is important that all staff are dealt with in the same way, otherwise the sense of injustice is great and trust is lost.

- **Build relationships**: As a manager, there is a distance between yourself and the staff, but leaders and managers who take the time to build relationships with staff will gain their trust. It is a wise manager who takes time to find out a little about their staff and to share a little about their own life. You are likely to remember a manager who takes an interest and asks about your family or is happy to share a few words.
- **Be honest**: Trust builds respect and it is this that gets results.
- **Provide constructive feedback**: This will enable staff to make the changes they need to. Highlighting achievements can empower your staff and motivate them to improve their practice even further.

The people using a service require staff who are confident and happy in their work, and this can be achieved only if managers are able to encourage this in their workforce.

Evidence opportunity

1.2 Developing trust and accountability within the team

Show your assessor how you develop trust and accountability and build positive relationships within your team(s), considering the topics discussed in this section.

Reflect on it

1.2 Developing trust and accountability

Reflect on the methods you use to develop trust and accountability within the team.

Think about a **critical incident** that demonstrates the way in which you maintain accountability and trust in your work. What have you learned from this?

KEY TERM

Critical incident: An unintended event that occurs when an individual in care is involved in something that results in a consequence to them; for example, a fall.

AC 1.3 Build and maintain team's commitment to the service/setting and its values

Here, you will need to show that you can build the team's commitment to the service and its values by consistently demonstrating your own commitment and expressing the vision.

As a manager your commitment to the vision and values within the service must be demonstrated by action and the way in which you behave. You must become a role model for your team if you are to help them to commit to the same values and vision. This will inspire the team to follow your lead.

Reflect on it

1.3 Mission statement

Reflect on your commitment to the vision and mission statement of the organisation for which you work. How might you demonstrate your commitment to the service to others?

Evidence opportunity

1.3 Leading by example

Show your assessor how you build your team's commitment to the service and its values by consistently demonstrating your own commitment and expressing your own vision.

AC 1.4 Support a positive values-based culture within a team by developing, implementing and reviewing strategies

Here, you will be required to develop, implement and review strategies that include:

- *action planning and reviewing of team(s) against service vision and related achievements*
- *commitment by all to a values-based team culture in support of the service vision.*

We are all familiar with companies such as Airbnb and Apple. One of the reasons they are all successful companies is that they deliver a service.

A major influence has been the development in these companies of a positive values-based culture, one in which employees share the whole ethos and vision of the company and are rewarded for it in diverse ways. These companies demonstrate real passion for what they do and engender this in their employees by involving them in decisions and providing significant time to help them to develop and be involved in change, and to be rewarded for their input.

Action planning and reviewing of team against service vision and related achievements

In devising an action plan and developing strategies, you first need to get together a planning group made up of individuals from the community that are involved in making the change. These can be the team in the setting and other stakeholders. You might also include family, carers, advocates and commissioning agencies. The first step is to describe the vision or what needs to be done and then say what success would look like.

Commitment by all to a values-based team culture in support of the service vision

Commitment by the team means that they can accomplish great things and move effortlessly towards the vision of the setting. Teams that self-manage and that are empowered to make their own decisions get the jobs done on their own terms and are willing to go the extra mile to support the service vision.

According to Skills for Care, workplace culture is the 'character and personality of your organisation' and having a positive one means quality care and support will be delivered.

Evidence opportunity

1.4 Strategies that support positive values-based cultures in teams

Show your assessor how you develop, implement and review strategies that include:

- ✔ action planning and reviewing of team(s) against service vision and related achievements
- ✔ commitment by all to a values-based team culture in support of the service vision.

Reflect on it

1.4 Strategies that support positive values-based cultures in teams

How do you intend to ensure that all of your staff are committed to a positive values-based culture?

Reflect on it

1.4 Positive values-based culture

Your organisation's leadership, values, beliefs, behaviours and the attitudes of the people all make up your culture.

How might you plan for a culture change in your own team to make it clear that you are developing a positive values-based culture?

AC 1.5 Demonstrate values and behaviours which recognise and champion diversity, equality and inclusion within the team

Here, you will be required to develop strategies that demonstrate methods of championing diversity and equality and implementing these in the setting.

The document 'Evidence review and sector consultation to inform Skills for Care strategy (Skills for Care, 2021) demonstrates a commitment to the development of inclusive cultures and workplaces free from discrimination. Demonstrating equality, diversity and inclusivity in the workplace is so beneficial to organisations as research shows that staff who are part of an equal and inclusive culture feel psychologically safe. This positive impact on workplace culture helps to decrease sickness absence and improve retention.

By creating genuinely inclusive workplaces and demonstrating a commitment to diversity and inclusion, your setting will communicate to the people using the service, to staff and to potential employees that the service is becoming more diverse and less exclusive.

Unconscious bias in the workplace can threaten practice and may hinder progress towards a truly diverse service. Looking at the way you currently interview for new staff and giving everybody a fair chance to succeed will be a step in the right direction.

You might also start to acknowledge religious and cultural holidays to ensure that employees are valued for their differences. Not everyone celebrates Christmas, so being flexible and enabling staff to celebrate their own religious holidays and events will demonstrate inclusion.

Staff should be asked to provide feedback about how inclusive they feel the setting really is. By encouraging discussion you will show staff that their opinions are important.

Take steps to address microaggressions – these are common but subtle behaviours that show bias against various marginalised groups. This is often unintentional, and some people may not realise that what they do and say is actually discriminatory. By ensuring that your setting values equality and inclusion and strives to respect all differences you will be able to create a positive culture that champions dignity and respect for all.

Reflect on it

1.5 Unconscious bias and microaggressions

Think about how you would tackle unconscious bias and microaggressions within the workplace and make notes on what you could do.

Evidence opportunity

1.5 Championing diversity, equality and inclusion

With other members of staff, undertake a small project to identify methods of championing diversity and equality and implementing these in the setting. What sorts of strategies will you use to show how you are creating a culture that celebrates inclusivity and diversity?

LO2 Be able to manage teamwork

AC 2.1 Engage team members in agreeing team objectives

Here, you will be required to show you can facilitate inclusion when agreeing team objectives to support strategy and vision.

Effective teams share a commitment to achieving the common objectives of the organisation and work well together. The overall objectives that need to be achieved should be clearly identified and defined in terms that each team member understands. Participation of each team member is encouraged, and they are given free rein to contribute ideas.

Evidence opportunity

2.1 Facilitate inclusion of team members when agreeing team objectives

Show your assessor how you facilitate inclusion when agreeing team objectives to support strategy and vision.

Alternatively, you could ask a team member to write a detailed testimonial for you to show how they were included in agreeing team objectives on a project.

AC 2.2 Encourage creativity and innovation in team members

Here, you will be required to show you can facilitate creativity and innovation when agreeing team objectives and plans.

Planning how to meet team objectives

It is essential to create a team culture where innovation and creativity are valued. In doing so, team members are more likely to speak up and to have the confidence to give their ideas freely. Staff need to feel that ideas they generate will be considered and that their contribution will make a difference to organisational objectives and goals.

Team objectives that are created with the team members enable them to feel connected to the organisation's larger goals. By setting up a team meeting with the whole staff, you can start to address this by discussing how the team feel they are progressing, their successes so far and where they would like to be in the future.

Objectives might then be planned which align with the wider organisation plans. This will enable staff to see how their individual work fits into the strategic plans for the setting. Creating objectives in this way ensures that staff feel ownership of the plans and trust and collaboration will develop as a result.

Agreeing a team plan

A team plan outlines the future direction of the team, setting out its objectives and how these will be achieved. It is a step-by-step guide that enables each staff member to work towards the objectives of the team.

By outlining the vision and objectives of the team, you can clearly state how the team's vision will affect the setting and help it to reach its goals.

Key performance indicators

Key performance indicator (KPI) measurements are used to gauge long-term performance. For example, you may set a KPI for your staff to undertake all mandatory training within a specific time frame. This can be measured by checking training records. You might also include KPIs within the plan to show the success of goals. By setting KPIs, staff have tangible goals to work towards that can be measured. For example, one of your teams' objectives might be to improve the experience of care. For this objective to be met, a time frame and a quantitative measure will need to be applied. You might look at satisfaction surveys of the individuals using the service from the last year and measure the level of satisfaction as a percentage. The target for the coming year can be set to exceed or match the level.

Staff can be involved in setting KPIs and time frames for completion. These need to be achievable and realistic goals for the whole team.

Encouraging creativity

There are a number of ways in which innovative and creative strategies might be used to encourage staff to contribute to change.

Kaizen and lean management philosophies

Kaizen is a Japanese business philosophy of continuous improvement of working practices. The expression comes from two Japanese words that translate as 'good change' or 'improvement'. As part of lean management, it now refers to rapid improvement processes to eliminate waste, improve productivity and achieve sustained continual improvement. The philosophies of Kaizen and lean management describe a culture of continuous improvement where all employees improve the organisation by being actively involved in the change.

Kaizen is part action plan and part philosophy and has been adopted by some hospital trusts in the UK to engage in continuous improvement in a meaningful way. It could be adopted in adult social care in much the same way as it has been used in hospitals.

The Virginia Mason Institute in Seattle, USA, provides training to enable care providers to introduce and develop this culture into their work to improve the quality and safety of their practice. Using the Kaizen approach, week-long Rapid Process Improvement Workshops (RPIW) where staff at all levels, particularly those engaged in the actual practice under scrutiny, take part in a process of change in a given area. At these events, an initial review of the current state of the practice is looked at and a plan for improvements developed. Initial visits and then follow-ups to the area are undertaken and staff are involved in implementing the improvements and reviewing and adjusting them to find out what works. When the changed process is in place, staff report their findings to the public with the results after 30 days, 60 days and 90 days. For example, a most successful RPIW was the reduction in the time it took to treat individuals with sepsis on arrival.

The same process can be implemented for adult social care. If a problem in the workplace exists, Kaizen methodology can be brought in to fix it. Once we acknowledge the problem, we can begin to act.

A Kaizen process:

1. identifies a problem or opportunity
2. analyzes the current process
3. identifies or develops an ideal solution
4. implements the solution
5. studies the results and if anything doesn't work then it is adjusted
6. standardizes the solution
7. repeats for the next problem.

The philosophy behind Kaizen is to build a culture where all employees become actively engaged in suggesting and implementing improvements to the setting.

> **Research it**
>
> **2.2 Lean management principles**
>
> Look at the Kaizen philosophy and lean management principles and make notes on them. How might you incorporate such an approach in your work?

AC 2.3 Agree roles and responsibilities, considering individual team member's strengths and developmental needs

Here, you will need to show that you acknowledge individual skill sets, interests, knowledge, expertise and development needs while motivating all individuals, including the topics covered here.

The success of a team will depend on bringing together people with diverse skills and knowledge and if they lack these, encouraging them to undertake training and education. As described in this unit in AC1.1, a multidisciplinary team can best meet the needs of the people using a service.

Recognising the diversity of skills within the staff will be a useful starting point. Some staff will have experience which they can pass on to others. They can also be asked to take on more responsibility to help and support their colleagues and can be a good source for coaching. It is also important for staff satisfaction that strengths are built on and opportunities for further training are offered.

Listen to what it is the employee wants and needs to help them to do their job and then acknowledge that by showing your appreciation. A simple word of praise for what they are doing may be all that is needed. If they require additional support or training, then this might be more readily available through redeploying other staff to help them. The point is to listen to the staff member and identify what it is they need. Only then might you be able to offer a solution.

Staff who are not assigned their first choice of role

Members of staff may apply for one role within the setting and then be offered another and this may fall outside their comfort zone. Discussion about what support they require and any additional training may be helpful here to re-motivate them.

Staff who might disengage with the process

These staff, also known as plateaued performers, have reached points in their work where they no longer engage well with work. They may feel bored by what they are doing or are showing less motivation and/or enthusiasm than others. A conversation about what is happening for them at work and how they believe they might feel more re-energised to find some motivation at work would be useful. They may simply feel unchallenged and need a new focus.

Staff who might demonstrate complacency and/or disengagement

Much like the above, these staff members may need a new challenge in their work to get them to re-engage with the team. Maybe they have been passed over for promotion or a training course and are finding it hard to continue in the same role.

What might you do? You can never overestimate the importance of good communication in such situations, and you will need to listen and get involved with staff to determine how to move forward.

All of the above categories show staff who have been demotivated in some way. Some may be disappointed about not being given an additional responsibility or a promotion. Others may simply be less enthusiastic about a project and may begin to disengage from it. These sorts of behaviours can quickly escalate and other members of staff may pick up on the mood and start to feel the same. As a manager you need to be aware of the mood of your team and deal with any negativity before it grows.

Reflect on it

2.3 Motivating your staff

As a manager, knowing what everyone in your team has to offer will aid the success of the team. You need to know what motivates each member of staff and how to ensure that they continue to give their best. How, though, might you deal with:

- staff who are not assigned their first choice of role
- staff who might disengage with the process
- staff who show less motivation and/or enthusiasm than others
- staff who demonstrate complacency and/or disengagement?

Evidence opportunity

2.3 Agree roles, detailing responsibilities and personal work objectives

How do you agree roles with team members and detail the responsibilities and personal work objectives with team members? Show how you acknowledge individual skill sets, interests, knowledge, expertise and development needs while motivating all individuals, for example:

- ✔ staff who do not get their first choice of role
- ✔ staff who might disengage with the process
- ✔ staff who show less motivation and/or enthusiasm than others
- ✔ staff who demonstrate complacency and/or disengagement.

AC 2.4 Support team members to work towards team objectives

Here, you will be required to show how you implement systems that enable team members to match their personal goals to the overall objectives of the service.

Adult social care workers are subject to performance reviews, supervision and appraisal, and a review or appraisal is the ideal time to set objectives for the coming year and for change in their workload or requests for training. SMART targets are a useful way of identifying personal objectives.

Case study

2.4 Workload and training and development

Meeting with Jasmine

Workload – Jasmine feels that currently her workload level is fine, and she is enjoying working with the individuals who have come to the service recently. She feels the changes the team made by allocating a named staff member to a group of individuals is useful. Jasmine feels her confidence has grown and she is relishing the more independent way of working. I commented that as her team leader I had noticed that she was making appropriate decisions for her group and was working well in the team.

Training and development

So far this year Jasmine has attended the health and safety update and two further in-house training courses. She seems very keen to undertake a foundation degree in Health and Social Care at her local university. We discussed what this would entail, and Jasmine mentioned that it was one day a week in college for two years with additional days off to undertake further work placement activity. We devised the following action plan:

- Jasmine to advise of fees and days required out of work by 17/10/23.
- Jasmine to approach the college and to get an application form and start the process of applying by 20/11/23.
- TT (the team leader) will approach the area manager to obtain permission in principle for attendance and to inform Jasmine of the decision by 20/11/23.

Further meeting to take place on 22/11/23 to discuss next steps.

Staff must remain 'fit for practice' by undertaking professional development activities regularly (training for example) and updating their own CPD records to show how they have developed. By undertaking this course and carrying out the activities throughout this book you are engaging in continuing professional development (CPD) and providing evidence through the activities you complete. Your staff also require development and in supervision or appraisal sessions you need to work with them to identify their own strategies for development.

Evidence opportunity

2.4 Implement systems to support team members to work towards objectives and monitor progress

Show your assessor how you implement systems that enable team members to match their personal goals to the overall objectives of the service.

Case study 2.4 shows one way in which you might set objectives. You may wish to show or discuss with your manager how you set your personal work objectives for the coming year. You could also discuss with them how you work with a member of your own team to identify opportunities for their development and growth.

AC 2.5 Review team progress against objectives

Here, you will be required to show how you review team members' progress in order to assist them in meeting their personal goals and the overall objectives of the service.

Having defined your team's work objectives and met with them to clearly explain the work and tasks to be performed, you now need to undertake a review of whether their performance has been successful. For example, perhaps one of your team objectives was to ensure that all staff undertake annual mandatory training as soon as previous training is out of date. This can be measured by checking the training schedule or by meeting with staff to ask for self-appraisal on this objective.

Evidence opportunity

2.5 Review SMART targets

Complete an appraisal of the recent SMART targets you set for the team. How have the team fared? What evidence have you collected?

AC 2.6 Facilitate opportunities for team members to reflect on progress

Here, you will be required to show that you use constructive evaluation and feedback to inform individual action plans for continued professional development and ongoing learning for the team(s) and how you recognise progress achieved towards team and personal work objectives through some of the topics discussed in this section.

Individual and team feedback

Feedback to the team should relate to the objectives set and to the work they are doing. This sort of feedback can be done at team briefings or in meetings.

Individuals' supervision – self and others

During supervision with individual staff members, you can highlight where the team is in achieving group goals and can then pinpoint how the staff member has been part of that achievement. This can be a good way to motivate staff as they can see that what they are doing is having a positive impact upon the team and the setting. This might also be an opportunity to praise and reward somebody for their good work.

Individual appraisal – self and others

As stated above, staff appraisal can be an opportunity for growth and self-development. Encouraging staff to reflect upon the objectives and then appraising their performance can be motivating if they can see how their work impacts the setting.

As the manager you need to recognise the progress that is being made and reward staff for their performance.

Individual/team observations – formal and informal

Observing the way in which a practice is carried out is a useful way to check progress of staff and to determine whether best practice is being employed. Informal observations occur when you happen to notice a member of staff carrying out their daily duty. Formal observations are those which are arranged in advance for a particular date and time.

Auditing processes and procedures

There are many types of audits, which are simply systematic reviews of care measured against criteria and are designed to improve care.

The effectiveness of policies within a care organisation can be checked if an audit is carried out. For example, you might trace an individual's complaint from the time the letter was received to the time it was dealt with. By going through the complaints policy, you can tell whether the stages have been followed or not. Other forms of audit are financial, internal and organisational.

Informal and formal inspection processes

The thought of undergoing an inspection is often an area of concern for staff but if informal inspections are part of a daily routine, where the conditions within the workplace are looked at for safety and efficiency reasons, this need not be the case. Formal inspections may be carried out by external bodies to check that the setting is fit for purpose and is doing what it should to protect the safety of those using the service.

Reflect on it

2.6 Individual development

Provide evidence of a meeting with a member of your staff (you should be mindful of the need for confidentiality and should anonymise the record). Describe how you prepared for the meeting and how you approached the subject of the individual's continuing development. Show how you used constructive evaluation and feedback to inform individual action plans for CPD and ongoing learning for them and the team.

Evaluate your own performance by writing a reflective account of what you did, why you did it that way and the outcome of the meeting.

Evidence opportunity

2.6 Recognise progress achieved towards team and personal work objectives

Provide evidence in your portfolio to show your assessor how you recognise the progress that has been achieved towards the team's and your personal work objectives, including that achieved through feedback and the topics covered in this section.

Feedback from those in receipt of care and support

In 2013, the NHS launched its Friends and Family Test (FFT) to help service providers to know whether the people who use their service are happy with the service provided or whether improvements are needed. A simple leaflet that is quick to fill in is given to individuals, friends and family.

Your care organisation may use a similar tool to measure satisfaction.

Sometimes individuals may not be able to complete paperwork, so other ways of monitoring satisfaction may be required. The Helen Sanderson Associate website (Helen Sanderson Associates, n.d.) provides a variety of tools that can be used to capture much needed information about your service.

For example, the person-centred thinking tools are a set of easy-to-use templates that give structure to conversations. They can be used to capture information from an individual using the service that feeds into care and support planning. The individual can sit with a member of staff and answer questions about their care and the support they need.

The 'What's working/not working' template also provides a visual tool to find out about the person's current situation: what they are happy with and what they would change.

Reflect on it

2.6 Inspection, observations, audit and feedback

How have you used constructive evaluation and feedback from staff to plan for continued professional development and ongoing learning for the team?

How do you recognise and celebrate the progress and objectives achieved?

AC 2.7 Provide feedback which recognises team performance against team objectives

In this section, you will need to show how you provide feedback and the methods you use, including, for example, the ones discussed here.

We all like to know what we are doing well and what we might be able to improve upon so being given some feedback is useful. Positive and negative feedback impacts the motivation and performance of staff so it is essential that it is planned. You need to consider how and why you are going to deliver feedback and also what outcome you want from it.

If you are delivering negative feedback and there is an issue that the staff member must address this must be clearly communicated to them. A relaxed atmosphere and a conversation that is friendly will help to prevent the staff member from feeling threatened or defensive. The issue needs to be explained in an objective manner and specific examples given.

Sensitive topics must be discussed in a private place which is free from distractions. You need to be specific and polite and make the focus the behaviour you wish to change, not the staff member's personal characteristics. Also make sure you listen to their responses.

Team-based feedback

At a team level this might be during meetings when organisational performance is looked at and feedback is provided to demonstrate how productive projects have been. Of course, feedback may also be negative, and the team made aware of improvements that must be made.

360-degree feedback

360-degree feedback is a method of performance appraisal which gathers feedback from a number of sources, including peers, direct reports, senior colleagues and individuals using the service. This variety of feedback can offer line managers a wide-ranging perspective and help them to make performance management a more objective and fair process.

Constructive criticism

Occasionally, it is necessary to give negative feedback to staff in order to address issues with unsatisfactory performance. This can inevitably cause conflict and can be quite uncomfortable. Individuals receive criticism in different ways and you need to ensure that you are sensitive to how they will be feeling at this time.

A good approach is to provide a positive point initially and to say clearly what was good about it. You can stress how well they did and what you liked about their performance. When critiquing their performance, you could highlight this as 'an area for improvement'. Again, you must specifically draw attention to what you expect the team member to do and give a clear indication of how they might achieve this. You can then constructively give advice on how they can change. Finally, by ending with a positive point you can do much to rebuild self-esteem in what can often be a rather uncomfortable situation.

Supervision(s) and appraisal

Supervision is a practice that provides regular, ongoing support for staff and, as such, time should be set aside for it. Staff need to be clear about what supervision is for and given space to discuss issues in a confidential and safe environment.

Supervision supports good practice, enabling staff to maintain and improve standards of care and to reflect upon their practice. Similarly, appraisal is about enabling staff to reflect on their work and learning needs in order to improve their performance. This can be achieved by discussing their development and feedback on their job performance in a way that is constructive and motivational. It should result in an effective personal development plan which can be revisited and updated continually.

Coaching and mentoring

Coaching and mentoring are very similar, so make sure you understand the difference. For more on coaching and mentoring, see Unit 500, AC2.1.

One-way communication

We often engage in one-way communication; this means the way in which information is transferred from one person to another with little opportunity to give feedback to the sender. Sometimes we do this to transmit a fact, or to instruct somebody to do something. One-way communication is not effective and there needs to be reciprocal methods by which individuals are able to give feedback about the process. Stakeholders and staff are entitled to personal, two-way communication, and face-to-face meetings are essential to ensure positive outcomes.

Evidence opportunity

2.7 Provide feedback on performance for individuals and the whole team

Using the headings in AC2.7, show your assessor how you provide and receive feedback on performance for individuals and the whole team.

LO3 Be able to support the wellbeing and resilience of team members

AC 3.1 Describe factors that influence the health and wellbeing of team members

Here, you will be required to show that you can identify and describe the potential health and wellbeing issues that may arise within the team.

Many internal and external factors affect the health and wellbeing of the team. A culture in which leaders do not provide clear team goals or fail to include staff in decisions in the development of the setting will lead to staff feeling pressured and out of control. Increased workload, pressure and poor communication all take their toll on staff wellbeing and can lead to a toxic work environment.

A toxic work environment is one in which staff experience mental and physical health problems such as stress, anxiety, depression and many other negative effects. This can result in increased staff absences due to ill health.

Organisational changes are common due to external legal factors and this can affect the trust in a team and diminish their sense of belonging. When leaders are unable to embrace change and new ways of working, staff are more likely to feel devalued and worthless.

In addition, the type of work that adult social care requires can result in distressing emotions and feelings, and if there is no outlet for staff to express these, they may turn to unhelpful coping strategies, such as alcohol or drug abuse.

Reflect on it

3.1 Factors affecting health and wellbeing of the work environment

Think about work environments you have been part of and consider the factors that made it negative and/or positive. Maybe you had a manager who micromanaged everything you did or perhaps you had a manager who trusted you and enabled you to make decisions? How did this affect you and your team?

AC 3.2 Explain own role in monitoring, assessing and promoting the health and wellbeing of team members

Here, you will be required to explain how you ensure that team members are aware of health and wellbeing issues and encourage better health and wellbeing within the setting.

Role modelling

As manager, you can make the necessary changes to ensure that staff health is promoted and monitored. You should role-model the behaviour you wish your staff to display. For example, you may encourage your staff to take regular breaks and to leave on time but if you do not follow this advice too, then staff will feel conflicted and you will not see positive changes.

Importance of supervision

Care work can sometimes be distressing, particularly when dealing with people who are very ill or may demonstrate behaviour that challenges. Ensuring that regular supervision is available, so that staff have opportunities to talk about events and critical incidents, as well as encouraging staff to engage in reflective practice are helpful strategies to open up conversations about wellbeing.

You may have heard of the term 'psychologically safe', which was created in 1999 by Harvard professor Amy Edmonson and means the 'absence of interpersonal fear', or the ability to speak up at work without fearing any reprisals. **Psychological safety** means that staff are able to ask for help, and to admit mistakes. They will feel at liberty to raise any concerns they may have about practice and will not think twice about suggesting ideas or challenging ways of working. This open and honest approach to work will improve outcomes and also staff motivation and trust.

Work–life balance

There is a lot of discussion about **work–life balance**, but how easy is it for staff to practice it? Family-friendly policies means that staff who are parents are able to enjoy flexible working so that they can take and/or collect their children from school, attend school events and attend other family commitments. Staff should not be made to feel guilty for taking a child or ageing parent to the doctor, for example. These types of event can produce much stress as staff may feel they are letting other members of the team down or are not seen to be pulling their weight. As manager, developing a flexible approach to hours worked will be useful for staff and make them feel more supported.

KEY TERMS

Psychological safety: The 'absence of interpersonal fear' or the ability to speak out at work without fear of reprisal.

Work–life balance: Giving equal priority to the demands of work and the demands of our personal life.

Fairness at work

Fairness and parity at work are also high on job satisfaction surveys. If staff feel they are dealt with fairly, this will build trust. If pay is fair and there are equal opportunities across job roles, staff will feel they are being treated with respect. As a manager you must be impartial with respect to promotions and not simply reward favourites. All staff need to believe that they are being treated fairly, regardless of personal characteristics, and need to be able to challenge unfair decisions.

Regular one-to-ones to check in with staff are a good way to monitor and assess the health and wellbeing of staff.

Mental health

Research has shown that poor mental health is a contributor to wider health inequalities, being associated with increased health-risk behaviours and increased morbidity and mortality from physical ill health. Promoting good mental health, therefore, has significant potential benefits – not only the improvement to health outcomes and life expectancy, but also improving educational and economic outcomes.

The Care Policy and Evaluation Centre and London School of Economics published a report entitled 'The economic case for investing in the prevention of mental health conditions in the UK' (McDaid et al., 2022), which shows that in 2019 mental health problems cost the UK economy at least £117.9 billion a year (£100.8 billion in England; £8.8 billion in Scotland; £4.8 billion in Wales and £3.4 billion in Northern Ireland). These costs do not include those associated with dementia, intellectual disabilities, alcohol or substance misuse and deliberate self-harm or suicide.

This research recognising mental health issues and its effects on physical health further highlights the impact this has on care settings. Additional resources will be required to ensure that mental health issues are not only recognised but are adequately resourced to manage the increased risk to physical health. This is likely to further impact already scarce financial and staffing resources.

Research it

3.2 Wellbeing at work

Skills for Care's 'Wellbeing at work' resources (Skills for Care, n.d. a and Skills for Care, n.d. b) recognise the impact of stress and burnout on adult social care staff. It is essential that people with care and support needs and their families receive good quality care to live independently, so supporting the health and wellbeing of the workforce is crucial.

Also provided are webinars and information about health and wellbeing hubs.

Evidence opportunity

3.2 Health and wellbeing of staff

Write a short report to explain how you currently monitor, assess and promote the health and wellbeing of your staff.

AC 3.3 Explain the process to follow when concerns have been raised about the health and wellbeing and resilience of team members

Here, you will need to explain how you implement systems to ensure that a culture within the setting exists to enable health and wellbeing concerns of team members can be addressed safely.

In 2022, there were around 1.5 million people estimated to be working in adult social care (Skills for Care, 2022). This shows how the population's health and wellbeing is dependent upon the commitment of adult care professionals to be able to carry out their duties safely.

As a result of the COVID-19 pandemic and the impact this had on social care, many adult care staff did significantly more than they were contracted to do. Without this effort, the quality of care provided to individuals would have suffered enormously. Such effort is not sustainable and now workforce burnout is becoming a widespread issue.

In May 2021, the government published a report addressing workforce burnout and resilience in the NHS and social care (House of Commons, 2021). The aim of the report was to test the resilience of the NHS and social care workforce and determine how resilience could be strengthened in the future. The scale of workforce burnout across NHS and social care and how it is assessed and caused was also to be addressed.

Before the COVID-19 pandemic it was becoming difficult to attract and retain skilled staff. Long hours, poor pay and lack of resources were often cited as reasons for burnout and staff leaving care roles. With the advent of the pandemic, this has been exacerbated with exhausted staff who have seen no real increase in salary and no let up with respect to long hours at work. This, together with the mandatory requirement to be vaccinated against COVID-19 in order to work in care has meant further staff have opted to leave, with replacements proving very difficult to find.

The importance of creating a culture across care sectors where staff feel supported to speak up when they see things going wrong has been highlighted in the report. The establishment of the National Guardian's Office (NGO) in 2016 provided a forum for staff to speak up through 'Freedom to Speak Up' Guardians. In December 2020, the NGO published data in its Annual Report 2020 (NGO, 2020) that indicated that a record number of cases had emerged and these included reports of concern for individuals' safety or quality of care, and bullying and harassment. There were also concerns raised about social distancing, personal protective equipment, redeployment of workers and general anxiety about the pandemic. At the time of the publication of the report, Freedom to Speak Up Guardians had yet to be established in social care and this was described as 'a yawning gap'. Workers in all settings should have the ability to speak up about their concerns and be secure in the knowledge that leaders and managers will listen.

In your own setting, a forum in which staff are able to speak up about whatever is on their mind will create a safe culture in which to work.

Although the regular team meeting might at first be considered an appropriate forum for this to occur, some staff may feel uncomfortable speaking out during a whole team event. If your supervision is a regular monthly event, this might be a preferred opportunity for adding a health and wellbeing discussion as part of the agenda.

Evidence opportunity

3.3 Workforce burnout and resilience

How are concerns for staff wellbeing raised in your setting?

What support and systems are in place to ensure that the setting can address the concerns of staff safely?

AC 3.4 Lead practice which develops resilience in team members

Here, you will be required to show how you implement systems that enable team members to match their personal goals to the overall objectives of the service.

We all experience stress and adversity, but some people are better at managing it than others. Resilience is not about avoiding stress but about facing it and learning to adapt your actions and behaviours to recover quickly from any difficulties.

Building a resilient team requires not just individual resilience but developing a culture of belonging, positive relationships and purpose in the setting. Good communication, transparency and listening to staff will help to build a team that trusts each other, which in turn will lead to greater team resilience.

Teams who feel supported and safe can effectively take on changes and challenges and this can be developed by ensuring that there are opportunities for staff to get to know each other to build connections. Having a resilient leader will help to maintain an optimistic outlook when challenges arise.

Finally, team resilience is enhanced by building psychological safety, where the team can take risks by offering creative ideas without fear of being criticised or ostracised. Resilient teams have respect for each other and can openly and honestly voice their ideas and opinions.

Stretch and challenge

3.4 Staff health and wellbeing checks

Review your staff records and add a health and wellbeing check to the format.

Monitor staff and determine how you might improve your current practice. How could you make your setting a more flexible and family-friendly one?

AC 3.5 Implement procedures which enable team members to access support/services to enhance their health, wellbeing and resilience

Here, you will be required to show how you implement systems that enable team members to enhance their health and wellbeing.

In April 2022, the Chartered Institute of Personnel and Development (CIPD) published the results of their annual health and wellbeing survey report, 'Health and wellbeing at work 2022' (CIPD, 2022). This provides data on mental health, managing attendance at work and the need to upskill managers to support wellbeing. A key finding of the survey was the lack of focus on health and wellbeing following the COVID-19 pandemic and that there has been a 'slip in attention' to employees' mental health and physical health. There was agreement, however, that employee wellbeing is still on senior leaders' agendas but the percentage tackling it had dropped since the last survey.

The survey commented upon **presenteeism** or working when unwell, with 81 per cent of organisations reporting this practice among staff working from home and 65 per cent reporting it for staff in the physical workplace. There was also evidence of staff using annual leave and holiday entitlement rather than reporting sickness.

KEY TERM

Presenteeism: Being at work for more hours than is required, or when ill, because of insecurity about one's job.

This practice of presenteeism is widely thought to be a sign of an unhealthy workplace and managers should look at the underlying factors for this and develop positive plans to tackle unmanageable workloads. Staff may be concerned about their jobs or even how taking sickness will be viewed by others in the workplace. The preference then is to go to work even though ill. This attitude of working when ill may also be seen in staff with mental health issues who do not want to take time off to get help for this.

With the rise in the number of reported mental health issues, managers need to recognise that mental as well as physical wellbeing in the workplace is of the highest importance. To support the physical and mental health of your staff, you should ensure that they have access to counselling services or employee assistance programmes (EAP) if required. As a manager, you need to support your teams and undertake sensitive conversations to help staff to access expert help when they need it. All staff should be encouraged to have a good self-care routine including a healthy approach to diet, relaxation and sleep.

The 2022 CIPD survey identified three top benefits for employers who have an increased focus on employee wellbeing:

- a healthier and more inclusive culture
- better work–life balance
- better morale and engagement.

Rather than being something that is 'nice to have', staff health and wellbeing should be central to all your organisation plans.

Evidence opportunity

3.5 Health and wellbeing at work

Discuss with your assessor how you implement systems that enable team members to enhance their health and wellbeing.

Legislation

Legislation	Key points
Equality Act 2010	This is an umbrella act bringing together legislation that deals with race, disability and gender. It highlights protected characteristics of age, gender reassignment, pregnancy, religion, marriage and civil partnerships, and sexual orientation in an attempt to end discrimination.

References

Helen Sanderson Associates (n.d.) 'One-page profiles'. http://helensandersonassociates.co.uk/person-centred-practice/one-page-profiles/

House of Commons Health and Social Care Committee (2021) 'Workforce burnout and resilience in the NHS and social care'. https://committees.parliament.uk/publications/6158/documents/68766/default/

McDaid, D., Park, A-L., Davidson, G., John, A., Knifton, L., McDaid, S., Morton, A., Thorpe, L. and Wilson, N. (2022) *The economic case for investing in the prevention of mental health conditions in the UK (summary)*. London: The Mental Health Foundation.

Mullins, L.J. (2010) *Management and Organisational Behaviour*, London: Financial Times/Prentice Hall.

National Guardian's Office (2020) 'Annual Report 2020'. https://nationalguardian.org.uk/wp-content/uploads/2021/04/NGO_AR_2020_Digital.pdf

NHS Digital (2022) 'NHS workforce statistics – July 2022'. https://digital.nhs.uk/data-and-information/publications/statistical/nhs-workforce-statistics/july-2022

Skills for Care (2021) 'Evidence review and sector consultation to inform Skills for Care strategy'. www.skillsforcare.org.uk/resources/documents/Adult-social-care-workforce-data/Evidence-review-and-consultation-analysis.pdf

Skills for Care (2022) 'The size and structure of the adult social care sector and workforce in England'. www.skillsforcare.org.uk/adult-social-care-workforce-data/Workforce-intelligence/publications/national-information/The-size-and-structure-of-the-adult-social-care-sector-and-workforce-in-England.aspx

Skills for Care (n.d. a) 'Looking after yourself'. www.skillsforcare.org.uk/resources/documents/Support-for-leaders-and-managers/Managing-people/Wellbeing/Digital-wellbeing-Z-Card.pdf

Skills for Care (n.d. b) 'Wellbeing for registered managers: A bite size practical guide'. www.skillsforcare.org.uk/resources/documents/Support-for-leaders-and-managers/Managing-people/Wellbeing/Wellbeing-for-registered-managers-a-bite-size-practical-guide.pdf

Tannenbaum, R. and Schmidt, W.H. (1973) 'How to choose a leadership pattern', *Harvard Business Review, May 3–12.*

Tilmouth, T. and Quallington, J. (2016) *Diploma in Leadership for Health and Social Care.* London: Hodder Education.

Tuckman, B.W. (1965) 'Developmental sequence in small groups', *Psychological Bulletin*, 63(6), 384–99.

Wheelan, S.A. (2005) *Creating Effective Teams: A guide for members and leaders.* London: Sage.

Useful resources and further reading

Cavazotte, F., Moreno, V. and Hickmann, M. (2012) 'Effects of leader intelligence, personality and emotional intelligence on transformational leadership and managerial performance', *The Leadership Quarterly*, 23(3): 443–55.

Department of Health, Skills for Care and Skills for Health (2013) 'The Code of Conduct in action: A user guide for healthcare support workers and adult social care workers in England'. **www.skillsforcare.org.uk/resources/documents/Support-for-leaders-and-managers/Managing-people/Code-of-conduct/Guidance-on-the-Code-of-Conduct-for-support-workers.pdf**

Goleman, D. (1998) *Working with Emotional Intelligence.* New York: Bantam Books.

Gopee, N. and Galloway, J. (2009) *Leadership and Management in Health Care.* London: Sage.

McGrath, J. and Bates, B. (2017) *The Little Book of Big Management Theories and How to Use Them.* London: Pearson.

Newton, R. (2011) *The Management Book: How to manage your team to deliver outstanding results.* Upper Saddle River, NJ: Prentice Hall/Financial Times.

Owen, J. (2015) *The Mindset of Success: From good management to great leadership.* London: Kogan Page.

Peters, S. (2012) *The Chimp Paradox: The mind management programme to help you achieve success, confidence and happiness.* London: Vermilion.

Reynolds, M. and Holwell, S. (eds.) *Systems Approaches to Managing Change: A practical guide.* London: Springer.

Skills for Care (2016) 'Manager Induction Standards'. **www.skillsforcare.org.uk/Support-for-leaders-and-managers/Developing-leaders-and-managers/Manager-induction-standards.aspx**

Unit 505

Leading team learning and professional development in adult care

GLH 30

About this unit

People receiving care services must be confident that they can trust those who deliver care to not only know what to do but also to know how to do it well. This requires you to continually update and extend your knowledge and skills and, as a manager, to ensure that your team is also equipped with the appropriate knowledge and skills to fulfil their roles effectively.

Personal professional development is a journey for the whole of your life; it does not end with the completion of a course or a specific activity but should, ideally, be an 'activity of daily living'. The secret of successful personal development is to learn to be reflective and questioning about both the things you know and the things you do not know.

This unit will help you to examine and assess your understanding of professional development, supervision and performance management, and the responsibilities that these concepts entail as a manager and leader. You will develop your reflective and individual planning skills to help you determine how you can most effectively support your own development and that of others.

Learning outcomes

By the end of this unit, you will:

1 Understand principles of learning and professional development in adult care.

2 Be able to lead learning and professional development practices.

Getting started

Before you study the unit, think about the following:

- What does professional development mean to you?
- Why is professional development important when working in adult care settings?
- What types of support and resources are available to staff teams to support their professional development?

LO1 Understand principles of learning and professional development in adult care

AC 1.1 Outline the range of required and recommended learning and development for teams in adult care

Here, you will be required to outline the range of requirements and other recommended knowledge for workers in the adult care sector.

Your teams will be made up of people with differing levels of skills and knowledge, and all will require some form of training to maintain standards.

As a minimum, all staff should adhere to the Skills for Care Code of Conduct, which state:

> *As a Healthcare Support Worker or Adult Social Care Worker in England you must:*
>
> 1 *Be accountable by making sure you can answer for your actions or omissions.*
>
> 2 *Promote and uphold the privacy, dignity, rights, health and wellbeing of people who use health and care services and their carers at all times.*
>
> 3 *Work in collaboration with your colleagues to ensure the delivery of high quality, safe and compassionate healthcare, care and support.*
>
> 4 *Communicate in an open and effective way to promote the health, safety and wellbeing of people who use health and care services and their carers.*
>
> 5 *Respect a person's right to confidentiality.*
>
> 6 *Strive to improve the quality of healthcare, care and support through continuing professional development.*
>
> 7 *Uphold and promote equality, diversity and inclusion.*
>
> Source: Skills for Care and Skills for Health (2013)

This Code, based on the principles of protecting the public by promoting best practice, ensures that all care workers are 'working to standard' and providing high quality, compassionate care. It describes the conduct, behaviour and attitudes of care workers that the public who use care services can expect.

The behaviours, attitudes and conduct of staff will be part of their personal values, so the staff you employ should have the right values to work in your setting and in social care. The setting will have its own set of values in order to embed a positive workplace culture and these values should be part of the learning and development strategy.

Care Quality Commission (CQC) requirements

Following the serious case review into the Mid-Staffordshire NHS Trust, the Cavendish Report (2013) recommended changes to the training of care assistants in hospitals, care homes and other provisions, and individuals' own homes to ensure that they provide the highest standard of care. The Report recommended that a training course in fundamental care should be developed that care workers must do before they can care for individuals unsupervised.

Professional development is further reinforced in professional codes and standards of conduct, which articulate the standards that the public can expect from those delivering care. Although not specifically required as care workers are not required to be registered, staff should be aware of the existence of:

- the Code of Conduct for Healthcare Support Workers and Adult Social Care Workers in England (2013)
- the Health and Social Care Act 2008 (Regulated Activities) Regulations 2014 (Regulation 18).

The Health and Social Care Act 2012 and the Care Act 2014 introduced the CQC as the lead inspection and enforcement body for safety and quality of treatment and care matters for people in receipt of a health or adult social care service. The CQC regulates all social care services in the UK, including those provided by local authorities, private and voluntary organisations, as well as the National Health Service. It also provides protection to people being treated or cared for under the Mental Health Act.

The CQC regulations ensure that providers have enough suitably qualified, competent and experienced staff to enable them to meet all the regulatory requirements described in the Health and Social Care Act 2008 (Regulated Activities) Regulations 2014. It also demands that staff must receive 'the support, training, professional development, supervision and appraisals that are necessary for them to carry out their role and responsibilities'. The CQC must refuse registration if providers cannot satisfy that they can and will continue to comply with this regulation.

Providing support, training, professional development, supervision and appraisals ensure that staff are able to develop and improve their knowledge. It is important that you as the manager also update your own knowledge along with that of your staff. For example, supervision and appraisals provide opportunities for staff to discuss the areas they would like to and need to develop, and areas where they need to improve their knowledge and practice. They can then find ways to achieve this, which may include attending a training course, for example. Supporting your staff to undertake further training and development is very important and you should ensure that they have regular supervision sessions and appraisals as well as training and professional development opportunities. This will ensure that all staff are equipped with the most up-to-date knowledge and practice which will enable them to provide the best possible support to those who use social care services.

Care Certificate

The Care Certificate was developed by Skills for Health, Skills for Care and Health Education England as part of the Cavendish Review (2013). Its primary aim is to ensure that social care support workers, care assistants, assistant practitioners and nursing associates have the knowledge and skills to provide safe care. The Care Certificate is an agreed set of standards detailing the knowledge, skills and behaviours expected of those new to the social care sectors. It describes what support workers must know and be able to do as a minimum when they work in care. For those new to care work it is a good course to start their career journey because it supplies a foundation for health and adult social care knowledge.

If this is not already happening in your setting, determine how you might use the Care Certificate to inform your induction training for new staff.

> **Research it**
>
> **1.1 Training resources**
>
> Visit the Skills for Care website and look at the resources for training (Skills for Care, n.d. a).
>
> Look at the Care Certificate Overview and familiarise yourself with the 15 standards required for new staff (see below for more information).

AC 1.2 Explain the differences between learning requirements and continuous professional development

Here, you will explain the role of continuous professional development and different types of learning requirements in adult care.

Induction

Skills for Care highlights the Care Certificate for apprenticeships at Levels 2 and 3 as required training. An induction programme for those new to care might include the 15 standards as outlined in the Care Certificate. The standards are as follows:

- Understand your role
- Your personal development
- Duty of care
- Equality and diversity
- Work in a person-centred way
- Communication
- Privacy and dignity
- Fluids and nutrition
- Awareness of mental health, dementia and learning disability
- Safeguarding adults
- Safeguarding children
- Basic life support
- Health and safety
- Handling information
- Infection prevention and control

Induction helps new team members to fit into your setting and also supports them to be safe in their role. It helps to reduce the risk of new staff feeling out of their depth and stressed. A number of activities can help with this such as shadowing, mentoring, buddying, peer support, values-based learning and additional training around core skills.

Skills for Care have a resource for buddying and mentoring that includes a clear explanation of the differences between the two roles (Skills for Care, n.d. b).

Buddying is an informal and flexible role provided by a peer who has no specialised training. They can assist new staff for a short period of time as they enter a new role and while they are undergoing formal training opportunities. This relationship enables discussions, advice and support.

Mentoring is a more formal, structured process. Often the mentor may be at a higher level in the setting or has previous experience. At the beginning of the process a partnership agreement is established to define structure and boundaries. The focus may be on achieving both short- and longer-term career goals for the mentee but for the mentor there is also a degree of personal and professional development. Any discussions between the mentor and mentee are confidential and there is an expectation that a mentor may provide coaching, advice or act as a facilitator.

Following the COVID-19 pandemic and the urgent need for care settings to recruit new staff, Skills for Care have introduced three packages of learning: Rapid induction programme, Refresher training and Volunteer programme. All three are available through endorsed learning providers and are described below.

Rapid induction programme

The rapid induction programme, completed within five days of starting a new job, requires the following standards to be covered:

- Assisting and moving people
- Basic life support
- Fire safety
- Food safety
- Health and safety awareness
- Infection prevention and control
- Medication management
- Safeguarding (specifically around isolation).

The rapid induction also includes the main knowledge elements from the Care Certificate Standards Self-Assessment Tool, which should be completed by apprentices. In regulated services, a full induction should also be carried out.

Refresher training

This course is for staff who require urgent refresher training which has expired or is due to expire, in order for them to continue to work safely. The eight topic areas are the same as those in the rapid induction programme.

Volunteer programme

This programme includes an introduction to adult social care, highlighting roles and responsibilities, whistle blowing, equality, diversity and person-centred values, telephone support and communication, pain and discomfort, infection prevention and control, food safety, fluids and hydration, and health and safety and stress.

Statutory learning

Statutory learning is training that is required by law. Statutory bodies instruct organisations to provide training on the basis of specific legislation. For example, the Health and Safety at Work Act 1974 and the Management of Health and Safety at Work Regulations 1999 are laws that all staff must be aware of, so health and safety training courses have therefore been developed to ensure that all staff understand their legal obligations in this area.

In adult care settings, all new staff are required to undertake core health and safety awareness and training. This usually includes the following:

- health and safety awareness training
- food hygiene/food safety
- manual handling and/or moving and handling of people
- safeguarding vulnerable adults
- infection prevention and control
- emergency first aid at work.

You might also be required to undertake training in:

- Control of Substances Hazardous to Health (COSHH)
- Reporting of Injuries, Diseases and Dangerous Occurrences Regulations (RIDDOR)
- fire safety awareness
- basic risk assessment.

Mandatory learning

Mandatory training will need to be undertaken by the relevant people, such as you and your staff, to ensure that the service is safe for everyone involved. Mandatory training is important and is needed to comply with legislation, local and national policies as well as agreed ways of working within the setting. Such training might, for example, be offered to comply with health and safety legislation and to reduce the risk of accidents in the setting. As a manager you must ensure that staff are given time to attend mandatory training and are compensated if they are attending in their own time.

Mandatory training might include safeguarding, record keeping, hand hygiene, infection prevention and control, and medicines handling and management. The training offered will depend upon the staff role, so some staff may be required to attend more sessions than others depending upon the role they undertake in the organisation.

Whatever mandatory training is offered, however, is unlikely to be sufficient to meet the responsibility and breadth of expectations for personal and professional development implied in the law and in codes of conduct.

Specific service specialist training

Specialist care training enhances a care worker's role but is neither mandatory nor statutory. It can include training for particular care conditions.

For example, a number of training providers offer accredited Positive Behaviour Support (PBS) training courses for professionals working in mental health and related areas. This sort of training would be invaluable to staff who support people who display challenging or distressed behaviours because this may be the only way they can communicate. Offering this sort of training will give staff a way of supporting people and a greater understanding of the reasons behind the behaviour. Additionally, the UK PBS Competency Framework provides a detailed framework of the things that you need to know and the things that you need to do when delivering best practice.

Such training enables staff to gain the skills and knowledge necessary to support individuals with more complex care needs such as mental health issues and physical and learning disabilities. For example, you might wish staff to have specialist knowledge in dementia care and therefore seek out specialist training, although this would not be considered mandatory.

Evidence opportunity

1.2 Learning and CPD

Explain the differences between mandatory and statutory learning. What constitutes continuous professional development in your setting? What courses are offered over and above the statutory required ones?

AC 1.3 Describe the purpose and benefits of workforce planning and development

Here, you will be required to describe workforce planning and how this is applied in your setting.

Workforce planning and development is an essential part of ensuring that the right people with the right attitudes, skills, values and experience are providing the care and support that the organisation is offering.

Role of a manager in workforce development planning

As a manager, you are responsible for completing a workforce development plan, which analyses the setting's current skill mix to ensure that staff can fulfil the needs of the individuals in your care.

Workforce planning is the way in which an organisation's short- and long-term objectives are achieved by employing the 'right people with the right skills in the right place at the right time'.

Linked to the strategic organisation goals of the organisation and the planning process, workforce planning covers activities such as succession planning and flexible working and can help you to develop work schedules and employee hours so that the setting can run productively. With a good plan in place you can ensure that the needs of the organisation are met and that any staff gaps are filled. Additionally, you may be required to rethink job roles that may require change. As a manager, one of your roles is to ensure that your employees are satisfied in their work, and this includes developing and putting into practice policies to help them carry out their roles in a safe and confident manner. In analysing your plans, you may need to upskill and retrain some staff to ensure that you are meeting current care needs and are also planning for future ones.

You should have a workforce development strategy and plan in place to identify and prioritise development goals and targets to meet standards and address and avert potential risks resulting from knowledge or skills deficits. This will enhance service delivery and develop the personal and professional capacities of your staff. It should be realistic and recognise any limitations but also strive to be ambitious. It is important to achieve a balance between what can properly be supported and devising creative strategies to achieve more.

The plan must be fair, with opportunities distributed across the team and across all levels of staff. It must result in tangible outcomes and, once completed, enable staff who are developed in their roles to share and/or implement their learning. Consequently, when designing your plan, you will need to build in evaluative measures to ensure that you are fulfilling these obligations and objectives.

Having identified strengths, deficits, training needs and ideas for service enhancements, it is important that these are transformed into tangible actions that can be articulated as objectives. Objectives are statements that describe what the end point of an activity will be. Objectives should be written with the SMART acronym in mind; that is, they should be Specific, Measurable, Attainable, Relevant and Timebound. Your plan must be able to deliver what you set out to do and you must evaluate how successful you have been.

You may find, however, that you meet barriers to your efforts, and these may be due to fear of change and the sort of negative thinking that stops people from moving forward. New ideas are often met with fear of change and as a leader you need to outline a clear strategy and enable others not only to be heard but to contribute to the discussions.

When developing change in an organisation, training may be arranged at venues away from the workplace. This reduces interruptions, work phone calls and participants leaving the meeting to attend to work-related situations.

For more information on workforce planning, see CIPD (2022).

Evidence opportunity

1.3 Workforce planning

What do you understand about workforce planning? Provide an explanation of it in a short written piece.

AC 1.4 Explain the importance of literacy, numeracy and digital skills in adult care

Here, you will be required to explain the requirements in literacy, numeracy and digital skills for workers in adult care.

The need for the UK to upskill the workforce in order to be able to compete in a global economy that was undergoing rapid change has led to changes in education to ensure that the future workforce is sufficiently skilled in literacy, numeracy and new developments. This, together with moves to extend training in the workplace, is ensuring that regular upskilling of the workforce occurs.

The UK Parliament POSTnote published in December 2021, entitled 'Upskilling and retraining the adult workforce', provides an overview of the national context of adult education and demand for skills. It discusses the key impacts of adult learning to address mismatches between supply and demand of skills in the UK workforce. Participation in adult education in England has fallen from 4.4m in 2003–04 to 1.5m in 2019–20 and this was marked also by a fall in the funding.

There are concerns that funding restrictions around Level 2 and 3 qualifications (GCSE and A Level), and a removal of some qualifications (such as BTECs), could create barriers to adult education. There is also a need to address the demand for skills as well as supply of skills with a more focused approach on progression routes for lower skilled and lower paid workers.

Staff in care are expected to have the core skills of English, numeracy, digital and employability skills, including teamwork and problem-solving. They ensure that all care workers can complete everyday tasks such as communicating with the individuals they support, counting medication, using a computer and completing a care /support plan.

AC 1.5 Describe how to develop literacy, numeracy and digital skills within the team

Here, you will be required to describe how team members can be encouraged to develop the necessary literacy, numeracy and digital skills.

Basic skills are the ability to read, write and speak in English and use maths in everyday life. Skills needed to use basic technology such as phones, laptops, tablets and computers to carry out a range of everyday activities are increasingly considered to be basic or core skills.

As care work becomes more reliant on the use of computers, tablets and personal devices to record care, digital skills will be vital. In addition, the complexity of administering medication requires a good level of numeracy as dosages require calculation. Communication with staff and the individuals using the service, some of whom may have their own difficulty in this sphere, also requires knowledge of verbal, non-verbal and written forms of communication.

At recruitment stage you may want to assess candidates to determine their level of ability in the core skills to check that they have the minimum level required to work safely and meet quality standards. To assess whether these skills are present, observation at a trial shift might prove useful, but if this is not possible then try setting a task at interview that will help the candidate to demonstrate these skills. At the recruitment stage, you might ask for a written covering letter or during an interview you could ask the person to read something and then answer questions on it. You can include numeracy in this comprehension exercise.

In the workplace you need to support literacy, numeracy a nd spoken communication skills with your existing staff by encouraging them to use the skills often in their day-to-day work.

From induction and through other training and development, staff need to be clear about exactly how to undertake tasks involving literacy, numeracy and spoken communication skills. Staff should know what effective communication, both verbal and written, looks like, and how they are expected to behave in the workplace. You can then check in with them at supervision and ask them to feedback to check outcomes.

Evidence opportunity

1.4 and 1.5 Staff development

Explain what the requirements are for literacy, numeracy and digital skills for workers in adult care. How will you ensure that your team members develop the necessary skills?

AC1.6 Evaluate the benefits of continually improving own and team's knowledge and practice

Here, you will be required to evaluate the importance of your own and your team's continuous professional development.

Care is a complex, multi-dimensional activity and encompasses more than simply performing a skill. While technical competence gained through developing knowledge and skills is important, it is not sufficient on its own. Excellent care can be achieved only when technical competence is accompanied by appropriate attitudes and characteristics that relate to feelings, values and the way activities are carried out.

Professional development is a continuous process and care workers need to develop up-to-date knowledge, understanding and skills to meet changing needs and demands. In striving to improve quality of service and positive outcomes for the individuals using a service, only the best possible practice will be acceptable. This can only be achieved with a workforce that continually updates knowledge and skills in line with any changes that occur.

Continuous professional development is not a new concept but has emerged as changes to the care system have developed. With moves to partnership working and new models of care which value personalisation and individualised care, professionals have had to ensure that upskilling of the workforce has been a top agenda item.

It is recognised that those organisations that embed personal, professional development into their culture are best able to respond to day-to-day challenges and pressures and are more resilient and able to transform in response to changing situations and requirements (Schön, 1983, Harrison, 2009).

Personal, professional development increases the capabilities of staff. If it is tailored to individual needs, it should bring about personal enhancements and opportunities as individuals expand their personal tool box of skills.

One way of thinking about professional development is to think about the continual movement of escalators between the different levels of a building. It generates the image of individuals having access to a range of education and development opportunities at different levels that can be individually selected and packaged in different ways. It supports the idea that professional development can be undertaken in a traditional, linear way, starting at the bottom and moving through the levels to the top, but that it is equally valid for an individual to get off the escalator at any point and move around on that level in order to access a whole package of different activities before re-joining the escalator. The direction of travel may take an individual up a floor to access new learning, or down a floor to extend previous knowledge. It also suggests that there should be no limit to opportunities, that even if you start at the bottom you can move to the top. As a manager it is important that you and your organisation capitalise on the benefits that professional development brings by ensuring that it is purposeful and planned to meet the individual needs of your staff and your organisation.

Evidence opportunity

1.6 Importance of continuously improving knowledge/practice

Undertake a discussion that evaluates professional development in relation to the areas discussed in this section. Look at the pros and cons and the importance of continuously improving your own knowledge and practice and that of the team you manage and lead.

You might want to explain how you undertake the process of professional development in adult care in relation to those you manage and your own professional development. You could evidence this by putting a copy of your professional development plan into your portfolio. Consider:

- ✔ the processes involved to manage learning and development
- ✔ how you undertake workforce development planning
- ✔ how you identify and provide mandatory training
- ✔ how you evidence that you support CQC requirements
- ✔ the relationship between training and positive outcomes.

Reflect on it

1.6 Training and positive outcomes

Write a reflective piece about the relationship between training and positive outcomes. How do you know this happens?

Reflect on it

1.6 The importance of continually improving knowledge/practice

What professional development activities have you and your team participated in over the last year?

- How do they reflect the changes that have impacted your work in adult care? Make a list.
- Were they planned, and if so, by whom?
- Were they part of a development plan for the organisation or focused on individual needs?
- What is the evidence that they have resulted in positive outcomes? Give examples.
- How have they helped to improve knowledge and practice?

Summarise the importance of improving knowledge and practice.

AC 1.7 Describe the ways to develop/improve own and team's knowledge and practice

Here, you will be required to describe the methods of progression development for yourself and your team.

Professional development is a process, and the development and improvement of your teams' knowledge and practice is an ongoing activity. It needs to be thought about as something that is incremental, with the different elements contributing to a larger whole. It is important that you have processes in place to manage and advance staff learning and development. For example, in developing your staff you need to have a clear idea about the strategic direction of the organisation so that you can determine what skills and competencies staff will need to support that plan. A **training needs analysis** is a process by which you can clearly compare your staff's capabilities with your organisation's skill requirements. This will then highlight skills gaps and further development can be put in place.

It has been said that the richest resource that any organisation possesses is the people who work within it. Individuals are interested in, and motivated by, different things and this includes their motivation to learn something. Consequently, everyone's knowledge base and skill set are different, even when similar levels of formal training have been undertaken. If you could pool and share this knowledge, everyone, including the organisation, would benefit. A key role for a manager is to utilise the existing skill set within a team in order to enhance the knowledge and skills of others. This is achieved by having in place a training needs analysis in which you clearly set out what training must be accomplished and how this is best achieved.

KEY TERM

Training needs analysis: Determines the current knowledge, skills and abilities of all staff and identifies the gaps that might need to be filled to strengthen the organisation. It is the process of identifying training needs to improve staff job performance.

If your staff are required to carry out different roles in the future, perhaps to move a project along, then the learning and development plan will need to include additional training and sometimes retraining to help staff to fill the gaps. Evaluation of training currently on offer needs to be undertaken to determine its effectiveness and value for staff.

Other processes include the need to prioritise some training and to allocate budget accordingly. Professional development and training enable an organisation to keep up to date and to change proactively so that its service is relevant and appropriate. It is important to note that to get the most out of investment in professional development it should be planned in line with an organisational vision. Ad hoc training can be useful but may only lead to staff undertaking a disparate set of activities that do not contribute to the greater whole.

Providing staff with a variety of skills-based training and one-to-one support is imperative if staff are to develop in a professional way. They are required to undertake mandatory training courses on an annual basis to ensure that their skills and knowledge remain up to date and this is all part of professional development.

The apprenticeship framework provides training at Level 2 and 3 in Health and Social Care and are ideal both for mature employees within the sector as well as younger people just starting their careers.

The Intermediate Apprenticeship (Level 2) provides a Level 2 Diploma in Health and Social Care (Adults) for England, which is the competency part of the qualification and essential to achieve the full apprenticeship. The Level 2 Certificate in Preparing to Work in Adult Social Care develops the necessary technical skills, knowledge and understanding of theoretical concepts, as well as knowledge and understanding of the relevant market and sector.

The Advanced Apprenticeship (Level 3) is suitable for those working in lone worker or supervisory care roles in social care settings and the Level 3 Diploma in Health and Social Care (Adults) for England is the part of the course that shows that competency in performing the skill, trade or occupation has been achieved. The Level 3 Certificate in Preparing to Work in Adult Social Care provides knowledge of the necessary technical skills, knowledge and understanding of theory, as well as knowledge and understanding of the relevant market and sector.

Evidence opportunity

1.7 Progression development

Describe the methods of progression development for yourself and your team. How do you determine what training you or your staff require to stay up to date?

AC1.8 Analyse the factors to consider when identifying, planning selecting and commissioning activities or learning and professional development

Here, you will be required to analyse the range of factors that impact the identifying, planning, selecting and commissioning of activities for learning and professional development within the work setting.

Identifying and planning development activities will be highlighted from appraisals, supervision and through the training needs analysis referred to in AC1.7.

Your training programme for staff must identify who needs to be trained, in which areas and the type of training needed to achieve this. If you undertook a training needs analysis in Evidence opportunity 1.7, you will be able to identify the gaps in your current staff skills and knowledge and you can then choose training to address this.

Some factors that may hinder the process of selecting and commissioning training include time, finance and availability of staff, so when commissioning activities you need to recognise these as potential barriers. Failure to keep up to date with training and a lack of investment in staff can lead to business failure, or you may find that individuals simply boycott your organisation.

Finance to support workforce development planning and delivery

Lack of finance can be a constraint in relation to professional development and is often the main reason for not supplying training. Inevitably, investing in opportunities to enable staff to keep up to date is costly and it would be unrealistic and irresponsible not to consider these costs seriously. However, the risk of not engaging in development activities may be very costly in terms of the long-term organisational plan and the workforce development plan, so it is important to balance these investment costs against this. While it might be tempting to see staff development as a luxury or non-essential activity when times are tight, in an environment in which treatments, practices and expectations are constantly changing, that would be a mistake. It is important to ensure that any development budget is spent appropriately and that key risks are prioritised over other less important activities. For example, failing to ensure that staff gain appropriate training in relation to manual handling would leave the organisation vulnerable to litigation and potentially expensive compensation claims from both staff and individuals. Some care work requires moving and handling individuals, so it is highly likely that an incident will occur, and it is also likely to have a significant impact. This would result in a high-risk score on a risk assessment chart, which should alert the manager that there is a need to do something urgently to rectify the deficit. Risks can be plotted on a chart so that it is easy to get a visual image of where key areas need to be addressed.

Financial contributions of staff to support the costs of training and return on investment

This is potentially a major barrier as staff may be unable or unwilling to pay for their own training, so effective methods to enable this need to be sought. Training that staff wish to undertake for their own professional development and career enhancement is usually paid for by themselves, and this should be made clear to them. However, they may be able to access bursaries or funding to support training. You might also agree to fund part of the training, particularly if you can see that upskilling a member of staff in this way would be a useful addition to the training portfolio of the team. Staff may be able to cascade their knowledge to others so investing in their training may provide a better service for individuals and improved training for other members of staff.

Impact on the setting of staff attending training

Time is a factor that must be considered if staff need to go off site to attend training since training days mean that staff are unavailable to work, and this requires cover staff to be paid. Additionally, staff may not always use the time in training sessions wisely and may see it as a day off from work. Any staff training that is provided must be good quality and you could ask those receiving training to evaluate or provide a reflective account of their learning to ensure that they are gaining the most from the investment. Staff who are undertaking apprenticeships are entitled to spend 20% of their working week on training activities.

Insufficient or high turnover of staff

With insufficient staff in the department or team you may find attendance at training becomes impossible. Staff may be denied training if the department is busy and the setting would prefer staff to be available in the setting than away attending a training course. Part of your workforce planning needs to address reasons behind the high turnover of staff in order to recruit sufficient numbers. A high turnover of staff may be due to workplace stress and excessive workload; knowing this means your recruitment process can look at introducing incentives to encourage staff to join your organisation.

Access to nationally recognised qualifications and/or apprenticeships

If staff are unable to access recognised qualifications, they may be unwilling to work for your organisation, and this is a potential barrier to developing a well-qualified, resourceful team. It would be good to be familiar with the apprenticeships and national awards available to staff in case they are interested in undertaking this level of training.

Internal and informal training

Informal on-the-job training is an important part of resourcing care work. Mentors and coaches in the workplace can provide support for staff in their daily duties so you may wish to invest in training for suitable staff to undertake these roles. This can also help to save on the cost of external training. Staff can cascade what they have learned to other staff members.

Personal motivation and impact on work–life balance

It is useful to know what type of learners your staff are to ensure that they are motivated and to understand how a course or training might impact their lives. A training course that might take three years of hard work with lots of written work and research may not appeal to staff who already work hard and have families to consider.

Individuals learn in different ways, and you should think about the method that suits their preferred learning style so that, where possible, you can select appropriate learning activities. Your understanding of what development activities suit each learning style means staff are likely to get more from their learning.

Lack of personal motivation can be a barrier and constraint if workers do not feel motivated in their roles, and this can impact their work greatly. You need to be watchful of staff becoming burnt out and ensure that during supervision and appraisal you discuss possible ways to support them.

Other factors include time and career goals and aspirations. Having a firm career plan in place can be an asset in terms of choosing appropriate training activities. As a manager it is your responsibility to ensure that staff development both meets organisational needs and priorities and supports and motivates individual team members' personal and professional development.

Levels of language, literacy and numeracy among workforce

Levels of language and literacy will affect how – and whether – staff learn. Everyone is different and professional development should be tailored to suit individual education levels, abilities, interests and experience. Think of the ways you prefer to learn. Do you like discussion and working with others? Do you prefer tutor guidance? Do you like exploring and learning on your own? Are computer programs a style of learning that you enjoy? If you enjoy the process of learning, you are more likely to stick with it, particularly if it is over a period of time. Staff may avoid learning and training courses if they struggle with literacy and numeracy and this will be a potential barrier to developing your workforce. Again, you should be mindful of how these staff might be helped by different technologies and ways of learning.

Level of IT skills

With new technology arriving all the time, new and possibly older staff may find this difficult to come to terms with. Time must be given to introduce new technology and staff who need help with IT skills must be supported in their learning.

Recommendations for practice

Guidelines for practice are available and need to be implemented into ways of working to deliver the best care possible. It is not possible to ignore recommended ways of doing things and staff must be encouraged to change when required to do so.

Evidence opportunity

1.8 Potential barriers and constraints for professional development

Provide a written account analysing the potential barriers and constraints in your working environment in accessing professional development, with consideration of the areas discussed in this section.

You might like to use the headings shown here to analyse how you have understood and can address each barrier to accessing professional development in your workplace. Suggested headings are:

- ✔ Workforce development strategy and planning
- ✔ Financial budgets to support workforce development planning and delivery
- ✔ Financial contributions of staff to support the costs of training
- ✔ Return on investment – financially, improved service delivery
- ✔ Poor time management and commitment of staff
- ✔ Quality of training delivery and support – in-house, external
- ✔ Insufficient or high turnover of staff
- ✔ Access to nationally recognised qualifications and/or apprenticeships
- ✔ Levels of informal training, internally
- ✔ Personal motivation and impact on life balance for individuals
- ✔ Levels of language, literacy and numeracy among workforce
- ✔ Level of IT skills

What recommendations for your own area of practice will you make?

AC1.9 Explain the importance of reflective practice in improving team's performance

Here, you will be required to explain reflective practice and how it can be applied to your setting.

Reflective practice is an essential element of personal development and provides an opportunity to stop and take stock. The term was first coined by Donald Schön (1983) and it involves analysing experiences and actions in order to achieve improvement and development in practice. For example, staff who experience a critical incident happening in the care setting can engage in reflective practice and start to think about what happened, how they reacted and what mistakes they may have made. By doing so and discussing this with others, staff may be able to avoid making mistakes in the future.

There are benefits to reflective practice. It can lead to gaining new knowledge and refining existing knowledge. It enables you to identify the connections between theory and practice. Staff can also start to understand the rationale behind their own actions, such as why they do the things that they do. Reflection also helps staff to experience increased feelings of autonomy, competence and control, which will lead to improved performance.

> *It is not sufficient simply to have an experience in order to learn. Without reflecting upon this experience it may quickly be forgotten or its learning potential lost. It is from the feelings and thoughts emerging from this reflection that generalisations or concepts can be generated. And it is generalisations which enable new situations to be tackled effectively.*
>
> Source: Gibbs (1988)

KEY TERM

Reflective practice: The act of stopping and thinking about what you are doing in practice and analysing the decisions you make in the light of theory and the things you have learned. By doing this you are more able to relate theory to practice, helping you to generate new knowledge and ideas.

Reflect on it

1.9 Reflect on work activities

Reflect on an activity you have undertaken this week at work. Choose something you do regularly and therefore take for granted. Think about the purpose of the activity, how you feel about it and how you might want to improve it.

AC1.10 Describe different models that support reflective practice

Here, you will be required to describe models of reflective practice and explain how they can be applied in the work setting.

Schön's reflective model

Donald Schön (1983) identified that learning in practice could be enhanced by two different kinds of activity: reflection in action and reflection on action:

- Reflection in action requires practitioners to 'think ahead', to critically reflect on what one is doing while one is doing it and to revise actions in the light of that reflection (Greenwood, 1993). This is sometimes referred to as 'thinking on your feet' and being able to look at the experience and to say how you feel about it at the time. For example, something new that surprises you may happen in the course of your duty and you therefore have to think about how you approach this unique event. In care work this may require you to move outside textbook-type responses and create new ways of doing things.
- Reflection on action is a retrospective activity that requires practitioners to interpret and analyse recalled information from activities that they have been engaged with (Boyd and Fales, 1983; Fitzgerald, 1994; Atkins and Murphy, 1994). Using the example above, this can be further explored by reflecting upon what you did in the new encounter and why you did it. In this way you start to develop questions and key ideas about the event and the experience. In doing so you are engaging with a critical evaluation of a situation and can then build upon your knowledge of the practice and your responses.

One major criticism of the reflection in- and on-action theory is that of time and the notion that sometimes you need to make decisions quickly without much thought or reflection. You have to fall back on routine practice and carry out the task as set. However, this may set up some questions about why you are doing certain things in certain ways and this sort of reflection then becomes useful not only in moving practice forward but also for your own knowledge.

Reflection is, therefore, the art of thinking back and examining the things that happened, learning from them and avoiding those same mistakes. Schön's model encourages you to explore thoughts and feelings to become more self-aware and by doing so you can develop your practice. You should try to make sense of your learning so that what you learn then becomes normal practice.

Kolb's learning cycle

David A. Kolb's (1984) cycle of experiential learning can be adapted well here. Kolb suggests that we need to recall our observation of an event, or the change in this case, reflect on those observations, develop and research some theories about what we saw and then decide on some action because of the process (Jasper, 2006).

Kolb's theory was based on the premise that learning is a process in which knowledge comes about through the transforming experience. Like Schön's theory, in this cycle the 'concrete experience' of the learning event (stage one) is followed by 'reflection' in which the learner thinks about what happened (stage two). Stage three is the process of thinking about how the learning can be used and, finally, in stage four the learner plans how to use the knowledge in the future.

Gibbs' six stages to reflective practice

Many models are constructed around the use of structured questions to prompt reflection in a logical and systematic manner (Johns, 1995). These questions are often focused on incident analysis as the key method of reflecting (Gibbs, 1988). Graham Gibbs' model was developed from Kolb's four-stage experiential learning cycle (1984) and is sometimes referred to as an iterative model or learning through repetition as opposed to Kolb's experiential learning model described as learning through experience.

Gibbs' reflective cycle has six stages:

1. Description – Asking oneself 'what happened?'
2. Feelings – What did I think or feel here?
3. Evaluation – What was good or bad about what happened at that time?
4. Analysis – What does it mean, and can I make any sense of it?
5. Conclusion – How else might I have dealt with it? What else could I have done?
6. Action plan – What will I do next time?

This approach entails practitioners selecting a significant incident, writing about it in detail and then analysing what happened, asking why, and identifying what additional knowledge would have enabled the practitioner to behave differently. It requires the reflector to explore what evidence there is that similar things have been addressed by others more effectively and to establish what learning can be drawn from the experience. It also enables practitioners to be better prepared when faced with similar experiences in the future, as well as providing an opportunity to identify shortcomings in knowledge or skills which can be rectified.

As a learning tool, this theory can make the structure of how you write about an event easier. Occasionally, you may write in a purely descriptive manner and sometimes confuse evaluation and analysis, which leads to repetition. By using the stages discussed, you can be sure that you are addressing each part of the learning cycle in a more constructive way.

Models of reflection are normally illustrated as cyclical activities, such as those depicted in Figures 11 and 12.

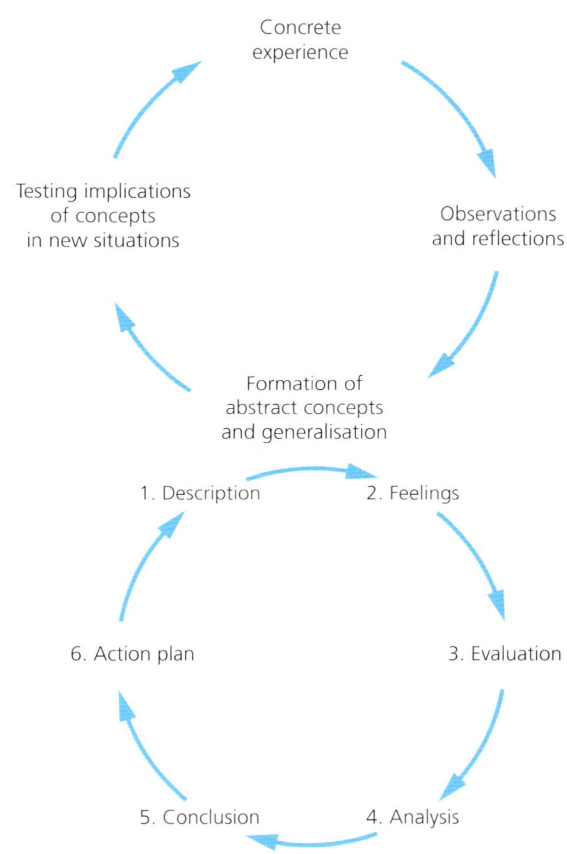

▲ **Figures 11 and 12** Models of reflection based on Kolb and Gibbs

Choose a model that suits your learning needs

Different models of reflection suit different learning styles and different purposes. A model is a tool to provide structure to an activity and it is important that you select one that suits your style. The significant thing to remember is that whichever model is selected, it is the learning that results from the activity that is the important thing; learning that is either confirmation that behaviour is appropriate or learning that suggests a need to gain more information or change practice.

Reflective practice improves performance because it helps you to challenge your assumptions about what you do on a daily basis. For example, it helps you to question why you practise in certain ways and do certain things and in doing so you can start to explore different approaches. You are also engaged in identifying your own strengths and weaknesses and are then in a position to address them.

Reflection for action, reflection in action, reflection on action

Schön's theory identifies reflection in action and reflection on action as described earlier, but some writers have added a further stage: reflection for action. Killion and Todnem (1991) refer to the stages in Schön's model as occurring during (reflection in action) and immediately after (reflection on action) an event. Their addition of reflection for action expects the learner to review the previous two processes and to reflect upon what has been accomplished and to identify guidelines to follow to succeed in the same task in the future. By undertaking this sort of reflection learners are encouraged to think about past experiences before rushing into completing the same actions in the future.

Professionalism, reflection and individual responsibility

Your fitness to work in adult care requires you to behave professionally and to do so means you need to demonstrate behaviour which shows you are open minded, reflective and take your duty of care seriously by engaging in life-long learning and self-improvement.

Professionalism is a core quality to be developed and demands that you work to defined standards within codes of conduct and demonstrate a responsible attitude towards how you manage individuals and their information. Your clinical judgement must be based upon evidence.

Relationship between professionalism and accountability

Being professional means behaving in ways that do not bring the profession into disrepute, and you can accomplish this by keeping your professional development up to date through supervision as well as reflection on your practice. You are accountable for how you practise and how you approach the individuals in your care and this accountability and professionalism comes through regulation and the duty of care you owe the people you care for.

When times are difficult it may be necessary to reduce the amount of development that can be supported. Trying to do too much runs the risk of creating additional stress for staff and possible loss of good will. It is your responsibility to be able to justify decisions. Sorting your activities into priority categories with identification of associated risks if an activity is not done is one way of prioritising development.

Barriers to effective reflective practice

It is not difficult to mount a convincing argument for integrating professional development and reflective practice into organisational culture, yet when times are busy and challenging, it can be the first thing to drop off the agenda. However, reflective practice and staff development are essential requirements for any service seeking to provide care for others. The challenge for the manager, therefore, is to find ways of identifying, recognising, overcoming and reducing any barriers to reflective practice and professional development. Barriers are hurdles to get around. While they may seem insurmountable, ingenuity, creativity and a positive attitude may be sufficient to overcome them. Barriers should be viewed as problems to be solved rather than as overwhelming obstacles.

Potential barriers to effective reflective practice

Boud and Walker (1993) classify barriers to reflective practice as being internal, or those coming from the learner themselves, and external, those coming from the environment and other forces that may impact the learner, such as stereotyping and culture.

Personal barriers may become evident when you experience stress because of negative events. In this case, you may avoid thinking about the situation and this then becomes a barrier because to revisit such raw feelings is painful. You may become more inclined to lock such feelings away rather than addressing the emotion and feeling inherent within reflection.

You may also be unaware of the existence of barriers. For example, journal writing is a major part of reflection and, for some professionals, group discussion, yet how many of your colleagues express their dissatisfaction with doing such activities, being unable to see the benefit of the activity? Getting down to writing the journal may also present a barrier as you may struggle to know what to write or how to write it. A further barrier is the environment in which to write because of potential interruptions, lack of space and time.

Staff need to feel that reflecting is an activity valued for its own sake and is not just another chore to be squeezed in around more important routine activities, so it's important to encourage them to put their reflection and learning into practice.

Evidence opportunity

1.10 Importance of reflective practice

Provide a written account describing the theories of reflective practice in improving individual performance, with reference to:

- ✔ Schön's reflective model (reflection for action, reflection in action)
- ✔ Kolb's learning cycle
- ✔ Gibbs' six stages to reflective practice
- ✔ Killion and Todnem's reflection on action.

Research it

1.10 Potential barriers to professional development

Research potential barriers to undertaking professional development and reflection in your workplace and then set up an action plan to overcome them. You may like to copy the table shown below to help you.

Potential barrier	Action to overcome barrier	Potential risk if not undertaken
Journal writing		

Reflect on it

1.10 Barriers affecting outcomes for individuals

Write a short reflective account of how the potential barriers to reflective practice affect the outcomes for the individuals using the service.

LO2 Be able to lead learning and professional development practices

AC 2.1 Evaluate available mechanisms and resources to support learning and professional development in adult care

Here, you will be required to evaluate a range of sources and systems of support for professional development for the manager and their staff, including areas discussed in this section.

Not all professional development will be achieved by attending formal training or education events. In fact, financial restraints often mean you need to be careful about how much money is spent on training and often other in-house activities can be just as valuable and sometimes more cost effective. There are various forms of informal and formal support that are of significant value in developing the capability of others.

Resources – internal financial support and publicly-funded training opportunities

Inevitably, investing in opportunities to enable staff to keep up to date is associated with costs and it would be unrealistic and irresponsible not to consider these costs seriously.

There will be a budget for staff training (including for yourself, as manager) set aside but often this is inadequate and staff may need to be prepared to fund some of the cost of training themselves. Sometimes funding can be accessed from external sources. For example, grants and bursaries may be available to help with fees.

However, the risk of not engaging in development activities may be very costly in terms of the long-term organisational plan, so it is important to balance these investment costs against this. While it might be tempting to see staff development as a non-essential activity when finances are tight, in an environment in which treatments, practices and expectations are constantly changing, that would be a mistake. It is important to ensure that any development budget is spent appropriately and that key risks are prioritised over other, less important, activities.

Other factors include time and career goals and aspirations. Time is a factor that must be considered if staff need to go off site to attend training. Having a firm career plan in place can be a valuable asset in terms of choosing appropriate training activities.

Resources – access to books and journals

Access to relevant books and journals may also be a source of learning for your staff, so a library of such might be a useful addition to the resources. In a small organisation, this may well be a luxury, but staff may be willing to donate books they no longer have any use for and you might also check with other stakeholders about access to their book resources.

Digital resources – e-learning

E-learning packages are an excellent way of ensuring that all staff undergo the same training, and they can access these either at work or in their own time. They are also able to build their own e-portfolios without having to store paper files of their work and can upload reflective accounts, certificates and test results as well as essays and other pieces of information. These can then be accessed by tutors and assessors at a distance.

Many organisations have their own system of online training. Some of the partnerships you have may have access to such training and this might be shared. Staff can access this learning at any time. They can do so from home or when in work by simply logging into the system and undertaking the online modules.

Mentoring, peer supervision, buddying and coaching

Mentoring

Mentoring is an invaluable tool for supporting staff development and is a powerful means of individual empowerment. Clutterbuck and Megginson (1999) describe mentorship as 'standing in front of a mirror with a trusted other, who can help you see things that you do not know how to see, or that have become too familiar for you to notice'.

Mentoring can be defined simply as a helping relationship between an individual with potential and an individual with expertise. The role of the mentor is to guide the mentee. Knowledge, experience and organisational perspective are shared candidly within a context of mutual respect and trust. It is an effective way of helping people to progress in their careers and is becoming increasingly popular as its potential is realised. Among the roles of the mentor are role model, enabler, teacher, encourager, counsellor, befriender, facilitator, coach, confidant, supporter and 'un-learner' (Bolton, 2010). We might also add peer supervision to this list and buddying. For more on mentoring see Unit 500 AC2.3.

Peer supervision and buddying

Peer supervision is an arrangement in which peers work together for mutual benefit to provide support and feedback to each other, while buddying is a more informal arrangement, which also involves support and advice for the care worker. For more on buddying see AC1.2 in this unit.

Coaching

Coaching is designed to help individuals fulfil their potential and is therefore an ideal strategy for some elements of professional development. It is a process of helping individuals to learn rather than teaching them. Coaching requires a belief that individuals are capable of addressing and resolving their issues and needs; not only are they capable but coaching implies that they are best suited to take responsibility for their decisions, actions and solutions. Coaching can, therefore, be described as a leadership style. Coaches use a range of tools and models to support their coachee. Coaching requires an attitude of positive regard and good communication skills to provide the right prompts to enable the coachee to reach their resolutions and conclusions. A coach may or may not have experience or expertise in the coachee's occupation. The skill of the coach is in asking the coachee appropriate prompt questions in order to enable them to think clearly and coherently about their issues.

Coaching enables control and development to remain squarely with the coachee, with the effective coach acting merely as a key to help them unlock their potential. For more on coaching, see Unit 500 AC2.2.

These roles, although useful, do have their drawbacks. Some require additional training and others require time, which is always a scarce resource.

Use of external training providers

External training providers can offer experience and often challenge entrenched ways of thinking in an organisation. They are also specialists in their field and so may offer greater depth of knowledge. Additionally, an external company will bring in staff who are able to train others in an effective way. Often, in-house training relies on people who might be great managers but who may not necessarily possess good teaching skills. Unfortunately, external training providers are expensive, and hidden costs, such as travel for the course trainers and possibly their accommodation, as well as the cost of the course itself, can all add up and need to be factored into the budget. Also, you will want to ensure that most of your staff attend the training, and this will then have an additional cost with staff needing to be covered for the duration of the training.

Personal development planning

Formal support for development is organised and has learning objectives, the intention of which is to gain knowledge and skills. Informal support, meanwhile, may not be organised or planned, but may happen because of experience in the workplace. Again, it is important to understand which style suits the individual by discussing their personal professional development.

Appraisal

Appraisals are a key strategy for managers to assess performance and needs against organisational requirements and aims. An appraisal is a formally constituted, annual activity that should be booked with all staff. Appraisals are normally conducted by a manager but can be conducted by peers if their focus is on developmental needs rather than role performance. Whichever model is adopted, individuals need to be warned about what it will involve so that they can prepare. Ideally, they should see examples of any documentation that will be used so that they can plan responses to the questions that will be asked.

Appraisal offers a vehicle for structured, personal development planning (PDP) that can have positive outcomes for both individuals and the organisation. It may help develop a strategy for an individual to meet personal goals and objectives, both short and long term. It will help the manager to match individuals and their training needs against organisational aims and will also enable managers to assess the fairness of the training and development allocation across the staff team. Where necessary, it also provides a process for managing staff performance, as it encourages managers to measure individual performance against role competency criteria.

Appraisal is a shared activity, which takes time and effort and must be planned if it is going to have any significant impact on PDP. PDP can have a number of different purposes and it is important that the method you select meets your needs as a manager, as well as the individual staff member's needs. It is important that the tool you design or utilise addresses those purposes that you have identified as important for your organisation. If you do not have an appraisal process in your organisation, you may want to consider writing a proposal to implement one.

> **KEY TERM**
>
> **Appraisal**: A process where employees and line managers discuss their performance, developmental needs and the support they need in their role. It is used to provide evidence and evaluation of recent performance and focus on future goals, opportunities and resources. Sometimes referred to as performance appraisal.

Of course, there are drawbacks to appraisals and if they are not carried out correctly they can be a negative experience, particularly as they may be somewhat subjective and potentially viewed as biased. Also, time is a major issue in carrying out this activity.

Support for staff with learning needs

You may have workers who have specific learning needs such as dyslexia or speaking English as an additional language. They may need extra help or different forms of learning. For example, some people with dyslexia report that text can appear to move or become blurred, and that white paper or backgrounds make print hard to read. Changing the colour of the paper and the font style used may help with this. For staff who have English as a second language you need to offer more creative ways to help them to continue to learn English but also the vocabulary that comes with care work. By using a more visual approach in training in the form of pictures and photographs, such learners can make sense of new information. You can also get learners to work with partners or in small groups to help them.

Older learners may prefer a different style of learning to those who have just left school; for example, online learning may come more naturally to younger learners who have grown up with the internet. It is a case of knowing what fits each member of staff best and working with it.

Your role as a manager

As a manager it is your responsibility to ensure that staff development both meets organisational needs and priorities and supports and motivates individual team members' personal and professional development. A good development plan will fulfil both requirements. It will identify and prioritise development goals and targets to meet the standards and will address and avert potential risks resulting from knowledge or skills deficits. It will enhance service delivery and develop personal and professional capacities. It should be realistic and recognise any limitations but also strive to be ambitious. It is important to achieve a balance between what can properly be supported and devising creative strategies to achieve more. It must be fair: opportunities must be fairly distributed across the team and across all levels of staff. It must result in tangible outcomes and staff who are developed must be enabled to share and/or implement their learning. Consequently, when designing your plan, you will need to build in evaluative measures to ensure that you are fulfilling your obligations and objectives.

See Unit 519 AC1.4 for more information. See also AC1.3 in this unit for more information on SMART objectives.

Evidence opportunity

2.1 Mechanisms and resources that support learning and development

Look at this range of sources and systems of support for professional development:

- ✔ Resources – internal financial support, access to publicly funded training opportunities
- ✔ Resources – access to books, journals
- ✔ Digital resources – e-learning
- ✔ Peer shadowing, coaching, mentoring, buddying
- ✔ Use of external training providers
- ✔ Training needs analysis
- ✔ Personal development planning
- ✔ Support for staff with learning needs (e.g. dyslexia, non-English speakers, older learners, younger learners).

Provide a written account evaluating a range of sources and systems of support for professional development for you as the manager and your staff, including the ones listed. Consider how you use each type of learning in your setting, taking into account how useful they are to staff members, which types particular staff would benefit from, how you can measure their success and how you can improve the planning and provision of systems of personal development.

Research it

2.1 Comparing different sources/ systems of support

Research sources and systems of support where you work. Think about which of the following functions of personal development planning are important within your organisation. You might like to think about it as a manager, or from a more general staff perspective.

Function of personal development planning	Tick	Does your PDP enable this function to be realised?	Comment here upon the strengths and weaknesses of these approaches
Assessment of competence to undertake a role against predetermined criteria (e.g. role descriptor)			
Opportunity to enhance effectiveness and performance			
Planning for the future (short, medium and long term)			
Clarification of values and behaviours			
Evaluation of service			
Means of enhancing service			
Increase staff motivation			
Opportunity for self-reflection			
Identification of strengths and areas for improvement			
Strategy to solve problems			
Provide a structure for and commitment to staff training and development			
Opportunity to manage and respond to change			
Increase team capabilities			
Manage underperformance			
Provide a structure for individual feedback			

AC2.2 Promote a learning culture within own team

Here, you will show different methods of promoting learning within the team and identify which will be effective in promoting continuous professional development.

If you are going to have knowledgeable and skilful staff, you need to create a culture in which learning is at the heart of their work, so continuous development of knowledge and competence must be encouraged as part of the organisation's culture.

You can do this by being supportive of independent learning and development and by encouraging staff to reflect on their work and share their learning. This might be an agenda item during each team meeting where staff are assigned a 'sharing good practice' item to discuss.

Having a growth mindset in which staff believe their skills and knowledge can be developed through hard work and input from others will foster a desire to learn. Effective learning takes place in environments where staff are supported and believe that their development is valued, with time given to it.

Reflect on it

2.2 Continuous development

Is continuous development encouraged as part of your team's work? Think about staff attitudes to learning. Might it be better? How can you encourage a 'culture of learning'?

AC2.3 Support team members to plan for, achieve and review their professional development goals

Here, you will show how you support team members through development plans and appraisal to achieve their professional aims and objectives.

During appraisal and supervision sessions staff must be encouraged to plan for their own development and set goals for their own professional needs.

A personal development plan can be a useful tool for this exercise. A PDP is a form of self-evaluation reflection where individual goals are outlined. Undertaking a SWOT analysis (see Unit 500 AC1.2) will enable you to identify strengths and weaknesses and these areas may form part of the PDP as you define what you need to improve upon or maintain and how you will do this.

Evidence opportunity

2.3 Personal development plan

Source a personal development template and conduct your own PDP. Now undertake the same activity with a member of staff to help them to plan their development goals and review these at a later date.

AC2.4 Facilitate the development of others to enable effective delegation

Here, you will explain the role of delegation in a team and show how this can be achieved effectively.

Delegating not only lightens your workload as a manager but also empowers your team and builds trust. It is also a great way to professionally develop your staff because they can undertake new skills and gain new knowledge in preparation for taking on more responsibility in the future.

Rather than simply the act of passing off work to another, delegating can enable workloads to become more manageable and provide valuable training opportunities.

Managers may be reluctant to pass on tasks as they feel they may lose control, so delegation requires confidence in the team and in the person to whom you are delegating. Your team will want to be successful and if your staff succeed, then so do you.

Managers sometimes complain that a job is easier to do and takes less time if they do it themselves. The first time you delegate to a member of staff, training them may take time but you will gain time when you do not have to do the task in future. For example, it may take you two hours a week to do the rota. It might also take you eight hours to show somebody how to do it. However, after eight weeks you will have recouped 16 hours that you can use for other tasks.

In determining what tasks you can delegate, think about what you do each week. Think about any tasks that you are not good at and check with somebody who is efficient at that task. For example, keeping the website up to date can be delegated to somebody who is adept at this. Time-consuming tasks can be broken down and aspects of them shared to other staff.

Delegation is a good opportunity to develop staff, to keep them interested in their roles and to show respect for their knowledge and skills.

Evidence opportunity

2.4 Delegation

Show how you facilitate the development of members of your team to enable effective delegation. Think about the last task you delegated and explain to your assessor how effective it was.

Legislation

Legislation	Key points
Health and Safety at Work Act 1974	This Act is the primary piece of legislation governing workplace health and safety in the UK. It defines the general duties of employees and employers, owners and managers for maintaining health and safety within the workplace.
The Management of Health and Safety at Work Regulations 1999	The Management of Health and Safety at Work Regulations 1999 makes clear that employers are required to carry out risk assessments, and to appoint competent people and arrange for appropriate information and training.
Health and Social Care Act 2012 Care Act 2014	These introduced the Care Quality Commission (CQC).

References

Atkins, S. and Murphy, K. (1994) 'Reflective practice', *Nursing Standard*, 8(39): 49–54.

Bolton, G. (2010) *Reflective Practice: Writing and professional development* (3e). London: Sage.

Boud, D. and Walker, D. (1993) 'Barriers to reflection on experience', in *Using Experience for Learning*. Buckingham: SHRE/Open University Press.

Boyd, E. and Fales, A. (1983) 'Reflective learning: The key to learning from experience', *Journal of Humanistic Psychology*, 23(2): 99–117.

Cavendish, C. (2013) 'The Cavendish Review: An independent review into healthcare assistants and support workers in the NHS and social care settings'. https://assets.publishing.service.gov.uk/government/uploads/system/uploads/attachment_data/file/236212/Cavendish_Review.pdf

Clutterbuck, D. and Megginson, D. (1999) *Mentoring Executives and Directors*. Oxford: Butterworth-Heinemann.

Fitzgerald, M. (1994) *Theories of Reflection for Learning*. Oxford: Blackwell Scientific.

Gibbs, G. (1988) *Learning by Doing: A guide to teaching and learning methods*. Oxford: Oxford Further Education Unit.

Greenwood, J. (1993) 'Reflective practice: A critique of the work of Argyris & Schön', *Journal of Advanced Nursing*, 27: 13–17.

Harrison, R. (2009) *Learning and Development*. London: Chartered Institute for Personnel and Development.

Health and Care Professions Council (2016) *Standards of Conduct, Performance and Ethics*. London: HPC.

Jasper, M. (2006) *Professional Development, Reflection and Decision-Making*. Oxford: Blackwell Publishing.

Johns, C. (1995) 'Framing learning through reflection within Carper's fundamental ways of knowing in nursing', *Journal of Advanced Nursing*, 22: 226–34.

Killion, J. and Todnem, G. (1991) 'A process for personal theory building', *Educational Leadership*, 48(7): 14–16.

Kolb, D. (1984) 'Cycle of experiential learning', in Tilmouth, T., Davies-Ward, E. and Williams, B. (2011) *Foundation Degree in Health and Social Care*. London: Hodder Education.

Nursing and Midwifery Council (2018) *The Code: Professional standards of practice and behaviour for nurses and midwives*. London: NMC.

Schön, D. (1983) *The Reflective Practitioner: How professionals think in action*. New York: Basic Books.

Skills for Care and Skills for Health (2013) 'Code of conduct for healthcare support workers and adult social care workers in England'. www.skillsforcare.org.uk/resources/documents/Support-for-leaders-and-managers/Managing-people/Code-of-conduct/Code-of-Conduct.pdf

UK Parliament (2021) POSTnote, 'Upskilling and retraining the adult workforce'. https://post.parliament.uk/research-briefings/post-pn-0659/

Useful resources and further reading

Chartered Institute of Personnel and Development (2022) 'Workforce planning'. www.cipd.org/uk/knowledge/factsheets/workforce-planning-factsheet/

Skills for Care (n.d. a) 'Care Certificate'. www.skillsforcare.org.uk/Developing-your-workforce/Care-Certificate/Care-Certificate.aspx

Skills for Care (n.d. b) 'Buddying vs mentoring'. www.skillsforcare.org.uk/resources/documents/Recruitment-support/Retaining-your-staff/Buddying-Vs-Mentoring.pdf

Unit 506

Professional supervision in adult care

GLH 20

About this unit

People receiving care services must be confident that they can trust those who deliver care to not only know what to do but also to know how to do it well. This requires you to continually update and extend your knowledge and skills and to seek out supervision. You also need to provide professional supervision to ensure that staff are supported in their roles and enhance their skills and performance.

This unit will help you to examine and assess your understanding of supervision and the responsibilities that this practice entails as a manager and leader. You will develop your reflective and individual planning skills to help you determine how you can most effectively support your own supervision of staff to aid their development.

Learning outcomes

By the end of this unit, you will:

1. Understand the purpose and practice of professional supervision in adult care settings/services.
2. Be able to provide regular professional supervision.

Getting started

Before you study the unit, think about the following:

- What do you think are the key principles of formal supervision?

LO1 Understand the purpose and practice of professional supervision in adult care settings/services

Here, you will be required to develop an understanding about the purpose and practice of professional supervision in adult care settings/services.

In the past, professional supervision has been likened to the apprentice system or the 'student learning at the feet of the master'. Today, professional supervision is recognised as a complex exchange between supervisor and supervisee, with models and theories developed to provide a framework for it. It is an ethical requirement of professions where one-to-one contact with the individuals using the service is an ongoing process and the models that have been developed lend themselves more to this type of process. The purpose of supervision is to provide support to care workers and enable the development of good practice.

Regular contact between a supervisor and a care worker is invaluable to monitor and reflect on practice. It provides an opportunity to gain feedback on work with individuals as well as guidance and support. It also helps to identify areas of work that need development.

As managers and members of care staff you are expected to 'Strive to improve the quality of healthcare, care and support through continuing professional development (CPD)' (Skills for Care, 2013).

To do this, there should be policies and procedures to enable such development to take place, as well as a vehicle for you to discuss your practice and to support you in changing any deficiencies in practice.

The whole purpose of this clear directive is to improve the quality of the work you do in order to achieve agreed objectives and outcomes. Your intention through supervision and CPD is to ensure that all people who use services in social care settings have the capacity to lead independent and fulfilling lives. It also ensures that staff themselves feel supported in their work and have recourse to a system of help should they require it.

The British Association of Social Workers Code of Practice to support social workers highlights the purpose of supervision as being,

> *to support social workers to provide good quality services. Social work is a complex and demanding profession. Effective supervision of social workers enables social workers to maximise their effectiveness.*

Source: British Association of Social Workers (2011)

Reflect on it

1.1 What does 'supervision' mean to you?

Write a short account to answer the following questions:

- What do you understand the purpose of supervision to be?
- What policies and procedures are in place for your own supervision and how does it help you in practice?

AC 1.1 Outline the requirements of regulation, codes of practice and agreed ways of working that influence and structure professional supervision requirements in adult care

Here, you will be required to outline how supervision is informed by current legislation, codes of practice and agreed ways of working, compliments and complaints.

Current legislation, codes of practice and agreed ways of working

Health and Social Care Act 2008 (Regulated Activities) Regulations 2014

Regulation 18 of the Health and Social Care Act 2008 (Regulated Activities) Regulations 2014 requires that not only are enough suitably qualified and experienced staff required for a setting, but that staff must also 'receive the support, training, professional development, supervision and appraisals that are necessary for them to carry out their roles and responsibilities' (CQC, 2022).

As the manager, it is your responsibility to ensure that staff are aware of the legislation that they must abide by in the setting. For example, this will include being aware of:

- Data Protection Act 2018
- Health and Safety at Work etc Act 1974
- Equality Act 2010
- Human Rights Act 1998
- Health and Social Care Act 2008 (Regulated Activities) Regulations 2014: Regulation 18

You will also need to ensure that your staff are up to date with changes to legislation, codes of practice and agreed ways of working.

The focus of supervision is for the care professional to practise in such a way as to meet legal requirements and to ensure that codes of practice and local policy are being followed. The policies and procedures within your own work setting will reflect the legal position and any guidelines that need to be followed and you need to make a thorough analysis of these policies to ensure that you understand how these may impact your work as a supervisor. Analysing your policies in line with legislation will ensure that staff are being given the best supervision experience in line with legal requirements.

Skills for Care offers a useful 'Effective supervision' guide (Skills for Care, 2020).

Supervision is seen as a monitor and review process in which standards can be set and training and learning needs identified. It is also an opportunity to update staff on news from the organisation.

SCIE Supervision Guide

The Social Care Institute for Excellence (SCIE) has some excellent guidance on supervision on its website. It sets out what effective clinical supervision should look like and provides a useful guide for all care sectors and settings.

The website explains the features of good supervision, including policy and practice and the challenges of providing supervision to people working in various settings which require shift work or even home care work. For more information see SCIE (2017).

CQC regulations

The CQC's regulations state the standards below which care must never fall. The fundamental standards relating to supervision are the requirement for suitably qualified, competent staff who have the support, training and supervision they need to help them do their job. In the Health and Social Care Act 2008 (Regulated Activities) Regulations 2014, Regulation 12 'Safe care and treatment' states that care and treatment must be provided in a safe way to prevent avoidable harm or the risk of harm. Paragraph 12(2) states: 'Staff should be appropriately supervised when they are learning new skills but are not yet competent.'

In your own care setting, the implementation of the CQC regulations will ensure that you are not only complying with the law but also monitoring staff performance to ensure that there are no breaches of standards in your setting. The CQC website has guidance for providers on meeting the HSCA 2008 (Regulated Activities) Regulations 2014 (Part 3) (as amended) and the Care Quality Commission (Registration) Regulations 2009 (Part 4) (as amended). For more information, see CQC (2015).

The Care Certificate

The Care Certificate identifies supervision as a key role for workers, insisting that it be supportive rather than judgemental.

The focus of supervision is for the care professional to practise in such a way as to meet legal requirements and to ensure that codes of practice and local policy are being followed.

Research it

1.1 CQC guidance and professional supervision

Look at the CQC document 'Guidance for providers on meeting the regulations: Health and Social Care Act 2008 (Regulated Activities) Regulations 2014 (Part 3) (as amended), Care Quality Commission (Registration) Regulations 2009 (Part 4) (as amended).

On page 3, the guidance states, 'Regulation 21 of the HSCA 2008 (Regulated Activity) Regulations 2014 (as amended) says that registered persons "must have regard" to this guidance.'

Demonstrate how you meet the requirements set out in these Regulations in your setting.

'Section 25(1) says that the CQC will take this guidance into account' when regulatory decisions are made. If your setting is already registered with CQC, consider this guidance in relation to the regulated activities you provide and demonstrate to your assessor what you do to meet the Regulations.

The policies and procedures within your own work setting will reflect the legal position and any guidelines that need to be followed and you need to make a thorough analysis of these policies to ensure that you understand how they may impact your work as a supervisor. Analysing your policies in line with legislation will ensure that staff are being given the best supervision experience in line with legal requirements.

Safeguarding procedures

A core responsibility of supervision is to deliver adult social care that is safe for all. As a manager of adult care services, you are responsible for the safety and wellbeing of the individuals using your service, but for those individuals who are less able to protect themselves from harm, neglect or abuse, or those with impaired mental capacity, there is a greater need for diligence. Safeguarding, therefore, prevents the harm and abuse of individuals through the provision of high-quality care. Additionally, any allegations of harm or abuse should be responded to effectively and according to policy.

Agreed ways of working

These are the ways in which your work setting wants you to work in accordance with policy or procedure. With supervision it is easy to forget the importance of this practice and sometimes it can become an activity that is not taken seriously enough or not given time to. As a manager it is, therefore, vital that you practise in accordance with the supervision policy and devote time to its implementation and use.

Compliments and complaints

A compliments and complaints systems will help you to identify where the practice is working and where it is falling short.

The intention through supervision is to ensure that all people who use services in social care settings have the capacity to lead independent and fulfilling lives. It also ensures that staff themselves feel supported in their work and have recourse to a system of help should they require it. By using the compliments and complaints system within your sessions you can start to address the failings and the successes of your work.

Reflect on it

1.1 Compliments and complaints

Write a short reflective piece about how compliments and complaints have informed supervision where you work. These could be compliments and complaints from those who use care services, or you may even like to think about compliments and complaints that you have received with regard to supervision, for example:

- How have these impacted supervision?
- Have they led to an improvement in supervision practice? How?
- Have they led to improvements in the care services that your setting offers to individuals? How?
- What did you do to address these compliments and complaints?

Evidence opportunity

1.1 Ways supervision can be informed

Outline how your supervision is informed by current legislation, codes of practice and agreed ways of working, compliments and complaints.

AC 1.2 Describe the function of effective professional supervision in adult care

Here, you will describe the key principles and functions of supervision, including the areas covered in this section.

What is professional supervision?

Supervision is a process whereby a manager or supervisor oversees, supports and develops the knowledge and skills of someone else (a supervisee). It is the way in which a manager can enable a worker to carry out their role in an effective manner.

Skills for Care (2020) defines supervision as 'providing support for staff members with different aspects of their role. The supportive function can help to address any emerging issues that may impact staff performance and/or wellbeing.'

It further defines supervision as 'a process that involves a manager meeting regularly and interacting with staff to review their work.' This regular meeting will include a review of workload, ensuring the expected standards are being met and the discussion of learning and development opportunities.

The Social Care Institute for Excellence (SCIE) website defines supervision as:

> *a process by which one worker is given responsibility by the organisation to work with another worker in order to meet certain organisational, professional and personal objectives which together promote the best outcomes for service users ... good one-to-one supervision has the following features:*
>
> - *it occurs regularly in a safe environment*
> - *it is based on a respectful relationship*
> - *the process is understood and valued, and is embedded in the organisation's culture.*

Source: Lambley and Marrable (2013) quoted on SCIE website

Carroll (2007) provides a fantastic potted history of the development of what we now know is supervision, from its inception during Freud's time to now:

> *At its simplest, supervision is a forum where supervisees review and reflect on their work in order to do it better. Practitioners bring their actual work practice to another person (individual supervision), or to a group (small group or team supervision), and with their help review what happened in their practice in order to learn from that experience. Ultimately, supervision is for better quality service.*

Research it

1.2 Models of supervision

The three primary models of supervision are:

- developmental models
- integrated models
- orientation-specific models.

You will also come across:

- managerial supervision
- clinical supervision
- professional supervision.

The first three models are those primarily used in a counselling or psychotherapeutic context. Research these various models and write down your findings.

As a care worker and manager, you will have your own ideas about supervision. It is important, though, to focus on the purpose of the activity as well as the main principles.

Function of professional supervision

The function of supervision is to provide professional support and learning for staff, to enable them to develop knowledge, skills and competence in their work. This enhances the experience of those using the service and in turn improves quality and safety in the care setting. As a manager, it is your responsibility to provide professional supervision for the staff to ensure that they are supported in their roles and to enhance their skills and performance.

It is a practice that should provide regular, ongoing support for staff and as such time should be set aside for it. Staff must clear about the need for supervision, what it is for and also given space to discuss issues in a confidential and safe environment.

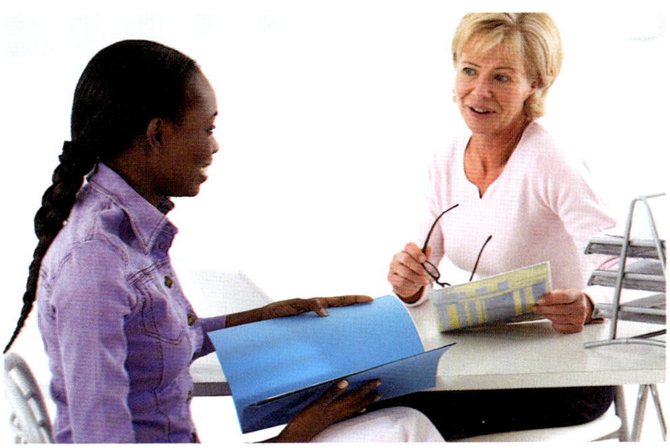

▲ **Figure 13** Professional supervision involves supporting care workers to carry out their roles effectively

There are three key functions of supervision.

Supportive supervision

This involves supervisors providing support for staff members which can help to address any emerging issues that may impact staff performance and/or wellbeing. Supervisors can support staff with challenges in their role and monitor staff health and wellbeing, ensuring that the organisation has the right support in place to address any issues. Any issues that need further investigation, for example if there are concerns regarding performance, can be dealt with in this role. Staff can also be informed about the wider organisation and any changes or developments.

Line management supervision

Line management supervision helps managers to maintain good standards of work by ensuring that staff are following policies and procedures. In a supervisory role the manager can manage team resources and delegate workload, using supervision to provide meaningful communication between managers and staff at all levels.

Setting targets and objectives and discussing performance and quality can also be a function of supervision. As a manager you have a duty of care to ensure that staff clearly follow the standards that are expected of them.

Educational and/or developmental supervision

The purpose of this type of supervision is to help staff to develop critical thinking and analysis skills, and also explore and develop their own learning needs. For supervisors, this function might include an assessment of staff skills and knowledge.

Supervision provides support to and enables the development of good practice for care workers, thus improving the quality of service provided by the organisation. It is a vital part of individual performance management.

In regulated care services, social care workers and managers are required to undergo supervision and meet standards and requirements. As a manager, you are accountable for the quality of the service provided and therefore need to have a good grasp of how staff are performing. Supervision is one way in which you can undertake this task.

Evidence opportunity

1.2 Supervision

Describe the key principles and functions of supervision in your setting.

AC 1.3 Explain different supervision activities and processes which can be used in adult care

Here, you will explain the different methods of supervision used in the work setting.

Supervision can occur individually, in threes (triadic) with two supervisees and one supervisor, in groups (of more than three) or as a whole team supervision and can also happen with different supervisors.

Some of the most common activities in supervision are described below.

- **Supervisee self-report**: This is when the supervisee discusses or brings case studies to include in the dialogue with their supervisor. The supervisee discusses incidents that may have caused them concern or areas of practice they felt went well. This gives the supervisor the opportunity to ask questions to enable the supervisee to reflect on practice. The supervisor can then give guidance and support.
- **Observation**: This can be live and on the job with the supervisor present, or it might involve a video recording.
- **Role-playing**: This involves acting out scenarios, with the supervisor and supervisee taking on the roles of counsellor and individual, or individual and care worker.
- **Modelling**: This is also a type of role-playing, but the supervisor takes on the role of counsellor or care worker, assuming their role as an aid to teaching a technique or giving an intervention to the supervisee.

Evidence opportunity

1.3 Conducting supervision

Provide an explanation about how you conduct your supervision.

AC 1.4 Describe how effective supervision supports and protects different groups

Here, you will describe the ways in which supervision can benefit the different groups in the work setting.

Supporting and protecting the supervisee and carers/volunteers

Effective supervision is about sharing experiences in a safe environment, whether you are a carer or a volunteer in a setting, and informality will enable both parties to feel comfortable and safe. It is important to set boundaries, such as how the session will be conducted and what can be discussed, as well as addressing confidentiality, at the outset of the process. In doing so the worker can feel confident that the session is being taken seriously and is not just a tick box exercise.

Without such a structure in place there is a danger that supervision sessions will not be viewed as meaning much and learning may not occur at all. The best way to impose structure on the proceedings is to first ensure that there is a supervision policy in place. If so, then you will be expected to undertake this aspect of staff development and there will be guidelines as to how you can do this.

The whole process of supervision needs to be 'owned' not only by the organisation but also by the supervisee. Everybody needs to feel part of the process if the merits of such an activity are to be appreciated.

Thompson (2006) writes:

> *Some people unfortunately adopt a narrow view of supervision and see it primarily ... as a means of ensuring that sufficient quantity and quality of work is carried out ... a broader view of supervision can play a significant role in promoting learning and developing a culture of continuous professional development.*

The support provided in supervision gives the supervisee the space to talk about concerns in their practice and to check in with how they are practicing. They can talk about certain processes and procedures in safety and discuss how they dealt with situations and how they might improve.

A possible framework

You may wish to adopt the following framework to manage your supervision sessions:

- Establish ground rules and boundaries, reminding the supervisee of these at the start of each session.
- Remind the supervisee of the need for confidentiality of information on both sides and agree the boundaries of such and areas that may have to be divulged.
- To ensure that the supervisee is confident that the whole process will take place in a calm and confidential manner, the room must afford privacy and you will need to ensure that mobile phones are switched off or landlines re-routed to another line for the duration of the meeting.
- Agree that the session will not be interrupted unless an emergency occurs and agree what constitutes an emergency. This will really help to confirm the importance of the process.

- Agree the appropriate reasons for cancelling the session.
- Identify the agenda for discussion at the start of each session and agree an action plan following each item discussed. Both you and the supervisee should agree on this. This should fit within the categories of:
  - clinical issues/reflections on role and accountability
  - what support is needed/professional issues
  - educational issues/workload discussions
  - management issues.
- Ensure appropriate allocation of time and agree that you, the supervisor, should act as timekeeper.
- A brief record of the contents of the session should be kept by the supervisor.
- Conduct the session in a non-judgemental/non-discriminatory manner.

Accountability, when it comes to confidentiality, means we need to take responsibility for personal data. Employees working in adult care are bound by a legal duty of confidence to protect personal information. This is a legal requirement. You and your setting will need to be aware of legislation such as the Data Protection Act 2018 and make sure you comply with it.

Supporting and protecting individuals and families

During supervision you may become party to knowledge about individuals in your care and brought into confidential discussions. You and the supervisee need to be clear that although in such cases the protection of individuals, their families and other carers is very important, if safety is compromised then the confidentiality of the supervision session may need to be breached. For example, your supervisee may express concern about the treatment of an individual by others in the team. In supervision, such discussion would be confidential, but in cases where there may be a safety issue it is your duty to ensure that the information is shared with the appropriate agencies and perhaps the family of the individual. This would need to be discussed with the supervisee.

> **Reflect on it**
>
> **1.4 Engaging with supervision**
>
> Think about how you and your staff currently engage with supervision.
>
> Describe the framework of these sessions and reflect on how they might be made more useful for both you and the staff.

AC 1.5 Describe how effective supervision can protect the supervisor and the setting/service

Here, you will describe how supervision is essential for you and your setting.

To provide effective supervision and to remain safe in that practice, supervisors must model high levels of good practice and must be competent and professional. They should work within ethical boundaries and develop good relationships. Safety for the practice is built into the clear management of personal boundaries and the confines of confidentiality. Supervisors need to be aware of conflicts of interest and avoiding exploitation.

By behaving with integrity and honesty and acting within the law, the supervisor will remain safe in the role. All communications and discussion that involve the individuals using the service and are divulged in supervision should remain confidential and compatible with policy.

> **Reflect on it**
>
> **1.5 Maintaining boundaries and acting honestly**
>
> How do you maintain your own safety with respect to the information shared with you in supervision?
>
> Give an example of how you behave honestly and in a confidential manner.

AC 1.6 Explain why the wellbeing of the supervisee should be included within effective supervision and supportive practices

Here, you will explain how supervision can benefit the wellbeing of all staff members and outline practices that will enable effective supervision.

The wellbeing of staff is not just about the absence of illness and the fact that they show up for their shifts on a regular basis. It combines physical, mental, emotional and social health factors. As a manager, you want staff to feel happy at work and satisfied with the job they are doing so staff wellbeing could be described as how they are feeling about themselves, their lives and their work.

Our lives are influenced by many factors which can impact our wellbeing. Our relationships with partners, friends and work colleagues, having enough money, having a career, being physically fit, optimistic and having some form of belief and belonging are all factors that can affect our self-esteem. The factors of wellbeing are interrelated. For example, a job provides not just money but purpose, goals, friendships and a sense of belonging. However, sometimes aspects of our work are difficult and may be less than fulfilling.

Supervision provides an environment in which staff can explore their own personal and emotional reactions to their work and their job and reflect on and challenge their own practice in a safe and confidential environment as well as receive feedback on their skills. Managers can check in on the wellbeing of their staff members and start to determine what they need for their professional development and their wellbeing. Effective supervision will develop a good working relationship which can provide the opportunity to discuss wellbeing and any social, physical, emotional and psychological needs of the staff member.

> **Evidence opportunity**
>
> **1.6 Managing wellbeing during supervision**
>
> How do you ensure that the wellbeing of staff is managed in supervision? Share an example but ensure that you are mindful of the confidentiality requirements – anonymise your example.

AC 1.7 Describe ways to enable and promote effective supervision and supportive practices

Here, you will assess different methods of effective supervision and supportive practices.

While there are a number of models for supervision, including one-to-one supervision, group supervision and peer group supervision, the approach chosen will depend on a number of factors, including personal choice, access to supervision, length of experience, qualifications and availability of supervisory groups.

Alongside supervision there will also be appraisals, one-to-one meetings, mentoring, counselling and coaching.

Appraisals

Appraisals, which may be an annual event, ideally discuss performance and should be a regular event at team meetings and on an individual basis. Regular updates on progress towards targets and goals that have been set are likely to be more meaningful than a yearly meeting. For more on appraisal, see Unit 505 AC2.1.

Mentoring

Skills for Care advocate the use of mentoring programmes for staff, who can access their mentor on a regular basis to support self-development through discussions. Staff will often have questions to which an immediate answer may be crucial. They cannot always wait for supervision, so having a mentor on hand to discuss their question is good practice which can help mentees to move forward. In such a partnership staff will be 'encouraged to take control of their own development, try things out, learn from mistakes and benefit from the advice and support of the mentor' (Skills for Care, 2019).

For more on mentoring, see Unit 500 AC2.3 and Unit 505 AC2.1.

One-to-one meetings

A one-to-one meeting takes place outside formal supervision or appraisals. There is no set way of doing these and they can be ad hoc. New staff may want more regular one-to-one meetings, but for established team members a monthly one-to-one may be enough for an opportunity to discuss priorities and provide updates on operational matters. You might also use the time to discuss support and learning requirements.

One-to-one meetings are informal but always require your full attention. This can be a good time to discuss feedback on performance and to receive feedback about how well you are supporting the team member too. It is also the time to check in on wellbeing, current workload and to pass on any information about the setting.

Counselling and support networks

During appraisals and one-to-one meetings, it may become apparent that a member of staff will require support that might be outside what you can offer. For example, you may become aware of a domestic issue which is impacting a member of staff's health and wellbeing. You will be responsible for escalating the issue to a safeguarding officer in your setting and providing your staff member with further help. Staff members who have mental health issues that are impacting their lives can be offered counselling services and your human resources team will be able to give advice on this.

Other support networks include employee assistance programmes or links to people in your own or partner organisations who have a mental health first aid qualification and are trained to support employee mental health.

Coaching

Coaching is a highly effective way to raise the quality and impact of management and leadership by guiding and supporting staff. As a result, staff develop self-confidence and increased motivation as they can focus on their own development aims and objectives.

However, it can be a costly exercise as coaches are usually external to the setting. Developing your own in-house team of coaches can be a way forward.

For more on coaching see Unit 500 AC2.1 and Unit 500 AC2.2

Evidence opportunity

1.7 Ensuring that staff are supervised

Describe the activity you undertake to ensure that your staff are supervised. Include one-to-one supervision, group supervision and peer group supervision, and describe factors that have affected your choice of approach.

AC 1.8 Explain how external and internal factors influence practice and can be used within professional supervision objectives

Here, you will explain how external factors, such as national polices, and internal factors, such as lessons learned from internal events, can be used to enhance supervision.

External factors, such as updates to national policy or local procedures and evidence of best practice, can be used in supervision sessions. This would be a good opportunity to share with the staff member changes that impact their own practice. Social movements and campaigns are also external factors that are useful for discussion in supervision as they may impact the work that is being done. Based on raising awareness of an issue to generate support, social movements typically strive for policy or cultural change. Campaigns are set up to generate support for the movement.

Internal factors, for supervision may include lessons learned/learning reviews, concerns or complaints, skills development/training or the emerging needs of individuals accessing services.

Lessons learned from practice are likely to emerge from supervisee self-reporting when the supervisee has reflected on their actions during a situation or incident and can see how they might change their practice as a result. This can then lead to a discussion about further development or training that might need to be undertaken.

Supervision can also be used to address complaints or concerns brought to the manager about the supervisee, where these areas can be addressed formally and again, development plans put into place. Further training may be needed for the staff member, and this can be planned with them at this time.

Evidence opportunity

1.8 Factors affecting staff practice

Explain the external and internal factors influencing the practice of your staff and how is this brought to supervision.

AC 1.9 AC1.9 Describe how supervision can be used alongside appraisals and professional development processes to enhance performance and aspirations of the supervisee

Here, you will describe how the interaction between supervision, appraisals and continuous professional development can be used to enhance the performance of the supervisee.

By using a performance management cycle, you impose structure and process on the management of staff, their training and development needs and supervision.

Performance management involves the use of appraisals and professional development activities. In any organisation, the aim is to produce and deliver high-quality services and to ensure that all opportunities for improvement, change and innovation are clearly identified and worked towards. To achieve that end, the organisation must realise its potential against performance targets and ensure that the performance management systems in place get the best out of people in the workplace and deliver the best for people who use the services. This can be monitored through the supervision process.

Existing systems and procedures

All adult care systems in the UK are required to provide safe and good quality care and support, as well as continually updating practice and systems in the light of evidence from research.

The scandal of the Winterbourne View hospital for adults with learning disabilities and the subsequent report from the CQC concluded that a systemic failure to protect people or to investigate allegations of abuse had been found. Staff did not appear to understand the needs of the people in their care, and those who had no background in care services had been recruited. References had not been checked and staff were not trained or supervised properly. The use of methods of restraint without considering alternatives was too readily sought. Additionally, the abuse experienced by older adults in care homes in Cornwall led to several Safeguarding Adults Reviews being undertaken with subsequent changes being ordered.

Performance management systems identify organisational goals, measuring the achievement of those goals through different systems, which control employee behaviour and performance. Target setting, 360-degree appraisal and personal development plans together with supervision are designed to measure staff performance. The advantages of these approaches are that they are less subject to personal bias and provide information and evidence. A disadvantage is that the collection of such information can be time consuming.

Standards and policies to support performance management

The essential standards of quality and safety consist of 28 regulations (and associated outcomes) that are set out in two pieces of legislation: the Health and Social Care Act 2008 (Regulated Activities) Regulations 2014 and the Care Quality Commission (Registration) Regulations 2009. Together with the apprenticeship standard, knowledge and skills, they are helping to change the performance management framework in the social care sector, and this is something to celebrate. The inspection process and even the supervisory framework you adopt should be seen as an opportunity to improve performance and service delivery rather than be used as a punitive or disciplinary measure to be feared. Critics argue that performance management is not a good thing for this very reason and there are also some people who do not value supervision. However, effective performance management and supervision can promote good quality service delivery and result in more highly motivated staff (SCIE, 2007).

As a supervisor, there is a need to measure performance against results and not merely focus on behaviours and activity. Think for a moment about the member of staff who always seems to have a lot to do but rarely accomplishes what should be done. In this instance, the employee needs to be made aware of the organisational goals together with methods by which those goals may be achieved. This can be done through good supervision, continuing professional development and effective line management.

The role of individual supervision and performance indicators

As previously stated, supervision is an important part of professional development and managing the performance of staff. Setting SMART objectives is key so that each member of staff can show they have reached the desired standards, and you, as manager, can be satisfied that the safety and wellbeing of those using the service is maintained.

A good way in which to do this is to have a set of performance criteria made up of measures and standards that clearly state the level of performance required in different areas. You need to ensure that the setting's organisational performance indicators are used to focus on what the organisation wants to achieve. These might be:

- deadlines or delivery
- cost or budgets
- the views of colleagues and of individuals using the service on your performance
- the quality that is expected
- how much is expected or the quantity.

You also need to ensure that the objectives you set are:

- consistent with the member of staff's job description
- consistent with the organisational goals
- clearly expressed
- supported by measurable performance criteria
- challenging.

Setting objectives is not an easy task by any means, but objectives that are specific, measurable, achievable, relevant and time bound, or SMART, are a useful way to start.

- **Specific**: Being specific means you have a much greater chance of success and the way to set such a goal is to plan with these questions in mind:
  - Who is involved?
  - What do I want to accomplish?
  - Where will this happen?
  - When – in what timescale?
  - Which requirements and constraints do I need to identity?
  - Why do I need to do this?

  Example: Tina Tilmouth to rewrite the Safeguarding Policy by the end of [date].

Although this example does not specify the reason for doing this, it can be assumed that safeguarding being a huge area in care work is a good enough reason.

- **Measurable**: To ensure that your target is measurable, you might ask questions such as:
  - How much?
  - How many?
  - How will I know when it is accomplished?

In the case of the example above, I will know it is done when it is written. I might also add how much I would expect to be written; I could, for example, specify a word count.

- **Achievable**: An achievable target for a member of staff is one which they agree is needed and one they can actually do. In helping a member of staff in this part of target setting, you could identify small steps towards a larger goal and outline dates by which they should achieve this.

- **Realistic**: To be realistic, the member of staff and you as the manager must believe that they can actually accomplish the task. It is wise to check that the individual has done something similar in the past and is given the opportunity to identify what they might need in terms of support to accomplish the target.
- **Time bound**: Without a timeframe, the target loses urgency and momentum. By setting a date for completion, there is a given point when the task is to be completed and delivered.

Having a large number of performance indicators will result in little progress being made and it is important to be aware of this. By measuring practice using SMART objectives, the information you obtain may then be used in staff appraisals. The facts obtained provide firm evidence for performance and will show improvement or limitations. As a manager, it is crucial to focus your staff on essential areas for improvement.

Setting organisational performance indicators to improve and monitor the performance of individuals

Your organisation's objectives are the starting point when it comes to setting targets for performance. You will also be aware of staff job descriptions and the competencies required to carry out certain roles. To maintain high-quality care in your organisation you need to create a performance management system which:

- identifies areas of best practice
- focuses on continuous improvement
- sets organisational and individual performance indicators to improve and monitor the performance of individuals.

For example, a performance indicator is a performance measurement that helps you understand how your organisation or team member is performing and whether you are achieving the strategic goals. You might need to know what percentage of your staff receive regular supervision, so a target will be set which may be measured against appraisal, supervision and personal development records when audited. This will help to:

- deliver better outcomes for those using the services
- improve care services by acting upon new initiatives and information
- ensure that organisational activities are linked to the overall goals of the organisation.

Helping individuals set and achieve meaningful goals in respect of their practice

One of the most important functions you have as a manager is to ensure that staff are fully aware of the organisational strategy and targets, and to link those with individual objectives. In supervising staff, performance management is an issue that needs to be part of the agenda. Staff must be clear about the aims and focus of their job role in relation to the wider aims of the organisation, and it is the supervisor's responsibility to ensure that staff are clear about how they can achieve these objectives.

Staff appraisals, performed at the end of an annual cycle for managing staff, are a vehicle for reviewing the goals set throughout the supervision process and planning for the year to come:

- Review the job description and role.
- Look at individual performance and achievement and reward (performance-related pay or other incentives).
- Plan ongoing professional development.
- Give feedback.

The object of appraisal is to set goals for the coming year and to identify ways in which the staff member can improve their performance over the next year. It should be a positive process in which the member of staff can be given details about their performance and can start to plan for the forthcoming year. Staff who have been underperforming should have been made aware of this during supervision and an appraisal will identify ways in which they can meet the required standards in the year to come. They should not be surprised to learn of the problems with their performance at this stage in the proceedings since they will have received feedback in the previous supervision sessions.

The process of appraisal is similar to supervision. For example, you could check in with how the staff member is going about their own CPD and whether the work they are doing is within their expertise or if they need to develop their skills further. You may also want to look at how the employee dealt with the workload and what they have achieved with the individuals using the service.

There is more information on appraisals in AC1.7 of this unit.

For individual staff in an organisation, one method of measuring performance may be management by objectives (MBO), developed by Peter Drucker, who was an influential writer and thinker on management theory. The process of MBO involves the manager and employee identifying employee goals together with a list of the resources and a timeframe necessary to achieve those goals. Meetings to evaluate the outcomes and to discuss progress are held regularly and during these meetings goals may be reset. The employee's performance is measured by how many goals have been accomplished within the timeframe. For more information, see Communication Theory (n.d.).

Research it

1.9 Drucker's management by objectives model

Research Drucker's management by objectives model.

How might you go about setting organisational performance indicators to improve and monitor the performance of your staff?

If you already set performance indicators, how does this support performance?

AC 1.10 Evaluate the factors which can result in a power imbalance in professional supervision

Here, you will evaluate power imbalances and how these can be addressed.

Factors that result in power imbalance

Being the manager means you invariably supervise the work of the team and this may lead to power imbalance and occasionally conflict. Supervision in care has become one of the ways in which it is possible to monitor employees' work, ensuring that performance indicators are being met. This can lead to conflict, so you need to look at ways to address the imbalance.

Evidence opportunity

1.10 Factors leading to power imbalance and how to address these

What factors might you see resulting in a power imbalance in professional supervision in your setting? How do you deal with power imbalance in your own setting? What action do you take, for example, when an important decision needs to be made which you know is likely to be unpopular? Evaluate an example from your workplace. Make sure that your example is anonymised.

AC 1.11 Describe how to address any power imbalance in professional supervision

Here, you will explore management supervision practice with regard to some of the areas we discuss in this section.

Addressing power imbalances in formal supervision

In most organisations, there will be people who have more power than others simply because they are in a higher position in the hierarchy. This may bring about a power imbalance in the adult care setting and may be a barrier to adult care and also to staff relationships. In formal supervision, staff need to know that, despite the existence of a hierarchical difference between supervisor and supervisee, their input is valued and shared decision making is possible.

Power that comes with positions in adult care can be used in a positive way, but often the concept of power has negative connotations of abuse and harassment, and this type of thinking can lead people to distrust anybody who is in a position of power. In this way, power can be perceived as influencing or controlling somebody negatively. This can affect supervision.

If you are the manager in a work setting, you are already in a position of power. It is possible that you may even have recruited the people you manage. You have influence and authority over those people.

Two main types of power, personal and organisational, are worthy of further investigation here. When we refer to personal power, we are noting the knowledge, skills and competence associated with an individual that make them an expert. As an expert, the individual can exert a certain amount of power in various situations. Think about the teacher–learner relationship.

According to Gopee and Galloway (2009), organisational power can be of four types:

- **Reward power**: The manager's ability to give inducements such as pay, promotion or praise to move an organisation forward.
- **Coercive power**: The use of sanctions such as disciplinary procedures.
- **Legitimate power**: That which comes with a rank in an organisation that gives authority.
- **Information power**: Based on access to information or data that is valued and not open to all.

Power imbalance is common between employer and worker and supervisor–employee relationships simply because we may be affected by a person who has greater authority than ourselves. But power imbalance can be healthy or not and conflict has the potential to arise when imbalance occurs.

How to address power imbalance in own supervision practice

If you recognise that a power imbalance exists in the supervision relationship, then you can start to address it. What do we mean by this? Look at the following case study.

Case study

1.11 Power imbalance

James was the manager in a large care organisation but found his role a difficult one. He always blamed the unpopular decisions he had to make on higher management with the line 'it's not my decision, it's what they have told me to do' and then took credit for the more palatable ones. In time, he lost credibility with staff who saw his lack of integrity.

What do you think was the problem here and how might James gain the staff's trust again?

James was clearly trying to be popular with the staff while failing to accept that he would sometimes have to make unpopular decisions. It seems he was not comfortable with that and did not want to adopt an authoritarian approach or an approach in which he would be seen to be dictating and directing matters. Unfortunately, staff are likely to lose confidence in this type of manager and then conflict arises.

As a manager with responsibility for the smooth running of a department or organisation, your staff will be looking to you to lead with respect for them and honesty. You will always have the power in the relationship because you are accountable for the actions of the staff, that is, the buck stops with you.

However, you are responsible for addressing power imbalances and there is no need to take an authoritarian approach to how you lead. Having a conscious awareness of how being 'in charge' can make or break a relationship means you can take control of decisions and set the tone for the work group. While it is good to be 'one of the team' and adopt a friendly manner towards staff, there is a fine line between this and taking control of a situation when you need to. It is always best policy to act with honesty, integrity, fairness and respect for others – this will help to ensure a positive relationship between the supervisor and the supervisee.

Managing difficult situations, disagreements and conflict during formal supervision

Difficult situations and conflict that arise in the workplace can cause the team to feel insecure and as their manager you need to establish stability. By reminding them about how you value their work, you should offer the opportunity to talk about concerns they have in a professional manner. By approaching conflict in this way, you are demonstrating how each person involved in the conflict should behave. By showing each other respect, conflict can be quickly diminished.

What is a conflict situation and why does it occur?

In supervision, the potential for conflict arises when there is a disagreement about a point of professional practice or the values and goals of the supervisor do not fit with those of the supervisee. For example, the supervisor may challenge the member of staff, and this could cause some opposition.

You may come across two types of conflict:

- **Task-based conflict**: Disagreements related to approaches to work, processes and structural issues within the team and the organisation.
- **Relationship-based conflict**: Conflicts between individual members of the team, usually caused by differences in personal values and beliefs.

Specific areas of conflict that you may come across during supervision include:

- lack of clarity around team roles and responsibilities
- unfair distribution of work
- lack of clear vision on the part of the supervisee
- lack of understanding of the role of others
- poor communication.

Effects of conflict

Conflict can disrupt performance but within teams it is a common occurrence. When the resolution of the conflict is effective, it can have a positive effect, leading to personal growth and development.

If managed effectively, conflict can be 'creative and productive and creative solutions to difficult problems can often be found through positive conflict resolution' (Tilmouth et al., 2011).

How to deal with conflict situations

Resolving conflict in a team is done most effectively by the people concerned having a constructive conversation. LaFasto and Larson's (2001) CONECT model for resolving conflict by conversation is useful – see Unit 509 AC3.4.

It would also be useful for you to read about Thompson's RED approach to managing conflict – see Unit 509 AC3.4.

In resolving conflict, when people's needs are discovered then a solution can be found. We may be tempted to compromise, but compromise means that people's needs are still not fully met, and this can lead to resentment (West, 2004).

Ensuring that conflicts are addressed in the right manner means that relationships are maintained and can function smoothly.

Reflecting on practice

A conflict situation is never pleasant but by reflecting on the circumstances that led to the event and thinking about how it might have been handled in a different way you can sometimes find more useful ways of managing conflict should it arise again.

In dealing with any challenging situation, your supervisees must be directed to the policies in the workplace and should be given the opportunity to undergo training. Challenging behaviour by an individual using the service, another staff member or a visitor can be frightening, and staff need to be given the opportunity to talk about the situation and to discuss the triggers that may have led to the outburst.

It is a good idea to discuss this with new staff and to remind experienced staff of the types of challenging behaviour your setting might come across and to ensure that they understand how they are to deal with such incidents. By reflecting on these incidents, staff can learn from challenging situations and start to be more aware of how they felt in such instances.

By evaluating the event in this way, staff can start to appreciate how they might have been affected by a situation and how others may also be affected. They will also see how circumstances at the time may have led to the event and this sort of examination can be useful in planning for a different reaction the next time it happens.

Reflect on it

1.11 Conflict areas in supervision

Identify an example of a conflict situation in supervision you have had to deal with and discuss it with your assessor.

Reflect on it

1.11 Challenging behaviour

Remind yourself of your policies with respect to how you would help staff to deal with behaviour that challenges.

Research it

1.11 Conflict management

For your next team meeting, add an item on conflict management to the agenda.

Collect information about how staff manage conflict with the individuals using the service and with other staff members. Use this information to provide a record of types of conflict experienced and ways in which it is managed.

Managing challenges arising during and after professional supervision

Occasionally, difficult situations within supervision and team management arise. You may have to deal with cases of poor individual or team performance or complaints from members of the public via commissioning agencies that deal with quality issues. It is likely that at times of staff shortages, you may have to respond to the worries or complaints of team members who are unhappy about the situation they are in.

The fact that conflict exists, however, is not necessarily a bad thing, because if it is resolved effectively, it can lead to personal and professional growth. If managed well, conflict can be creative and productive, and creative solutions to difficult problems can often be found through positive conflict resolution. However, conflict within the team or among staff should not impact the wellbeing of the individuals using the service.

Support systems available to staff after formal supervision

Staff need to be aware that they can receive support after formal supervision should they so wish. They can be directed to your manager if they wish to discuss a grievance or can simply talk to a mentor or a peer to discuss what happened. In an organisation that values and respects its employees, everybody should feel able to discuss challenging situations in a responsible and open manner.

Current appraisal processes used alongside supervision to manage and improve performance with those they manage

See ACs 1.7 and 1.9 for more information on appraisals.

Task-based and relationship-based conflict was covered earlier in this unit, but there can also be conflict with carers and the individuals using a service over service decisions. Whatever the cause of the conflict, the related emotions can be damaging to the care being delivered. People may start to avoid each other, with rifts developing as teams take sides. In the midst of this, the individuals using the service will suffer as care starts to disintegrate into ineffectiveness.

One of the crucial things to remember here is that behaviour may be the only way a person can communicate at that time, and it is important for you as manager to find out what the 'function' of that behaviour is. For example, a member of staff in a supervision setting may start to lose their temper and shout at you. This can be because they are frustrated in some way or cannot articulate well enough what they are feeling. Although the behaviour is potentially threatening to you, by trying to understand the reason for that behaviour you can help to change the situation. It is easy to shout back or to manhandle somebody, but by standing back and trying to determine what led to the behaviour and what is being communicated by that behaviour you can work towards defusing the situation.

If you describe behaviour in a negative manner, you are likely to deal with it as such. But if you view it as a way of getting attention to a problem, you might have a different reaction to it. By working out what the 'function' of the behaviour is and what it helps the person to achieve in a given situation you can then start to help the individual to deal with the situation they find difficult in more constructive ways.

You might use the following as a guide:

- Get the facts first and ask questions – it's common to race to find a solution, but it is more useful to gather information and ask questions to really understand what is happening.
- Ask questions that get to the core problem and try to stop the person going into too much detail.
- Listen carefully.
- Reflect on the answers you are given and do not be too quick to jump in with a solution. Do not be tempted to think you know the answer and pre-judge the person. Avoid making such a judgement, as it may be wrong.
- Act professionally.
- Aim for a balanced solution. You do not want people to feel that they have lost a battle and that management has won! Negotiate to find a mutually acceptable solution where both parties feel listened to. This may not always be possible but careful negotiation can be useful.

Case study

1.11 Dealing with challenging situations

Nadia is a member of staff who has worked in the same role for three years. She is currently experiencing some issues at home and has recently been off sick for at least one span of duty per fortnight. There seems to be a pattern developing and you are wondering what is going on. In your regular supervision session, Nadia becomes very defensive and starts to lose her temper with you. You remain calm – you are aware that this is uncharacteristic but is something you need to address.

How will you deal with this situation?

Reflect on it

1.11 Behaviour that challenges policies

Remind yourself of your policies with respect to how to deal with behaviour that challenges shown by a member of your staff and how a power imbalance might be addressed.

Reflect on it

1.11 Managing and reflecting on conflict situations

What sort of conflict have you managed in your own practice? Identify an area of conflict you have been involved in with a member of staff and write a short piece showing how you managed that situation.

Evidence opportunity

1.11 Factors that can result in a power imbalance

Describe the management supervision practice in place in your setting and describe how power imbalances are addressed.

AC 1.12 Describe ways to address any challenges that might arise during professional supervision

Here, you will describe the challenges that may occur because of supervision and methods of addressing those challenges.

Common examples of supervision challenges might be the result of workplace challenges. You may give constructive feedback but find it is not well received. This might be due to a misunderstanding either of intentions, expectations or job priorities. Poor communication between employees, leadership and employees might also result in challenge in the supervision session.

Staff may also be challenged by a lack of planning in the workplace, which can lead to high levels of stress. Low staff levels and dealing with other staff who are not the right fit for the setting or who are not pulling their weight will also negatively impact the overall morale of the workforce.

Whatever the challenge or conflict, feedback needs to be provided on a regular basis and should be a daily part of your work as a manager but occasionally it is received defensively and may be challenged.

Occasionally, we are very critical about what we do, and it is therefore nice to hear some positive praise for how we have completed a particular job. Positive feedback is often not forthcoming and yet it is motivating when it is genuinely felt. Thanking somebody at the end of the day for a job well done or acknowledging a person's work during a shift builds respect and ensures that the member of staff is secure in their work.

Think about the following: Your manager wants to give you some constructive feedback and has called a meeting for that purpose. How are you feeling? You are probably approaching the meeting in a negative way, thinking that you are about to be criticised in some way. The term 'feedback' is often confused with criticism and how we might have done a job in a better way, and for that reason we view the whole concept less than positively.

If that is how you feel about it, it is likely your staff and supervisees share the same negative feelings. We cannot go through life without making mistakes and without requiring some guidance on aspects of our work, and although the content of feedback may be negative, it can always be given in a constructive and encouraging manner. When done this way, you can help the member of staff to solve a problem, or even to address an aspect of their behaviour and work towards organisational goals.

Constructive feedback must be based upon what you have observed about somebody's performance, and you should not fall into the trap of giving praise or criticism, which comes from a place of personal judgement. Instead, you should provide information that is specific to the issue in question. You need to give the message clearly and get right to the point and not give mixed messages. What you want to be done needs to be clear to the person receiving the message. For example, telling a colleague that she 'needs to improve her handover reports' is vague – she will need to be told *how* she can improve. Also, informing her that her handover was 'quite good' on Monday and adding the word 'but' or 'however' is not clear. She hears the praise but may fail to hear the real message, which is that she needs to improve. You need to give clear, constructive feedback. Emphasise the positives but be clear on how the supervisee can improve.

Unambiguous feedback that clearly sets out any issues

If you need to give negative feedback it should be done in such a way that the person is clear about what has to be done. The tone of voice in such a delivery is important, showing concern but never anger or frustration. The message needs to be helpful to the person and they need to know that it is sincere. Focus on what you have observed and be clear, concentrating on the facts of the situation. This shows a non-judgemental approach and means the issue does not become personal. For example, 'I have noticed that you are not using the hand gel on patients' bedsides before you approach them, and our guidelines specify that we should be doing this every time. Please make sure that you build this into your routine.' It is clear what you require as a manager and the member of staff is left with a clear message about what needs to improve.

> **Evidence opportunity**
>
> **1.12 Providing constructive feedback**
>
> Describe how you dealt with a challenge from a member of staff regarding constructive feedback you gave that was not well received. How did you deal with the challenge?

LO2 Be able to provide regular professional supervision

AC 2.1 Establish understanding and agreement with supervisee on key areas

Here, you will outline polices needed for supervision and how these can be agreed with the supervisee to ensure that supervision is effective.

Agree the purpose, frequency and location of supervision activities

As a manager, you must ensure that there is clarity about when supervision is to take place, how often, where it will be held and how the environment is to be managed. For example, it should be a quiet, well-lit place where there are no interruptions and any enquiries should be directed elsewhere. You also need to be strict about the duration of the session. Some of the more 'practical' roles and responsibilities of each party must also be established. For example, you must agree on the frequency and location of the supervision. How often you meet will depend upon the policy in your organisation, but you may agree to meet regularly on a fortnightly or monthly basis for 1–2 hours.

Both of you need to be prepared for each session and topics for discussion may be arranged in advance. An action plan may require the supervisee to do something before the next meeting and to bring it with them. For example, the supervisee may require some support in course work, and so they could bring with them copies of work, course content and reflective accounts of their learning so far, which you could discuss during the meeting. However, you will need to ensure that you do not fall into the trap of becoming a 'surrogate course tutor' for the supervisee but enable them to reflect on how their learning is affecting or changing their practice.

Agree actions which support preparation for supervision

In preparing for the supervisory meeting, staff need to be aware of the agenda set at the previous meeting. If this required work to be completed, they should get into the habit of bringing with them evidence to support the work done.

Prior to a supervision session, the supervisor and supervisee must have records in place and have taken time out of their day to be present. As a supervisor you should be mentally prepared to listen and respond to concerns and challenges from the supervisee. Additionally, you will want to discuss previously set goals and how the person is performing to reach those goals. You might also expect the supervisee to come with written summaries or records, which help them to discuss certain cases. Having the necessary records to hand and any agenda you need will also help.

Agree sources of data and evidence used to inform supervision

The evidence you require a member of staff to bring to supervision will depend on the agreement you have made and the agenda set at the last meeting. The evidence will be linked to the supervisee's objectives and may include reflective accounts of critical incidents that have occurred, assessments undertaken, observations and surveys of the individuals using the service.

All of this will be recorded in the supervisee's personnel file and will become part of their personal development plan.

Agree need for confidentiality, respecting boundaries, roles and accountability and action planning

Confidentiality is a requirement, so that the supervisee feels they are able to discuss with you things that are troubling them. Breaching confidentiality can lead to a lack of trust and a workforce that fails to give care that is of high quality. The assurance of confidentiality needs to be established at the very first session, with boundaries being set and accountability clearly shown. With a policy in place, together with a supervision agreement, you can then look at the roles and responsibilities in more detail.

The supervisor, who is likely to be you in your own area, is usually a skilled professional who assists staff to develop their skills and helps them to attain knowledge and professional values. You are also required to give advice in supervisory situations and to counsel staff on practice guidelines and policy. Supervisors require training in the process and should provide a good role model for the supervisee.

The person being supervised, or the supervisee, is a practitioner who receives professional advice, support and guidance from a supervisor who is engaged in observing and assisting staff in delivering good quality care and then giving feedback. In the case of an experienced person, the supervisor may impart support and guidance on reflective practice. You may occasionally manage people who have more experience than you and in this case you may be used more as a source of support in their practice.

Research it

2.1 Your supervision policy

Obtain a copy of your supervision policy. Discuss with your assessor how you might change it to fit what you have learned about supervision to date.

Evidence opportunity

2.1 Establishing agreement with the supervisee on key areas

Show your assessor how you gain agreement from your supervisee on key areas.

Reflect on it

2.1 Supervision meetings

Write about the way you set boundaries, ensure confidentiality and agree location and times for meetings. Ensure that you first have your supervisee's permission, and that names and other identifying details are changed.

In your supervision meetings, what actions do you take to prepare? What factors do you consider in terms of how often you have the meetings and where you have the meetings?

AC 2.2 Use information from a range of sources to build an understanding of the supervisee's performance

Here, you will be required to support supervisees to reflect on their practice using the range of information available and their own insights, to include the areas discussed in this section.

Sources of data and evidence and staff insights used to inform supervision

The evidence that a staff member brings to supervision may include reflective accounts of critical incidents, assessments undertaken, observations and surveys of individuals using the service.

In preparing for the supervisory meeting, staff need to be aware of the agenda set at the previous meeting. If this required work to be completed, they should get into the habit of bringing with them evidence to support the work done.

Building an evidence-based understanding of the supervisee's performance to date

In order to analyse information, the supervisee needs to be able to undertake the process of reflection. This is extremely important since it enables an individual to bring together practice and theory. Reflection on practice enables us to take a step back from what we are learning and assess what was good and what we might have done differently in any one situation.

In helping your staff to be more reflective about their work, there are a number of useful reflective tools, such as Gibbs' six stages to reflect practice (1988). See Unit 505 AC1.10 for more information on Gibbs.

By using a range of information available from other sources and from any learning they have undertaken, supervisees can reinforce their own insights that they have gained from reflecting. For example, when they engage with the art of reflecting in a meaningful way, reflection can clarify the learning that they have gained from a training course and also from situations that arise in experience gained in the workplace. Following a training session, a member of staff may have learned some new skills, for example emergency first aid. In developing these skills, they need to practise and reflect upon the successes and failures they may have when undertaking them. In this way, they gain a better insight and can build evidence about their own performance.

Evidence opportunity

2.2 Supporting supervisees to reflect on their practice

Paying attention to the following areas, how can you support supervisees to reflect on their practice?

- ✔ **Reflection** helps you to achieve a better understanding of yourself and the roles you carry out. It involves actively analysing experiences, attempting to 'make sense' or find the meaning in them.
- ✔ **Stand back**. It can be hard to reflect when you are caught up in an activity. 'Standing back' gives a better view or perspective on an experience, issue or action.
- ✔ **Undertake repetition**. Reflection involves 'going over' something, often several times, in order to get a broad view and check nothing is missed.
- ✔ **Gain a sense of deeper honesty**. Reflection is associated with 'striving after truth'. Through reflection, you can acknowledge things that you find difficult to admit in the normal course of events.
- ✔ **'Weigh up'**. Reflection involves being even-handed or balanced in judgement. This means taking everything into account, not just the most obvious.
- ✔ **Achieve clarity**. Reflection can bring greater clarity, like seeing events reflected in a mirror. This can help at any stage of planning, carrying out and reviewing activities.
- ✔ **Gain understanding**. Reflection is about learning and understanding on a deeper level. This includes gaining valuable insights that cannot just be 'taught'.
- ✔ **Make judgements**. Reflection involves an element of drawing conclusions in order to move on, change or develop an approach, strategy or activity if your assessor agrees with this and is happy to accept.

Evidence opportunity

2.2 Support supervisees to reflect on their practice

Show you support supervisees to reflect on their practice using the range of information available and their own insights, to include the areas discussed in this section. Demonstrate this to your assessor or obtain a witness testimony if your assessor agrees with this and is happy to accept.

AC 2.3 Support a supervisee to review their own wellbeing, including a range of strategies and support available

Here, you will be required to effectively support a supervisee and outline the strategies that may be used in order to ensure that supervision is effective.

Staff wellbeing is more than just not being ill but is about lifestyle and having a good work–life balance. Staff need to be aware of the support that might be available to them with respect to any physical or mental health issues they have, for example help to quit smoking, increasing exercise and even nutritional advice.

Staff may be concerned about how to stretch their salaries to support their family so innovative means of doing this could be to provide help with childcare, a cycle to work scheme or even free meals while on duty. For more on staff wellbeing, see Unit 504 AC3.1–3.4.

AC 2.4 Support a supervisee to address work challenges

Here, you will be required to support supervisees to explore different methods of addressing challenging situations in their work practice, agree suitable methods in any actions to be taken forward, reflect on own strengths and resilience in addressing challenges, and understand own responsibilities and own role when facing work challenges.

Explore different methods of addressing challenging situations in work practice

There is a saying that goes, 'If we always do the same thing, we will always get the same results'. Occasionally, those results are not what we need or want, but we repeat the behaviour and get into a spiral of non-achievement.

In challenging situations involving staff members, you need to address the incident quickly to ensure that it does not become practice. Some ways to do this may include:

- Describe the behaviour: 'I noticed you did …' or 'I noticed you did not do …'
- Say how this feels or how it impacts the team: 'I felt …' or 'This means the team cannot do …'
- Say what needs to be done: 'Instead of… I need you to …'
- Gain commitment: 'Do you think you can do this?' or 'Is there anything I need to help with?'

By undertaking a simple approach like this you deal with a situation in a factual and non-emotive way.

Agree suitable methods in any actions to be taken forward

Agree with staff the way in which you wish to handle any situations that may be challenging. You may decide to adopt the simple strategy shown above.

Reflect on own strengths and resilience in addressing challenges

Think about how you handle challenges and the feelings that emerge when something happens. What are you good at in these situations and how might you improve where you have weaknesses?

Understand own responsibilities and own role when facing work challenges

Each member of staff needs to be clear about where their authority ends with respect to challenging situations. For example, a complaint from a relative may be dealt with at a higher level than the team and this needs to be made clear. Staff must be aware of their limitations in dealing with certain areas of challenge.

Evidence opportunity

2.3 and 2.4 Support supervisees addressing challenging work situations

Show your assessor how you support supervisees to explore different methods of addressing challenging situations in their work, taking into account the topics discussed in this section.

Additionally, show how you enable staff to build their resilience and work to their strengths.

AC 2.5 Provide constructive feedback to the supervisee that can be used to improve and develop performance

Here, you will be required to show how to provide feedback in a manner that will ensure that the supervisee will benefit from it.

In a formal supervision session, the best way to approach feedback is to ask the supervisee how they perceived their performance of a task before you launch in with your assessment. By linking the feedback to their professional development, the member of staff will be able to focus more on what they need to change. In this way, you can see what they understand about how well they are doing their job and you are also encouraging them to be reflective about their performance.

AC 2.6 Support a supervisee to identify, plan and achieve their own learning and professional development needs

Here, you will be required to provide feedback to the supervisee, which covers the areas discussed in this section.

Ongoing staff development is just one discussion you will have with your supervisees during the supervision session. These needs are likely to reflect their job role and the long-term goals of the organisation. Supervisees should be encouraged to reflect on their practice with respect to this and their future career development.

If the member of staff is seeking new responsibilities in the work setting, they may be helped to identify courses to enable them in a new role. It is important that you as a manager and supervisor are up to date with policy changes, national initiatives and legal requirements for the setting in order to specify the sort of training they need.

Support supervisee to identify their own development needs

As a manager, you will support staff to identify their professional development needs in different ways, such as appraisals and the setting of SMART objectives as discussed in AC1.9.

Reflect on it

2.5 and 2.6 Positive and constructive feedback

1. Reflect on an example of positive and constructive feedback you have used to help improve the performance of a member of staff.
2. How did you support a supervisee to identify their own development needs? How have you provided feedback that is unambiguous and clearly sets out any issues?

Evidence opportunity

2.5 and 2.6 Providing constructive feedback and supporting supervisee

Produce evidence, possibly through a witness testimony, that you can provide feedback to a supervisee that can be used to improve performance and covers the areas discussed in this section. You will also need to show that you can support your supervisee(s) to identify their own development needs.

AC 2.7 Use supervision to meet objectives of the work setting and individual objectives of the supervisee by agreeing, reviewing and revising targets

Here, you will be required to review and revise targets with the supervisee that meet objectives of work settings and the individual.

It is not enough to set targets; you should also plan when to review progress. Review is about reflecting upon experience, making sense of it and determining what has been learned from the outcomes. Without reviewing targets, you cannot move on with development, as you will not be able to clarify what has been achieved or be able to measure the success or failure of a project. Also, the supervisee will lose interest in the plan and may start to feel devalued as a result. Time needs to be spent on going over what has happened since the target was set and what has been achieved. Through the review you can then help to make revisions to targets and set new objectives.

Meet objectives of work settings

In supervision, the objectives of the work setting should be part of the targets that are set for each individual. For example, one of the organisational objectives may be to ensure that all new members of staff be made aware of the values of the settings and a target may be that your supervisee is involved in training to help new staff understand the work of the setting and its values.

Meet the objectives of the individual

In addition to working towards the organisation's objectives, your supervisee may have their own individual objectives. For example, they may wish to undertake further courses to improve their career prospects. Professional development requirements attached to various roles and required by regulatory bodies change over time and your supervisee may want to undertake their own further development to ensure that they keep up to date.

Reflect on it

2.7 Development needs

1. Reflect on how you support supervisees to identify their own and the organisation's development needs.
2. What do you think is good about the system you are using? Is it fit for purpose? How might you improve it?

Evidence opportunity

2.7 Review and revise targets to meet objectives

Show your assessor that you can agree, review and revise targets with the supervisee that:

- ✔ meet objectives of work settings
- ✔ meet the objectives of the individual.

Reflect on it

2.7 Your review process

Using the same evidence from AC2.5 and 2.6, critically evaluate your own review process. Was it successful? Or do you need to make a change to ensure that it is? Make some notes about how you might improve this aspect of your supervision.

Evidence opportunity

2.7 Development needs, objectives and challenging situations

Describe how you support supervisees to identify their own development needs and how you work with them in challenging situations. How have you reviewed and revised targets to meet objectives of work settings and individual objectives of supervisees?

AC 2.8 Record outcomes of supervision activities in line with agreed ways of working

Here, you will be required to show that you are able to record supervision meetings and decisions agreed in line with workplace policies and procedures.

All supervision meetings need to be properly recorded to identify and support agreed actions and their completion within agreed timescales. Without records you cannot be sure you have actually set tasks and actions, and this can lead to confusion. You will need to record the decisions and plans made in line with your organisation's policies and procedures.

However you choose to record the meeting, you should consider the following points:

- Record decisions and actions which you agree on and ensure that these are signed and dated.
- Have clear timescales.
- Detail responsibilities.
- Ensure that copies are filed in a safe place and supervisees know that other managers may have access to them.

AC 2.9 Store outcomes of supervision activities in line with agreed ways of working

Here, you will show how the records of supervision meetings are securely stored.

In your setting, there may be a specific system by which supervision is recorded, perhaps in staff files or online using software, and such procedures must be followed.

The supervisee may have a personal development plan which is stored on their online continuous professional development training system or you could simply undertake to record their sessions in a way they prefer.

However records are kept, there needs to be mutual agreement as to how they can be accessed and measured. Any records made of the supervision must be stored appropriately and in line with confidentiality and the Data Protection Act 2018.

Reflect on it

2.8 and 2.9 Supervision feedback

How do you ensure that the information you have about supervision is confidential and how long do you keep the records?

Who else has access to these records?

Legislation

Legislation	Key points
Health and Social Care Act 2008 (Regulated Activities) Regulations 2014	This Act requires all providers of 'regulated activities' in England to register with the Care Quality Commission (CQC) and to comply with the requirements and fundamental standards set out in regulations made under the Act.
Data Protection Act 2018	The Data Protection Act 2018 controls how personal information is used by organisations, businesses and the government and is the UK's implementation of the General Data Protection Regulation (GDPR). Everyone responsible for using personal data has to follow strict rules called 'data protection principles'.
Equality Act 2010	An umbrella Act bringing together legislation that deals with race, disability and gender. It highlights protected characteristics of age, gender reassignment, pregnancy, religion, marriage and civil partnerships, and sexual orientation in an attempt to end discrimination.
Care Act 2014	Sets out the key responsibilities of local authorities in meeting the needs of individuals who require help and support to promote their wellbeing. Its main aim was to provide integrated care and to introduce the right to an assessment for all.
Health and Safety at Work Act 1974	This Act is the primary piece of legislation governing workplace health and safety in the UK. It defines the general duties of everyone from both employees and employers, owners, managers and maintainers of work premises (etc.) for maintaining health and safety within the workplace.
Human Rights Act 1998	This Act may be used by every person resident in the United Kingdom regardless of whether or not they are a British citizen or a foreign national, a child or an adult. The Act enables them to defend their rights in UK courts. It compels public organisations to treat everyone equally, with fairness, dignity and respect.

References

Care Quality Commission (2022) 'Regulations for service providers and managers: Regulation 18: Staffing'. **www.cqc.org.uk/guidance-providers/regulations-enforcement/regulation-18-staffing**

Carroll, M. (2007) 'One more time: What is supervision?', *Psychotherapy in Australia*, 13(3), May.

Communication Theory (n.d.) 'Management by objectives (Drucker)'. **www.communicationtheory.org/management-by-objectives-drucker/**

Gibbs, G. (1988) *Learning by Doing: A guide to teaching and learning methods*. Oxford: Oxford Further Education Unit.

Gopee, N. and Galloway, J. (2009) *Leadership and Management in Health Care*. London: Sage.

LaFasto, F.M.J. and Larson, C.E. (2001) *When Teams Work Best: 6,000 team members and leaders tell what it takes to succeed*. Thousand Oaks, CA: Sage Publications.

Lambley, S. and Marrable, T. (2013) *Practice Enquiry into Supervision in a Variety of Adult Care Settings Where There Are Health and Social Care Practitioners Working Together*. London: SCIE.

NHS Employers (2022) NHS Health and wellbeing framework. **www.nhsemployers.org/publications/nhs-health-and-wellbeing-framework**

Skills for Care and Skills for Health (2013) 'Code of Conduct for Healthcare Support Workers and Adult Social Care Workers in England'. **www.skillsforcare.org.uk/resources/documents/Support-for-leaders-and-managers/Managing-people/Code-of-conduct/Code-of-Conduct.pdf**

Skills for Care (2019) 'Developing opportunities through mentoring'. **www.skillsforcare.org.uk/About/Blog/Blog/Developing-opportunities-through-mentoring.aspx**

Skills for Care (2020) 'Effective supervision: A practical guide for adult social care managers and supervisors'. **www.skillsforcare.org.uk/resources/documents/Support-for-leaders-and-managers/Managing-people/Supervision/Effective-supervision-guide.pdf**

Social Care Institute for Excellence (2007) *Providing effective supervision. A workforce development tool, including a unit of competence and supporting guidance*. London: SCIE.

Thompson, N. (2006) *People Problems*. Basingstoke: Palgrave Macmillan.

Tilmouth, T., Davies-Ward, E. and Williams, B. (2011) *Foundation Degree in Health and Social Care*. London: Hodder Education.

West, M. (2004) *Effective Teamwork: Practical lessons from organizational research*. London: Wiley and Sons.

Useful resources and further reading

British Association of Social Workers (2011) 'Code of Practice to support social workers'. www.basw.co.uk/resources/february-2011-%E2%80%93-code-practice-support-social-workers

Care Quality Commission (2015), 'Guidance for providers on meeting the regulations, Health and Social Care Act 2008 (Regulated Activities) Regulations 2014 (Part 3) (as amended) and the Care Quality Commission (Registration) Regulations 2009 (Part 4) (as amended)'. www.cqc.org.uk/sites/default/files/2015024%20Guidance%20for%20providers%20on%20meeting%20the%20regulations.pdf

Skills for Care: www.skillsforcare.org.uk

Social Care Institute for Excellence (2017), 'Effective supervision in a variety of settings'. www.scie.org.uk/publications/guides/guide50/

Unit 507

Safeguarding in adult care

GLH 35

About this unit

The purpose of this unit is to enable you to understand and engage with issues related to the safeguarding of adults.

The unit will introduce you to the legal framework and best practice with respect to handling situations where danger, harm, abuse or exploitation is known to have taken place or is suspected, as well as systems and processes that safeguard vulnerable adults. You will gain a better understanding of the role and responsibilities of adult care practitioners in ensuring the safety and wellbeing of adults and how to promote health and safety in the workplace.

Learning outcomes

By the end of this unit, you will:

1. Understand requirements for safeguarding in adult care settings/services.
2. Be able to lead the implementation of practices, policies and procedures to support safeguarding in adult care settings/services.

Getting started

Before you study the unit, think about the following:

- What do you understand by the term 'safeguarding'?
- How much do you know about wider aspects of danger, harm, abuse and/or exploitation?
- How are you supporting all work colleagues to be vigilant?
- Why is it crucial that managers in adult care services have an understanding of their responsibilities in safeguarding adults?

LO1 Understand requirements for safeguarding in adult care settings/services

Safeguarding and protection, while often used synonymously, are different concepts and since the introduction of the personalisation agenda, perceptions have changed. The main difference between the two concepts is that safeguarding is the practice of preventing harm associated with vulnerable people whereas protection is the action we take to safeguard those at risk of harm or who are already experiencing serious harm. If the individual using the service has the capacity to make decisions about their care, then they should be enabled to safeguard themselves and to make calculated risks if they choose to do so.

Anyone can be vulnerable, but certain definitions are specific. A vulnerable adult is defined as an individual aged 18 or over who:

- depends on others for assistance with respect to the performance of basic functions, or
- has a severe impairment in their ability to communicate and, therefore, reduced ability to protect themselves from assault, abuse or neglect.

There is a debate about the differences in definitions that seem to surround this subject.

These definitions seem to identify groups of people who are considered vulnerable to abuse, harm or exploitation, such as older adults, as being vulnerable and we may find this unacceptable. We might also include those people who indulge in risky behaviour, have chaotic lifestyles, substance misuse issues or illness leading to some sort of impairment. Additionally, there may also be people in domestic arrangements where there is a power imbalance, causing them to become vulnerable. It is, after all, the situation in which the person finds themselves that makes them vulnerable, not the actual individual. There are many older adults who would be most upset to be termed vulnerable just because they happen to be aged over 65, for instance.

The lack of clarity with respect to the terms used may lead to confusion over the roles and responsibilities of care workers. As there does not seem to be a commonly accepted definition for 'safeguarding adults', your own policies need to clarify the term for your staff in order to ensure that a shared understanding is at least possible for your workplace.

> **KEY TERM**
>
> **Safeguarding**: The CQC defines this as 'protecting people's health, wellbeing and human rights, and enabling them to live free from harm, abuse and neglect. It is fundamental to high-quality health and social care'.

AC 1.1 Describe the current legislative framework and national guidance that underpins the safeguarding of adults

Here, you will provide evidence of key aspects of legislation which apply to safeguarding in adult care services in your management and leadership role.

Your work in the care system is governed by the legal system and you will be familiar with the laws under which you work. The following legislation and reports relate to the safeguarding of adults.

Health and Care Act 2022

Although not particularly referencing changes to safeguarding, this new legislation has introduced measures to make it easier for care settings to deliver joined-up care for people who rely on multiple different services. This includes a new Provider Selection Regime (NHS England, 2022), giving a wider range of options when commissioning services. The Care and support statutory guidance document (Department of Health and Social Care, 2022) does, however, refer to the principle of wellbeing in section 1 of the Care Act 2014 (see next page).

Domestic Abuse Act 2021

This Act provides enhanced protection for those who have suffered domestic abuse and places obligations on local authorities to provide accommodation for those at risk.

Revisiting safeguarding practice report

'Revisiting safeguarding practice' (GOV.UK, 2022) is an independent report commissioned by the government to standardise adult safeguarding best practice and to raise service quality and increase positive outcomes. It sets out the roles and responsibilities in adult safeguarding and includes reference to the statutory duties which social workers and others must fulfil.

The guidance stresses that more than simply keeping people safe, you need to respect and protect individuals' needs and aspirations, both mental and physical, and make sure that all the support services around them do the same.

Care Act 2014

This Act highlights adult safeguarding as an important part of public services, with key responsibilities placed on local authorities (LAs) in partnership with the police and the NHS. This was a major move to put adult safeguarding into a legal framework. Under the Care Act 2014, LAs are responsible for:

- setting up local Safeguarding Adults Boards (SABs), with core membership from the local authority, the police and the NHS Clinical Commissioning Groups and other relevant bodies
- arranging independent advocates to represent and support adults who are the subject of a safeguarding enquiry or Safeguarding Adult Review (SAR)
- following up any concerns about actual or suspected adult abuse.

The key message of the legislation highlights six principles of safeguarding:

- **Empowerment**: The emphasis is on person-led decisions and informed consent.
- **Prevention**: Taking action before harm occurs.
- **Proportionality**: The need to risk assess and apply proportionate and least intrusive responses.
- **Protection**: Support and advocacy for those with the greatest needs.
- **Partnerships**: To seek local solutions through services working with their communities.
- **Accountability**: Accountability and transparency in delivering safeguarding.

This law advocates a person-centred approach and a move away from process-led care. In addition, there is a recognition of the key role of carers in relation to safeguarding.

The whole concept of partnership working to achieve safety for vulnerable adults is a key part of the Act, recognising that safeguarding requires joint working with police, the NHS and other key organisations as well as awareness by the wider public. The statutory guidance also introduces Designated Adult Safeguarding Managers (DASMs) in organisations concerned with adult safeguarding.

Local SABs came about as a result of the Care Act 2014 and are in place to safeguard adults with care and support needs by ensuring that local safeguarding arrangements are in place and that the safeguarding practice offered is person-centred and outcomes focused.

Safeguarding Vulnerable Groups Act 2006

This Act introduced changes to the reporting system by the introduction of the Vetting and Barring Scheme ('the Scheme'). The changes followed the publication of the Bichard Inquiry (2004), which was commissioned following the well-publicised murders of Holly Wells and Jessica Chapman in 2002 and revelations that certain checks had been missed. The inquiry recommended a new scheme under which everyone working with children or vulnerable adults should be checked and registered.

Recognising the need for a single agency to vet and register individuals who want to work or volunteer with vulnerable people, the Independent Safeguarding Authority (ISA) was set up and the Criminal Records Bureau (CRB) was made responsible for managing the system and processing the applications for ISA registration. The Bichard Inquiry also led to the Safeguarding Vulnerable Groups Act 2006 and the Safeguarding Vulnerable Groups Order (Northern Ireland) 2007, which set up the scheme.

While these policies were instrumental in ensuring that all people working with children and vulnerable adults undergo strict checks if they are to work with these groups, they were criticised for being expensive and time consuming. It led in some cases to potential staff in these sectors deciding not to volunteer as the checks required are too onerous and costly to undertake.

The Disclosure and Barring Service (DBS) replaced the CRB and ISA in 2012. The DBS helps employers make safer decisions regarding recruitment and prevents unsuitable people from working with vulnerable groups, including children. It acts as a central access point for criminal records checks for all those applying to work with children and young people.

Mental Capacity Act 2005

The main aspects of the Mental Capacity Act (MCA) can be found in Unit 508.

With respect to safeguarding, the MCA 2005 protects and restores power to vulnerable people over the age of 16 who lack capacity. It empowers those in social care to assess their capacity in order to decide the best interests of the individual concerned.

Mental Health Act 1983 (amended 2007)

The Mental Health Act 1983 (amended 2007) gives health professionals the powers to detain, assess and treat people with mental disorders in the interests of their health and safety or for public safety and thus ensures that appropriate treatment is arranged to safeguard individuals who suffer with mental health problems. The main aspects of the Mental Health Act are covered in Unit 501, AC1.1.

Liberty Protection Safeguards 2019

In 2019, the Liberty Protection Safeguards were introduced into the Mental Capacity (Amendment) Act. These replaced the Deprivation of Liberty Safeguards (DoLS) system.

These will deliver improved outcomes for people who are or who need to be deprived of their liberty and have been designed to put the rights and wishes of those people at the centre of all decision making. Originally planned to come into force in April 2022, their introduction has been delayed at the time of writing (May 2023) and there are suggestions that they may not change at all.

The new bill broadens the scope to treat people, without gaining prior authorisation to deprive them of their liberty, in a medical emergency. You should keep up to date with the changes and most recent legislation. For more information, see SCIE (2022).

Sexual Offences Act 2003

This Act revised the law of sexual offences in order to safeguard a wider range of society, to address the growing concern about child sexual abuse and to provide clarity about new forms of sexual abuse. Individuals who lack capacity may be vulnerable to sexual abuse and this act added several different offences which may apply where consent was not given by them. Individuals who suffer with mental disorders are also safeguarded under this Act.

Health and Social Care Act 2012

This Act introduced the role of the Care Quality Commission, set up to ensure that the Essential Quality Standards were being implemented and regulated. Safeguarding and protection of individuals are specifically mentioned in these laws to address concerns about abuse. One of the intentions of this Act is to safeguard people who use care services from suffering any form of abuse or improper treatment while receiving care and treatment. To meet the requirements under this Act, providers must demonstrate zero tolerance of abuse, unlawful discrimination and restraint.

Court of Protection

The Court of Protection is in place to ensure that decisions on financial or welfare matters for people who lack mental capacity are fair and just.

The Court is available to:

- decide whether someone has the mental capacity to make decisions for themselves
- appoint deputies to make ongoing decisions
- give people permission to make one-off decisions on behalf of someone else who lacks mental capacity
- handle emergency applications when a decision must be made on behalf of someone else
- make decisions about a lasting power of attorney or enduring power of attorney
- consider applications to make statutory wills or gifts
- make decisions about when someone can be deprived of their liberty under the Mental Capacity Act.

Source: GOV.UK (n.d.)

Prevent duty 2015

The Prevent duty is part of the Counter-Terrorism and Security Act 2015 and places a duty on certain bodies to have 'due regard to the need to prevent people from being drawn into terrorism'. While counter-terrorism is ultimately the responsibility of the UK government, health, education and local government are included in the authorities that also have a role to play.

The Prevent duty aims to stop people from becoming terrorists or supporting terrorism. There are three specific strategic objectives:

- Respond to the threat and challenge of terrorism from those who promote it.
- Prevent people from being drawn into terrorism or 'radicalised' and ensure that they are given appropriate advice and support.
- Work with sectors and institutions where there are risks of radicalisation that we need to address.

This is to be done through effective leadership and working in partnership with specified authorities, to establish strategies for understanding the risk of radicalisation and ensuring that staff understand the risk and build the capabilities to deal with it.

Modern Slavery Act 2015

This Act was introduced to deal with the trafficking of human beings into the UK and to ensure that people who are enslaved, exploited and forced to work in the UK can seek help through this law. Additionally, there are cases of slavery with respect to vulnerable adults in this country who find themselves being forced to work in inhumane conditions and for little gain. Adults with additional care and support needs, as well as children, are vulnerable too, and can become victims of modern slavery. Safeguarding these people requires carers to recognise signs that might indicate a person is in need of help. For example, care workers should be alert to warning signs such as adults who do not seem to have access to their legal documents such as passports and bank account details, who are withdrawn, frightened, unkempt or malnourished in appearance and have old untreated injuries.

You can find out more at legislation.gov.uk (n.d.).

Public Interest Disclosure Act 1998

This Act is also known as the whistle blowers Act. It enhances the safeguarding of individuals in care. Any care worker who is concerned about individuals in their care, who exhibit signs of neglect or abuse which they believe is ongoing at the hands of relatives or other staff members, for example, must be able to voice such concerns in a safe environment without feeling they will be victimised because of that **disclosure**. This is known as '**whistle blowing**'. Additionally, concerns about other staff members who are exhibiting signs of being radicalised in any way are covered here and staff must be able to report their concerns.

KEY TERMS

Disclosure: Making new or secret information known.

Whistle blowing: Making a disclosure or revealing information that is in the public interest.

Other legislation that is relevant to protection and safeguarding includes:

- Safeguarding Adults – A National Framework of Standards for good practice and outcomes in adult protection work
- Equality Act 2010.

As a manager of a care setting you are duty bound to ensure that the setting complies with legislation and that staff are compliant with it. It is imperative that staff are regularly updated with respect to change and are aware of and are complying with their legal duties with respect to safeguarding.

National guidance

Dignity in Care 2006

The Human Rights Act 1998 had a direct impact on the way in which care is delivered in this country and in meeting the fundamental rights of individuals. Rights that relate to dignity in care include:

- the right to life
- the right not to be subjected to inhuman or degrading treatment
- the right to a family life.

These rights were first recognised by the European Court of Human Rights (ECHR) when it acknowledged that the protection of human dignity was 'inviolable' and had to be protected and respected (Dupre, 2011).

The Dignity in Care campaign started in 2006 as a response to negative media reports about how people were being treated in social care services. It is led by the National Dignity Council. The 10 Point Dignity Challenge states that high-quality care services that respect people's dignity should (among other things):

- 'treat each person as an individual by offering personalised services
- enable people to maintain the maximum possible level of independence, choice and control'.

Source: Dignity in Care (n.d.)

In practice, enabling people to have more independence is not an easy option in care but it can be achieved through simple changes to practical care. For example, you should be ensuring that people are fully involved in all decisions that affect their care. These could be personal decisions about what they want to eat, wear and what time they wish to go to bed. They might also be included in making decisions about the wider functions of the place in which they are resident. If they are in a care home, for example, they could be included in decisions about the menu or activity planning or even the home décor. People need to feel that they have a purpose in life and must be able to participate as fully as they can at all levels of the service. As a manager, you will need to ensure that staff are aware of and implement person-centred care.

Adult Social Care Outcomes Framework

The Adult Social Care Outcomes Framework (ASCOF) collects data on the outcomes for adult users of local authority-funded social care and support (including carers) for each local authority area. ASCOF measures care and support services and how well they achieve the outcomes that matter most to people. It is used locally and nationally to set priorities for care, to measure progress and strengthen transparency and accountability. It includes statistics taken from the Survey of Adult Carers in England (SACE), which seeks opinions of carers aged 18 or over and who care for a person aged 18 or over to assess how their unpaid caring role impacts their life.

ASCOF draws on several sources of data including SACE and the Adult Social Care Survey (ASCS) and looks at such issues as:

- the quality of life score reported by carers
- the proportion of carers who have as much social contact as they would like
- how satisfied carers are with their local social services
- the proportion of carers who say they are consulted on decisions about the person they care for
- how easy it is for carers to find information about support.

Evidence opportunity

1.1 Legislative framework and guidance

Describe the current legislative framework and national guidance that underpins the safeguarding of adults.

Reflect on it

1.1 Your setting and legislation

Think about and evaluate the impact of legislation and policies on your work in your care setting and how it affects the standards by which you work.

Research it

1.1 Legislation

Choose two of the following legislation or policy documents and find out more about them. How do these laws shape care work, particularly with reference to safeguarding?

- Human Rights Act 1998
- Mental Capacity Act 2005
- Equality Act 2010
- Care Act 2014
- Health and Care Act 2022

Evidence opportunity

1.1 Impact of policy documents and legislation

All of the legislation and guidelines described in this section changed the way in which care was being delivered by recognising the real threat of abuse and its impact.

Describe the key aspects of legislation that applies to safeguarding and whistle blowing in adult care services in your management and leadership role, including examples of relevant legal requirements and provisions such as those discussed in this section.

AC 1.2 Describe local systems, procedures and agencies relating to adult safeguarding and own role within these

Here, you will be required to describe current national and local guidance and agreed ways of working in respect of safeguarding in adult care services.

Care Quality Commission fundamental standards

The CQC Fundamental Standards are the standards that care must never fall below. Every individual using a care service has the right to expect the following:

- **Person-centred care**: This is the right for people to have care that is tailored to their own needs and preferences.
- **Dignity and respect**: This means that every person using the service in your setting has a right to expect to be treated with dignity and respect at all times, having privacy when they need it and being treated as an equal. They must also be supported to remain independent and involved in their local community.
- **Consent**: This means that before any care or treatment is given, the person or anybody acting on their behalf must give consent.
- **Safety**: Any person in your care must be cared for in a safe manner. This means that all care providers need to assess the risks to health and safety and ensure that staff are qualified, competent and have the right skills and experience.
- **Safeguarding from abuse**: In the care setting, neglect or degrading treatment are outlawed and freedom should not be limited.
- **Food and drink**: Making sure that adequate food and drink (nutrition/hydration) are provided and that any dietary requirements are met is vital.
- **Premises and equipment**: All equipment in the care setting must be clean, cared for and used properly.
- **Complaints system**: This must be in place so people are able to complain about inadequate care or service so that service can be improved.
- **Good governance plans**: Plans that ensure that standards are met should be in place and there should be systems to check on the quality and safety of care to ensure that the service can improve and any risks may be reduced.
- **Staffing**: Staff must be suitably qualified, competent and experienced to meet these standards and should be given support, training and supervision to help them.

- **Fit and proper staff**: Recruitment procedures must be in place to enable the employment of people who can provide care and treatment appropriate to their role. Safeguarding checks must also take place at this time.
- **Duty of candour**: The adult care provider needs to be open and transparent about all care and treatment, and if something goes wrong you have a duty to report what has happened, provide support and apologise.
- **Display of ratings**: The CQC rating must be displayed in the setting as well as on the service's website.

CQC Regulations

The CQC provides guidance on how providers may meet the fundamental standards within the Health and Social Care Act 2008 (Regulated Activities) Regulations 2014 and Care Quality Commission (Registration) Regulations 2009 (Part 4).

This guidance was developed in response to Section 23 of the Health and Social Care Act 2008 (HSCA 2008), which made it clear that the CQC should produce guidance to help providers to comply with the regulations made under this Act.

The fundamental standards are similar to the idea of a national minimum standard. If an inspection finds care falling below a standard, the service will be required to take the appropriate actions to become compliant with the standards. This then requires the care setting to readdress its ways of working.

Nothing ventured, nothing gained: risk guidance for people with dementia

This report provides guidance on best practice in assessing, managing and enabling risk for people living with dementia. *Nothing Ventured, Nothing Gained* (Department of Health and Social Care, 2010) presents a framework for managing the risk in a positive way by enabling and supporting people with dementia and their carers and helping settings to agree ways of working that focus upon improved outcomes for people living with dementia.

Domestic violence and abuse guidance

The government definition of domestic violence and abuse describes controlling, coercive and threatening behaviour as well as physical, sexual, psychological and financial abuse and recognises that young people aged 16 and 17 can be victims of domestic abuse.

The recognition in law of coercive and controlling behaviour extends previous legal powers to bring to justice individuals who inflict this sort of psychological control over others.

The Domestic Violence Disclosure Scheme (often referred to as 'Clare's Law') gives individuals the right to ask police to check whether a new or existing partner has a violent past. Disclosure by the police can be made if the records show that there may be a risk of domestic violence from a partner.

Care workers may become aware of people who are exposed to domestic abuse and need to respond in an appropriate way, by listening and empathising with the person, validating their decision to come forward and disclose, and indicating their willingness to help. The safeguarding policy in the setting will identify how to work in such situations and informing the designated safeguarding officer should be an agreed way of working.

Care Certificate

Standard 10 of the Care Certificate relates to the principles of safeguarding adults and describes ways of working to safeguard adults in the setting. The Care Certificate is a response to the need for upskilling staff in care work to ensure that vulnerable people have access to qualified and skilled staff. As a manager, you need to ensure that your policies and procedures meet the Care Quality Commission's Fundamental Standards of Quality and Safety and that your care staff follow the Code of Conduct for Healthcare Support Workers and Adult Social Care Workers in England. For more information, see Skills for Care (n.d. a).

SCIE – whistle blowing guidance

SCIE supplies a useful video to help staff to raise concerns about issues in the workplace: see SCIE (2014).

Importance of partnership working

Multi-agency working refers to an approach that involves professionals from various agencies working together to provide support for those who have been affected by issues such as abuse or neglect.

An example of this is a multi-agency risk assessment conference (MARAC), which is a meeting held to share information and respond to domestic abuse cases. It involves representatives from the local police, probation service, health, child protection and housing practitioners. Independent Domestic Violence Advisors (IDVAs), and other specialists from the statutory and voluntary sectors are also invited. Increasingly, adult safeguarding representatives from local authorities are also invited.

Under the Care Act 2014 every local authority is required to establish a Safeguarding Adults Board (SAB) for its local area to help and protect adults from abuse and neglect. This is to be achieved through co-ordinating and reviewing a multi-agency approach across all member organisations.

Boundaries are in place in care work to ensure that there is clarity about what your role and responsibilities are. With clear boundaries, all members of staff in the partnership will understand where their roles begin and end.

- **Information sharing and recording information**: There must be a safe way of sharing information and confidentiality must not be breached. Systems need to be in place to ensure that all partners are aware of how they may accomplish this. Record keeping should also be standardised where possible across the partnership so that records are consistent.
- **Limits of authority**: As with boundaries, all partners must know where their authority ends and is taken up by another service.
- **Decision making**: Clarity with respect to who makes final decisions in certain areas of the service should be established at the outset of the partnership.
- **Areas of responsibility**: Like boundaries, each partnership member needs to be clear about what they are responsible for with respect to the care an individual requires. You will need to understand all of these areas.

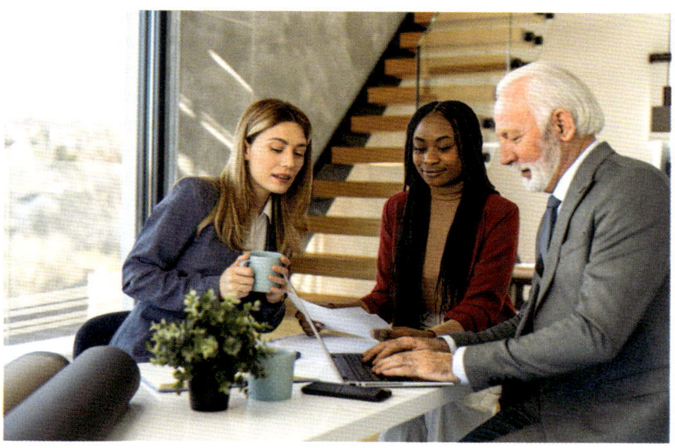

▲ **Figure 14** You will need to agree ways of working when working in partnership

The established partnership then brings together an executive management team to oversee strategic development of the work in the form of a strategic/forward plan. The strategic plan includes:

- safeguarding adults' policy – development and review
- safeguarding adults' procedures for reporting and responding to concerns of abuse or neglect – monitoring, development and review
- equal access strategy
- information-sharing agreement – development and review
- training strategy for all staff and volunteers
- training strategy for the people using the service and for carers
- strategy to disseminate information about adult abuse and safeguarding adults to staff, volunteers, the people using the service, carers and members of the public
- a commissioning strategy for services for people who are at risk of/have experienced abuse or neglect
- a commissioning strategy for responses to and services for perpetrators of abuse/neglect
- strategies for reducing risk of abuse and neglect across a range of settings, including care settings and the community
- review of the strategic plan and publication of an annual report

Source: ADSS (2005)

Vulnerable Adults Risk Management

The Vulnerable Adults Risk Management (VARM) protects adults who are suffering with severe self-neglect or for whatever reason are refusing to engage with services. It is also for people who are being targeted by an unknown third party; so, for example, a carer who cares for a vulnerable person may believe that abuse is happening at the hand of another person, a family member or a neighbour.

Local safeguarding boards are required to produce policy statements which provide agencies with a framework to help them work with adults who have mental capacity but who are at risk of serious harm or death through self-neglect. This may also include individuals who engage in risky behaviour, such as self-harm. You may find it useful to refer to guidance on how to work within VARM procedures provided by your local safeguarding board.

Multi-Agency Safeguarding Hubs

It is important to note that not everyone will use the MASH system, but these were set up as a result of a government report published in 2014, which highlighted several cases of child abuse including the death of four-year-old Daniel Pelka. The report identified the risks involved in information not being shared between care agencies and resulted in the establishment of Multi-Agency Safeguarding Hubs (MASHs) to address the risk of anyone slipping through the safeguarding net (Home Office, 2014).

MASHs include police, local authorities and other agencies that work together to ensure that safeguarding agencies and their data are located in a single secure research and decision-making unit to enable effective information sharing.

Safeguarding Adult Boards

Safeguarding Adults Boards were set up as a result of the Care Act 2014. Section 43 of the Act specifies the need for Safeguarding Adults Boards in each local area and outlines their objectives. Membership of SABs involves many agencies and key partnerships as well as consultancies of specialist advisers when needed. The needs of the local community must be considered when forming SABs and selecting the agencies needed for partnership working.

Shared training opportunities

You can read more about the potential for shared training opportunities in Unit 505 Leading team learning and professional development in adult care and Unit 504, AC2.4.

With partnerships, shared training for staff will ensure that all parties are aware of the protocols to protect people in care. Failures in the past where information has not been shared have led to untimely deaths of children and adults.

Research it

1.2 Agreed protocols

Research the agreed protocols for working in your partnerships and write notes documenting your findings.

Reflect on it

1.2 Policies in your setting

Review the policies in your setting now and reflect on how you might need to change them in light of legislation such as the Health and Social Care Act 2022.

Evidence opportunity

1.2 National and local guidance and agreed ways of working

Look at the headings in this section and describe current national and local guidance and agreed ways of working in respect of safeguarding in adult care services.

You might, for example, think about how current national and local guidance affects and informs the agreed ways of working with regard to safeguarding in your setting. How can you make sure that the policies and procedures in your setting reflect and are informed by the national and local guidance, and your setting follows these? Write down your responses.

AC 1.3 Explain how national and local guidelines, policies and procedures for safeguarding affect different groups

Here, you will explain the main legislation and guidance that affect work with individuals, team members and your own work.

Day-to-day work with individuals

Safeguarding adults is about the safety and wellbeing of all individuals using the service and providing additional measures for those who may be unable to protect themselves. Your responsibility as a manager is to ensure the safety and wellbeing of individuals in your setting and to comply with legislation and regulations in delivering care.

Safeguarding legislation and guidance will inform the policies in place in your work setting and you will need to regularly review your policies and ways of working to ensure that they still meet the requirements of the Care Act 2014. This will include ensuring you have a safeguarding system which prevents abuse and neglect and, if it happens, it is addressed immediately. You therefore need to ensure that your staff fully understand what they need to do if they believe an adult with care and support needs may be at risk of abuse or neglect.

See AC1.1 for more information on legislation and AC1.2 for information on current national and local guidance and agreed ways of working.

The establishment of Safeguarding Adults Boards may require you as a manager to represent your setting alongside members of the local authority, NHS and police. You may also be required to carry out **Safeguarding Adults Reviews**.

KEY TERM

Safeguarding Adults Reviews: Previously known as serious case reviews, these take place after a person is seriously injured or dies, particularly if abuse or neglect is thought to have been a causative factor. It looks at what might be learned from the occurrence in order to help prevent similar incidents from happening in the future.

Safeguarding Adults Reviews

Safeguarding Adult Boards (SABs) were introduced as a result of the Care Act 2014. SABs are required to carry out a Safeguarding Adult Review (SAR) if an adult in its area dies as a result of abuse or neglect, or the SAB knows or suspects that the adult has experienced serious abuse or neglect. The SAB must investigate partner agencies if there are concerns that they have not worked together effectively to protect an adult.

A SAR is a multi-agency review which investigates what might have been done differently to prevent serious abuse, neglect or death.

Own responsibilities towards individuals, their families and carers

Your responsibilities when working with individuals, their families and team members are to work in a way that prevents abuse and protects the individuals. All staff must be aware of the signs of abuse and neglect. Recording procedures and how to report concerns and incidents should be part of staff training.

As a manager, you must follow the six safeguarding principles set out in the Care Act 2014:

1. **Empowerment**: Personalisation and the presumption of person-led decisions and informed consent. The individual is central to all decisions about their care and as the care manager you should be ensuring that person-centred care is at the heart of your work.
2. **Prevention**: This states that action should be taken before harm occurs. Staff, individuals and their families should all be aware of what abuse is, how to recognise the signs and what they can do to seek help.
3. **Proportionality**: The least intrusive response appropriate to the risk presented should be taken to ensure that staff work with the individual's best interests.
4. **Protection**: This requires that staff support and represent those individuals in greatest need, provide them with help to report abuse and enable them to take part in the safeguarding process.
5. **Partnership**: Communities have a part to play in preventing, detecting and reporting neglect and abuse and individuals need to feel confident that professionals will work together to get the best result.
6. **Accountability**: There must be accountability and transparency in safeguarding practice.

Team members

For staff and anybody who comes into your setting, the safeguarding agenda needs to be clearly outlined and the setting has a duty to ensure that the care given is safe and of a high standard. All staff must have completed induction training which clearly outlines how they are expected to behave towards people in the setting and how they can recognise poor care, neglect, abuse and exploitation. They need to be clear about what they can do should they experience or see anything that detracts from a person's wellbeing and follow the policies and protocols which translate legislation into agreed ways of working.

Staff training and development

Staff require training in safeguarding, and this should be updated on an annual basis. They also need to be aware of what it means to whistle blow and how and when to do so. Policies must clearly address the agreed way of working with respect to both areas.

Individuals who use adult care and support services

Those people who use the service and those who support them should be clear about how staff will work with them to meet safeguarding needs. The policies should be made available to them in a format they can understand and must be transparent with respect to how they can expect to be treated and cared for. Any concerns must be dealt with through a complaints procedure that is both robust and fair.

External workers or visitors to the organisation

Stakeholders, partners and other agencies, as well as families who work alongside you, should all be aware of how the setting handles safeguarding and how it promotes transparency and openness in its approach to dealing with issues. The current legislation and guidance affect how you as a manager work with others in the setting, ensuring that anybody who enters the premises is fully aware of the behaviour expected of those who care for the individuals using the service and the ways of working in the setting. A zero-tolerance policy towards neglect, abuse or mistreatment must be promoted and monitored.

Working in the community requires employers to put policies into place to protect lone workers. As an employer you need to provide protection and safeguards for your staff working the community so that they will feel safe.

Evidence opportunity

1.3 Legislation, guidance, agreed ways of working and how they impact your practice

Provide a written account explaining how current legislation, guidance and agreed ways of working impact your day-to-day work, your own responsibilities and your team members within your work setting.

You might like to show evidence from policies in your setting.

Reflect on it

1.3 Improving ways of working

Following on from the activity above, say how you might improve ways of working and policies to ensure that the legislation surrounding safeguarding is promoted. For example, what might your setting do better? How has it improved? How might it improve further?

AC 1.4 Explain how investigations into serious failures to uphold individuals' rights to live free from abuse and neglect have impacted national policy

Here, you will explain the main cases that have affected the way in which care and safeguarding are legislated for on a national level.

A number of cases showing serious failures with respect to care and upholding safeguarding principles have led to policy and legal change.

Orchard View, West Sussex

Between November 2009 and October 2011 there were 19 unexplained deaths at the Orchid View nursing home, owned by Southern Cross Healthcare in West Sussex, and an anonymous alert to the police was made concerning this. An investigation found that, in the case of five of the people who had died, neglect was a contributory factor and several deaths were attributed to poor care. An insufficient number of staff compromised safe care and resident records were falsified, and in some cases shredded, to hide overdoses, errors in medication administration and neglectful care.

The contributory factors to the abuse and neglect identified by the Serious Case Review (SCR) were:

- insufficient checks and visits on the service to ensure that it was safe
- the absence of a registered manager so the level of monitoring was insufficient and poor practice was unchecked
- failure to check qualifications and professional registration of nurses working at the home
- insufficient staff training
- poor information sharing, which led to poor safeguarding investigations by the local authority when concerns of abuse were reported
- lack of information sharing with ambulance services, which might have prompted them to gain a better understanding of circumstances in the home
- visiting professionals did not act on their concerns, assuming that the CQC were already dealing with them.

This case highlights the need for quality assurance, staff training and shared information procedures to be in place and monitored to ensure that safeguarding is foremost in your care giving.

As a manager, you may find that you are expected to run a service with smaller budgets and fewer staff, and this is where good practice may suffer. Your role is to be vigilant and to challenge poor practice before it results in abuse or neglect.

> **Research it**
>
> **1.4 Safeguarding Adult Reviews**
>
> Research Safeguarding Adult Reviews in your local areas. Reflect on what happened in the cases covered by the reviews and how the care services may have failed to protect the individual. Analyse how your care setting will address any shortfalls in your own practice.

AC 1.5 Describe legal provisions in relation to whistle blowing and information sharing

Here, you will describe the main legal provisions that affect how team members share information and how whistle blowers are protected.

Whistle blowing

Whistle blowing refers to a staff member passing on information concerning wrongdoing. This may be something they have witnessed at work.

Whistle blowing is covered by the Employment Rights Act 1996 (as amended by the Public Interest Disclosure Act 1998) and provides the right for staff to take a case to an employment tribunal if they have been victimised at work or they have lost their job because they have 'blown the whistle'.

To be covered by whistle blowing law, a member of staff who makes a disclosure must be acting in the public interest and must reasonably believe that their disclosure shows past, present or likely future wrongdoing. These might be criminal offences, failure to comply with law, a miscarriage of justice, endangering of someone's health and safety or damage to the environment.

The policies in place which define the agreed ways of working, together with additional training, need to be available to staff to ensure that they are aware of their responsibility with respect to safeguarding and whistle blowing.

Staff training on safeguarding and whistle blowing

Staff training should be available to all staff to ensure they are aware of their responsibilities in regard to safeguarding and whistle blowing. This should be delivered on an annual basis to update them on any new legislation and guidance.

Open door approach for whistle blowing and safeguarding concerns

Staff need to feel secure in the knowledge that they can approach you as their manager at any time with concerns about a safeguarding issue. Having an open-door policy for this type of thing will make it easier for staff to voice concern and know that it will be dealt with appropriately.

Information provided on how to raise a concern or make a complaint

A complaints procedure must be available in the setting, in a format that the individuals using the service can understand. This will ensure that all who enter can raise concerns should they need to.

Information sharing

Where there are safeguarding concerns, everyone has a duty to share information. In regard to the most serious case reviews described earlier in this unit, a lack of information sharing was a significant contributor to things going wrong.

Information should be shared with consent when possible but a person's right to confidentiality may be overridden where there is evidence that sharing information is necessary to support an investigation or where there is a risk to others, for instance in the interests of public safety, or a police investigation.

The Data Protection Act, far from being a barrier to sharing information, provides a framework to ensure that personal information is shared appropriately.

> **Evidence opportunity**
>
> **1.5 Whistle blowing and information sharing**
>
> Describe your whistle blowing and information sharing policies. Do you need to update these in light of current legal provision?
>
> How will you ensure that staff are informed? Add an item to your next team meeting agenda to discuss this and keep evidence of this for your assessment.

AC 1.6 Describe own role in leading a response to suspected or disclosed abuse or neglect

Here, you will describe your role and responsibilities when allegations of abuse in the setting have been made.

The safety and wellbeing of the individual and others is the most important consideration when an allegation of abuse or neglect is made. As a manager your role will be to implement the safeguarding policy, engaging others in the policies and procedures.

When an allegation is made, action must be swift. Your role is to ensure that the investigation is carried out in a professional manner and that each part is dealt with according to the policy and procedures your own setting outlines. Discussing the case with others in your team who are not involved is not helpful and may damage the investigation, but you may need to inform the team of what has happened without giving any specific details. It is important at this time to ensure that team morale is not damaged in any way, and you need to be available to support staff.

Table 3 has been compiled from Standards 6, 7, 8 and 9 of the Safeguarding Adults (ADSS, 2005) document. It includes examples of actions to take and the time frame for these when there are concerns about abuse or neglect. Again, this is just guidance, and you should refer to your setting's agreed ways of working.

Table 3 Guidelines from the Safeguarding Adults document

	Action	Time frame
Alert	Report concerns of abuse or neglect which are received or noticed within a partner organisation. Any immediate protection needs should be addressed. Ensure that the individual is safe. Seek medical attention if needed.	Immediate action to safeguard anyone at immediate risk.
Referral	Ensure that other agencies are given information and made aware of the concern.	Within the same working day.
Decision	Deciding whether the 'Safeguarding Adults' procedures are appropriate to address the concern.	By the end of the working day following the one on which the safeguarding referral was made.
Safeguarding assessment strategy	Formulate a multi-agency plan for assessing the risk and address any immediate protection needs.	Within five working days.
Safeguarding assessment	Co-ordinate the collection of the information about abuse or neglect that has occurred or might occur. This may include an investigation, e.g. a criminal or disciplinary investigation.	Within four weeks of the safeguarding referral.
Safeguarding plan	Co-ordinate a multi-agency response to the risk of abuse that has been identified.	Within four weeks of the safeguarding assessment being completed.
Review	Review the plan.	Within six months for first review and thereafter yearly.

Source: Adapted from ADSS (2005)

What to do if a colleague has an allegation made against them

Sometimes, an allegation may be made against you as the manager or against a colleague. If this happens, it is recommended that you involve your own manager as soon as possible, if you have one, or the safeguarding team in your area. You might go to the local authority or the adult care trust to document the complaint. Taking yourself out of the situation (removing yourself from that specific situation) will help and discussing it with your next in line will be most useful. In the case of a colleague, you will need to ascertain the facts and start an inquiry. It may be that you take the colleague out of the situation by reassigning them or perhaps giving them leave until the investigation has been dealt with. It is imperative that claims like this be dealt with sensitively and in privacy. Your colleague must not feel that any blame is being apportioned but that an allegation has been made which requires investigation. They need to be reassured that the situation will be dealt with in a confidential manner and as swiftly as possible.

Reflect on it

1.6 What would you do?

What would you do if you or a colleague had an allegation made against you?

Reflect on it

1.6 Effective support for team members where danger, harm or abuse is suspected or disclosed

Highlight how as a manager you address cases of suspected abuse. Be sure to detail the measures that you take with your staff to avoid abuse taking place as well as the steps taken in the case of suspected or alleged abuse. How do you make sure that you provide information on all these areas to individuals, staff and families?

Think about how you would deal with situations where allegations are made against you or a colleague.

AC 1.7 Explain how and when to engage others in relation to responding to safeguarding concerns

Here, you will explain approaches to ensuring that safeguarding is embedded in the setting among team members and other stakeholders.

All staff (including people from other services, team members and supervisors), family and friends are responsible for the safety and wellbeing of the people using the service and colleagues.

It is a fundamental human right to live a life that is free from harm and abuse. One of your roles as a manager in a setting is to raise public awareness so that everyone can contribute to preventing, identifying and responding to abuse and neglect. To this end you need to ensure that all roles and responsibilities are clearly laid out and there is a strong multi-agency framework for safeguarding.

The safety and wellbeing of the individual and the establishment of the individual's views and wishes about the safeguarding issue and procedure must be made clear. Any evidence that arises must be maintained.

Everyone involved in the event must be sure to follow local procedures for reporting incidents/risks. You need to help everybody to remain calm, not showing shock or disbelief.

After listening carefully and acknowledging concern for what has happened, the person must be informed that you are required to share the information, explaining what and why, and that a written record recording of what the person has said, using their own words, will be taken, as well as recording what you have seen and what actions you will undertake. Sometimes the person will be unable to express what is happening to them so you need to be able to observe changes to their behaviour and their body language, which will give you an indication that something is amiss.

Evidence opportunity

1.7 Safeguarding the people using the service

What are the procedures in your setting for reporting a safeguarding issue? Who will you contact and how?

Think also about what you should **not** do in the case of somebody divulging abuse.

AC 1.8 Explain issues relating to consent to share information

Here, you will explain issues around confidentiality relating to information sharing.

Good care demands that confidentiality is central to the relationship. Without this, individuals may be reluctant to get medical treatment or to provide information needed for staff to give good care.

Sharing information, however, is required in cases of protecting vulnerable people. In these cases confidentiality is not an absolute duty and information may be shared in certain situations. If, for example, the law requires the information or there has been a court order issued then information can be given. If the person the information relates to gives their consent to share the information, then it is also justified to do so. You may also give information if the benefits to the vulnerable person outweigh the public and the individual's interest in keeping the information confidential.

AC 1.9 Describe own responsibilities to share information about suspicions or disclosures of abuse or neglect

Here, you will describe your responsibilities when allegations or suspicions of abuse are raised in the setting.

Any suspicion or discovery of abuse or complaint made which indicates abuse is suspected or happening must be dealt with immediately. An individual may also approach you or a member of your staff and say that they are being abused. This is called 'disclosure'. You are duty-bound to believe what you are being told and to act on it. If the person wants to tell you in confidence, you need to inform them that if they are at risk of harm, you have a duty to put a stop to it and will need to inform others in order to help them. You cannot keep abuse a 'secret'. In addition, reviewing care/support plans and assessments may highlight issues with respect to care and may raise questions relating to potential neglect and abuse. In the Winterbourne View care home case, abuse was suspected and disclosed to higher management, the local authority and the CQC, but there was a failure at each stage to take the allegations seriously. There have since been reviews to ensure that this failure never happens again.

As a manager, a disclosure of abuse sets in motion a time-consuming process of meetings and writing reports, and this can distract you from the day-to-day running of the setting. It is very important, therefore, that you have processes in place to deal with this that comply with legal regulation and that staff fully co-operate with these processes.

The Care Act 2014 sets out a clear framework for how local authorities should deal with abuse and you as a manager must comply with the processes set out by your local Safeguarding Adults Board.

Your responsibility as a manager is to tell an appropriate agency, such as your local authority, if you are concerned that individual is at risk of or is suffering abuse or neglect. When telling the appropriate agency, the information should include the identity of the person and the identity of any other person(s) who may pose a risk to them, the reasons for your concerns and any relevant information about their parents or carers.

You should ask for consent before sharing confidential information. If this is not given, you must still share the information but inform the person that you will support them through the process.

If you do go ahead and share information without consent, an explanation as to why this has been necessary should be provided and this should be recorded.

Evidence opportunity

1.8 and 1.9 Sharing information

Go to the SCIE website and download a copy of the report 'Safeguarding adults: sharing information' (SCIE, 2019).

Describe your responsibility with respect to sharing information and confidentiality. Read and reflect on one of the case studies in the report.

AC 1.10 Describe local systems, procedures and agencies relating to children's safeguarding and own role within these

Here, you will describe the legislation relating to the safeguarding of children.

Safeguarding children and adults is a requirement within the Health and Social Care Act 2008, so all regulated providers of social care services have a key role in safeguarding children and adults receiving care or treatment who may be at risk of abuse and neglect. There are, however, some significant differences in the laws and policies in safeguarding children compared to how we safeguard adults.

The statutory framework that provides information for safeguarding children is Working Together to Safeguard Children 2018, the Children Act 1989 and the Children and Social Work Act 2017, while for adults it is the Care Act 2014. The overarching objective for both is to enable people to live a life free from abuse or neglect.

Your role in safeguarding children is to have effective systems and processes in place to help keep children safe and to make sure the right people act at the right time to help keep them safe. The following principles should be a guide in all care settings:

- All children and young people have a right to be protected from abuse and neglect, and care workers have a duty to act on any concerns they have about the safety of a child. The overarching principle is that the needs of the child are paramount.
- The needs and wellbeing of children must be considered by staff.
- Children and young people are individuals with rights and there must be no discrimination against a child for any reason.
- Children have a right to be involved in their own care and this includes the right to be heard and the right to be involved in major decisions about their care.
- Decisions made about children must be made in their best interests.

Decisions about child protection should be made in consultation with colleagues and other agencies whose expertise will protect and promote the best interests of the child.

Evidence opportunity

1.10 Safeguarding children

Although you may be working in an adult care setting, you are still duty bound to ensure that any children are safeguarded. Your staff and the individuals using your service will be in contact with children, and you therefore have a duty to ensure that safeguarding extends to them.

Describe local systems, procedures and agencies relating to children's safeguarding and your own role within these. You may need to contact the Local Authority Designated Officer (LADO), who is responsible for co-ordinating the response to concerns that adults who work with children may have caused them or could cause them harm.

AC 1.11 Analyse tensions between maintaining the safety of colleagues and others, with the duty of care to individuals known to be a potential risk to children/adults

Here, you will be required to analyse the potential tensions between maintaining the safety of team members and others with the duty of care to adults who are known to have abused children and young people.

Keeping the people in our care and in the team safe does bring tension. We sometimes need to manage individuals who are aggressive or who have perpetrated crimes or acts that are difficult to understand or to come to terms with. We might also have to deal with abuse happening between individuals or even visitors. Whatever is happening, we have a duty to treat everyone fairly, with respect and with kindness.

One area of concern may be the treatment of staff by some individuals. To be kicked or bitten is a risk but is it really to be expected and therefore accepted as part of the job? Or do we manage this risk in different ways? Perhaps we will warn staff of the risks and manage it by increasing staff ratios.

Tension and conflict are likely, particularly if we are caring for somebody who is on the sex offenders register. Staff must be able to carry out their work safely, whether working in an adult care setting or in the community.

The concept of unconditional positive regard (UPR) is one that you need to adopt. A term coined by Carl Rogers (1951), it describes the acceptance and support of a person regardless of what the person says or does and requires you to set aside your personal opinions and biases. This is used extensively in counselling therapy. Rogers believed that by approaching individuals in this way you can help them to accept and take responsibility for themselves. UPR is dependent on your ability to isolate the behaviour from the person. In other words, while you disagree with their behaviour, it is the person you are caring for. You may, for example, have a person in your care setting who has served a prison sentence for a crime against a child. Some staff may find it difficult to treat the person with compassion but as a manager you have to ensure that the person is safe and is receiving the care required. It is important, therefore, to enable staff to talk to you about their feelings and to reassure them of their duties, of the **6Cs** in social care, and your support. It is a good idea to have a risk assessment in place to ensure that the individual is kept safe from opportunities to harm others.

KEY TERM

6Cs: These are the values that underpin social care – care, compassion, commitment, communication, courage and competence.

Reflect on it

1.11 Unconditional positive regard (UPR)

Reflect on how you could help staff understand the importance of UPR.

Evidence opportunity

1.11 Tensions between maintaining the safety of team members and others and your duty of care to adults who have abused

Explain the potential tensions between maintaining the safety of team members and others with the duty of care to adults who are known to have abused children, young people and others. Analyse actions you might take to protect staff in these circumstances.

Reflect on it

1.11 Tensions between maintaining the safety of team members and others and your duty of care to adults who have abused

Have you come across situations in your setting where you had a duty of care to someone who had abused another individual or a child, but you had to balance your duty with maintaining the safety of staff and others? What did you do? What kinds of things did you have to consider? If you have not been in this situation, what would you do? Discuss your thoughts with your assessor and make notes to document your discussion.

LO2 Be able to lead the implementation of practices, policies and procedures to support safeguarding in adult care settings/services

AC 2.1 Ensure that all policies, procedures, systems and processes used in the work setting comply with legal requirements, local and national guidance

Here, you will be required to provide evidence of how your setting's policies and procedures to support safeguarding and whistle blowing reflect national and local requirements and how these are reviewed to ensure currency.

A policy statement makes it clear to everyone in the setting – staff, individuals using the service, stakeholders and others – what you and your organisation will do to keep people safe. There are many policies available online that might be of use if you are updating or re-writing your own policy, for example you may like to look at the websites for Quality Compliance Systems (www.qcs.co.uk) or Care UK (www.careuk.com).

Any sample policy statement can be used as a guide, and with amendments you can personalise the policy to fit your own setting. All safeguarding policies need to acknowledge the duty of care your setting has to safeguard and promote the welfare of the individuals in your care. The agreed ways of working within the setting must reflect legal responsibilities, government guidance and guidance of your regulatory body.

The policy should be reviewed annually and changes made according to current guidance and practice. The policy may also need to reflect changes to working practices which have emerged as the result of experience. Consider also how you present your policies, particularly in settings for people with learning disabilities or dementia where understanding may be compromised. You might depict your policies in a more visual way using pictures or undertake to use a system such as EasyWrite, which advocates using simpler words to aid understanding. The Autism Research Centre and the British Institute of Learning Disability may offer some advice on how this can be accomplished.

Evidence opportunity

2.1 Safeguarding policies and procedures that reflect legal, national and local requirements

Provide evidence to your assessor of how your policies and procedures to support safeguarding and whistle blowing reflect national and local requirements and how you review these to ensure that they are current.

Reflect on it

2.1 Your setting's policies

Identify the policies in place in your setting which ensure that safeguarding procedures and prevention of abuse are addressed.

How do your setting's policies and procedures supporting safeguarding and whistle blowing reflect national and local requirements?

AC 2.2 Embed safeguarding principles throughout all practices, policies and procedures

Here, you will explain how safeguarding should be embedded in your own and team members' work.

Safeguarding practice must be at the core of what you and your staff do each day. Employees have a duty to ensure that everyone is working within policy and is up to date with agreed ways of working in the setting.

Unintentional abuse such as racial comments, sexist remarks or even rushing the care carries the same consequences for individuals as intentional abuse. If, however, we work towards a culture of compassion in the setting, with staff recognising the suffering of the people they care for then safeguarding will follow.

Staff may also be asked to be part of the review of policy and this is something you as a manager may wish to instigate within the course of appraisal sessions or team meetings. Staff should be encouraged to reflect upon how policies are working and whether and how changes can improve the quality of care. Family and other agencies may also be a useful source of information about how a policy change might improve the care being given.

All care providers are required to have comprehensive safeguarding policies which form part of staff or volunteer induction. All partnerships with external organisations are also required to comply. Safeguarding policies are needed to protect vulnerable people who are either suffering abuse, or who are at risk from abuse, but they need to be part of the day-to-day running of the setting to be fully embedded in practice. Staff must be trained to ensure that they fully embrace safeguarding practice and, as a minimum, they could be offered an introductory level of safeguarding training.

Safeguarding also applies to the use of the internet for daily operations in the setting. Computers and the internet are now used widely so users are at risk of viewing harmful content. Within the setting, internet filters can be set to block any potentially dangerous content and this could include the use of social media, but if the individual has capacity then they cannot be banned from watching what they want. In this case, staff need to advise and guide. Staff training and induction should include safeguarding protocols and internet safety to ensure that staff know what acceptable use is.

It is not only staff who need to practise safeguarding but all people who come into the setting, such as volunteers, individuals and external partners. All staff who work in the community must be aware of the safeguarding policies and practices and be well informed about what to do if any safeguarding concern is raised. It is good practice to make the safeguarding policy available to all parties by sending out email bulletins and making your safeguarding policy visible to the public. As changes to practice and law come about, the policy should be reviewed at least every two years.

Finally, you should have an equality and diversity statement that prohibits any discrimination, targeted harassment or bullying based on ethnicity, gender, age, ability, religion or sexual orientation. Practicing equality ensures that everyone has equal opportunities and is treated the same, regardless of their characteristics. Diversity, on the other hand, is more than this and is about valuing those differences.

Evidence opportunity

2.2 How individuals and/or families are included in reviewing policies and procedures

Provide evidence to your assessor of how you embed the practice of safeguarding in your setting. How do you ensure that others are involved in reviewing and/or updating the adult care service safeguarding policies and procedures, including those in receipt of care and support, employees and others?

Reflect on it

2.2 Reviewing and updating policies

Write a short report which shows how you include individuals or family members when it comes to reviewing policies and procedures about the care of vulnerable adults in your care. Describe the process. For example, sometimes the individuals you care for may exhibit behaviour that challenges, so how do you build relationships and provide positive support to help them to avoid behaving in challenging ways? It might be that you have been trained to use approved methods of physical intervention or have put in place support plans that will detail the de-escalation strategies for each individual. Include some examples in your report. How did you involve individuals and family members to improve the policies and was this helpful?

AC 2.3 Support team members to develop the knowledge and skills they need to safeguard adults at risk

Here, you will provide evidence to show how you support team members when dealing with issues of safeguarding.

A vulnerable adult is anyone aged 18 or over who is at risk of harm, because they are unable to take care of themselves or protect themselves. Staff who undertake care work need to understand how various conditions put people at this risk.

People with mental health problems, learning or physical disabilities and age-related physical or mental disabilities may need additional support and so they are at a greater risk of harm, abuse and exploitation than others. Dementia and sight or hearing impairments are also conditions which might make a person vulnerable simply because they rely on others to assist them with their day-to-day living. This immediately puts carers into a position of power, which can be positive but also negative if used to take advantage. It is essential that staff look out for people with vulnerabilities and know when and how to report any cases of vulnerable adult abuse.

Annual safeguarding training will ensure that staff update their knowledge and understand how they are expected to behave with respect to this area of work. Many organisations focus on safeguarding by including it in their values or a mission statement. Annual performance review requires staff to demonstrate how they implement their knowledge into their practice and to give examples of having done so. Nurses, for example, are required to reflect upon practice and to give examples of how they safeguard the individuals in their care.

Evidence opportunity

2.3 Staff safeguarding training

Review the training for your staff to show how you develop the knowledge and skills they need to safeguard adults at risk. Undertake an appraisal and address safeguarding with a staff member. Keep evidence of this for your assessment.

AC 2.4 Ensure team members understand their role in responding to concerns about the safeguarding of a child or young person

Here, you will provide evidence to show you have supported team members with safeguarding issues concerning young people.

Team members need to have clarity about how to deal with concerns about suspected abuse. In your day-to-day work you have a duty to safeguard and promote the welfare of every individual you care for and this means you need to be very clear about the organisation's policy and procedures for safeguarding. When concerns are expressed about the welfare of anybody in your care, you must report these concerns immediately to the designated safeguarding officer. If a member of staff reports concerns to you, as the manager you will be required to make a written and dated note of their concern and inform the safeguarding officer as soon as possible. This person will then take the matter forward. For concerns related to historical abuse or cases where there has been inaccurate recording of safeguarding issues you need to be aware that any allegation of abuse or neglect might lead to a criminal investigation and, therefore, you as the manager and your staff must not do anything that may jeopardise a police investigation.

No attempt must be made to investigate the allegations yourself as this sort of action in the past led to cases that did not result in court action.

When a child discloses details of abuse, all disclosures should be taken seriously. It is vital that anyone who works with children and young people is able to provide support. Children may be reluctant to disclose abuse for fear of getting into trouble, so sensitivity when dealing with them is essential. Staff should notice signs of distress in a child and should ask skilled and appropriate questions about what might have caused this.

Concerns can then be taken to the organisation's designated safeguarding lead, or to the police if the danger is imminent.

The NSPCC's 'Speak out Stay safe' is an online safeguarding programme for children aged 5 to 11-years-old. It is designed to help children understand:

- what abuse is and how to recognise signs of abuse
- that abuse is never their fault and that they have the right to be safe
- where to get help and the sources of help available to them, including the Childline service.

If a child tells a member of your staff they are experiencing abuse, they need to be reassured that this has been the right thing to do. Accurate and detailed notes on any concerns the staff member has must be implemented and shared with the nominated child protection/safeguarding lead. If you actually witness the abuse or suspect it is happening, you must report it immediately as you have a legal and moral responsibility to protect the child.

Information sharing is key to promoting the welfare of the child, so staff need to be clear about the purpose of sharing a child's personal information. Keeping records of the reasons why you are sharing or requesting information about a child or their family is best practice. There also needs to be assurance that the child's safety and welfare is not being put at risk by sharing information about them.

Consent to share information about a child and their family must be sought but if not given, under certain circumstances, for example if you are protecting a child from significant harm, information may still be shared.

The Data Protection Act 2018 and the General Data Protection Regulation (GDPR) do not affect this principle and you need to ensure that the information shared is accurate and clear as to what is factual and what is based on opinion.

Evidence opportunity

2.4 Safeguarding information and the people you work with

Provide evidence to your assessor of how you ensure that safeguarding information with respect to children and young people is disseminated safely to employees, non-care staff and those in receipt of care and support services, such as families and carers.

How do you check your team members' knowledge, understanding and expected behaviours which apply to their roles and practice in safeguarding?

Finally, provide evidence of how safeguarding information is actioned in the event that knowledge in relation to care/practice was not current and/or inaccurate.

AC 2.5 Review person-centred practices, policies and procedures to ensure continuous improvement in safeguarding of adults at risk of abuse or neglect in own setting/service

Here, you will understand how Safeguarding Adults Reviews are used to improve safeguarding in settings.

Outcomes from safeguarding reviews and investigations

Safeguarding Adults Reviews (SARs) have shown that abuse in care has been ongoing for a number of years and, despite a number of government initiatives, it continues today. This includes abuse occurring in institutional settings and in the home by care staff, relatives and friends in the form of:

- sexual and financial abuse
- abuse of medication to control and sedate
- physical abuse
- neglect
- behaviour designed to degrade and humiliate.

This has been highlighted through media coverage and reporting.

For example, Orchid View was a nursing home registered as a care home with nursing for up to 87 people in the categories of old age and dementia. Opened in November 2009, it closed in October 2011 following revelations of a number of safeguarding alerts and investigations and possible criminal offences. In October 2013, an inquest found that five people had *died from natural causes attributed to neglect' and that several other people 'died as a result of natural causes' with 'insufficient evidence before me [the reviewer] to show that this suboptimal care was directly causative' of their deaths ... this suboptimal care caused distress, poor care and discomfort to residents and the families of people who were not the subject of the Inquest.*

Source: WSASB (2014)

The Care Act 2014 introduced SARs. See AC1.3 for more on SARs.

The purpose of an SAR in adult care is to determine whether any lessons could be learned from the case about the way in which professionals and organisations work together to safeguard vulnerable adults. The main aim is not to apportion blame but to promote learning and improve practice.

While it is not a statutory requirement to publish reports, it is recognised as good practice and demonstrates transparency and accountability to enable lessons to be learned as widely as possible. The main aim has been to prevent the same incidents occurring again.

Trauma informed care

Experiencing a traumatic event will trigger a negative impact on anyone in a care setting and new trauma-informed models of care address this. Serious case reviews from children's services have shown how trauma is one of the possible outcomes of some experiences which are so overwhelming for children that they create helplessness in the short term and can lead to mental health issues later in life.

Research it

2.5 Serious case reviews

Look at some of the serious case reviews such as the Orchid View case, the Francis Report or Winterbourne View and describe what you have learned from such cases.

How have these cases brought changes to local or national safeguarding requirements in adult care services?

Reflect on it

2.5 Analyse how the findings from recent Safeguarding Adult Reviews have impacted the provision of adult care services

What lessons have been learned from a recent national or local inquiry or Safeguarding Adult Review? Show how these have brought changes to local or national safeguarding requirements in adult care services. For example, the Francis Report recommended that care workers should undertake training and the Care Certificate is one response to this. Other changes include the need for transparency when dealing with individuals and if mistakes are made health professionals are now duty bound to tell the individual what has happened and to apologise.

How do you think this will ensure that care is improved? What changes have been made in your own setting and have they been useful? What else will you need to do to bring your setting up to the required standard?

Trauma-informed care seeks to understand and address the impact of trauma and set up pathways for recovery. More geared towards children's services, it seeks to ensure that traumatic events in a child's life do not limit their growth and development. Rather than asking a young person 'what is wrong' with them, it reframes the question to 'what happened to you' and recognises the signs and symptoms of trauma, integrating that knowledge into policies, procedures and practices. This actively avoids re-traumatisation.

Current guidance arising from safeguarding adult reviews relating to adult care and its relevance to own organisation

Local authority safeguarding duties have changed as a result of SARs and the Care Act 2014. These require that local authorities must:

- lead multi-agency local adult safeguarding systems to prevent abuse and neglect
- make enquiries, or request others to do so, when they think an adult with care and support needs may be at risk
- establish Safeguarding Adults Boards which include the local authority, NHS and police, to develop, share and implement a joint safeguarding strategy
- carry out SARs when someone with care and support needs dies as a result of neglect or abuse. This is done when there is concern that the local authority or its partners could have done more to protect them

- arrange for an independent advocate to represent and support an individual who is the subject of a safeguarding enquiry or review.

Source: Adapted from SCIE (2023)

Organisational culture

Organisational culture is the collection of values, expectations, beliefs and practices that guide your setting. It is not just about the organisation's policies and procedures but also about the behaviours of the staff and how they align with these values.

Culture affects all aspects of the setting and if, for example, one of your values is to 'support person centred care in everything we do' then it will be evidenced in the way your staff behave with individuals, how they approach each individual in their care, and how they promote independent living. When workplace culture aligns with your staff, they will feel supported and valued.

Trust is a key aspect for building a culture that is positive and supportive. Where there is trust, staff will feel able to express themselves and to find support when needed. Change occurs rapidly in care work and can have an unsettling effect. External influences such as new legislation and guidance will impact internal practices. For example, during the COVID-19 pandemic, rapid changes had to be implemented in order to secure safe working environments and safe care practices. A positive workplace culture is one that can handle adverse situations and this requires strong connections between team members, so communication and collaboration is very important. To develop this sort of culture all staff members must feel appreciated and valued so it is important to regularly provide recognition and thanks for the contributions of others. One key advantage of having a positive workplace culture is that people will be drawn to work for you.

Every organisation's culture is different, and you need to know what it is that makes yours unique. High-performing organisations consistently show the following qualities:

- **Alignment**: This happens when all the workforce is pulling together to meet the same goals.
- **Resilience**: A key requirement, particularly when change is continuous.
- **Teamwork**: When the whole team support each other, more will get done and staff will feel happier doing it. Collaboration, communication and respect between team members will build a trusting and happy team.
- **Honesty and transparency**: This is critical to building a trusting team culture as staff will feel they can they rely on each other for support.

AC 2.6 Evaluate the outcomes of the review of person-centred practices, policies and procedures to plan developments to ensure safeguarding of adults at risk of abuse or neglect in own setting/service

Here, you will be required to show how you effectively disseminate and implement safeguarding policies and procedures.

Internal policies and procedures relating to all aspects of management and non-management practice

This has been covered in earlier sections, specifically AC1.3 and AC2.1.

Your organisation's strategic plan will specify how safeguarding will be practised and the policy will ensure that abuse and neglect are prevented and will explain how the individuals using your service will be protected. The policy should include details about effective joint working and identify the agencies and professionals with whom you share this responsibility. There must be clear lines of accountability within the organisation for safeguarding and staff need to be aware of the role of the local Safeguarding Children Boards' and Safeguarding Adults Boards' strategies.

The policy should also identify the arrangements for staff training and continuing professional development as well as safe working practices with respect to recruitment and vetting and barring procedures. You need to check that the policies and procedures for safeguarding and person-centred practice are effective and relevant.

Whistle blowing guidance for staff

The expectation in any organisation is that individuals should raise challenges and concerns, but they must be able to do this in a supportive and protective environment. Most challenges or complaints should be dealt with inside the organisation, which should, with appropriate guidance, enable you to resolve the situation or support sanctions. However, there are occasions when a practice is so widespread and resistant to change or of such a serious nature that a more radical approach is required. In such circumstances, staff who witness such activities will be protected by law for making this public. However, this does not mean that the individual has a right to go to the press or other public forum to expose an organisation without trying to resolve issues internally first.

The policies and systems discussed below apply to staff as well as to the individuals using the service.

A whistle blower is protected by law for disclosure if they:

- are a 'worker'
- believe that malpractice in the workplace is happening, has happened in the past or will happen in the future
- are revealing information of the right type (a 'qualifying disclosure'), which refers to information that the worker believes is a criminal offence, a miscarriage of justice or failure to comply with a legal obligation. This may have taken place in the past, or may happen in the future
- reveal it to the right person and in the right way (making it a 'protected disclosure'). This is where workers bring information about a wrongdoing to the attention of their employers or a relevant organisation, and in doing so they are protected in certain circumstances under the Public Interest Disclosure Act 1998.

As the manager of a care setting you need to ensure that you have created an environment where staff can report concerns knowing that you will act upon them and investigate. Staff must be confident about this so having an open culture will help. Your whistle blowing policy should be promoted to staff to make it clear that they can go outside their normal line management to raise concerns and that they will have the protection of the Public Interest Disclosure Act if the disclosure is not untrue or malicious. As a manager you may also wish to raise such concerns and can make disclosures to report concerns.

Without a whistle blowing policy, there is a possibility that bad practice will go unchallenged as staff will not feel confident about their rights to make a disclosure.

Your whistle blowing policy might cover the following points:

- The identity of the person the whistle blower made the disclosure to (e.g. disclosing to a relevant professional body may be more likely to be considered reasonable than, say, one made to the media).
- The seriousness of the wrong doing.
- Whether the wrong doing is continuing or likely to occur again.
- Whether the disclosure breaches the employer's duty of confidentiality (e.g. if information made available contains confidential details about an individual).
- If the whistle blower made a previous disclosure and whether they followed any internal procedures then.

It is important to note that the term 'worker' includes agency workers and people who aren't directly employed but are in training with employers. Some self-employed people may be considered to be workers for the purpose of whistle blowing if they are supervised or work off-site.

Making a disclosure

For a disclosure to be protected by the law, it should be made to the right person or authority and in the right way. Disclosures must meet the following criteria:

- The disclosure must be in good faith (honest intent and without malice).
- The whistle blower must reasonably believe that the information is substantially true.
- The whistle blower must reasonably believe they are making the disclosure to the right 'prescribed person'.

If a qualifying disclosure is made in good faith to an employer, or through a process that the employer has agreed, the whistle blower will be entitled to protection.

If a worker feels unable to make a disclosure to their employer, there are other 'prescribed people' to whom a disclosure can be made. Disclosure can be made to the person responsible for the area of concern, such as a team leader or mentor.

To make a protected disclosure to 'others' rather than the employer, the whistle blower must:

1. Reasonably believe their employer would treat them unfairly if the disclosure was made to the employer or a prescribed person.
2. Reasonably believe that the disclosure to the employer would result in the destruction or concealment of information about the wrong doing.
3. Have previously disclosed the same or similar information to the employer or a prescribed person.

Whistle blowers should not become the subject of an internal investigation or be ridiculed or dismissed as a result of raising concerns. In health and care organisations, the law requires a **Duty of Candour**, which protects individuals from poor or unsafe care. The Duty of Candour (2014) requires transparency about failures or lapses in respect of care.

KEY TERM

Duty of Candour: Requires providers to be open and transparent with individuals about their care and treatment. If treatment goes wrong, the care provider must inform the individual about the incident, provide support and offer an apology.

Reflect on it

2.6 Your own person-centred working practice policy

Take a critical look at your person-centred working practice policy. What might be improved? As a manager, what is your specific role with respect to person-centred practice? What is the role of your staff with respect to how they are involved with person-centred practice? How does it link to effective safeguarding practice?

Evidence opportunity

2.6 The effectiveness of safeguarding and whistle blowing policies, procedures and protocols

How effective are your person-centred practices, policies, procedures and protocols? Show your assessor how you effectively disseminate and implement person-centred policies and procedures and consider the topics covered in this section.

Reflect on it

2.6 The effectiveness of safeguarding policies, procedures and protocols

Look at the systems and processes that promote safeguarding and whistle blowing in your workplace and comment on how effective they are and how they fit into person-centred practice. How do the protocols relating to person-centred practice link to those of safeguarding?

AC 2.7 Implement revised person-centred practices, policies and procedures relating to safeguarding in own setting

Here, you will show how safeguarding can be developed and improved in the setting.

Person-centred care demands that each individual is central to their own care and that the care and support given matches the needs of the individual rather than trying to make a person fit existing procedures. There is a fine balance between person-centred care and safeguarding. Having revised the policies and protocols, it is important to ensure that they are implemented and used. When you work with individuals in a person-centred way, planning their care and support to meet their own unique needs, the risk of unfair or harmful treatment and neglect is minimised and increases safeguarding of the person.

When providing care and support, staff need to be mindful that a 'one size fits all' approach does not work. Promoting an individual's independence means looking at what they can do for themselves. In this way they are empowered to do things for themselves as much as possible.

In implementing your care practices and policies you should ensure that person-centred values inform your working. These values include:

- individuality
- independence
- privacy
- partnership
- choice
- dignity
- respect
- rights.

For more information, see The Care Certificate Workbook Standard 5 (Skills for Care, n.d.).

Changes to practice and information about safeguarding must not be restricted to policy but need to be actively shared and implemented among employees and those who work in partnership with your setting. You might schedule safeguarding as a permanent agenda item for discussion at team meetings, ensuring that all staff are firmly aware of their role in practice. For non-care staff, support services, families and individuals using the service, the information must be made available on the setting's website and perhaps in hard copy by means of a prospectus about the setting.

You can obtain feedback about how safeguarding information is being disseminated and received through appraisals and supervision sessions. Additionally, when working in partnership with other agencies, families and carers, information must be recorded and shared safely, and confidentiality must not be breached. Systems need to be in place to ensure that all partners are aware of how they may accomplish this. Record keeping should also be standardised where possible across the partnership so that records are consistent.

As the manager, you need to ensure that everyone connected to the service is supported in their efforts to apply safeguarding policies and procedures. Training and guidance may be required to help the people involved in the care of individuals to understand policies and to question the content if they need to.

Reflect on it

2.7

Draw a diagram or mind map to show how you can promote the values of individuality, independence, privacy, partnership, choice, dignity, respect and rights in your day-to-day work and, at the same time, ensure that they are safeguarded.

AC 2.8 Promote practices that encourage and empower adults at risk, and those who are important to them, to share concerns

Here, you will show how individuals in the setting can be encouraged to share their concerns with yourself and team members.

Ensuring that staff and individuals using the service are able to complain when necessary

People receiving care or support are vulnerable because they rely on others for support. They may be reluctant to speak up about incidents that happen because they do not want to 'upset' anyone or 'rock the boat' in any way. They may avoid making complaints for fear of this resulting in poor care or support being withdrawn. Individuals and their families must be made aware of organisational policies regarding safeguarding and whistle blowing, which show clear routes for escalation and how to respond appropriately to a safeguarding concern. Policies need clear information about how confidential information will be shared between departments in the same organisation and externally. You will need to retain evidence of reported concerns and record any incidents and allegations made.

It is crucial that you operate a system of transparency so that staff and the individuals using your service feel confident that you will not only take them seriously if they make a claim of abuse but will also support them in their decision to do so. You can do this by ensuring that your setting is open about the complaints procedure and that this is available on notice boards, for example; that your staff know how they can support individuals in the complaints procedure; and that individuals feel that they can make a complaint or discuss issues that are concerning them.

Recommendations to improve management practice

Any allegation of abuse made by an individual using the service or anyone outside the setting against a member of your staff, or by a member of staff against another member of staff, will have an impact upon you as a manager. You may feel upset or angry about what has happened or is alleged to have happened and want to put a stop to this immediately. The way in which you respond may affect outcomes, so you need to adopt an objective approach to the incident and follow procedure to the letter. Putting aside your emotions can be hard to do but a professional approach must be developed here and gossiping or discussing the incident will be damaging to the team and the investigation. You may want to seek supervision to discuss how you are feeling about the incident or seek advice from higher management or the HR team, although not all adult care setting will have an HR team.

Reflect on it

2.8 Promote practices that encourage and empower adults at risk, and those who are important to them, to share concerns

What practices are in place in your setting that encourage individuals and their families or friends to share concerns when they feel at risk?

Whistle blowing

Whistle blowing or raising concerns about something harmful happening is a difficult action to take, particularly if the person taking action feels they will not be listened to. Your organisation's policy must therefore help individuals to report safeguarding concerns internally in the first instance or be directed to other routes if they feel unable to do this.

You must designate a safeguarding lead, and this may be you or a deputy. Good practice demands that everyone in the organisation knows who is accountable for safeguarding and how to contact them.

By developing a positive culture of open communication, staff and individuals using the service will feel more able to speak about safeguarding concerns. Staff, family and friends should be encouraged to look out for changes in an individual's mood or behaviour, which need to be recorded and shared as soon as possible. These could be indicators of abuse or neglect and immediate action must be taken.

Finally, by checking in with individuals and their families about their experience of raising safeguarding concerns, you will be able to make any changes in response to this feedback.

Evidence opportunity

2.8 Providing support when abuse is suspected

How can you, as a manager, provide support for team members, employees and volunteers when they suspect abuse, or if they have disclosed this?

How can you, as a manager, provide support for those who receive care when you suspect abuse, or if they have disclosed this?

Why might an individual not complain?

What recommendations to improve your management practice might you make to ensure that when there are allegations of danger, harm or abuse you support staff and the individuals using your service?

AC 2.9 Follow agreed protocols to participate in inter-agency, joint or integrated working in order to achieve the best outcomes for adults at risk

Here, you will show your assessor how you develop working relationships across different agencies to achieve the best integrated working in order to achieve the best outcome for an individual.

Inter-agency and joint working involves staff and social workers from different organisations working collaboratively to bring about change. This is a key part of supporting individuals and families who are identified as safeguarding risks and it is an effective method for improving their lives.

There are different kinds of inter-agency partnerships, and a variety of different organisations and professionals can be involved in working in this way. Practitioners may come from the justice system (police and probation staff), care workers, local authorities, mental health services, social care and the voluntary and community sector.

Working with partners reduces the risk of abuse and this was very much the finding from the Bichard Inquiry (see AC1.1). Different information is often shared with different care workers and bringing this information together can give a fuller picture of what might be happening to an individual. Having this level of knowledge and information means responses to safeguarding concerns can happen much more quickly and bring together more perspectives to support good outcomes.

You can also gain different perspectives when you work with people from different professional backgrounds. Care professionals can bring different experiences and ideas so where an individual may be at risk, this additional knowledge and information can lead to swifter action.

Working as an individual practitioner in cases of abuse is difficult and stressful. Inter-agency working shares the workload and responsibilities involved in protecting vulnerable individuals.

The most important thing you can do to develop effective working relationships is to build your reputation as a professional who is trustworthy and inspires confidence and respect in your team as well as between all team members. In this way, you can show that you provide other professionals with information, advice and support within the boundaries of your role and expertise and as such can develop protocols for partnership working that are fair to all parties involved.

Keep records of issues raised and action taken in line with agreements and legislative bodies

It is important that any action taken or any disclosure made is documented accurately and as soon as possible after the event. You need to inform human resources (HR) of this, and they can advise on the legal agreements and protocols. However, many smaller settings do not have an HR department. Here, you will need to act upon policy that is in the setting, or you can obtain further information from Citizens Advice or other settings. Your stakeholders may also be able to provide information for you, as can the Care Quality Commission.

Maintain clear processes for raising concerns and making complaints

Policies need to be available to all staff and stakeholders which clearly describe the process of making complaints and disclosure in the event of malpractice. Staff must be made aware through their induction process and training of how they can action this and what process they need to go through.

Evidence opportunity

2.9 Safeguarding protocols

How has your setting agreed protocols with partners to safeguard adults at risk? Collect evidence of inter-agency working to show your assessor.

Legislation

Legislation	Key points
Children Act 2004	This act places a duty on local authorities in England to promote co-operation with key partners and local agencies, with a view to improving the wellbeing of children in the authority's area. It places a duty to safeguard and promote the welfare of children on a range of agencies: local authorities, the police and health services. The roles and responsibilities of safeguarding partners are established in this law .
Children and Social Work Act 2017	This Act makes provision for looked after children, in relation to the welfare of children, and regulates the work of social workers. The main purposes are to improve decision making and support and to improve joint work at the local level to safeguard children. It promotes the safeguarding of children by providing for Relationships and Sex Education in schools and enables the establishment of a new regulatory regime for the social work profession in England.
Health and Care Act 2022	This Act introduced new legislation to make it easier for health and care organisations to deliver joined-up, integrated care for people who rely on different services. It builds on the recommendations put forward by NHS England and NHS Improvement.
Domestic Abuse Act 2021	This Act aims to increase awareness of and inform the response to domestic abuse. It provides statutory guidance for all organisations working with victims and aims to promote best practice.
Care Act 2014	Sets out the key responsibilities of local authorities in meeting the needs of individuals who require help and support to promote their wellbeing. Its main aim was to provide integrated care and to introduce the right to an assessment for all.
Safeguarding Vulnerable Groups Act 2006	This Act aims to help avoid harm or risk of harm by preventing people that are considered unsuitable to work with children and vulnerable adults from gaining access to them through their work. The Act established the Independent Safeguarding Authority.
Mental Capacity Act 2005	This act informs individuals about what they can do to plan and ensure that someone else can make decisions for them if they ever lack capacity to do so for themselves.
Mental Health Act 1983 (amended 2007)	The Mental Health Act 1983, amended by the Mental Health Act 2007, is designed to give health professionals powers to detain, assess and treat people with mental disorders in the interests of their health and safety or for public safety. The legislation also provides safeguards for individuals to ensure that they are not inappropriately treated under the provisions of the Act.
Sexual Offences Act 2003	This Act covers the offences of rape, assault by penetration, sexual assault and causing a person to engage in sexual activity without consent. It also sets out presumptions about consent.
Health and Social Care Act 2012	This Act introduced the role of the Care Quality Commission. Safeguarding and protection of individuals are specifically mentioned in these laws to address concerns about abuse. The Act aims to safeguard people who use care services from suffering any form of abuse or improper treatment while receiving care and treatment. To meet the requirements under this Act, providers must demonstrate zero tolerance of abuse, unlawful discrimination and restraint.
Counter-Terrorism and Security Act 2015	This Act aims to prevent people from being drawn into terrorism. Also known as the Prevent duty.
Modern Slavery Act 2015	This Act consolidates existing offences of human trafficking and slavery and all forms of exploitation.
Public Interest Disclosure Act 1998	This Act protects whistle blowers from detrimental treatment by their employer as a result of making a public interest disclosure.
Human Rights Act 1998	This Act sets out the fundamental rights and freedoms everyone in the UK is entitled to, as contained in the European Convention on Human Rights (EHCR).
Equality Act 2010	An umbrella Act bringing together legislation that deals with race, disability and gender. It highlights protected characteristics of age, gender reassignment, pregnancy, religion, marriage and civil partnerships, and sexual orientation in an attempt to end discrimination.

References

ADSS (2005) 'Safeguarding adults: A National Framework of Standards for good practice and outcomes in adult protection work' www.adass.org.uk/adassmedia/stories/publications/guidance/safeguarding.pdf

Department of Health and Social Care (2010) *Nothing Ventured, Nothing Gained: Risk guidance for dementia*. London: TSO.

Department of Health and Social Care (2022) 'Care and support statutory guidance document'. www.gov.uk/government/publications/care-act-statutory-guidance/care-and-support-statutory-guidance#using-the-care-act-guidance

Dignity in Care (n.d.) 'The 10 dignity do's'. www.dignityincare.org.uk/About/The_10_Point_Dignity_Challenge/

Dupre, C. (2011) 'What does dignity mean in a legal context?', *The Guardian*, 24 March.

GOV.UK (2022) 'Revisiting safeguarding practice' independent report www.gov.uk/government/publications/revisiting-safeguarding-practice

GOV.UK (n.d.) 'Court of Protection'. www.gov.uk/courts-tribunals/court-of-protection

Home Office, *The (2014) Multi Agency Working and Information Sharing Project Final Report*. London: TSO.

Rogers, C. (1951) *Client-centered Therapy: Its current practice, implications and theory*. Boston, MA: Houghton Mifflin.

Skills for Care (n.d. a) 'Care Certificate'. www.skillsforcare.org.uk/Developing-your-workforce/Care-Certificate/Care-Certificate.aspx

Social Care Institute for Excellence (2023) 'The Care Act: Safeguarding adults'. www.scie.org.uk/care-act-2014/safeguarding-adults/

West Sussex Adult Safeguarding Board (WSASB) (2014) 'Orchid View Serious Case Review'. www.westsussex.gov.uk/media/5168/orchid-view-scr-final-report.pdf

Useful resources and further reading

Community Care (2015) 'Government scraps designated adult safeguarding manager role'. www.communitycare.co.uk/2015/11/03/government-scraps-designated-adult-safeguarding-manager-role

legislation.gov.uk (n.d.) 'Modern Slavery Act 2105'. www.legislation.gov.uk/ukpga/2015/30/contents/enacted

Owen, T. and Meyer, J. (2009) *Minimising the Use of Restraint in Care Homes: Challenges, dilemmas and positive approaches*. London: SCIE.

Skills for Care (n.d. b) 'The Care Certificate: Work in a person-centred way. What you need to know: Standard 5'. www.skillsforcare.org.uk/resources/documents/Developing-your-workforce/Care-Certificate/Care-Certificate-Standards/Standard-5.pdf

Social Care Institute for Excellence (2014) 'Whistleblowing: Improving organisational practice'. www.scie.org.uk/contact/concerns/whistleblowingvideo

Social Care Institute for Excellence (2019) 'Safeguarding adults: Sharing information'. www.scie.org.uk/safeguarding/adults/practice/sharing-information

Social Care Institute for Excellence (2022) 'What are Liberty Protection Safeguards?'. www.scie.org.uk/mca/lps/latest

Unit 508

Understanding mental capacity and restrictive practice in adult care

GLH 20

About this unit

The Mental Capacity Act 2005 states that all adults have the right to make their own decisions and that 'a person must be assumed to have capacity unless it is established that he lacks capacity.'

In this unit you will learn about the legislation and codes of practice and policy regarding mental capacity and how they relate to adult care services/settings, together with your roles and responsibilities.

You will look at the support available for individuals when mental capacity needs to be assessed and determine how to assess risk in situations where an individual's capacity is a concern.

Restrictive practice, restraint and deprivation of liberty will be addressed, and you will be encouraged to consider your own responsibilities in relation to restrictive practices and deprivations of liberty. Additionally, you will look at how person-centred, outcomes-based practice must be encouraged as a way to mitigate the use of restrictive practices. Ultimately you must act in the individual's best interests when making decisions on behalf of a person who lacks capacity. The Mental Capacity Act states, 'Before the act is done, or the decision made, regard must be had to whether its purpose can be as effectively achieved in a way less restrictive of the person's rights and freedoms'.

Learning outcomes

By the end of this unit, you will:

1 Understand mental capacity and consent.
2 Understand the use and impact of restrictive practices in adult care.

Getting started

Before you study the unit, think about the following:

- What is your current understanding of the Mental Capacity Act?
- What restrictive practices do you currently have in place and how do they safeguard staff and the individuals using your service?

LO1 Understand mental capacity and consent

AC 1.1 Explain how current legislation, codes of practice and policy regarding mental capacity relate to adult care settings/services

Here, you will explain the main legislation that teams will need to know in relation to mental capacity and deprivation of liberty standards.

Mental Capacity Act 2005

The Mental Capacity Act 2005 (MCA) is an important piece of legislation that protects the rights of people to plan for their future in the event of becoming incapacitated. The Act clarifies and strengthens the rights of those who lack capacity to make decisions about their care. Capacity refers to the ability to make a decision and this can vary depending upon an individual's circumstances and health conditions at the time. Capacity is therefore decision-specific and time-specific, so an individual can only have capacity or lack capacity to make a specific decision at a specific time.

Five principles are set out in this Act:

- 'A person must be assumed to have capacity unless it is established that he lacks capacity.
- A person is not to be treated as unable to make a decision unless all practicable steps to help him to do so have been taken without success.
- A person is not to be treated as unable to make a decision merely because he makes an unwise decision.
- An act done, or decision made, under this Act for, or on behalf of, a person who lacks capacity must be done, or made, in his best interests. Before the act is done, or the decision is made, regard must be had to whether the purpose for which it is needed can be as effectively achieved in a way that is less restrictive of the person's rights and freedom of action.'

Source: Mental Capacity Act 2005

The Act also provides guidance for people who are acting on behalf of someone who cannot make decisions for themselves and includes a 'best interests' checklist of the person's wishes, feelings, beliefs and values as well as advance statements. These statements will have been prepared when the person had capacity and will take into account the views of their friends and family.

The Mental Capacity Act 2005, which provides a statutory framework for people who lack capacity to make decisions for themselves, is supported by a Code of Practice to guide anyone who works with or cares for adults who lack capacity to make particular decisions. The code focuses on those who have a duty of care to individuals who lack the capacity to agree to the care being provided and further describes their responsibilities when acting or making decisions on their behalf. For more information, see Department for Constitutional Affairs (2007).

Your knowledge of the MCA will be useful when managing decision making for individuals. The Act enables people over the age of 16 to appoint a proxy decision maker who has the legal power to give consent to medical treatment when the individual loses the capacity to consent. In the case of a person who is detained under mental health legislation, the principles of consent continue to apply, and care staff must ensure that the individual is aware of the circumstances and safeguards needed for providing treatment and care without consent. The decision as to whether the individual lacks capacity must be made with the staff providing the support and in consultation with family and care staff. In an emergency situation when an individual requires treatment but is unconscious, treatment to preserve life may be given, as long as it is in the best interests of that individual.

Refusal of treatment by a person with capacity should be respected and a record made. If the person who has refused treatment or care is confused or mentally incapacitated in some way, care staff must make a full and frank assessment of their care and ensure that the individual is safeguarded.

A referral to court to obtain permission to treat may sometimes be necessary.

There are a couple of exceptions where a capable individual may be treated without first obtaining their consent. For example, a magistrate can order detention in hospital if a person has an infectious disease that presents a risk to public health, for example rabies, cholera or anthrax (Public Health (Control of Disease) Act 1984).

Mental Capacity Act (Amendment) Act 2019 and Liberty Protection Safeguards

This Act is an amendment to the Mental Capacity Act 2005 and follows recommendations made by the Law Commission around mental capacity and deprivation of liberty. The Act also created the **Liberty Protection Safeguards (LPS)**, which are due to replace Deprivation of Liberty Safeguards (DoLS). The DoLS were inserted into the MCA to provide authorisation and safeguards for deprivation of liberty in care homes or other provisions and hospitals but were heavily criticised in 2014 by a House of Lords Select Committee as being 'poorly drafted, overly complex' and 'far from being used to protect individuals and their rights, they are sometimes used to oppress individuals'.

KEY TERM

Liberty Protection Safeguards (LPS): Introduced in the Mental Capacity (Amendment) Act 2019, these will provide protection for people aged 16 and over who lack the capacity to give consent to arrangements for their care or treatment and who need to be deprived of their liberty in order for that care or treatment to be given. They will replace the DoLS and provide a less bureaucratic system.

Under the terms for LPS, 'responsible bodies' can authorise deprivation of liberty provided there is medical evidence of 'unsoundness of mind' or the person lacks the mental capacity to consent to the arrangements to deliver care or treatment. The arrangements for care must be 'necessary and proportionate' in relation to the risk to the person or to others (GOV.UK, 2022a). Responsible bodies include hospitals, health bodies or local authorities who are responsible for arranging or delivering the person's care and treatment.

Other relevant legislation that you need to be clear about to ensure that a person's rights are upheld include the:

- Human Rights Act 1998
- Disability Discrimination Acts 1995 and 2005
- Equality Act 2010
- Care Act 2014.

Research it

1.1 Impact of MCA Code of Practice

Read the consultation document 'Changes to the MCA Code of Practice and implementation of the LPS: consultation document' (GOV.UK, 2022).

How will the changes in law and guidance affect your setting? What changes will you need to make with respect to consent, DoLS and the implementation of LPS?

AC 1.2 Explain own role in applying and upholding key principles of mental capacity legislation, internal policy and codes of practice

Here, you will be required to explain your own role in relation to the Mental Capacity Act and Liberty Protection Safeguards.

The key principles of the Mental Capacity Act 2005 and Mental Capacity Act (Amendment) Act 2019, outlined in AC1.1, require a person-centred approach to decision making and must underpin plans and monitoring arrangements to ensure that your service meets the needs of a range of adults to promote their rights, autonomy and independence.

Your responsibility as a manager is to ensure that the principles are embedded into your policies and practices in the setting. You must ensure that you and your staff understand the Act, so that assessments of capacity can be carried out appropriately and any decisions made on behalf of incapacitated people are made in their best interests.

Reflect on it

1.2 LPS

What is your role in LPS and how will you apply this?

AC 1.3 Outline the support available when mental capacity needs to be assessed

Here, you should outline the main sources of support when assessing mental capacity in an individual.

Support in determining whether a person lacks capacity can be found on government websites and guidelines produced by various organisations. You may find the following resources useful:

- Making decisions on behalf of someone: GOV.UK (n.d.).
- Assessing capacity: SCIE (n.d.).
- Mental Capacity Act 2005 Code of Practice: Including the Liberty Protection Safeguards 2022: GOV.UK (2022c).

If you think that an individual needs support in terms of their capacity to make a decision, or if their mind is affected by illness or disability, you may wish to involve a family member or an advocate before you take steps to assess their mental capacity. Lack of capacity may not always be permanent so all assessments of capacity should be time and decision specific.

In determining a lack of mental capacity, the care professional needs to be able to demonstrate that the person lacks the capacity to make a specific decision when they need to. Such an assessment must never be based on factors such as age, appearance, physical disabilities, learning disabilities or temporary conditions such as drunkenness. The decision must be clearly documented together with the rationale for the decision you have made.

The role of the independent mental capacity advocate (IMCA) was introduced in the Mental Capacity Act 2005 to represent individuals when there is nobody else to do so. They provide a legal safeguard to aid decision making when a person lacks capacity to do so and has nobody close to them to help.

Where an individual has no family or friends to represent them, but does have an attorney or deputy who has been appointed solely to deal with property and affairs, then it is a requirement to involve an IMCA. An IMCA must also be appointed if the personal welfare attorney or deputy is not authorised to make the specific decision in question.

'Best interests' assessments

The Mental Capacity Act 2005 states that '[a]n act done, or decision made, under this Act for or on behalf of a person who lacks capacity must be done, or made, in his best interests'.

What the Act does not do, however, is to prescribe in detail what 'best interests' means and therefore it lacks clarity. It does supply a checklist and a process to apply to ascertain an individual's capacity, but when applied in this way it is possible that two people may come up with very different views about what a person's best interests actually are.

In the case of *P v Cheshire West and Chester Council*, a landmark Supreme Court ruling threw out previous judgments that had defined deprivation of liberty more restrictively. Under the Deprivation of Liberty Safeguards, strict control of a person's living space had meant that many individuals might have been deprived of their liberty unlawfully and without safeguards in settings including care homes or other provisions and supported living placements.

P had lived in a supported living bungalow with other residents since 2009, receiving substantial one-to-one care and supervision. His behaviour, which was to tear his incontinence pads and put the pieces in his mouth, was managed by physical intervention. In 2011 the Court of Appeal had ruled that this was not a deprivation of liberty because P's life was as normal as possible for someone with his level of disability and he would require the same level of supervision in any other setting.

However, this ruling was rejected by the Supreme Court, which said that people with a disability should not face a tougher standard than people without a disability. Being constantly monitored and not being able to go out without supervision was depriving the person of their liberty.

Reflect on it

1.3 Your own practice

What do you think about the information on 'best interests' assessments? How might it change the way in which you work?

Evidence opportunity

1.3 Outline the support available when mental capacity needs to be assessed

In assessing mental capacity what support is required?

Reflect on your understanding and application of the legal requirements and implications relating to restrictive practice in your adult care setting.

AC 1.4 Explain how to access support available for a mental capacity assessment

Here, you will be required to explain the sources of support when assessing mental capacity in an individual.

Technically, anybody can make an assessment of somebody's capacity, so you and your staff may find yourselves having to make a decision about this. In order to do this properly and fairly you need to have access to the Mental Capacity Act Code of Practice and make this available for relevant staff.

Make sure that your staff has a good understanding of this Code of Practice and knows where they can find it. Everyone who makes decisions on behalf of others needs to recognise their role and responsibilities under the Code of Practice. The MCA 2005 is underpinned by five key principles in relation to determining whether someone lacks capacity. These are explained below.

- Principle 1: A person with mental capacity can make their own decisions, so when decisions need to be made regarding care or treatment, you need to start from the assumption that the person has capacity.
- Principle 2: Every effort must then be made to encourage and support the person to make the decision themselves.
- Principle 3: Even if a person makes a decision which you consider to be a little eccentric or even unwise, this does not automatically mean that the person is lacking in capacity.

- Principle 4: This principle requires that if it is decided that a person does NOT have mental capacity, then decisions made must be in their best interest. There is, however, no legal definition of best interest but there is a procedure set out in section 4 of the Mental Capacity Act which should be followed.
- Principle 5: Finally, if a decision is made on behalf of a person who does not have mental capacity, it should be the least restrictive option of the person's rights and freedoms.

Two-stage functional test of capacity

The two-stage functional test of capacity is one that will support you to make a good decision.

Stage 1 – Is the person unable to make a particular decision (the functional test)?

Stage 2 – Is the inability to make a decision caused by an impairment of, or disturbance in, the functioning of a person's mind or brain? This could be due to long-term conditions such as mental illness, dementia or learning disability, or more temporary states such as confusion, unconsciousness, or the effects of drugs or alcohol (the diagnostic test)'. (From SCIE)

If the person is unable to make their own decision because they do not understand the information being given to them, or they cannot retain that information long enough to be able to make the decision, then that may require support under the MCA. If they are unable to weigh up the information to make the decision or to communicate their decision – this could be by talking, signing or even simple muscle movements such as blinking an eye or squeezing a hand in the case of severe disablement – then this also warrants MCA support.

Source: Adapted from SCIE (2022)

1.4 Research it

SCIE offers support and resources to assess mental capacity. Go to the SCIE website and familairise yourself with the MCA support resource (SCIE, n.d.).

AC 1.5 Explain own role in the assessment of risk in situations where an individual's capacity is a concern.

Here, you will explain your role in assessing risk and the development of positive risk taking within a setting.

Risk and risk-averse culture and practice

Care settings vary in type and as such the risks associated with them will differ. The rights of individuals in your care can occasionally be in conflict with health and safety issues and you need to be prepared to address such occasions. For example, an individual new to a care home may wish to go out shopping by themselves or may wish to go along to the local pub in the evening. They are clearly not imprisoned in the home and there should be no reason to deny them that right, but at the same time the staff may well have some concerns as to their safety when they are not in the home. The document *Rights, Risks and Restraints: An exploration into the use of restraint in the care of older people* (CSCI, 2007), is useful. Concerned mainly with how some older people have been restrained in some care settings, and also with some references to laws that are not current, the article makes some useful points:

> *Respecting people's basic human rights to dignity, freedom and respect underpins good quality social care. People may need support in managing their care and making decisions but they have the right, whether in their own home or in a care home, to make choices about their lives and to take risks.*
>
> *Social care services have responsibilities to keep people safe from harm and to ensure their safety. It is this need to balance people's rights to freedom and to make choices with ensuring people are safe that is at the heart of this exploration into the use of restraint in the care of older people.*

It is a case, then, of balancing your duty of care and the individual's safety while also respecting their rights. The individual is at the forefront of any decision made and the risk assessment should enable rather than hinder. While workers might be afraid that they are neglecting their responsibilities when it comes to risk assessment, by putting measures in place and enabling risk, care can be transformed. One way in which this has been addressed is through the setting up of 'risk enablement panels'. The emphasis for the panel is on supporting **positive risk taking** while maintaining duty of care.

KEY TERM

Positive risk taking: Identifying the potential risks and then developing plans and actions that reflect the potential benefits and harm of exercising one course of action over another. It is a way of seeing the risk in a positive way that enhances the quality of life for an individual.

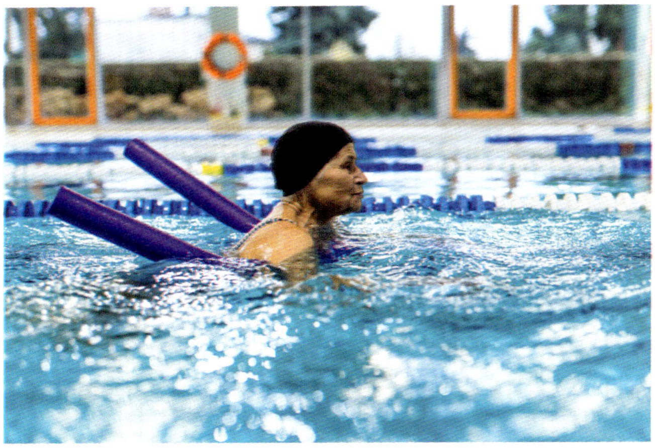

Figure 15 It is important to assess the environment for risks to individuals

Positive risk taking

Think about the risks you take on a daily basis. Did you pull out into a busy road in the path of an oncoming car? Perhaps you had to run to catch the bus and didn't look carefully at the road? Maybe you stood on a chair in order to retrieve something from a high cupboard?

Your attitude to risk is likely to be different when it comes to your work as a care professional. In this role, you are bound by law and have a duty of care to the individuals using your service and this is likely to affect your attitude to risk management. You may be more careful when dealing with individuals and take the view that as 'vulnerable adults' they need to be protected in some way. But is this a fair assessment of the people you care for or merely a stereotypical view? Titterton (2005) takes the view that care workers tend to focus on what individuals cannot do and therefore take what he calls a 'safety first approach' to risk.

This type of approach focuses on the person's physical problems and disability and tends to ignore other needs. This leads to loss of self-esteem and denies the right to choose and to an increase in independence. There is a danger that the care worker becomes more controlling of the individual and person-centred approaches become less of a reality.

Risk in this instance is thought of in terms of danger, loss, threat, damage or injury and the positive benefits of risk taking are lost. Therefore, a more balanced approach needs to be adopted.

SCIE offers a quick guide to help social care workers to understand how to gather evidence to identify and assess risks normally gathered through observation. It offers a risk assessment tool and suggests a four-stage process to discuss risks with people with dementia and their families. These stages are adaptable for other groups of people coming into contact with social care:

1. Identify risks in the life-context of the individual and their circumstances which impact quality of life.
2. Identify risk perspectives from all people involved.
3. Identify weighting of risks whether high or low together with the impact on emotional, social and psychological wellbeing.
4. Identify current and past strategies for managing risks.

Source: SCIE (2023)

An intelligent option is that proposed by Titterton (2010) in his positive risk approach. In this approach, risk is seen as positive and enhancing, and recognises the needs of individuals. It demonstrates that choice and autonomy are important and promotes the rights of vulnerable people. Steve Morgan (2004) summarises the approach:

> *Positive risk-taking is: weighing up the potential benefits and harms of exercising one choice of action over another. Identifying the potential risks involved, and developing plans and actions that reflect the positive potentials and stated priorities of the service user. It involves using available resources and support to achieve the desired outcomes, and to minimise the potential harmful outcomes. It is not negligent ignorance of the potential risks … it is usually a very carefully thought-out strategy for managing a specific situation or set of circumstances.*

If you are to provide real choice and control for the individuals using your service you need to enable them to take the risks they choose, with support from staff. This means that they can define their own risks and then plan and monitor any activity they wish to undertake that may entail some form of risk.

Evidence opportunity

1.5 Risk taking

Explain your role in assessing the risk of individuals where mental capacity is of concern.

AC 1.6 Describe ways of working which support individuals' ability to provide valid consent

Here, you will be required to describe the importance of obtaining consent from the individual.

Practitioners can support an individual's ability to make decisions and provide valid consent by:

- tailoring the information provided to the individual's specific needs
- accounting for any reasonable adjustments
- making information accessible and using communication, visual or hearing aids if needed

- involving advocacy services to support decision making
- referring to other services, such as a speech and language therapist, if specialist support is required
- choosing the best time to approach the individual to present the questions, e.g. are they better able to deal with things in the morning or evening?
- choosing a time when the individual isn't feeling anxious or distressed
- allowing enough time for the individual to make decisions and communicate.

Evidence opportunity

1.6 Consent policy

What is your policy on how you gain consent? Provide evidence.

AC 1.7 Evaluate development needs relating to mental capacity for self and team members

Here, you will evaluate your own and your team members' development needs in assessing mental capacity.

You and your team are responsible for providing health or social care interventions and these must adhere to the requirements of the Mental Capacity Act 2005 and the Code of Practice.

Where possible, individuals who lack capacity should be involved in the decision-making process, with family, carers and Independent Mental Capacity Advocates (IMCAs) being involved to establish their known wishes, preferences and values. In cases where there are complex needs or issues, a meeting should be arranged to identify appropriate responses to any disputes and to action plan next steps.

In order to make a best interests decision, a best interests assessor will be helpful. Best interests assessors are trained to assess capacity and are responsible for making an 'age assessment,' to ensure that the person is 18 or over and a 'no refusals' assessment, which assesses whether there are any lawful decision makers who object to what is proposed. If the best interests assessor also has training in Approved Mental Health, they are able to carry out the eligibility assessment, which decides whether the person's rights should be protected by the use of the MHA or the MCA, via the safeguards (SCIE, 2017).

You and the team will conduct a capacity assessment, and this will record that a person lacks capacity to make the decision. You also need to ensure that everyone involved in the best interests decision-making process knows and agrees who the decision maker is.

The National Institute For Health And Care Excellence (NICE) Guideline NG108 Decision making and mental capacity (2018) includes recommendations on best interest decisions and best interest decision maker responsibilities, and as a manager you should have knowledge of the requirements you and your team need to follow.

The NICE guidelines also focus on key areas such as advance care/support planning, supporting decision making, assessment of mental capacity to make specific decisions and best interests decision making for individuals who are assessed as lacking capacity. It shows it is important to ensure that individuals' input to decision making is paramount.

Evidence opportunity

1.7 Evaluate development needs relating to mental capacity for self and team members

Determine what training might be useful for staff or yourself with respect to the best interest assessor role.

LO2 Understand the use and impact of restrictive practices in adult care

AC 2.1 Explain what is meant by restrictive practice, restraint and deprivation of liberty

Here, you will explain the circumstances in which restrictive practice may be used in a setting.

Restrictive practice, restraint and hidden restraint

Restrictive practice is defined as any practice which restricts a person's right to choose, or restricts their privacy or freedom. An example would be sectioning under the Mental Health Act or locking doors to prevent people from leaving a building. Skills for Care identifies the use of restrictive practice as something that must be used only to prevent serious harm and must be ethically and legally justified.

Restrictive practice or any form of restraint of an individual must always be carried out with dignity and respect. You can find guidance in the Skills for Care documents on restrictive practice and restraint (www.scie.org.uk). Its definition of such practice is: 'Making someone do something they don't want to do or stopping doing something they want to do' (Skills for Care and Skills for Health, 2014) and it defines restrictive interventions as 'deliberate acts on the part of other person(s) that restrict an individual's movement, liberty and/or freedom to act independently' (Department of Health, 2014).

The publication of *A positive and proactive workforce: A guide to workforce development for commissioners and employers seeking to minimise the use of restrictive practices in social care and health* (Skills for Care and Skills for Health, 2014) advocated the use of a framework designed to 'radically transform culture, leadership and professional practice to deliver care and support which keeps people safe, and promotes recovery' and to ensure that restrictive practice was being used safely and not being misused, as seen in such cases as the incidents at Winterbourne View Hospital.

New approaches, then, are to reduce the use of restrictive practice where possible. The Mental Capacity Act 2005 states that anybody who uses or threatens to use force to make someone do something they are resisting is using restraint measures.

You can restrain people in a number of ways, such as through the use of medication, or through the use of keypad systems so they are unable to leave premises. You might also see physical restraint being used, but staff must be trained and aware of what they are able to use.

Restraint refers to anything that stops an individual doing what they appear to want to do. It is important to ensure that staff understand what restraint is, when it is right to use some of the physical methods and when it would be counterproductive. Some forms of restraint are:

- restricted escort, where an individual is moved from one area of a unit to another
- standing restraint, where the individual is restrained in a standing position
- seated restraint, where the individual is held in a seated position
- supine restraint, where the individual is held on their back.

SCIE (2009a) offers e-learning on 'Managing risk, minimising restraint', which explores restraint, the decision-making process and creating a positive culture.

You may also restrain somebody unintentionally, such as leaving an individual without means to mobilise and this might be termed hidden restraint. Hidden restraints are those activities that restrain somebody without actually seeming to do so. For example, putting an older adult into a chair that is low to the ground may make it more difficult for them to mobilise since they are unable to get up from the chair. While not physically restraining the individual, you are still preventing them from moving freely.

In some circumstances restraint is the right thing to do but it should always be consensual, part of a care package and used only if the individual lacks capacity and is unsafe.

Evidence opportunity

2.1 Explain what is meant by restrictive practice, restraint and deprivation of liberty

What is your understanding of restrictive practice, restraint and deprivation of liberty? Explain to your assessor what you use in your setting.

Deprivation of liberty

It is important to understand what restraint means and to enable staff to recognise the situations in which it would be safe to use. MCA 2005 and its Code of Practice introduced Deprivation of Liberty Safeguards. These are due to be replaced by Liberty Protection Safeguards (LPS) – for more information see AC1.1 and below.

AC 2.2 Describe own responsibilities in relation to restrictive practices and deprivations of liberty

Here, you will be required to describe the managerial role in decisions about restrictive practices and deprivation of liberty.

Under the Mental Capacity (Amendment) Act 2019, Deprivation of Liberty Safeguards (DoLS) were due to be replaced in April 2022 by Liberty Protection Safeguards (LPS). The amendment Bill to the MCA in July 2018 introduced Liberty Protection Safeguards (LPS), which will provide a streamlined process for authorising deprivations of liberty. However, at the time of writing (May 2023) the introduction of LPS has been delayed so the DoLS authorisations and process continue.

LPS are designed to protect the rights of individuals receiving care in a hospital, care home or other provision, who may become deprived of their liberty, due to lack of mental capacity to consent. This might happen if the person is unable to understand and retain information in relation to a decision when it needs to be made. It is then that a 'best interests' decision needs to be made to protect the individual from harm.

In this situation, you as the manager must currently apply for a DoLS authorisation from a 'supervisory body' or the local authority. You have responsibility for applying the safeguards and must therefore follow the Deprivation of Liberty Safeguards Code of Practice ('the Code'), which supplements the Mental Capacity Act 2005 Code of Practice.

In December 2021, the Department of Health and Social Care published the Mental Health Units (Use of Force) Act 2018 to ensure better accountability and transparency over the use of force in mental health units. The use of force can sometimes have serious consequences, as evidenced by the case of Olaseni (Seni) Lewis, who died as a result of being forcibly restrained in a mental health unit in 2010. This law is also known as Seni's Law and sets out clear guidance to ensure that NHS trusts comply with the law and that individuals in mental health settings are protected from inappropriate use of force.

However, restraint is used in some care settings as an acceptable form of positive behaviour support. The Challenging Behaviour organisation provides a practical guide (The Challenging Behaviour Foundation, n.d.) to help carers to reduce challenging behaviour, explaining what positive behaviour support is and what a positive behaviour support plan is.

Although your setting may not be one in which mental health is necessarily an issue, it is useful to know how these new guidelines might be adapted for your own area.

Reflect on it

2.2 Roles and responsibility in restraint use

What is your role and responsibility in ensuring that staff understand what is and is not allowed in the use of restraint?

AC 2.3 Explain how the use of the following practices are managed in own work setting for restrictive practices, restraint and deprivation of liberty

Here, you will be required to explain the use of restrictive practices in your setting.

Evidence opportunity

2.2 and 2.3 Maintain safe practice during restrictive practices, restraint and DoLS/LPS

Write a short report showing how you:

- ✔ monitor and maintain safe practice during restrictive practices, restraint and deprivation of liberty
- ✔ communicate your policy for restrictive practice in your setting.

Consider also coercion, seclusion, close supervision, limiting access and mechanical restraint. How do these practices impact your role?

Reflect on it

2.2 and 2.3 DoLS and LPS

How does your setting manage DoLS and the new LPS guidance?

AC 2.4 Analyse the current legal and ethical considerations of restricting an individual's rights and freedoms

Here, you will be required to analyse your understanding and application of the legal requirements and implications relating to restrictive practice in adult care services and be aware of recent case law and codes of practice, including the ones discussed in this section.

The 'Human rights framework for restraint: principles for the lawful use of physical, chemical, mechanical and coercive restrictive interventions' was published in 2019 by the Equality and Human Rights Commission and reflects the requirements of the Human Rights Act 1998.

It was produced to support work on tackling the unlawful use of restraint in education, care and detention settings and is informed by discussion with regulators, inspectorates and ombudspersons.

It sets out the key principles of the European Convention on Human Rights (ECHR) and provides examples from a range of settings to illustrate the principles.

The framework is intended to be used for building consensus and consistency on the use of restraint and for developing more comprehensive sector-specific guidance and training on restraint.

Additionally, in October 2009 SCIE published its guidance, 'At a glance 16: Managing risk, minimising restraint' (updated April 2021), which examines the use of restraint in care homes and other provisions. The key messages identified the different actions which constitute restraint and how to minimise their use. It also describes a five-step framework to help with making informed decisions in situations where the use of restraint might be appropriate:

Step 1: Observe

Step 2: Do some detective work

Step 3: Consider options and make a decision

Step 4: Implement the plan

Step 5: Monitor and review the plan.

Source: Adapted from SCIE (2009b)

Concern for safety is a common reason for the use of restraint in settings as well as a response to agitation. Making good risk assessments and planning the care needed will mean staff are more able to support residents and this will help to reduce the use of restraint.

By helping staff to understand what restraint means and supporting them to recognise its correct use in certain situations and how it might be wrong in other situations, you can then consider what will help to improve practice and staff development. You should investigate the types of training that is available and possibly arrange for specialist training. This will mean that staff can support one another and share their learning. It is also good practice to involve the individuals using the service in discussions about how they feel about a particular practice being used for their safety. Do they feel restrained in any way?

They may also wish to consider how they feel if restricted in public areas so there is a dignity and privacy issue to consider here too. There is also an ethical issue to be aware of as when we restrain somebody we risk increasing their vulnerability to neglect and harm, and this can have psychological consequences. If we value respect for individuals and the principle of do no harm, there may be conflict when physical restraints are used.

Stretch and challenge

2.4 Restricting freedoms

Do you ever have to restrain or limit your sevice users in any way? Consider how this is managed.

Access the SCIE's 'At a glance 16: Managing risk, minimising restraint' (SCIE, 2009b) and write short notes on the definition of restraint and what type of actions might constitute restraint. Also consider the five-step framework and how your own setting may need to adapt this.

AC 2.5 Evaluate appropriate and proportionate responses to restrictions on an individual's rights and freedoms

Here, you will evaluate your response to whether restrictive practices are proportionate.

Reflect on it

2.5 Case study

Read the case study and provide a reflective account.

Case study

Adam is living with dementia in a care setting. He is 72 years old and a former deputy head teacher of a local secondary school. He often wakes early in the morning, and is agitated that if he doesn't leave soon, he will be late for the staff briefing.

Staff in the care home are aware that Adam cannot just leave as he may be a safety risk to himself. It is therefore appropriate to restrict or divert him lawfully.

How can the staff restrict or divert Adam appropriately and proportionately? First the staff need to recognise that restraint may be needed but diversion will be the first step. The MCA describes restraint as 'the use of force to make someone do something that they are resisting, or restricting freedom of movement, whether they are resisting or not.'

People lacking mental capacity to make the decision to go out may be restrained by locked doors and it is important to recognise that this restraint is not always an incorrect one. In Adam's case, this type of restraint is being used completely in his best interests. However, having dementia and wanting to leave the building is not grounds for restricting freedom of movement, so other ways of diverting Adam's attention and encouraging a different type of activity will be better.

As a care manager, you will want all of the people using your service to live as they choose so you should always seek out the 'least restrictive option'. The MCA explains that there are two extra conditions that must be met for restraint to be lawful. These are:

- The person taking action must believe that restraint is necessary to prevent harm.
- The amount or type of restraint used, and the amount of time it lasts, must be a proportionate response to the likelihood and seriousness of that harm.

For Adam, an assessment of his capacity to decide to 'go out for the staff briefing' must be made. He has dementia, so staff know that he meets the first part of the test for capacity. They now need to check that he understands his decision and can communicate his decision.

If, during discussions, Adam is still insistent that he is the deputy head, this delusion means he cannot understand and therefore lacks capacity for this decision so staff must make a decision in his best interests.

Relatives and friends may have been consulted about what they felt would be the best action to take in this instance. However, taking Adam out for a walk might be helpful as he may forget that he wished to attend a staff briefing. Alternatively, he might be distracted, and so another activity can be offered to calm him.

AC 2.6 Describe the potential impacts of restrictive practices on individuals and others

Here, you will be required to describe the potential impact and outcomes of applying restrictive practices, and cover the topics discussed in this section.

Impact of restrictive practice on those in receipt of care and support services

A restrictive practice is designed to keep individuals safe, but it may make them feel trapped or without choice. Sometimes when individuals become distressed or confused they may lack understanding of their situation and may need restrictive interventions to keep them or other people around them safe. The impact of this may be disturbing to them or to their loved ones, but a carefully planned restriction can be explained and carried out in a compassionate and caring manner.

The need to restrict the person must be fully explained where possible and justified as being necessary to prevent harm to the person. Your staff must show empathy and compassion during such procedures. The safety of the individual and the protection of their dignity should be watch words for staff undertaking restraint.

Impact of restrictive practice on all staff

For staff, the decision to use restrictive practices will involve assessing whether the person has the mental capacity to make a specific decision and they must be sure that what they are proposing to do is necessary to prevent harm and not merely for staff convenience. While restricting the liberty of a person may go against the person-centred ethos for some staff and will be a difficult choice to make, they must be reassured that any restrictive practice is legal and ethical. Staff must be supported to undertake restrictions in an ethical and legal way.

Impact of restrictive practice on others such as families, carers

For families and carers, to see a loved one being restrained can be a very distressing event, so they need to be clear about what is happening and how the practice will be of help. If the use of restrictive practices can be planned in advance and involve the individual and their family, this will reduce the stress. For example, a person with increasing dementia may require safety in the near future and may need to be restricted in their movements. A discussion about what will happen to ensure safety in the future will be positive and useful.

> **Evidence opportunity**
>
> **2.6 Impact of restrictive practice on individuals**
>
> Describe how you might use restrictive practices with the individuals using your service and what effects this might have on:
>
> - ✔ safety
> - ✔ dignity
> - ✔ relationships
> - ✔ wellbeing of individuals.

Impact if restrictive practice is used incorrectly

People must be treated with compassion, kindness and dignity so any restrictive practice that falls short of this is unethical and legally wrong. The impact upon the individual, their family and staff in the setting is likely to be damaging and might be seen as abusive and neglectful.

> **Evidence opportunity**
>
> **2.6 Impacts of restrictive practice**
>
> Explain the potential impact and outcomes of applying restrictive practice for those in receipt of care and support services, for all staff, and for others such as families and carers.

AC 2.7 Explain how person-centred, outcomes-based practices can mitigate the use of restrictive practices

Here, you will be required to explain how person-centred practice can help to minimise the use of restrictive practices, including the areas discussed in this section.

By creating a positive person-centred environment, you can minimise the need for restrictive practice and the use of restraint. Person-centred care requires that the rights of the individuals you care for are paramount, the individual's needs and wishes are at the centre of the care you offer and that as a care worker you respect them and nurture them. The behaviour of the individuals using your service is a form of communication and can change and be influenced by medication, how they may be feeling, the people they are with or even the environment in the setting. While you aim to develop care/support plans that offer choice and control, sometimes it may not be possible for an individual to make a decision. It is then that a 'best interests' decision should be made and restraint may be required in the interest of safety.

The reason for the use of restraint is the risk to an individual's safety and that of others. By ensuring that the environment is supportive and offers activity and variety, such risks are minimised. For example, if the physical space within a care setting is pleasant to be in, with colourful decoration and good seating areas, offering some outside space and a variety of activities for the enjoyment of the residents, this will instill a sense of wellbeing and will reduce the need for restraint.

In the community, and when working in people's homes, we need to respect the choices and preferences of individuals. Applying the main principles of empowerment is a positive way of enabling individuals to make shared decisions about how they wish to live their life at home, ensuring that they have a choice in all aspects of their care and support.

Comply with legislative and organisational requirements at all times

Restrictive practices are still evident and necessary in care work. Restricted access to food, knives and other potential weapons is common and acceptable to keep staff and individuals safe. Your risk assessments and policies need to be up to date and clear, covering all aspects of the practices for your staff. There are legal guidelines that apply, and your own setting policy will give details of your practice guidelines. If, for example, your setting opts for no restrictive practice then to implement restraint would be against policy and may result in sanctions being taken against you.

Demonstrate/role model how an individual's behaviour is understood and valued

In your use of restrictive practice you need to ensure that you are a good role model and that you have the best interests of the individuals using your service at the forefront of the care given.

A role model is someone whose behaviour is seen by other people as a good example. In modelling good behaviour, high standards are set and passed on to others to guide their behaviour.

The National Autistic Society believes that support should always be guided by each individual and their strengths, challenges and interests. Positive Behaviour Support (PBS) is a person-centred approach that identifies and meets a person's support needs, and focusses on the challenging behaviour that some people who are distressed and at risk of harming themselves or others may exhibit.

The framework is most commonly used to support practitioners in delivering good quality support to people with learning disabilities, some of whom may also be autistic. Support must be person-centred and promote autistic people's dignity, enabling them to do the things they love doing and keeping them healthy and happy.

By working with individuals and learning why they sometimes experience distress, staff can provide tailored support. For example, knowing that a specific environment impacts a person's happiness means that the practitioner can adapt their support accordingly.

Demonstrate/role model how to value an individual's unique needs, aspirations and strength to enhance their quality of life

'Unique needs' refer to needs that are different from everybody else's. Each person we meet in our daily lives has their own identity, beliefs and values that enhance the quality of their lives and care professionals need to respect and value this. When it comes to providing support for the individuals using your service, a 'one size fits all' approach to care shows a disrespect for others' needs and aspirations and this is the same in determining if restrictive practices are required. A situational approach needs to be taken.

Demonstrate/role model how to effectively involve and enable active participation of individuals, their families, carers and advocates

Person-centred values are the principles that put the interests of individuals at the centre of their own care journey. By actively engaging people in a partnership where choice and participation in their care are encouraged, you can ensure that staff and those cared for retain their individuality and dignity.

Demonstrate/role model how to treat individuals with compassion, dignity and kindness

Care professionals have a responsibility to provide care that is respectful and compassionate. This is more than just providing care with a successful outcome or performing a procedure to a high standard. While people will be grateful for the skill of the care worker, they gain much more when the care worker has treated them with compassion. You should never forget the significance of events for the individuals using your service, which for care workers are just a daily routine. You need to consider ways in which you can show your respect for the people you care for by offering them kindness and dignity in the care you give.

Demonstrate/role model how to support and protect positive relationships between the people who deliver services and the individuals they support

Positive relationships are built by accepting that everybody is different and celebrating those differences. Work relationships are important to finding job satisfaction. Developing positive work relationships requires a willingness to listen to others and to communicate openly. You must show respect and offer support to those who may require it.

Evidence opportunity

2.7 Explain ways of minimising restrictive practices through person-centred practice

Explain to your assessor how person-centred practice can help to minimise the use of restrictive practices, including the areas discussed in this section.

Reflect on it

2.7 Minimising restrictive practices through person-centred practice

Take a critical look at your environment and ask yourself, would I be happy to live here?

What might you change to ensure that the space is a good one?

Make notes on how the use of person-centred practice can help to minimise the use of restrictive practice.

AC 2.8 Evaluate development needs relating to the use of restrictive practices for self and team members

Appropriate training in restrictive practices was discussed earlier in AC2.4. Ensuring that the physical space within a care setting is a positive one can help to promote wellbeing and may even limit the situations that result in the use of restraint. For example, individuals should ideally have a good view of outside space and the opportunity to use it. An inviting interior décor with good lighting and a colour scheme that is calming with comfortable chairs will help them to feel valued. For people with learning disabilities, the creation of a cool-down room for use when an individual is feeling agitated gives a safe space in which to de-escalate the situation. The Autism Society suggests minimal furnishings with soft objects in the room and windows covered with plexiglass. The use of sensory objects, relaxing music and calming items should be available. Clear signs and activities in the living area can help to make the space inviting and calming. Additionally, a calm, comfortable setting may also prevent individuals from wanting to leave the setting, further minimising such risk.

Many staff working in the community will need development and training for new roles that cover both health and adult social care as integrated care models are introduced. Key training in positive behaviour support to deal with behaviour that challenges should be offered to staff working in the community.

As a manager you should spend some time looking around your setting to get a feel for how the environment is used and to check in with staff to understand some of the challenges they have. In this way you can build up a picture of what staff need to support them and what training might be useful.

Legislation

Legislation	Key points
Mental Capacity Act 2005	This act informs individuals about what they can do to plan and ensure that someone else can make decisions for them if they ever lack capacity to do so for themselves.
Mental Capacity Act (Amendment) Act 2019	Amends the MCA 2005 in relation to procedures where a person may be deprived of liberty because they lack the capacity to consent.
Mental Health Units (Use of Force) Act 2018	Sets out measures to prevent the inappropriate use of force and to ensure accountability and transparency in regard to the use of force in mental health units.

References

Commission for Social Care Inspection (2007) *Rights, Risks and Restraints: An exploration into the use of restraint in the care of older people*. London: CSCI.

Department for Constitutional Affairs (2007) *Mental Capacity Act 2005: Code of Practice*. London: TSO.

Department of Health (2007) *Independence, Choice and Risk: A guide to best practice in supported decision making*. London: HMSO.

Department of Health (2014) 'Positive and proactive care: Reducing the need for restrictive interventions'. https://assets.publishing.service.gov.uk/government/uploads/system/uploads/attachment_data/file/300291/JRA_DoH_Guidance_on_RH_Summary_web_accessible.pdf

GOV.UK (2022a) 'Changes to the MCA Code of Practice and implementation of the LPS: Consultation document'. www.gov.uk/government/consultations/changes-to-the-mca-code-of-practice-and-implementation-of-the-lps/changes-to-the-mca-code-of-practice-and-implementation-of-the-lps-consultation-document

Morgan, S. (2004) 'Positive risk-taking: An idea whose time has come', *Health Care Risk Report*, 10(10): 18–19.

Skills for Care and Skills for Health (2014) 'A positive and proactive workforce: A guide to workforce development for commissioners and employers seeking to minimise the use of restrictive practices in social care and health'. www.skillsforcare.org.uk/resources/documents/Developing-your-workforce/Care-topics/Behaviours-which-challenge/A-positive-and-proactive-workforce.pdf

Social Care Institute for Excellence (2017) 'Deprivation of liberty safeguards (DoLS)'. www.scie.org.uk/mca/dols/practice/assessments/best-interests#:~:text=Best%20interests%20assessors%20are%20often,of%20the%20best%20interests%20assessment

Social Care Institute for Excellence (2022) 'Care Act: Assessment and eligibility'. www.scie.org.uk/care-act-2014/assessment-and-eligibility/

Social Care Institute for Excellence (2023) 'Risk assessment process and key points to risk identification in virtual interactions'. www.scie.org.uk/care-providers/coronavirus-covid-19/social-workers/risk-identification

Titterton, M. (2005) *Risk and Risk Taking in Health and Social Care*. London: Jessica Kingsley Publishers.

Titterton, M. (2010) *Positive Risk Taking*. Edinburgh: Hale.

Useful resources and further reading

Challenging Behaviour Foundation, The (n.d.) 'Information sheet: Positive behaviour support planning: Part 3'. www.challengingbehaviour.org.uk/wp-content/uploads/2021/02/003-Positive-Behaviour-Support-Planning-Part-3.pdf

GOV.UK (2022b) 'Changes to the MCA Code of Practice and implementation of the LPS'. www.gov.uk/government/consultations/changes-to-the-mca-code-of-practice-and-implementation-of-the-lps/changes-to-the-mca-code-of-practice-and-implementation-of-the-lps-consultation-document

GOV.UK (2022c) 'Mental Capacity Act 2005 Code of Practice: Including the Liberty Protection Safeguards 2022'. https://assets.publishing.service.gov.uk/government/uploads/system/uploads/attachment_data/file/1080137/draft-mental-capacity-act-code-of-practice.pdf

GOV.UK (n.d.) 'Make decisions on behalf of someone'. www.gov.uk/make-decisions-for-someone/assessing-mental-capacity

Owen, T. and Meyer, J. (2009) *Minimising the Use of Restraint in Care Homes: Challenges, dilemmas and positive approaches*. London: SCIE.

Social Care Institute for Excellence (2009a) 'Managing risk, minimising restraint e-learning course: Challenges, dilemmas and positive approaches for working with older people in care homes'. www.scie.org.uk/e-learning/managing-risk-minimising-restraint

Social Care Institute for Excellence (2009b) 'At a glance 16: Managing risk, minimising restraint'. www.scie.org.uk/publications/ataglance/ataglance16.asp

Social Care Institute for Excellence (n.d.) 'Assessing capacity'. www.scie.org.uk/mca/practice/assessing-capacity

Unit 509

Leading and managing partnerships in adult care

GLH 35

About this unit

Working in partnership defines a joint working arrangement where partners from different services all aim to achieve a common goal for the individuals in a care setting, despite being independent bodies. In the setting, and in your leadership role, this means sharing relevant information and creating a culture of shared ownership and common working arrangements across organisational and professional boundaries.

One of the aims of government in recent years has been to ensure that care services work together to provide care that is integrated and personalised. This requires services from a variety of settings to work as partners to ensure that individuals receive the best possible care. It also means that building good relationships between the services is imperative.

Joint health and care managed networks have been put forward as best practice for ensuring that individuals with complex health needs benefit from services that share information and work towards common goals. In this unit, you will look at how you can promote effective partnership working by establishing good working relationships with all of the care services you deal with, as well as with your colleagues, the families of the individuals you care for, advocates and the individuals themselves. You will cover the ways in which legislation and regulation influence your working partnerships and how the relationships you have with stakeholders underpin person-centred practice and the achievement of positive outcomes.

Learning outcomes

By the end of this unit, you will:

- Understand the context of relationships and partnership working in adult care.
- Be able to lead effective relationships with individuals, carers and families.
- Be able to manage working relationships with colleagues in own setting to achieve positive outcomes for individuals.
- Be able to work in partnerships with professionals and other agencies.

Getting started

Before you study the unit, think about the following:

- How many different agencies/individuals does your teamwork with on a daily basis? For example, dental services, physiotherapy or support groups such as Age UK.
- What percentage of these interactions do you think are positive?
- What, in your view, are the roles and responsibilities of managers in developing good working relationships?
- How do you think innovative procedures can be developed to engage colleagues and promote effective partnership working? Innovative procedures might include new and improved ways of working.

LO1 Understand the context of relationships and partnership working in adult care

AC 1.1 Outline the range of partnerships within adult care

Here, you will be required to outline the range of organisations with which partnerships may be necessary in a setting.

Separate organisations from a variety of multidisciplinary teams bring with them expertise and resources and so partnership working is a powerful way to enhance the quality of service provision.

Integrated care partnerships bring together the care providers and health organisations in a given area to work as one. Care providers working with local councils, education, planning, housing, environmental health and leisure services can help to reduce health inequalities and improve life expectancy. For example, partnerships can design and deliver services to meet the needs of the local population's needs and are able to focus services on areas of greatest need.

> **Evidence opportunity**
>
> **1.1 Partnership working**
>
> Outline the partners and organisations your own setting works with.

AC 1.2 Explain the complexity of different relationships within partnership-working

Here, you will explain the different types of partnerships that may be necessary with the organisations identified in the previous section.

Formal and informal partnerships

An informal partnership occurs when your setting works with another based on a verbal or written agreement but not a formally drawn-up partnership agreement. This might be a partnership with a local hairdresser who provides a service for the individuals in your care. Although such arrangements are often mutually beneficial, informal arrangements can experience difficulties when conflict occurs and partners have differing opinions about what is and isn't agreed.

A formal partnership has an agreement in place clearly showing management and operational plans and how the partners will work together. The aim is to combine different resources and expertise to achieve the shared goals for the setting. You might decide to set up an agreement to enable your own setting and another nearby to share some resources such as a minibus or other equipment. A formal agreement would be drawn up. This is similar to an integrated care partnership where services or equipment are brought together.

Integrated and multidisciplinary teams

Integrated partnership working describes the support of an individual from a number of different partners, with the individual at the centre of the process. Everyone involved in supporting the individual works together in an effective way to meet their needs and improve their quality of life.

A multidisciplinary team is one where organisations share resources to deliver work jointly. A partnership agreement describes the working relationship. In all partnerships there should be common goals, similar belief systems and respect and trust.

Organisation relationships refer to the relationships and connection between the various stakeholders in any partnership network. Like partnerships, agreed goals and systems are built into the ways of working.

> **Evidence opportunity**
>
> **1.2 Partnerships and organisation relationships**
>
> Using the list above, explain the different partnerships and organisation relationships you are aware of. Explain to your assessor about how the needs of each relationship must be considered, particularly with respect to their different priorities and systems.

AC 1.3 Explain how legislation and regulation influence working relationships with others

Here, you will be required to explain national, local and your own organisation's guidelines, legislations and policies that relate to partnership working.

The idea of partnership working developed as a result of acknowledging that it was impossible for one care provider to provide all of the care needed for an individual. Partnership working therefore describes the relationships between services that have a responsibility for supplying a variety of care services. In order to work as partners, services need to create new organisational structures or processes that are separate from their own organisation and in which they plan and implement a jointly agreed programme, sometimes with joint staff or resources.

To work effectively as a partnership there are certain features that need to be in place:

- joint agreement that the individual is the central figure in the process and must be empowered throughout the process
- good communication
- strong leadership
- adequate resources
- trust between partners
- shared policies and guidelines.

There are numerous national, local and organisational guidelines, legislation and policies that relate to partnership working. As a manager, you must be aware of these and how they may influence your relationship with others.

For more details about current UK legislation and statutory frameworks, see Unit 501, AC1.1.

Working in partnership – the Health and Social Care Act 2012 and reforms to adult social care

The Health and Social Care Act 2012 brought new structures and working arrangements for the NHS in England. Primary care trusts (PCTs) and strategic health authorities (SHAs) were dispensed with and new bodies such as NHS England (previously known as the NHS Commissioning Board) and Clinical Commissioning Groups (CCGs) were brought in with responsibility for commissioning NHS services. Local authorities took on the task of new public health commissioning. These have now been replaced with integrated care systems (ICSs), which are partnerships of organisations who plan and deliver joined up care services. The Health and Care Act 2022 recommended that 42 ICSs were established across England on a statutory basis from 1 July 2022.

Additionally, adult social care was also subject to reforms. Reforms to adult social care were rolled out in September 2021, when the government set aside £5.4 billion to fund the reforms between 2022/23 and 2024/25. £3.6 billion was to be used to reform how people pay for social care (charging reforms) and this included £1.4 billion to help local authorities move towards paying a 'fair cost of care' to providers. £1.7 billion would be used to support wider system reform.

The changes in social care were one aspect of a wider government drive to reform across all public service and reflected three key beliefs:

- that everyone has a contribution to make
- that everyone has the right to control their own lives
- that people using public services should be able to influence and change them to ensure that their needs are met.

The 'Putting People First' paper published in 2007 set out a detailed action plan for implementing the personalisation agenda at a local level and formally introduced the idea of a personalised adult social care system in which individuals would have maximum choice and control over the services they receive.

Working in partnership with other professionals has significantly changed the experience of individuals, putting them firmly at the centre of the care given, with greater access to shared resources, improved communication between teams and a more streamlined care service.

The influence of the changes in the law and the more structured inclusion of VCSE organisations means that more effective relationships have been forged between statutory and voluntary services, private providers and charities. This has resulted in better outcomes for individuals who have complex needs. Access to specialist expertise in the community and a focus on early action enable preventative services to contribute to improving health outcomes and takes pressure off secondary care services. Complex needs are being met in the community in which the individual lives, helping to prevent unnecessary hospital admissions. This ultimately provides a cost-effective way in which to treat people and relieves pressure on much-stretched services in the statutory sector.

Examples of statutory services working in partnership with adult social care include the NHS and local government, while voluntary services include charities such as the Red Cross, Age UK or faith-based organisations that provide support. Private providers such as nursing or residential care homes are also included here, and charities often provide care homes and hospice care. For example, the charity Marie Curie has numerous hospices throughout the UK.

Examples of guidelines, legislation and policies relating to partnership working

Partnership working has improved the quality of the service offered and has proved to be more cost effective. In 2020 (updated 2022) the CQC published a report on 'Promoting partnership working to drive experiences and outcomes for people' (CQC, 2022). This focused on how providers are responding to existing challenges and how they work together across different pathways and services. The report highlights how lack of collaboration between local services is a barrier to people getting good care. It also describes the importance of a shared and agreed local vision and shared governance arrangements together with joint approaches to ensure that there are enough staff with the right skills to meet the needs of all people locally.

By recognising common goals, a 'whole person' approach to care can be taken; there has been a growth in the understanding of other care professionals' roles and mutual respect is therefore built. The personalisation agenda has put individuals firmly in charge of ensuring that the care and support they require has been designed with their involvement to meet their unique needs.

'Expected ways of working between integrated care providers and adult social care providers' was published in 2022 and sets out a series of advisory principles for integrated care partnerships (ICPs) and adult social care (ASC) providers to help them work together. This guidance, developed by the Department of Health and Social Care (DHSC), Local Government Association (LGA) and NHS England (NHSE), in partnership with the Care Provider Alliance, recognises that ASC providers are critical partners in the health and care system with over 1.5 million people working in the sector. Most of these workers are employed by small and medium-sized independent providers including voluntary and community providers, and along with commissioners and people with lived experiences of care or unpaid carers among others, have valuable contributions to make to service planning across England.

Research it

1.3 Working with people and communities

Go to Department of Health and Social Care (2022) and review the principles of partnership, inclusion, subsidiarity and knowledge sharing. Explain how this will improve partnership working within your setting.

Case study

1.3 Working in partnership

Skills for Care have published a guidance document showing 'Practical approaches to working in partnership' (Skills for Care, n.d.). Read this and explain how your service and people could benefit from different partnerships.

Evidence opportunity

1.3 How legislation and regulation influences relationships with others

Think about how legislation and regulation influence relationships with others. Explain how national, local and your own organisation's guidelines, legislation and policies relate to partnership working. Which legislation are you required to follow and which is advised? You might like to consider how these have enabled partnership working and affected care outcomes overall. How do you manage these partnerships?

AC 1.4 Explain how relationships with individuals, families and carers underpin person-centred practice and affect the achievement of positive outcomes

Here, you will be required to explain the association between person-centred care and positive outcomes with the ability to engage in partnership working. This should include effects on a range of stakeholders relevant to own area of provision.

The importance of partnership working with the individuals using the service, colleagues, other professionals, families, carers and advocates should not be underestimated.

Individuals receiving care

For the individuals receiving care, partnership working has meant a more 'joined up' approach to their care. For example, having a single assessment process instead of multiple assessments by different agencies has been well received by individuals and extends their choice. The Single Assessment Process is a way in which social care organisations work together to assess and plan care for people in need of a care service. This care must be person-centred, effective and co-ordinated.

Individuals using a service are ultimately customers, and they are at the centre of designing and delivering social care. The Department of Health and Social Care has actively promoted the involvement of individuals and the public in decisions about the planning, design, development and delivery of local services, and individuals see themselves as having a particular role to play, not least because they are 'experts in their own experience'.

Colleagues and other professionals

Establishing good relationships in the workplace between adult care staff and other services underpins good person-centred care. For example, the housekeeping or catering teams may have little to do with the physical care of individuals, but they play an important part in ensuring that the environment is clean and well-resourced and that individuals are well-nourished. They are an important part of the holistic approach to care and the positive outcome for individuals is that they are being cared for in safe, clean environments. Additionally, those adult social carers who work in the community will need to establish good relationships with others who also visit the individual and may have some part in their care.

As a manager, your role is to recognise the part that other teams and services play in care delivery. Your leadership role does not stop with the team of people who deliver the care but extends to others in the work setting who all have a job to do. By establishing good relationships with these services the team will work together to ensure that the individual in the setting has a good experience.

Family and other carers

Family and carers also play a huge role in supporting their family members and are a major part of the partnership in care. It is important for care professionals to recognise and respect the role of family, particularly those who are also carers, and to support the role. Over the last 20 years or so, there has been greater recognition of the benefits of family members providing care, particularly if it helps to keep the family member in their own home. With detailed knowledge of their loved ones' preferences, illness, culture and value systems, these informal carers (i.e. those with no care qualifications) are better equipped to provide the loving support the individual needs. In the past, however, informal carers were rather neglected and felt isolated and unsupported. Care professionals therefore need to ensure that the relatives of individuals using the service are involved in care/support planning processes and assessments.

Better outcomes

Your role as a manager and leader in adult care is to ensure that every person your organisation cares for has a good experience of care and experiences good outcomes from the service.

Partnership working enables the strategic goals and vision of the organisation in which you work to be jointly discussed and understood. It enables agreement to be reached on how an individual's care can be implemented in the best interests of the individual and their family, as well as staff.

The Social Partnership Forum (Department of Health & Social Care and Social Partnership Forum, 2022) highlights the benefits of good partnership working as:

- trust and mutual respect
- openness, honesty and transparency
- top-level commitment
- a positive and constructive approach
- commitment to work with and learn from each other
- early discussion – no surprises
- confidentiality when needed.

Working in partnership therefore provides safe, quality care from a range of providers who have the individual at the centre of the whole process.

Outcome-based practice

You will find it useful to read Unit 515 AC1.1 on outcome-based practice before you read this section.

A different approach

The idea of 'outcomes' in care was seen to be focused on achievement and was regarded as a more meaningful way to assist with care. In using this approach, the care worker takes on the role of assisting the individual to identify immediate, medium-term and long-term goals. Rather than leading the individual's care, the health professional:

> *steers, guides, (and) pronounces the identification of 'needs' and the proposed 'intervention' towards practice driven by the service user, who is encouraged and facilitated to identify their 'outcomes', a set of immediate, medium- and long-term goals that they wish to achieve. The focus on outcomes overcomes many of the deficiencies of the 'needs' model described above.'*

Source: Qureshi et al. (2000) quoted in Barnes and Mercer (2004)

Care work becomes target driven and specific, with a goal in mind, and it is the individual in this type of care who sets review dates and monitors their achievement, thus moving away from the care professionals' assessment of the individual's needs.

The individual remains in complete control of the entire process, from the identification of outcomes to their achievement and evaluation of the success or failure of the venture. In this type of approach, the role of the care professional is to assist the individual in the achievement of their outcomes only.

While this approach would seem to provide the ultimate in person-centred care, it is not without its critics and a critical evaluation of the approach by Qureshi et al. in 2000 for York University highlighted some of the issues with it, as outlined below.

Care professionals seemed to struggle with the concept of outcomes as they lacked understanding of what the outcomes' focus actually was. A further area of concern was with the notion of 'expert power'. Putting the individual at the centre of the assessment process, identifying their own aims and objectives in negotiation with care professionals, meant that the professional felt their role had been reduced to one of facilitator as the control and responsibility for the achievement sat very much with the individual. For some professionals this did not sit well with the belief that as experts, they should have a bigger part in the decision-making process.

This somewhat radical approach to care meant that professionals needed to change their perceptions of care and embrace a newer way of working. The move to using the term 'outcome' rather than 'need' was one which helped to change perceptions, although the research showed this was not easy.

Helen Sanderson approaches outcomes with an eight step process to develop person-centred outcomes. She defines a good outcome as building on something that is working well but changing something that doesn't work and addressing needs and moving the person towards their future aspirations. A person-centred outcome is described as personally expressed and specific to the individual being within their control and influence. (See Helen Sanderson Associates, 2015.)

The role of the care professional

Further issues with this type of approach seemed to stem from the care professionals' need to reach a service solution instead of listening to the individual's desired outcomes. This was reported as a need to take responsibility on the part of the professional and was also linked to pressure of work. A number of professional practice issues were noted in Qureshi et al.'s research and the challenge of introducing an outcomes approach was raised. These were:

- the tendency of care professionals to fall back into a provider service mode instead of thinking and acting creatively with individuals
- the inability of care staff to grasp the outcomes concept.

Interestingly, the research showed that individuals valued the outcomes approach and 'appear comfortable with setting goals and working towards them'.

How outcome-based practice can result in positive changes in individuals' lives

By putting the person firmly at the centre of the care service, meaningful care can be delivered to individual outcomes. Go to Unit 515, AC1.1 to read about how a results-based accountability culture can lead to positive changes in individuals' lives, and what the key benefits of this care are.

Reflect on it

1.4 Person-centred care, stakeholders, positive outcomes

How has person-centred care affected the work of the partners you work with?

How do you and your partners work together to improve individuals' care? For example, you may wish to comment on how you work with the housekeeping team in your setting or perhaps an external partner such as the GP service.

You could refer to a change in policy which included your partners, such as how your service manages 'winter pressures' that affect the number of people coming to your service. Perhaps you have made changes to the assessment process of individuals that have affected other partners' work with those individuals. Analyse the association between person-centred care, working in partnership and the outcomes of this.

Stretch and challenge

1.4 How relationships with individuals, families and carers underpin person-centred practice and affect the achievement of positive outcomes

Explain how you encourage families, carers and individuals to adopt person-centred practice to achieve the outcomes the individual wants.

AC 1.5 Describe how networking and working collaboratively with other agencies and community groups, benefits those using the service

Here, you will be required to describe the impact of working with other agencies and community groups within the local area and relevant to the service. This will include a description of a range of potential benefits to both those accessing adult care services and the organisation.

In person-centred care, adult social care professionals work collaboratively with the individuals using services, supporting them to make informed decisions about their own health. By working with other partners and understanding and prioritising the needs of the individual, mutually beneficial and respectful relationships can be maintained, with a clear focus on the individual's own desired outcomes and needs.

Networking is the process of linking with professional contacts and sharing information with them. It can be a formal or informal process, with meetings being set up or simply having a conversation with another professional.

An important benefit of networking is that solutions to problems can be shared if everybody works towards a common purpose or goal. For example, you may notice that the satisfaction of the individuals using your service has started to fall but the solution is far from easy as there are many stakeholders who feed into the service that have an impact on the individuals using it. You discuss the issue with others in the network and they agree to work towards a common goal, that of reversing the current trend. Your first step might be to invite interested parties, such as other care professionals from various settings, individuals using the service in the setting and their families, and community members such as councils or other settings similar to your own, to a meeting to share their experiences and to discuss possible ways forward. Once established, this group can then feed into other groups in the local area to gain more data about the problem and bring their findings back to the core group. By working in such a way you can access many more people who will all have ideas about how the quality in the service can be improved.

Benefits of networking to those accessing adult care services

The benefits of working in this way will mean that those accessing care services in the future will experience a more informed quality service that is at the heart of a community network. The organisation itself will be able to work through its problems by accessing expertise from others external to the setting.

Look back at the Social Partnership Forum's list that highlights the benefits of good partnership working in AC1.2 of this unit.

Evidence opportunity

1.5 Benefits of networking

Describe how working collaboratively with other agencies and community groups within your local area would be beneficial to the individuals using your service.

You might, for example, like to consider how you have engaged with networking to ensure that you are able to access the expertise of a wide group of settings. If you work in the statutory care sector, say how working with partners in the voluntary sector has helped individuals in your setting to have better outcomes of care.

Include an example from your own practice which shows how partnership working has delivered better outcomes.

AC 1.6 Describe how networking and working collaboratively with other agencies and community groups benefits the sustainability and reach of the organisation

Here, you will be required to describe the benefits of integrated working.

Integration of care and working collaboratively is seen as the assimilation of organisations and/or services into single entities, enabling greater transparency between partners as well as enhanced benefits for the individuals using the service (Tilmouth et al., 2011).

Sustainability is a core issue for many settings and is about being able to meet current needs without damaging the future needs of generations to come. Currently the issue of global warming and reducing our carbon footprint to protect the planet are sustainability issues we are confronted with daily.

Within partnerships there can be an agreement to work together to reduce waste and energy consumption wherever possible to increase the sustainability of an organisation. Partners can collaborate and share waste disposal arrangements or perhaps pool funds to change to renewable energy sources in order to reduce energy costs.

The benefits of integrated working can be seen in the delivery of better all-round care for individuals. 'Integration' means working together to achieve better outcomes and it ensures higher levels of satisfaction. Effective integration, for example, means that you analyse, plan and deliver fully integrated services with colleagues from other disciplines, which reduces the overlapping of services, thus reducing costs and delivering a more seamless care package.

Evidence opportunity

1.6 Benefits of sustainability

Describe the benefits of being a sustainable organisation and how working with other agencies can deliver on this agenda.

AC 1.7 Explain how effective systems leadership supports integrated working with other agencies, overcomes barriers and delivers better outcomes for individuals

Here, you will be required to explain features of effective partnership working that minimise barriers.

The concept of systems leadership brings together the three elements of the individual, the community and the system to form and support change by using the skills and capability from each element. It is a collaborative approach to change, requiring a clear understanding of the issues at stake, together with the ability to engage with a diverse range of stakeholders to achieve shared goals.

The government white paper 'Health and social care integration: Joining up care for people, places and populations' (GOV.UK, 2022) highlights the way in which multi-agency community hubs, integrated neighbourhood teams and other local organisations and partnerships tackled the delivery of the COVID-19 vaccine roll-out. It applauds the way in which local partners made flexible use of resources across services to ensure that people got the support they needed.

The white paper states, 'Successful integration is the planning, commissioning and delivery of co-ordinated, joined up and seamless services to support people to live healthy, independent and dignified lives and which improves outcomes for the population as a whole' (GOV.UK, 2022). It suggests that these services should now be developed further and firmly identifies an agenda for building integrated health and care services with joined up care to make the best use of public resources and services.

Effective partnership working requires a commitment to sharing expertise and knowledge with colleagues in order to deliver services to those who need them. Some of the barriers to effective partnership can be reduced if a good partnership agreement is in place. This agreement should state the features of effective partnership working, such as a clear shared vision, clarification of role descriptions and lines of accountability, and details of reporting and complaints procedures.

All these features can minimise the barriers to effective partnerships. However, you are likely to come across barriers when you work with others. Some barriers to effective partnership working are described below.

Barriers to partnership working

Lack of role clarity

The various roles that come together in partnerships can make joint working difficult, particularly where there are perceived differences in status between occupational groups.

Joint employment

Joint employment, or co-employment, refers to the employment of a person in two related companies that are separate entities. It also applies to companies that provide employees to others even though they are financially separate and pay workers individually. Barriers may arise when working conditions between organisations are different, particularly where new patterns of working are being requested at the same time. In order for a partnership to work, it may require changes to an employee's terms and conditions or to the hours they work, and the employee may well perceive this as unfavourable. This can lead to resistance to change, resulting in poor morale among staff and other partners, particularly those people using the service, other professionals and colleagues.

Financial barriers

When professionals who work in partnership have different pay scales according to their professional group and their role within it, this can cause conflict. Additionally, there may be resentment if staff notice that money is used to employ staff from one group to provide a service normally provided by their own staff. Staff shortages can also damage interaction and the groups will start to withdraw from partnership working in an attempt to limit demands that are being made. If money is in short supply, establishing budgets and costs for various initiatives across partnerships can cause problems as there may be costs involved. Expenses, mileage payments and overtime all need to be found; this can be frustrating and may also become a barrier.

Difficulties in sharing information

There may be reluctance to share data and also difficulties in linking incompatible IT systems and the way in which records are kept in each organisation.

Limited time

With increasing numbers of partnerships developing, the time spent in meetings and travelling can be significant, so that less time is spent in practice. This may lead to the outcomes being far less successful than originally planned.

Different priorities and cultures

Staff working in different disciplines prioritise the care they give in a variety of ways. If you lack understanding about how a service works and constantly question the way staff carry out care, this can lead to barriers forming. Staff who must spend time explaining themselves may become resentful. In addition, your whole ethos of working may be vastly different to that of the partner and this can lead to you questioning the care they give. An underlying lack of understanding about how care can be delivered in different ways could damage the partnership.

Overcoming barriers

Overcoming barriers requires a commitment to working together in a professional way and this might be achieved by looking at the following.

Improving communication systems

Poor communication is an area that is consistently cited as a reason for underperformance and can also lead to conflict (Yoder-Wise, 2007). Therefore, as a manager and leader of a team, you need to hone these skills and improve any deficit or shortfall where you can. It is also important to communicate a clear vision to staff, and what teams are expected to achieve in their timeframes, a point that West (1994) emphasises.

A key factor in developing good teamworking and overcoming challenges is the manager's ability to develop positive relationships with the wide range of staff from different disciplines. This requires the ability to communicate effectively with people at all levels within the organisation.

Successful collaboration depends on open and transparent discussion. Traditionally, communication has relied on written formats such as referral forms, feedback forms, case notes, care/support plans, letters and emails. However, while quality record keeping and evidence-based policies and procedures are necessary, there does need to be one-to-one collaboration and **active participation** via regular meetings with partners.

KEY TERM

Active participation: In this context, this refers to enabling individuals to be included in their care and to be able to voice how they wish to live their life and obtain their own care.

Engaging families and putting interests of individuals first

Engaging the individual's family in all decision making and supporting families in their aims to help their loved ones means barriers to the partnership can become a thing of the past because everyone is working towards a common aim and purpose. The Care Act 2014 encourages person-centred care and this requires complete recognition of the needs and choices of the person receiving care. By ensuring that support is available to families and the individual, and by listening to those on the receiving end of care, a better quality of life can be expected.

Families are partners in the care process as much as professionals, and as such need to be informed and clear about their role.

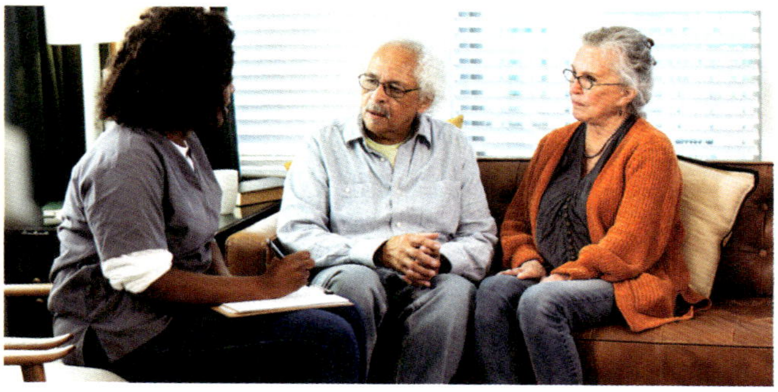

▲ **Figure 16** What methods do you use to overcome barriers to effective partnership working?

Retaining momentum

Effective partnerships work because they comprise groups of people who complement each other in the roles they undertake within the service.

In order to overcome barriers, it is important to retain momentum, and to ensure that everyone knows where the project is heading and what they need to do to get there. As a manager you need to be aware that any partners in the groups that fall behind schedule or fail to complete a task will have a negative effect on the team's momentum as a whole. Task sharing is one way this can be reduced. Time allocation is also important in maintaining momentum: too little and team members can get stressed, too much and the momentum can flag.

Engaging different professionals and working as a team

There is also a potential for conflict in partnerships between adult care staff working alongside medical staff, for example, who may be separated by geographical boundaries. Working in external settings, communication barriers and status inequalities may frustrate things and make the completion of tasks difficult. In addition, the mismatch of cultures, behaviours and understanding of services as well as a lack of understanding of each other's roles in the setting can be challenging and may affect the work you do. In order to overcome such challenges, joint working between professionals is critical and meetings need to be set up on a regular basis with members of the multidisciplinary team to jointly plan and deliver services.

One key factor in developing good partnerships is the manager's ability to develop positive relationships with the wide range of staff from different disciplines. This requires the ability to communicate effectively with people at all levels within the organisation.

Reflect on it

1.7 Features of effective partnerships and barriers

Think about a partnership you have set up in your setting and reflect on the effective features within it. What did you find particularly difficult? How have you worked to improve the barriers you experienced, if any?

Evidence opportunity

1.7 Effective partnership working and overcoming barriers

Explain how effective partnership and integrated working reduces barriers and leads to positive outcomes.

AC 1.8 Describe different communication methods used to forge relationships and partnerships with other professionals and agencies

Here, you will describe different methods of communication and when their use would be suitable in different partnership relationships.

Communication methods

The means of communication you have at your disposal to build relationships and forge partnerships include verbal and non-verbal. These may be:

- written
- electronic/digital
- pictorial
- signs
- social media.

The information may be:

- personal
- organisational
- formal
- informal
- public (information/promotional).

In the study of communication, you might come across the following three terms:

- **interpersonal communication**, which involves non-verbal, paralinguistic and verbal communication
- **environmental communication**, which involves the way in which our environment affects our interactions
- **intra-personal communication**, which takes place within ourselves, or 'self-talk'.

Before discussing written, electronic, pictorial, sign and communication through social media, it is worth exploring the different communication methods generally, and what they may mean in practice.

Verbal communication

Verbal communication can be complex since the meaning of words changes between cultures and generations. We can never be sure that a word has the same meaning for two people, especially when talking about feelings.

Choose words carefully: you need to be careful not to use jargon, abbreviations and language that is too complex, which the people in your care or your staff may not understand. Keep in mind the person you are speaking to and tailor your language to them. You need to be aware of cultural differences in language and conscious of the diverse nature of individuals. Similarly, you should avoid euphemisms, such as saying someone has 'passed away' instead of died.

- **Avoid clichés and alienating language**: One of the things that might alienate your staff is the use of cliché and 'management-type' speak. Terms such as 'thinking outside the box', 'blue-sky thinking' and 'scoping' can sound overused and inauthentic and may also be misunderstood.
- **Be culturally sensitive and speak clearly**: For example ensuring that you are not covering your mouth or turning away from a person when speaking will help those who need to lip read or listen carefully due to hearing problems. It is also important to consider cultural sensitivities around communication.
- **Be aware of paralinguistic communication**: When you moderate your speech, for example changing the pitch, volume, rhythm, tone of voice and timing, using occasional grunts, 'ums' and 'ahs', you are using paralinguistic communication. The way you say something can affect how your message is perceived. Yawning, sighing, coughing, tutting, laughing and groaning are also forms of paralinguistic communication. How do you communicate these aspects of language in non-verbal written communication though? In such cases you may change the colour or size of the font, or use

capital letters and exclamation marks. Paralinguistic communication can offer you a clue to how a person is feeling and this can help in your dealings with them.

Language, pitch, tone, inflection and its potential impact on others

Burnard (2005) argues that we must be careful of making assumptions about how someone is feeling and paralinguistic communication can offer us clues. It can also impact others and cause them to feel differently about our message. As a manager, you need to be aware of your paralinguistic signals, for example when giving feedback to a member of staff. Even if the words are positive, the person may feel they are being criticised if you haven't taken into account your tone and inflection.

Table 4 Paralinguistic communication

Tone of voice	Your tone of voice carries information about your feelings. It can add emphasis to the words you use.
Speed of speech	Speaking quickly can indicate that you are nervous. However, speech that is particularly slow may communicate that you are unsure about how you are being received by the listeners.
Volume	You may intentionally speak at a low volume (quietly) so that only the person closest to you hears. A person may mumble a reply when leaving the room so that you know they disagree with you but are unsure what they have said.
Inflection	Inflection is the movement of your voice. The emphasis you place on certain words can change the meaning of your sentences. For example, saying 'Do you WANT a drink?' can sound impatient and suggest that the person being asked is slow to respond, whereas 'Do you want a DRINK?' could suggest that things other than drink are on offer, such as food.
Pitch	A high pitch may communicate nervousness whereas a low pitch can be associated with authority.
Hesitations	Ums and ahs sometimes communicate uncertainty or fear, or can be used as clues that the other person wants to take a turn in the communication.
Accent	This communicates where you are from. It is important for a care worker to be understood so you may have to learn to modify a strong regional accent if recipients are unused to it.

Source: Adapted from Tilmouth et al. (2011)

Non-verbal communication

Table 5 shows types of non-verbal communication.

Table 5 Non-verbal communication

Facial expression	Your facial expression communicates emotions unless you train yourself to mask your feelings. If you say you are angry while smiling, it gives a confusing message.
Eye contact and gaze	If you can hold eye contact with another person throughout a conversation, it can communicate a level of confidence and willingness to communicate fully. Some of the people you communicate with will have a low level of eye contact, which might indicate a lack of ease with the conversation or a lack of confidence. It is a good idea to reduce the level of eye contact to reflect theirs, otherwise it can feel threatening. The appropriateness of maintaining eye contact differs according to culture.
Gestures	Gestures are movements of your arms and hands that accompany speech. Gestures can help communication – for example, pointing in the direction in which a person needs to go can add emphasis to the communication. However, too much gesturing can be distracting.
Body position, posture and movement	The body position of an individual can tell you a lot about how they are feeling – if they are hunched over, with arms and legs crossed, they are probably feeling quite anxious. Rogers (2002) recommends you try to maintain a relaxed posture, as it is important not to appear too formal and distant. However, if you are too laid back in your posture, you could appear uninterested. Sitting with your arms and legs crossed can appear closed off and defensive. In some circumstances, it may be a good idea to mirror the body posture of the person you are with.
Personal space and proximity	Two to three feet in distance between chairs is about right for many people; however, you may notice that some people push prearranged chairs back as soon as they sit down in them. This may be because the space does not feel comfortable to them. People seem to have their own invisible boundaries, which change according to who they are interacting with and how comfortable they feel.

Clothes	The clothes you choose to wear say a lot about you. Dressing too informally or too formally may alienate you from the people in your care.
Therapeutic touch	Touch can be a contentious subject. On the one hand, there is evidence of touch having therapeutic benefits; on the other, it can be misinterpreted and seen as an invasion of a person's personal space. Bonham (2004) suggests it may be appropriate and supportive for staff to use touch when an individual is distressed as it may validate the degree of their suffering. He suggests that appropriate places to touch in this situation are hands, forearms, upper arms and shoulders.

Source: Tilmouth et al. (2011)

Written communication – record keeping and reports

Working as a manager in an adult setting means you will be responsible for keeping records and reports. Accurately documenting events and care provides an account of what actually took place. Records form an account of the individual's experience, and this helps to provide continuity of care. You will rely on these records if, later on, you need to remind yourself of what was done at the time. Records must be:

- clear
- legible
- accurate
- honest
- in English
- signed and dated.

Records may be handwritten, or computer based, but staff must comply with whichever method the workplace requires. They should know how to use the systems and tools in the workplace and how to maintain confidentiality. Records must comply with legal requirements such as the General Data Protection Regulation (GDPR).

Written reports, notes, email and other forms of electronic communication are all important and being able to maintain clear and accurate records is a legal requirement. Written communications should be accurate, detailed, up to date, non-judgemental and legible so that others are able to read and understand them. Confidentiality guidelines and all forms of written communication must be kept safely and should conform to the requirements of GDPR.

Electronic/digital

Email is a quick and convenient method of communication with the bonus that people can respond immediately if they wish. As a written record of a communication, it can be accessed afterwards for evidence in a way that a telephone call cannot. You can also send attachments and links with the email, enabling the respondent to go straight to the information. There is no postage and it can save on journey time to and from meetings.

There are disadvantages with emails, however, due to their impersonal nature and the inability to pick up paralinguistic and non-verbal signals. Short and to-the-point emails can sometimes appear rude, and people tend not to reply to emails they do not understand, so you could be waiting for an answer for a while.

Confidentiality is another important consideration, with the potential for confidential information going to the wrong person by mistake or accidentally forwarded on by the respondent to someone else.

These documents are formal and therefore any colloquial or 'chatty' language needs to be avoided.

Pictorial

Pictorial (or assisted) communication refers to the use of aids such as picture and symbol communication boards and electronic devices, which help individuals who have difficulty with speech or language problems to express themselves.

Sign language

Sign language, Braille, Makaton, assisted technology and other non-verbal methods of communication are useful aids for those individuals who cannot communicate verbally. You need to ensure that staff are equipped to support individuals who may use these methods. Everyone in the setting also need to know the meanings of signs such as those displayed at fire exits or in smoking areas.

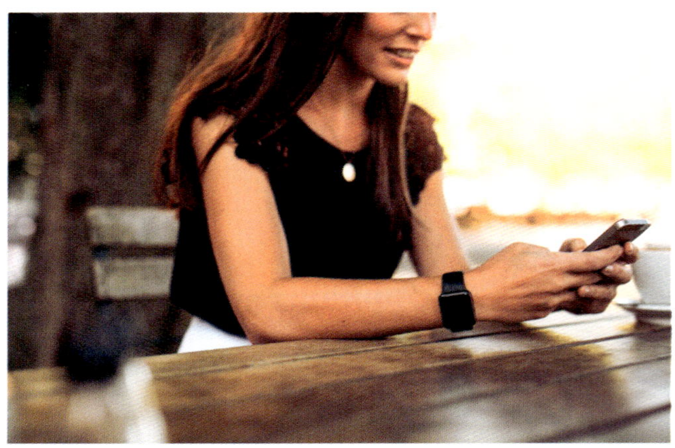

▲ **Figure 17** Mobile phones have made it easier to access social media and communicate using various social media websites and platforms

Social media

Facebook, Twitter, WhatsApp and blogs have changed the way in which we communicate. Businesses and settings use these methods for marketing and informing others about what they do. While these are useful tools for getting your message out there, you need to be aware of what you write and who might read your posts. As a manager, you may wish to restrict your personal accounts to friends and family only and not enable your staff to access them. These forms of media can never be deleted, and an unprofessional post or personal opinion may be viewed by staff or others and could prove detrimental to your own setting or the way in which you are perceived as a manager of staff.

Evidence opportunity

1.8 Methods of communication and their importance

Provide a written account explaining the effectiveness of communication models and methods within the practice and their impact on service delivery to include:

- ✔ written
- ✔ verbal and non-verbal
- ✔ electronic/digital
- ✔ pictorial
- ✔ signage
- ✔ social media.

Communication protocols

Effective care is provided in collaboration and partnership with others, either in the same team (internally) or across a range of agencies and disciplines within the care sector (externally).

You will spend time building personal and organisational or partnership relationships and trust within those relationships matter. The success of your setting or team depends upon the ability to collaborate and build effective working partnerships with both internal staff and those who work outside the organisation. Building sustainable relationships is also a useful indicator of how successful you are as a leader because good relationships will motivate staff and others to do their best.

All partnership working depends on effective communication and good working relationships. As part of a care team that goes beyond the boundaries of your own organisation, you need to be aware of the need to build team links with external bodies.

Partnership working

Partnership working is an important means of making improvements in adult social care. It depends on effective partnerships between the different professions and organisations involved in commissioning and delivering services and interventions. It requires shared communication systems, including shared databases, records and files, to ensure that consistency in care is maintained and decision-making processes are clear.

The Care Act 2014 and the Health and Care Act 2022 simplified and improved the existing legislation in care and the changes mean that more people are now able to access care and support from local councils or other organisations in the community. They also have more choice about the type of support and care they need. In addition, different ways to pay for care and support are now available. This means that communication between partners must be firmly established to ensure that all parties are talking to each other and have the individuals using the service at the heart of the care.

Communication limitations

Different communication systems are likely to be used within working environments. For example, you might find that different staff carry out record keeping in different ways, or some staff may present nursing or care assessments differently to others. This can lead to communication limitations, particularly if staff do not clearly understand how records are being stored and shared. Confidentiality may be compromised when there is confusion about how the records are sent between several partners.

The actual setting may be a form of environmental barrier. For example, excessive noise, poor layout or even the way in which people work in a setting can be detrimental to communication. These issues can be addressed by making changes to the fabric of the environment and improving the layout of the place in which communication occurs.

Also, the use of acronyms and abbreviations should be avoided as this can lead to misunderstanding. For example, ABC in a healthcare setting refers to airway, breathing and circulation, but you may understand it to mean antecedents, behaviour and consequences, as in the promoting positive behaviour model.

As a manager, you should critically examine the environment where you and staff engage with visitors and other staff, when you communicate bad news for example, or where supervision and team meetings are held. If you feel uncomfortable and unsettled in this setting, then the chances are that your staff and visitors will too.

Reflect on it

1.8 Communication with partners

Consider the partners you work with and identify the ways in which you communicate with them. How might you improve the methods you use to ensure that a more standardised approach to communication is used? How might this enhance the relationship?

AC 1.9 Explain potential conflicts within partnerships with other professionals and agencies

Here, you will identify and explain potential areas where there may be conflict between different organisations and examine methods of resolving conflicts.

When you come across a situation that is causing some conflict, this may cause you to have negative feelings about a person, which in turn may become a barrier to communication.

Conflict is often viewed as a negative issue and it becomes a problem when it affects your work, causes inappropriate behaviour and lowers morale, impacting the workforce and the individual using the service. John Adair, in his book Effective Teambuilding (2000), came up with the following five strategies for dealing with conflict:

1. Competing – forcing your own ideas through because you believe your way is right.
2. Confronting/collaborating – bringing all the issues into the open and exploring all feasible options you are showing an openness to change.
3. Compromise – negotiating to meet halfway.
4. Avoid – opting out altogether and avoiding taking up any position.
5. Accommodate – allowing the change to happen so as not to hurt feelings.

Issues can arise in partnership working. For example, different leadership styles may present a problem, particularly if they are at opposite ends of a spectrum. Some partnerships where a task-oriented, get-things-done approach is used may clash with those adopting a more laissez-faire or collaborative style.

Conflict can also arise in the way in which the partnership is split. There may be a major partner who is taking the lead, and finances can become problematic. Guidelines must be clear in these situations, and this can be done by setting boundaries, ensuring that decisions are made together.

Commitment is also a challenging area and if one partner feels that the other is not willing to put in the time and dedication this can provoke ill feeling.

Finally, job roles and responsibilities must be clearly outlined and any disparity in either pay or working conditions must be remedied.

Evidence opportunity

1.9 Dealing with conflict

Explain how potential conflicts may arise in your setting. How might you deal with it? Explain to your assessor the possible reasons for the conflict arising in the first place.

AC 1.10 Evaluate features of effective, collaborative partnership working across agencies

Here, you will evaluate the methods by which different agencies can work together effectively for the benefit of the individual.

Sharing information openly and honestly

Effective partnership working demands excellent two-way communication that is open and honest. When the workplace operates in a transparent way, employee engagement is high. Building trust between management and staff by open, honest conversations, having a no-blame culture, recognising achievements and hard work leads to a positive and effective collaboration.

Creating psychological safety within partnerships and teams

People in the workplace come with a variety of skills and different perspectives and ideas. Psychological safety means they are able to express themselves without fear that others will think less of them or dismiss their ideas. You should value the diversity of different skillsets and encourage staff to speak up, share ideas, ask questions, openly disagree, feel able to express concerns and, most importantly, to own up to mistakes. Such an environment enables staff to feel comfortable and develops a climate of trust and mutual respect.

Understand and prioritise the needs of others without compromising on desired outcomes

The best partnerships set goals for each of the partners at the beginning of the year. In this way all are working to the same agenda and are not prioritising their own needs over that of others. Each partner knows their role on the team.

Evidence opportunity

1.10 Working collaboratively with partners

Evaluate a feature of effective collaboration.
For example, one feature of a collaborative workforce is working together as a team, looking beyond your own personal agenda and recognising that each staff member has a role to play in meeting the common goals and outcomes.

AC 1.11 Describe own role and responsibilities in establishing positive relationships within and beyond the organisation/service

Here, you will be required to describe your own role as a leader in adult care services to ensure that the service creates and maintains positive relationships with all those that come into contact with the service.

The Authentic Leadership approach developed by Bill George (2003) focuses on characteristics of good leaders. He found that authentic leaders have a strong desire to serve others and demonstrate five basic characteristics:

1. They have a purpose.
2. They have strong values and are clear about the right thing to do.
3. They establish trusting relationships.
4. They demonstrate self-discipline.
5. They are passionate about their mission.

Respect other roles

Working in partnership means working alongside different people from a variety of disciplines, as well as colleagues within your own team and the families of the individuals using the service. One of the responsibilities you have is to maintain an open mind about the way in which other services work and to respect the roles of others in the care they give. For your colleagues, you also need to create a working environment which promotes national policies with respect to partnership working.

As a leader in adult care services, you must evaluate the way you carry out your own role to ensure that the service creates and maintains positive relationships with all those that come into contact with it.

Create a positive working environment

You need to create a working environment for your colleagues that promotes national policies with respect to partnership working. All partners need to be reminded that working together brings better outcomes for the individuals using the service and that is at the heart of the initiative.

Prioritise person-centred care

An emphasis upon collaborative working will ensure that the individuals in your care are provided with the support they require to live the lives they want with dignity. This is stressed in the Care Act 2014.

Link stakeholders

Effective teamwork enhances care and safety because members of the team co-ordinate and communicate their activities with the common aim of ensuring that the individual is at the centre of the care. One of your main roles will be to act as a link person in the partnership, whether it is with families or other professionals, and also to develop a climate of trust between all partners.

Build trust

Trust is such an important issue in management and leadership and is at a premium in today's working climate. If partnerships are to work, you need to ensure that you have created trust in your organisation by being open and reliable in your decision making and by articulating a commitment to the way in which the partnership is to work.

A lack of trust leads to fear, suspicion and insecurity and a lowering of morale in general, resulting in resistance to change and reduced productivity.

George (2003) noted that individuals wanted their leaders to be open with them and to become more transparent, thus softening the boundary between roles. A trusting relationship with the leader creates greater commitment to the mission and also loyalty.

Open communication

Communication is important and, in an atmosphere where trust is central to the workings of the team, individuals will feel free to contribute fully. Staff should feel able to be part of negotiations within an organisation. External stakeholders and partners are also part of the communication process and must be invited to engage in discussion about the work that is being done.

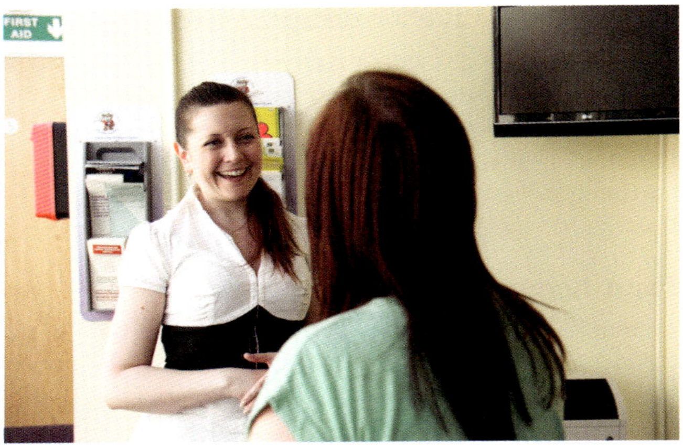

▲ **Figure 18** How do you ensure that there is open communication when working in partnership?

Evidence opportunity

1.11 Your role and responsibilities in establishing positive relationships

Find and describe evidence for your portfolio to show that, as a leader in adult care services, you ensure that the service creates and maintains positive relationships with all those that come into contact with the service.

You might like to include the ways in which you ensure that there is open communication when working in partnership. For example, say how you communicate with external partners and what methods you use. How do you ensure that all partners are kept informed of changes?

It might be useful for you to ask partners how they feel the work they are doing with you is helping the individuals in their care. You might also try to gauge whether they feel some change might be useful.

LO2 Be able to lead effective relationships with individuals, carers and families

Stephen R. Covey's *The 7 Habits of Highly Effective People* (2004) continues to be a popular choice for leadership development today, focusing on the principles of fairness, integrity, honesty and human dignity. Covey believed that the adoption of seven habits would make the difference for personal and team success and organisational effectiveness, as outlined below.

Habit 1: Be proactive®

A common damaging trait is one of reaction or the tendency to firefight issues or go into blame mode when something goes wrong. Some people react to situations that may be out of their control and start to behave like victims. Being proactive means taking a responsible approach to a situation. Covey breaks this down into response and ability, explaining it as '"response-ability" or the ability to choose your response. Highly proactive people recognize that responsibility. They do not blame circumstances, conditions, or conditioning for their behavior.' (Covey, 2004)

Proactive people focus their efforts on things that they can do something about and if a mistake is made, they recognise and acknowledge it, then apply corrective measures if possible. The main thing is they learn from it and do not apportion blame. Reactive people allow their feelings to control the situation and their actions, but in a negative way.

Habit 2: Begin with the end in mind®

Covey talks about the need for a 'principle-centred' basis to all aspects of life. By clearly establishing your own principles, you can define clear measures of success and a plan to achieve them. As a setting, this is also about having a clear strategic plan. Having principles central to your life means you can be better organised and balanced.

Habit 3: Put first things first®

Using his matrix, of which there are many iterations, Covey showed how you should prioritise and achieve the most important goals instead of constantly reacting to urgencies.

Time Management Matrix

	Urgent	Not Urgent
Important	**1. Quadrant of urgency** - Crises - Pressing problems - Deadline-driven projects, meetings, preparations	**2. Quadrant of quality** - Preparation - Prevention - Values clarification - Planning - Relationship building - Empowerment
Not Important	**3. Quadrant of distraction** - Interruptions, some phone calls - Many pressing matters - Many popular activities - Some emails, reports and meetings - Often deceptive and highjacks time	**4. Quadrant of waste** - Trivia, busy work - Junk emails - Some phone calls - Time wasters - 'Escape' activities

▲ **Figure 19** Covey's matrix of time management, adapted from Accounting Solutions Ltd (2020)

By breaking down all your activities you can clearly see how you can manage your time effectively.

Quadrant 1 – 'Urgent and important' is the quadrant of urgency and is for the unexpected things that happen and which need to be dealt with immediately. You should not always be working in this way, as doing so will lead to stress and the possibility of burnout.

Quadrant 2 – 'Not urgent, but important' is the quadrant of quality and is for planning and relationship-building. This is the place where you should aim to spend most of your time, because it will enable you to deal with important tasks.

Quadrant 3 – 'Urgent but not important' is the quadrant of distraction and relates to interruptions and the meetings you need to attend. Losing this time might feel as though you have loss of control and are suffering because of circumstances. It is a good idea to try to minimise or eliminate these unimportant but urgent items.

Quadrant 4 – 'Not urgent and not important' is the quadrant of waste and is where time wasting happens. You can eliminate a lot of what happens here, such as scrolling through social media or surfing the internet. If somebody spends a lot of time here then they are showing a level of irresponsibility and might even be unsuitable for employment.

Habit 4: Think win-win®

Collaborate more effectively by building high-trust relationships. Covey distinguishes between what he called a 'scarcity mentality' and the 'abundance mentality'. The first is similar to the fixed mindset and is the belief that there is only a finite amount of success that can be shared and so there is not much point in trying to achieve goals. Some people find it difficult to celebrate the success of others and this comes from the scarcity mentality belief. Our exam system has conditioned us to accept win/lose mentality, and even approval from teachers and parents is often related to 'success'. We therefore grow up believing that we need to compete in the workplace rather than collaborate.

The opposite or the 'abundance mentality' growth mindset is the belief that there are unlimited possibilities for growth and development and that if we can share in the success of others, we can achieve a win/win solution. This mindset teaches us that the possibility for growth is available for everybody.

Habit 5: Seek first to understand, then to be understood®

Actively listening and seeking to understand what the other person is truly communicating can be influential as you develop an understanding of their needs. Covey defined different levels of listening, such as hearing but ignoring or pretending to listen and making the right noises – 'Yes', 'Oh', 'I see ...', or selectively listening and choosing only what we want to hear. Attentive listening is when you concentrate on what is being said without making any judgements.

Empathic listening requires a deeper level to truly understand the other person but when you do feel that someone is genuinely seeking your point of view and listening, you feel more open to negotiate a win/win situation.

Habit 6: Synergise®

When you develop innovative solutions that take account of differences and satisfy all key stakeholders, you have synergy. You may have a different agenda, but if you value the other person you will seek to come to a solution using teamwork and a spirit of open-mindedness. This in turn leads to new insights and better results than can be achieved singly.

Habit 7: Sharpen the saw®

This final habit is about you as a person and the need to increase motivation, energy and work–life balance by making time for renewing activities.

Covey uses the metaphor of a woodcutter with a blunt saw. When asked why he doesn't stop trying to cut the tree down and sharpen the saw, his response is, 'I can't stop – I'm too busy sawing down this tree.' You can become so bogged down in a task that you fail to notice when the tools are not working well. A poor work–life balance may lead to stress as you neglect your basic needs. Your social and emotional self will suffer if you pay no attention to your relationships and personal development.

Source: Adapted from Covey (2004)

Nolan et al.'s senses framework

Nolan et al. (2006) developed the 'senses framework', which comprises six senses that are seen as prerequisites for good relationships within the context of care and service delivery. The basic concept of Nolan et al.'s relationship-centred care model is that best practice involves the creation of a set of senses or experiences for older people, for family caregivers and for staff working with them. These senses are security, belonging, continuity, purpose, significance and achievement.

For example, in developing 'a sense of security for older people', attention needs to be paid to physiological and psychological needs, so individuals feel safe and free from threat, harm, pain and discomfort. Additionally, carers, family and staff need freedom from physical threat, have secure conditions of employment (where appropriate), be recognised that the work they do is emotionally demanding and to work within a supportive culture.

The senses framework suggests an inclusive vision of dementia care practice. Services have traditionally worked with individuals with dementia separately from their carers and family, but this framework seeks to contextualise the care within significant relationships.

The Butterfly Model of Care, formally 'Dementia Care Matters', focuses on delivering emotion-focused care. It is a holistic approach that addresses individuals' needs, supporting the quality of life of those living with dementia across the whole of their lived experience. Using a 'feeling-centric' approach to care, eight key components are highlighted:

- BEING: rather than doing tasks for the individual, staff shift their focus to person-centred approaches to reach people on the inside.
- ENABLING: seeing, hearing and feeling the lived experience of people and measuring the minute by minute experiences of individuals can aid quality of life and improve the moment.
- INSPIRING: moving away from detached management to attached leadership is where people lead from the heart and not just by the hand.
- NURTURING: nurturing staff emotions in dementia care will lead to more positive team relationships.
- GROWING: training that focuses on the development of staff's emotional intelligence through reflection, modelling and coaching.
- ACHIEVING: achieving real outcomes is all about focusing on what is important. Rather than being led by policy, procedure and systems, the primary focus should be on measuring the quality of service and quality of life.
- SUPPORTING: by restoring compassionate cultures of care, staff in dementia care can be developed to lead and model person-centred care and relationship-focused support.
- MATTERING: involves the core skills in staff of feel, look, connect and occupy while creating a culture change through developing a community based on share, reach, relax and matter.

Source: Primacare Living Solutions (n.d.)

AC 2.1 Model open, respectful and supportive relationships with individuals, their families, and carers

Here, you will be required to show that you model open, respectful and supportive relationships and communicate to establish effective partnership working.

Individuals using the service

Individuals must be treated in a respectful manner. One way in which this might be done is to ensure that all staff respectfully address the individuals they care for using their chosen name and promote choices about their care. As a manager you can help staff to do this by ensuring training sessions are available and arranging supervision sessions where ways of working can be checked and discussed.

Families

Families, carers, advocates and friends are an important part of the care team surrounding the individuals using a service and so must be included when setting objectives for care. These people are usually at the heart of the individual's life and as such can often see things like imbalances in the care being planned. They should be aware of the way in which each part of the team communicates and the relationship between the specialists and other workers involved in the care. They can then see where the boundaries between partners lie and who is accountable for the care in the setting.

You will need to ensure that both you and your staff establish open and transparent relationships so that everyone who comes into the organisation can see that this way of working has been adopted and is practised by all staff. You will need to effectively communicate information and ensure that staff are willing to listen and put into practice actions that have been agreed. You and the staff you manage will need be respectful, not only to the individuals using the service, but to all who come into contact with the organisation and with each other.

When working with families and carers, individuals and their advocates, there are a number of ways that adult social care organisations develop their procedures to ensure that they meet the needs of carers. These include:

- identifying a key worker within the organisation who will be the first point of contact for carers and who will take primary responsibility for making sure that carers' needs are considered
- providing 'carer awareness' training for all staff to ensure that they understand what role the carer will be taking
- developing links to local carers' organisations to explore ways of working together

- developing a carers' charter to ensure that best practice guidelines for working with carers and staff are identified and that staff are aware of these
- starting up a staff–carers' network
- making sure information for carers is available and well-publicised
- involving carers in service planning and development
- providing training for carers in areas such as lifting and handling, intimate care, use of equipment, stress management and maximising their own health and wellbeing.

> **Evidence opportunity**
>
> **2.1 Model open, respectful and supportive relationships**
>
> Show your assessor how you model open, respectful and supportive relationships, and how you communicate to establish effective relationship with carers and families.

AC 2.2 Embed co-production within day-to-day practices of team

Here, you will be required to engage the team in a way that enables them to understand the values and importance of co-production.

Co-production

As a manager, you must engage your team in a way that enables them to understand the values and importance of co-production. Co-production refers to an equal relationship between the individuals accessing a service and the people responsible for providing the service. It recognises the knowledge and experiences that both have that can be used to help make services better.

The Social Care Institute for Excellence (SCIE) website defines co-production as 'A relationship where professionals and citizens share power to plan and deliver support together, recognising that both have vital contributions to make in order to improve quality of life for people and communities'.

The Care Act 2014 introduced the concept in its guidance to define a more meaningful relationship with care/support planning for the individual than just involvement. It is about moving the power to change things for the individual.

The values within co-production are as follows:

- Equality: Everyone has assets and no one person is more important than another.
- Diversity: Inclusivity and the efforts of groups who are from diverse backgrounds and who may be underrepresented in care should be heard.
- Accessibility: Equal opportunity for all to participate in any way they can.
- Reciprocity: Getting something back for putting something in.

Source: Adapted from SCIE (2022)

In the past, failure to listen to the people using the services and their carers has led, in some cases, to abuse and neglect. There have been numerous inquiries into such abuse and recommendations to develop more equal and meaningful relationships with people who use services. Co-production describes ways of working in partnership with people who use services, carers and citizens to improve services and to find a shared solution to the problems individuals face. For example, those who use a service need to be consulted and included at the start of any project that affects them.

Staff and partners need to be clear that a meaningful care relationship is one in which professionals and the individuals using the service are all empowered to plan and deliver support together. Everyone in the care partnership has contributions to make and co-production values this approach.

> **Reflect on it**
>
> **2.2 Co-production**
>
> Think about the term co-production and what it actually means for you. Can you come up with examples that show how you, in your role, have shared this concept with your staff? For example, using the four bullet point headings in this section, say how you have demonstrated this in your setting.

> **Evidence opportunity**
>
> **2.2 Support others to recognise the values of co-production**
>
> Show your assessor how you engage the team in a way that enables them to understand the values and importance of co-production and the expertise of those using adult care services and relevant others.

> **Research it**
>
> **2.2 Co-production**
>
> Read the recommendations in the Co-production guide published by SCIE (see SCIE, 2015).
>
> For each heading (Culture, Structure, Practice and Review), describe at least one way in which you can engage your team to enable them to understand the importance of co-production.

Reflect on it

2.2 Values of co-production

Think about the values of co-production. Write about the values to the team of this way of working.

You might use these headings:

- Equality and diversity
- Accessibility and equal opportunity
- Reciprocity.

How have these been embedded in adult care? For example, for equality and diversity you might discuss how individuals from different backgrounds who may be underrepresented in care have been given a voice.

AC 2.3 Implement measures to ensure that individuals, carers and others are aware of their rights in partnership working

Here, you will be required to implement procedures to ensure that everyone is aware of their statutory and legal rights. These could include procedures based on aspects of the following pieces of legislation and areas discussed in this section.

As the manager of a setting, it is important to ensure that everybody is aware of their statutory rights. Staff, individuals using the service, visitors and partners need to be fully informed of how your setting demonstrates an awareness of the legal aspects of care work and operates within the legislation. The policies you develop in the setting will reflect the legal requirements and help to make the legal aspect more accessible. The setting website should have a section that demonstrates to others your commitment to the law, and staff induction needs to include reference to the importance of working within policy and what this looks like in your setting.

It is especially important that individuals, their carers, families, advocates and any other people involved in their care are aware of their legal rights that are designed to protect them when using services. For example, many people who come into care settings are not aware of their rights with respect to data protection and consent and so need to be shown what they can expect from you as a care provider.

You might take the opportunity to issue the relevant forms when individuals first come into your care setting and to ask them to appoint people with powers of attorney if they have not already done so, and also to determine who they wish to have designated as their next of kin and nearest relatives.

During your admission procedure you might discuss rights and responsibilities with the individuals so that they can be more informed of these.

There are a number of pieces of legislation that individuals should be aware of, some of which are discussed in this section.

Mental Capacity Act 2005

The Mental Capacity Act (MCA) 2005 protects and supports people who do not have the ability to make decisions for themselves. For further information on this Act, refer to Unit 508.

Mental Health Act 1983 and 2007 (amended)

The 1983 Mental Health Act laid down provision for the compulsory detention and treatment of people with mental health problems in England and focused upon strengthening individuals' rights to review their treatment. The Act was amended in 2007 and focused on public protection and risk management. For more information on this Act, refer to Unit 501.

Liberty Protection Safeguards

Liberty Protection Safeguards (LPS) are designed to protect the rights of individuals who receive care in a hospital, care home or other provision who may become deprived of their liberty, due to lack of mental capacity to consent. They will replace Deprivation of Liberty Safeguards (DoLS) but, at the time of writing (May 2023), their introduction has been delayed. See Unit 508 for more on DoLS and LPS.

Equality Act 2010

The Equality Act 2010 brought together four major EU Equal Treatment Directives and replaced previous anti-discrimination laws, simplifying the law and making it easier to understand. For information on this Act, see Unit 501.

Power of attorney

Anyone making a decision on behalf of a person they believe to lack mental capacity must do so in that person's best interests. The Mental Capacity Act 2005 introduced a new type of power of attorney known as a Lasting Power of Attorney (LPA). An LPA enables people to choose someone who can make decisions about their health and welfare, as well as their finances and property, if they become unable to do so for themselves. Often a person chooses a member of their family or a close friend, but whoever is chosen, this should be done before the loss of capacity occurs and must be documented with the individual's knowledge and consent long before it might be used.

Care Act 2014

This Act put people in control of their care and support, and highlights adult safeguarding. It also specifies that individuals have the right to an assessment of their needs. For more information on this Act, see Unit 507.

> **Evidence opportunity**
>
> **2.3 Statutory rights and making sure everyone is aware**
>
> Show your assessor how you implement procedures to ensure that everyone is aware of their statutory rights. These could include procedures based on aspects of the following:
>
> - ✔ Mental Capacity Act 2005
> - ✔ Mental Health Act 1983 and 2007
> - ✔ Deprivation of Liberty Safeguards/Liberty Protection Safeguards
> - ✔ Equality Act 2010
> - ✔ Power of Attorney
> - ✔ Care Act 2014.

LO3 Be able to manage working relationships with colleagues in own setting to achieve positive outcomes for individuals

AC 3.1 Develop systems and procedures which facilitate effective working relationships with a range of colleagues

Here, you will be required to develop procedures to facilitate effective working relationships with colleagues.

Developing an effective team

Effective team performance requires the development of procedures that enable a positive and supportive culture and good relationships between staff in the organisation. Only in this way can you expect staff to be supportive of a shared vision to meet the agreed objectives for a care setting. The most important person in your team will be the individual using the service and they need to be central to any teamworking.

Imagine a group of footballers who have little idea about the rules of the game, what the objectives of the game are and how the position they play works with the rest of the team. Picture the first match and guess the outcome. Of course, it is likely to be a mess, isn't it? With nobody working together and without any direction, the game will be lost.

In total contrast to the example above, effective teams in your setting work together towards common goals and objectives and it is important that you know what the features of effective team performance are.

The reality of modern adult care services is that the care available depends as much on how social care employees work with each other as on their individual competence within their field of expertise (Tilmouth et al., 2011).

All teams need to go through a development process and well-established teams have to be motivated to perform in roles in which they fit comfortably. Effective teams are those which comprise people who complement each other in their roles and who are managed and led in an efficient way.

Staff relationships within the team should be nurtured to encourage a cohesive atmosphere at work. A key factor in developing good teamworking and overcoming challenges is the manager's ability to develop positive relationships with the wide range of staff from different disciplines. This requires the ability to communicate effectively with people at all levels within the organisation.

Trust within the team

In an atmosphere where trust is central to the working of the team, open communication is important and individuals should feel free to be able to contribute fully. Staff should feel able to be part of negotiations within an organisation. One way to encourage this is for you, as the manager, to be a role model for encouraging mutual support and respect. For example, the way you treat your staff will be under scrutiny by others who come in to work in the service. If they observe a lack of respect, there may be some resistance to communicating with you.

The most important thing you can do to develop effective supportive working relationships is to build your reputation as a professional who is trustworthy and inspires confidence and respect in your team, as well as between all team members. In this way you can show that you provide other professionals with information, advice and support within the boundaries of your role and expertise and, as such, can develop procedures for partnership working that are fair to all parties involved.

By being honest and open with staff you can develop a more co-operative way of working. Actively listening to the problems your staff and others have and attempting to come to a mutual resolution when conflict arises will go a long way to ensuring that the workforce remains positive. Your policy on communication, for example, can help effective working relationships by being robust and up to date.

Colleagues

You will be familiar with the notion of setting objectives in order to achieve aims. Part of your role as a manager and leader will be to educate your staff and, as such, you set objectives as to what you hope the people attending your session will gain from being there. So, too, with partnership working – there needs to be a good balance between developing the partnership and its objectives in order for it to be successful. You must recognise and respect the differences that might exist between all concerned and not make assumptions about the way in which other organisations or individuals work and lose sight of what you are actually there for. By being open and respectful in the relationship, you can improve the trust among the wider partnership and thus enable a more effective way of working.

Procedures

Teams are formed because having people work on shared goals interdependently will lead to improved performance and co-operation and interaction. In other words, individuals who work together can achieve more than individuals who work on their own.

Effective teams display certain features and the following are eight characteristics identified by Larson and Lafasto (1989) in their book *Teamwork: What Must Go Right/What Can Go Wrong*. According to Larson and LaFasto, the team must have:

- a clear goal
- a results-driven structure
- competent team members
- unified commitment
- a collaborative climate
- high standards that are understood by all
- external support and encouragement
- principled leadership.

To sum up, goals, roles, procedure, relationships and leadership are the essential pre-requisites for effective teamworking (McKibbon et al., 2008). The members of a team need to be able to communicate and collaborate to function effectively. If you co-ordinate the work of a group of people and develop shared goals, working towards a common aim, then you are almost there.

It is important to be able to measure how effective each of your work partnerships is and to do so requires appraisal systems and outcomes measures.

Work performance appraisal systems can be used to assess how effective the partnership is as well as the quality of the work produced. The evaluation methods used can take various forms and largely depend on the type of career professional being appraised. In adult social care, performance may rest on several basic techniques, such as supervision and performance appraisals.

In evaluating your working relationship with your staff, it might be useful to use a self-assessment tool in which staff are able to provide anonymous feedback about various aspects of the working relationship.

In evaluating procedures outside assessment, other professionals and teams may be asked to observe the workplace on a formal and informal basis, providing independent feedback. This can then be measured against the in-house evaluations by staff and the individuals using the service.

Evaluation can also be gained using written comment forms, telephone surveys or online questionnaires. Families and friends and others who may be supporting an individual may be included in evaluation and asked to comment upon the service provision. You may also ask advocates to evaluate the service and comment on whether and how they have been included in discussions and planning regarding the individual.

Undertaking such measures can identify the successes of teamworking as well as the failures and can provide evidence for change. By making an evaluation of the way in which partnerships are working it is possible to assess the effectiveness of the care provided and make changes accordingly.

Develop processes to accommodate different types of working relationships and a range of colleagues

The different people you come into contact within the course of your work may include visitors, ancillary staff and also those who may be called in from other disciplines. These diverse groups of people will bring different ways of working to the setting and you may be required to develop new sets of procedures.

All relationships are different, but it is easy to forget this and expect people to think and behave like we do, which is not always the case. Respecting the differences brought to the setting by diverse groups of people will not only enrich the process, but will also help to create a rapport.

Develop and lead the implementation of communication strategies when working with all internal stakeholders

Communication strategies play a role in developing high-performance partnerships and are necessary for change and improvement to take place. Effective strategies include ensuring that clear and consistent messages are sent to all parts of the organisation in a simple and direct way. As a manager in the setting it is wise to spend time thinking about what it is you want to say and how you will say it, as this can set the tone for developing an atmosphere of trust and openness.

Demonstrate trustworthiness when colleagues divulge personal confidences

To divulge a personal confidence takes a lot of courage and as the manager you need to be able to show you can be trusted with the information and that you will deal with it appropriately. If the confidence is troubling and you are concerned about any consequences to the person, you will need to discuss this with them and encourage them to open up further to others. For example, a person who may be being abused at home may require further support from other agencies and you should encourage them to seek out support with your help.

Demonstrate a range of communication skills for effective working relationships

Verbal skills

Verbal skills involve more than just talking. How you deliver messages and feedback and how you receive them requires an ability to speak clearly and effectively. Interpreting messages and acting upon the information gained is a skill. The ability to empathise, summarise, paraphrase and speak in a calm way is a skill that engages people and encourages them to open up in conversation.

Active listening

This involves asking questions, rephrasing the conversation to gain better understanding and paying attention to what the other person is saying. Sometimes you just need to remain silent, and this can be a difficult thing to do. Develop skills to listen and try not to jump in with a solution. Look at the other person's body language and learn from their actions. A good listener will do only that and not try to formulate their next question or their next response. In doing so you are not listening actively.

Questioning

Questioning in an open way is more effective than asking a lot of closed questions that require only a 'yes' or 'no' response. More information can be gained if the person is asked to expand on their response.

Written/electronic means

Emails and texts are good ways to send and receive messages, but you need to be aware of the tone and the way in which the message might be received. Because you cannot convey emotion within a text or show your body language, you must prepare the message in a clear and professional way. Some messages should not be delivered in this way as they can be perceived as cold and may damage a relationship.

Manage meetings to explore different aspects of working relationships and team meetings

People who attend a meeting need to know it will not drag on and that their time will be well spent. By setting out ground rules you can ensure that the meeting will be well run, and you can then keep control of proceedings. If the attendees are aware of how the agenda will be set and addressed and how long they are going to be in the meeting, you can ensure that the relevant aspects of the working relationship can be explored in a timely and efficient way. In team meetings you may need to ensure that everyone has an opportunity to respond if they need to and you may also have to keep general chat to a minimum.

Face-to-face meetings

These are most useful in imparting information that is too important to leave to an email or is sensitive in nature. If you are giving feedback to a member of staff or are meeting with a visitor or an individual using your service, this is the most appropriate way to talk. You then engage with verbal, non-verbal and listening communication, which enables you to gain a greater amount of information.

Digital conference/webinar

These are a useful way to keep in touch with external stakeholders and partners in other locations. The same advice applies here as for meetings but prior to this sort of meeting you will need to make additional checks to ensure that the Wi-Fi is working and you have the correct equipment in place to participate.

Evidence opportunity

3.1 Develop procedures to facilitate effective working relationships with colleagues

Discuss with your assessor how you develop procedures to facilitate effective working relationships with colleagues. Consider the topics you have covered in this section.

Research it

3.1 Procedures to facilitate effective working relationships with colleagues

Study the team you work with over the next couple of days and try to get to know the members in a little more detail. How do the features of effective team performance present themselves in your team?

Evaluate the effectiveness of current procedures in your setting that relate to working relationships with colleagues. For example, look at the appraisal systems and measures you have in place and use within supervision sessions. What do you think is good about the procedures and what might you change?

Think about how these were developed and say how they enable staff to develop effective working relationships. Supply evidence of this for your portfolio using relevant examples.

AC 3.2 Develop common objectives when working with colleagues ensuring they are agreed to

Here, you will be required to develop and agree common objectives when working with colleagues.

Agree objectives that are SMART when working with colleagues

See Unit 506, AC1.9 for more information on SMART objectives.

Use negotiation skills to ensure that colleagues agree with work-based targets to achieve objectives

Not everybody will agree with objectives or work targets that have been set so you will need to develop skills of negotiation to help in any situation where this happens.

Negotiating requires a planned approach, so to ensure that colleagues are in agreement with the targets set, you will need to meet with them to discuss and clarify the objectives, then look for a solution in which both parties are happy with the outcome.

Maintain focus on the overall aim of the working relationship

It is important to remember the reasons why you are in a working relationship and to focus staff on the need to provide a care service that puts the individual using the service first and staff issues second. Reminding your colleagues about the setting's commitment to the provision of a quality service may help.

Evidence opportunity

3.2 Develop and agree common objectives

Show your assessor how you develop and agree common objectives when working with colleagues, addressing the areas we have discussed here.

AC 3.3 Implement systems and practices that allow colleagues to make appropriate contributions using their specific expertise

Here, you will be required to implement systems and practices that demonstrate to colleagues that their expertise is valued and how their skills can be utilised.

Demonstrate that you value time taken to discuss issues

Meetings may be viewed as wasting time and taking staff away from the jobs they are doing. There may be some truth in this if the meetings are not well run, are lengthy and seem to achieve nothing. As the manager, it is important to ensure that your meetings are valued by staff. This is achieved by having a regular time set for discussion and an agenda that is specific and achievable in the time allocated. If you say the meeting will last one hour it is important to ensure that this happens. By setting boundaries, colleagues will start to value the time spent and will be more willing to contribute.

Demonstrate flexibility around working styles

Quality in the work you do is essential and must never be compromised. However, occasionally a creative approach can be offered that may prove to be a useful solution to a care issue. Sometimes your immediate reaction to a suggested change is to dismiss it and carry on with previous practice. However, just because somebody does the work in an alternative way does not make it wrong and you need to have some flexibility to accept individual expression and working style.

Show respect for contributions made by colleagues

No contribution should ever be dismissed even if it does not fully meet the objective. Too often new ideas are ignored simply because we are focused on the objective we need to achieve. Colleagues may be expressing excellent ideas and a good leader and manager will respectfully consider these and ask for clarification on them. Even if an idea is not immediately moving an objective forward, it may prove useful later.

Demonstrate acceptance of other's expertise

The humility to accept that there are colleagues who have expertise in certain areas is a quality in good leaders and managers; seeking input from colleagues to help with a decision is good practice. You should respect the fact that your colleagues have a wealth of experience from other employment and from the training and education they have undertaken, and as such can be a source of ideas and solutions. Their help to make decisions should not be underestimated or missed.

> **Evidence opportunity**
>
> **3.3 Enable colleagues to make appropriate contributions**
>
> Show your assessor how you implement systems and practices that enable colleagues to make appropriate contributions using their specific expertise. You could address, for example, the topics covered in this section.

AC 3.4 Work in ways that address conflicts or dilemmas constructively

Here, you will be required to show that you can manage conflicts or dilemmas that occur among colleagues.

Conflict

Conflict within teams is not uncommon but it can be unpleasant and can lead to disruption in performance. Badly managed conflict leads to ineffective teamwork as people start to avoid each other and rifts develop. This inevitably leads to ineffectual or weak care. However, when resolved effectively, conflict can be creative and productive, leading to personal and professional growth. It is important to be assertive and provide fair feedback on problems or areas of conflict.

Conflict should not always be viewed as a negative occurrence, however, as it may highlight an important issue and lead to a better outcome for all concerned. For example, in adult social care settings conflict between partners may arise if resources are threatened due to the introduction of another service. If staff feel that their role is undermined in any way by another service, this can lead to conflict. The main aims in any conflict resolution are to communicate, listen and keep an open mind about the situation.

The Research Briefing 41, 'Factors that promote and hinder joint and integrated working between health and social care services' commissioned by SCIE (2012) is a useful read and comments upon the findings from a large study about integrated (partnership) working. As this was published in 2012, although it may not reflect current policy, it still provides valuable guidance.

The factors that cause conflict include some of the following:

- lack of understanding about joint aims and objectives or failure to establish a shared purpose
- lack of clarity about roles and responsibilities
- confusion about policies and procedures underpinning the new service or way of working
- organisational difference or competing 'organisational visions' and lack of agreement about which organisation should lead
- absence of a pooled or shared budget and differences in resources and spending
- communicating across professional or agency boundaries, particularly when they are not located on the same site
- information sharing – difficulty sharing information, lack of access to information and incompatible IT systems
- lack of strong and appropriate managerial support (thought to undermine attempts to work across agencies and professional boundaries)
- different professional philosophies
- lack of trust, respect and control
- difficulties in role boundaries
- constant reorganisation
- financial uncertainty
- difficulty in recruiting staff.

Occasionally people involved in an individual's care, such as family members or members of the wider multidisciplinary team, may disagree about something in the setting and this needs to be dealt with in a sensitive and professional manner. There may be disagreements among other professionals or the family about the way in which care is given and this may be due to a lack of understanding about certain features of the care role. For example, the family or others involved in care may not understand the risk involved in certain lifestyle choices, such as eating unhealthily or the importance of ensuring that medication is given on time. This can lead to the individual being compromised and could cause conflict. The way in which this is handled needs to be specific to the person you are dealing with and will require a different approach to one you would use for care professionals.

Dealing constructively with conflicts or dilemmas

A conflict may fall into one of two categories:

- Conflict that revolves around disagreements in relation to approaches to work.
- Conflict that arises between individual members of the team stemming from differences in personal values and beliefs.

Thompson's (2006) RED model suggests an effective way of solving and managing conflict. He suggests:

R – Recognise the conflict; do not sweep it under the carpet.

E – Evaluate the conflict to see how detrimental it would be if it was allowed to develop.

D – Deal with the conflict; keep communication open.

The two destructive extremes, either pretending the conflict does not exist or overreacting to the situation, are best avoided, according to Thompson.

The most effective way of solving conflict in a team is for the people concerned to have a constructive conversation (LaFasto and Larson, 2001). By doing so, each person will be helped to see the other person's perspective and will gain some understanding about the way the other person feels about the situation. The conversation must result in each party committing to making improvements in the relationship (Tilmouth et al., 2011). These conversations might be initiated by the staff members themselves or they may require the services of a neutral facilitator or another person to mediate in the situation. This can be set up during supervision.

LaFasto and Larson's (2001) CONECT model for resolving conflict by conversation is useful:

- Commit to the relationship by discussing the relationship and not the problem causing concern. Each person should say why they feel change should occur and what they hope to gain.
- Optimise safety, with both parties committing to maintain confidentiality and create an atmosphere of trust.
- Neutralise defensiveness, with each person explaining what they have observed, how it made them feel and the long-term effects of the other person's actions.
- Explain each perspective or each side of the argument.
- Change one behaviour and ask each person to change.
- Track the change and decide how improvements will be measured. Agree to meet to discuss whether changes have been successful (Tilmouth et al., 2011).

Appropriate ways in which to deal with any barriers and conflicts that arise can be on a one-to-one basis or in group discussion. Providing information to enable individuals and the team involved in their care to make informed decisions may also help the process and reduce the conflict. Conflict may sometimes be the result of lack of information, which causes distress and may lead to angry outbursts.

You might also instigate contracts between people to highlight expectations with respect to roles and behaviour. This can then help to resolve potential conflict areas.

Another way in which conflict may be managed is through a mentoring system. By allocating a mentor to each staff member, conflicts can be brought to them for discussion and mediation.

The way in which you deal with and resolve conflict comes from your favoured leadership approach. The skills approach developed by Mumford et al. (2000) lists, within its five components, social judgement skills as one of the competencies required in dealing with conflict. The capacity to understand people and social systems serves to enable leaders to work with others to solve problems and to implement change. Part of this competency is social performance, and this refers to persuasion skills when communicating with others. Most conflict can be resolved if the leader acts as a mediator in the process.

Poor communication is often cited as a reason for underperformance and can also lead to conflict. Therefore, as a manager and leader of a team, you need to hone your communication skills and improve any deficit or shortfall where you can.

One aspect of communication is that of negotiation. Much of a manager's day is spent in negotiation with other people and it can become an almost unconscious activity. You may simply be setting up a meeting or planning care with a member of staff, but the way in which this is carried out can mean the difference between an effective outcome or a failed one. Successful negotiation is linked to assertiveness, and you should aim to negotiate in an open and flexible manner in order to achieve a positive outcome.

Conflict can also arise when staff are faced with dilemmas. When an incident occurs that goes against your own values and beliefs, you are faced with an ethical dilemma. For example, a dilemma may arise when you feel obliged to break confidentiality. You may feel that a member of the team is acting in a way that is not respectful to the individuals using the service. The dilemma you have is what to do with this information. You need to safeguard the individuals and you will be required to follow your organisation's vulnerable adults' procedure, but this means that the member of staff in question will need to be held accountable and this can have a detrimental effect on team morale.

Another example may include actions taken when you observe poor practice in the setting. While it is the correct course of action to report such matters, it may be difficult to do so if you believe somebody may lose their job because of this.

The dilemma that you as a manager need to reconcile is how far someone's right to make decisions for themselves can be supported when it conflicts with a professional obligation. The duty of the care worker is not to control others' lives, but to inform and support them in order that they can make good decisions for themselves, whether they are staff members or individuals using the service.

You might consider the following points when addressing a challenge to the team's effectiveness, whether it be due to a conflict or an ethical dilemma:

- Are you empathetic? Have you really considered what it feels like to be in the shoes of the particular team member with a problem?
- Can you seek clarification to make sure that you fully understand the other person's position and their needs?
- Are you calm or taking things personally?
- Are you prepared to support your case?
- Can you keep to the point and not allow yourself to be side-tracked?
- Can you offer a compromise?

Demonstrate calmness and acknowledge the feelings of colleagues

You may feel that you have little or no control over conflicts that arise and are faced with a colleague who is angry or upset that you will react with the fight or flight response, as you might with any kind of perceived threat. Your body will flood with adrenaline, and this will make it more difficult to remain calm. By taking a moment to breathe you start to control and calm those hormones and can make a more considered response.

Respond promptly when requested to provide support

To prevent a situation escalating you need to respond quickly and to treat all parties with respect. Care should be taken not to display behaviours that suggest you are criticising the parties involved or showing a lack of concern about them.

Take time to establish the causes of the conflict

Arguments may arise because of simple misunderstandings or poor communication. Listening to both parties helps you to understand how each person is feeling.

Demonstrate a non-judgemental approach

It is important to remain impartial and not to take sides. You need to listen to both parties' explanations and take care to keep your judgement to yourself until fully explored.

Case study

3.4 Deal constructively with conflicts or dilemmas

Here are some examples of situations where duty of care and responsibilities come into conflict. How might you deal with each of these dilemmas? Should they be supported and on what basis is this justified?

- An individual does not want confidential information to be shared with his daughter.
- An individual you see being treated disrespectfully by one of your colleagues does not want the incident reported.
- A staff member wants time to attend Mass when on duty on a Sunday.
- A carer refuses to undertake any further training on the basis that she has little time to do so.

Support colleagues to come to an amicable outcome

If you can get your colleagues to look at the bigger picture, they may start to gain a different perspective. They may begin to see the other person's point of view in a disagreement, and this can then lead to a solution that is agreeable to both parties. Reminding colleagues of their duty of care to the individual using the service and to the organisation may help them to reprioritise the way they are dealing with the situation and to look again at what has led to the conflict.

Show leadership when conflicts or dilemmas cannot be resolved amicably

If a solution is not agreeable to both parties, you may need to escalate it to another person. If you have a Human Resources department, they can help to negotiate a solution. Otherwise you will need to look at what can be agreed on, and then ask the parties to either agree to differ or negotiate a plan to move forward in some way.

Reflecting on practice

According to West (2004), in resolving conflict when people's needs are discovered, a solution can be found. We may be tempted to compromise, but compromise means that people's needs are still not fully met and this can lead to resentment.

Ensuring that conflicts are addressed in the right manner means that relationships are maintained and can function smoothly.

A conflict situation is never pleasant but by reflecting on the circumstances that led to the event and thinking about how it might have been handled in a different way you can sometimes find more useful ways of managing conflict should it arise again.

Evidence opportunity

3.4 Deal constructively with conflicts or dilemmas

Show your assessor how you manage and deal constructively with conflicts or dilemmas that occur. Address the topics discussed in this section.

Collect a piece of evidence or a witness testimony to show how you have handled a recent conflict in your area. What actions might you take or change next time?

Reflect on it

3.4 Conflict with colleagues and other professionals

Write a reflective account about a conflict or a dilemma that has arisen in the workplace, detailing how you dealt with it and what solutions you put forward. Did you experience any conflict throughout the process of working with others? Reflect on what you learned from this. Alternatively, write a reflective account about how you would use the following approaches to address conflicts and dilemmas that may arise between individuals, staff, carers, families and significant others:

- one-to-one discussion
- group discussion
- using contracts
- providing information to inform choices
- mentoring for conflict resolution.

Reflect on it

3.4 Managing conflict between colleagues

Explain how you have managed conflicts or dilemmas that occur among colleagues within the work setting and evaluate the impact of your style of conflict resolution. Describe how a different way of dealing with the same conflict might have changed the outcome.

How might you apply Thompson's RED model in relation to how you dealt with your situation?

AC 3.5 Evaluate own working relationships with colleagues

Here, you will be required to evaluate your own working relationships with colleagues.

Demonstrate self-reflection on performance in work role and engage in self-appraisal

Taking a step back and reflecting upon your aims and objectives, and occasionally on the way you do your job, can be refreshing and help you to gain a better picture of yourself. Self-reflection and appraisal are ways of gaining a better insight into your thoughts and behaviours and your performance and motivation. It helps you to look at the experiences you have and learn from them, making changes where necessary.

Engage colleagues in providing feedback on your performance and value feedback

Encouraging colleagues to give you feedback on how you are performing is a useful way to check your own evaluations. In teams where a culture of trust operates, your colleagues will be honest and you can accept the feedback and work it into future plans. Sometimes it may be a challenge to accept negative feedback but in reflecting upon what has been said you benefit from making changes that will lead to better working relationships.

Evidence opportunity

3.5 Evaluate working relationships with colleagues

Evaluate your own working relationships with colleagues.

LO4 Be able to work in partnerships with professionals and other agencies

AC 4.1 Negotiate with professionals in external agencies to agree objectives, roles and responsibilities, procedures, and ways of working for a specific task or area of work

Here, you will negotiate with professionals in other agencies to agree a specific task or area of work, including the topics we cover in this section.

There are a number of people with whom you will work in your role as manager. External to your own setting will be voluntary agencies and community network groups. You may also be involved with educational settings and sometimes expert user groups.

Understand the range of professionals and other agencies you may work with

You will work with many different people in the course of your duties including health professionals such as GPs, community nurses and care workers, physiotherapists and pharmacists, the local council, advocacy services, mental health workers and also charitable organisations such as Age UK or Citizens Advice.

Formal partnerships

This includes formal care professionals who are contracted and paid. These may be community care workers, community nurses or hospital nursing staff, physiotherapists or care home staff as well as other paid and contracted health professionals. Your partnerships with other paid professionals such as the GP service also come under this heading. These partnerships are in place by law and the way in which you relate to and communicate with these people will be more structured and bound by policy and procedure. Community facilities such as leisure centres and museums are also a good source of partnership working.

Informal partnerships

These are people who provide care but are unpaid. These include family members or friends. They could also be voluntary carers, support groups or faith groups that provide care for no fee. Commissioning agencies are also partners in adult social care services. The informality of the partnership means a different relationship is experienced and the way in which you communicate here will differ from your communication with formal partners. For example, it is unlikely that an informal carer will be expected to attend many meetings or be subject to audit and appraisal. Your relationship is likely to be more friendly and supportive.

Work collaboratively to agree partnership objectives and allocation of tasks and responsibilities

All partnerships thrive on effective communication and good relationships. Collaborating with professionals from external agencies should include agreeing shared objectives and responsibilities and tasks so that there is no overlap of duties, and each partner has a clear idea of what is expected of them.

Ensure that objectives are SMART

For an objective to have a successful outcome, it should be SMART. SMART objectives define the required result in a clear manner and the way in which this can be reached. Being specific about what is wanted and having a measure by which to check the outcome means that everyone will have a better understanding of what is required to achieve the goal. See Unit 506, AC1.9 for more information on SMART objectives.

Work with professionals and other agencies to agree timelines for monitoring progress

Alongside SMART objectives, clear timelines will show exactly when a project is to end and where progress needs to be shown at various points along the way. In this way, success of short-term targets can be celebrated as well as final ones, and the achievement of the project so far can be evaluated.

> **Evidence opportunity**
>
> **4.1 Negotiate with other agencies for a specific task or area of work**
>
> Show your assessor how you negotiate with professionals in other agencies to agree a specific task or area of work. Include the topics covered in this section.

AC 4.2 Use agreed ways of working within partnerships with professionals in external agencies to carry out own role and support others to carry out their responsibilities

Here, you will be required to use agreed ways of working to carry out your own role and support others to carry out their responsibilities.

Establish agreed ways of working that meet agreed objectives

As stated in AC4.1, when working with other professionals it is important that agreed ways of working are established at the outset so that consistency may be maintained.

Establish boundaries of role and responsibilities and agree timelines

While you are the manager in your setting, you may well be working alongside the manager of another similar setting and this will therefore require boundaries to be set as to the role and responsibility each of you will have for a project. These need to be agreed at the outset when you are setting the agenda and review dates for the work. Doing so will aid the process to clearly describe each person's part of the management of the project.

Open and respectful relationships with your partners will ensure that all involved will feel valued and want to make the partnership work, and as the manager you need to model this type of behaviour. For example, engaging with joint objectives and acknowledging the potential areas of conflict within a partnership may be useful and is one way to achieve co-operation to work towards a common goal. Your role will be to ensure that conflict is dealt with effectively and that you manage the partnership workers respectfully.

Reflect on it

4.2 Open communication and respectful relationships with partners

How do you ensure that there is open communication when working in partnership? Supply some evidence to demonstrate how you do this in your setting.

How can you model open, respectful and supportive relationships with partners? Make a list and provide this as evidence for your portfolio.

Evidence opportunities

4.2 Use agreed ways of working

Show your assessor how you use agreed ways of working to carry out your own role and support others to carry out their responsibilities, addressing the topics covered in this section.

AC 4.3 Work in ways that address challenges constructively to promote change

Here, you will show methods by which the challenges of partnership working can be addressed.

As already stated, the primary purpose of partnership working is to improve the experience and outcomes of people who use services, and this is achieved by minimising organisational barriers between different services. In addition, partnerships work by:

- delivering co-ordinated packages of services to individuals
- reducing the impact of organisational fragmentation
- bidding for, or gaining access to, new resources
- meeting a statutory requirement.

Partnership working is central to the care of individuals and brings together a variety of other services such as those in the voluntary sector. The King's Fund report 'Volunteering in health and care: Securing a sustainable future' describes volunteers as an important group who add significant value to the work of care professionals (The King's Fund, 2013). The research shows that volunteers help to improve people's experience of care, and also build stronger relationships between services and communities. The research suggests that volunteering could be an important part of a new and closer relationship with health services, so their critical role should be acknowledged.

You may also be working with other agencies within the wider multidisciplinary team such as advocacy agencies or other care teams. An advantage of working closely with other organisations is that they may be able to offer advice on specific issues. A disadvantage of relying purely on other organisations is that some may be affected by lack of funding, which may make it difficult for the sector to finance its work. Whatever challenges you face, as a manager it will be your responsibility to manage these.

Challenges

While partnership working has many advantages, its success depends on dealing constructively with challenges. With more formal partnerships such as with medical professionals, the challenges will be different than those with family members and may involve difficulties with time and scheduling meetings to suit everybody involved. There may also be professional challenges in which procedures or practice are questioned. For example, it might be difficult for a nurse to challenge the practice of, say, a GP even though the nurse may have more knowledge about the practice. The hierarchy within some services may, therefore, be a challenge.

Reflect on it

4.3 Challenges

Think about your own job role and that of one of your partners. It might be an external partner or even a partnership within your own service. It might be a member of a faith group or the local leisure centre. How do you feel when you need to challenge a decision they have made or when a support worker challenges a practice you have put in place?

Dealing constructively with challenges within partnership working

Systems leadership may be a starting point for addressing the challenge of partnership working. Changes to the NHS and to adult care over the last 50 years have meant that a different approach to leadership must be employed. One of the changes is that care organisations and their staff must work across services to meet the needs of the growing older population and the number of people with complex medical conditions who need care and support from different services.

KEY TERM

Systems leadership: How the best resources from other settings and disciplines can be used to bring about improvement and beneficial change across partnership systems in other organisations. The style of leadership is characterised by a belief that leadership is the responsibility of teams, rather than individuals, and is collaborative in nature.

The King's Fund has researched the value of systems leaders, which describe a type of collective leadership with 'everyone taking responsibility for the success of the organisations and systems in which they work' (Timmins, 2015).

This approach focuses on the belief that leadership is the responsibility of teams and not just the managers in an organisation.

The report shows that effective systems leaders are people who lead through influence and persuasion and who recognise the need to engage their peers in decision making. They recognise that improvements take time and that obstacles and resistance occur. One of the leaders interviewed stated that systems leaders succeed by 'being comfortable with chaos' (Timmins, 2015).

Timmins described systems leadership as 'an act of persuasion that needs to have an evidence base for change'. He stated that leaders can achieve anything as long they 'give away ownership' and 'don't want to take the credit for it' (Timmins, 2015). This approach may cause conflict with some partners or other professionals who are not fully in tune with a different way of working.

By entering into dialogue and taking time to explain how such a system may work you can deal constructively with some of the criticism that you may receive.

Agree ways of working to establish common ground

Your aim will be to provide a service that achieves a positive outcome for the individuals in your care, so you need to work towards establishing a mutual understanding about what is best for all.

Identify the causes of conflicts in a non-judgemental manner

Trying to establish common ground may lead to conflict and as a manager you may be required to take a step back and identify what is the cause and how it is best managed. Laying blame on one party will be destructive, so a non-judgemental and impartial approach must be taken.

Acknowledge the feelings of professionals and other agencies

Working in a calm, respectful manner with other agencies and professionals enables you to identify the information needed to support the outcome. You need to recognise that sometimes feelings run high, particularly when it comes to ways of working, and people may want to defend their profession's input into a project. This will require careful and considerate handling, acknowledging how others feel while negotiating a shared outcome.

Research it

4.3 Timmins Report

Read the Timmins report published by The King's Fund (Timmins, 2015). Explain how you could integrate systems leadership into your own style of leading the staff through partnership working.

Evidence opportunity

4.3 Dealing with challenges

Show your assessor how you deal constructively with challenges to partnership working. Consider the topics covered in this section.

AC 4.4 Deal constructively with poor practice, or failure to work in agreed ways

AC 4.5 Work in ways that address poor practice, or failure to work in agreed ways constructively

Here, you will be required to challenge any poor practice or failure to work in agreed ways and work in ways that address this constructively.

Agree ways of working that support the duty of care in line with legislative requirements (law of tort)

As a care professional, you have a duty to provide a standard of reasonable care, and failure to do so is punishable in law. In English tort law, the duty of care is a legal obligation and the absence of it must be established to proceed with any action in a claim for negligence. Anybody claiming against a care professional for negligence must be able to show a duty of care has been breached. As a manager you must determine with other care professionals that the duty of care is clearly understood and that any poor practice is dealt with quickly and efficiently.

Agree ways of recording and reporting poor practice

There should be agreement among partners over standard ways of reporting poor practice across all organisations and partners.

Challenge actions that could cause harm

Any poor practice needs to be challenged and brought to the attention of the manager. Therefore, whistle-blowing policies must be agreed. An agreement as to how poor practice will be dealt with should be drawn up. For example, a designated safeguarding officer who works with all the partners and to whom everyone can come with issues might be a way forward.

> **Evidence opportunity**
>
> **4.4 and 4.5 Challenge poor practice or failure to work in agreed ways**
>
> Show your assessor how you constructively challenge any poor practice or failure to work in agreed ways.

AC 4.6 Use communication and recording systems that comply with current legislation for information sharing between agencies

Here, you will be required to use communication and recording systems that comply with current legislation for information sharing between agencies.

Establish shared ways of working to support effective communication

Effective communication among partners needs to have a clear statement of purpose that outlines to all how it will help to achieve overall organisational objectives and how it will engage everybody effectively.

Support a problem-solving approach to communication issues

As a manager you will appreciate that communication problems can be detrimental to effective care delivery so will want to minimise these. Adopting a problem-solving approach, where transparent communication processes are preferred, enables all staff to freely express themselves. Effective communication facilitates dialogue between people in an environment of trust and safety.

Ensure that all professionals meet current legislative requirements for the recording and storage of information

Care work demands the keeping of records and their safe storage. When you are working with partners across locations this may become difficult. It is important that each partner agrees on the best way to record and store data and that this meets legislative requirements.

Establish regular meetings with professionals and other agencies

A regular meeting when all partners can discuss the objectives and the current achievement of objectives against performance indicators will ensure that the focus remains firmly on the individuals using the service. The meeting, which may be fortnightly, monthly or quarterly, should be one in which representatives from all areas of the partnership can contribute and then feed back to the wider team. Digital technology makes this process a lot easier. By setting up regular meetings online using a virtual meeting platform or conference calls, remote teams can meet more easily.

Evidence opportunity

4.6 Implement communication and recording systems

Show your assessor how you use communication and recording systems that comply with current legislation for information sharing between agencies.

AC 4.7 Evaluate the effectiveness of partnership work and the processes that underpin it

Here, you will be required to evaluate the effectiveness of partnership work and processes that underpin it and see agreement for improvements.

Agree timelines for evaluating work objectives with professionals and other agencies

Evaluation is an essential part of quality improvement and is how you determine the merit or value of the care being given. In evaluating objectives, you engage in a process to improve the care and to enhance decisions being made, and this needs to be done at regular times throughout the work rather than at a single end point. As the manager in a setting, it is useful to agree a timeline with other agencies to check this is done.

Agree processes for evaluating work objectives and the impact on individuals

Agreeing the type of evaluation to be carried out will impact the way in which the evaluation data can be used. For example, a summative evaluation 'sums up' the effect of the intervention and comes at the end, helping the team to determine whether the objective has been met or not. It is useful for judging the overall worth of an intervention. Alternatively, you may decide that formative evaluation should be used, as this approach provides information about how things are developing as the project is happening and helps the team to see whether improvement has been achieved. It also helps to see how it has occurred in their particular environment.

Agree how reflection from all parties will contribute to any evaluative process

Evaluating the ways of working with partnerships is a crucial process to ensure that quality improvement in care is ongoing. Successful care can be celebrated, and lessons can also be learned from mistakes that may have happened. Poor evaluation can undermine care. It should be agreed with professionals and other agencies that the outcomes of evaluations and reflection will be recorded and reported to all parties.

Evidence opportunity

4.7 Evaluate the effectiveness of partnership work

Speak to your assessor or provide a written account evaluating the effectiveness of partnership work and the processes that underpin it and how you seek agreement for improvements.

AC 4.8 Negotiate agreement for improvements for the effectiveness of partnership work

Here, you will be required to work with other organisations to best support the needs of the individual in an effective way.

Clarify how staff will work with individuals and the partners

Partnerships must ensure that individuals are able to make their own decisions about the care they receive. Occasionally, staff may find it difficult to step back from giving the care that they deem necessary, but which disempowers the individual. For example, it might speed up the process if staff simply step in and carry out the care the individual needs, but this may not be in the best interest of the individual. As a manager you will need to support your staff in this and recognise that sometimes more time for care may be needed. Partners should also be aware of this and work together.

You may need to develop a plan of action to give staff access to training to ensure that they fully appreciate all the issues surrounding outcome-based care.

Individuals and their families must have correct information on the rights of the individual in care and who is going to provide the care. During the admission process, it is useful to engage with the individual and their family and inform them of the various acts that may have a bearing on the individual's wellbeing. For example, you may like to discuss the concept of capacity and what might happen should the individual be unable to make a decision about their care in the future. You also need to talk about the partners who will be involved in the care giving.

All organisations coming together to deliver care must be clear about why they are doing this and what the vision of the partnership is. This process is important so that each participant understands what they are signing up to and are able to buy into the vision of the partnership. There should be an agreement in place to formally sign up to the partnership on behalf of their respective boards, staff and beneficiaries. It is essential that governance arrangements are clearly defined and built into any agreement.

Strong leadership is required to support people through the discomfort of change. Even if partnership working is clearly improving services, there may still be unease with some staff and key stakeholders so continual negotiation and collaboration must be ongoing.

Research it

4.8 Negotiate agreement for improvements for the effectiveness of partnership work

Find out about the systems in place in your setting that encourage and enable partnership working. Add notes to your portfolio.

Evidence opportunity

4.8 Negotiate agreement for improvements for the effectiveness of partnership work

Show your assessor how your partnerships encourage and enable engagement in decision making and reviews.

Legislation

Legislation	Key points
Health and Care Act 2022	This Act introduced new legislation to make it easier for health and care organisations to deliver joined-up, integrated care for people who rely on different services. It builds on the recommendations put forward by NHS England and NHS Improvement.
Health and Social Care Act 2012	This Act introduced the role of the Care Quality Commission. Safeguarding and protection of individuals are specifically mentioned in these laws to address concerns about abuse. The Act aims to safeguard people who use care services from suffering any form of abuse or improper treatment while receiving care and treatment. To meet the requirements under this Act providers must demonstrate zero tolerance of abuse, unlawful discrimination and restraint.
Care Act 2014	Replaces previous laws to provide a coherent approach to adult social care. It set out duties for local authorities and partners, and rights for individuals and carers. It aims to ensure that: • fairer care and support are given to individuals • support for physical, mental and emotional wellbeing is offered to the person needing care and their carer • prevention and delay of the need for care and support are avoided • people are in control of their care.
Health and Social Care (Safety and Quality) Act 2015	Confers a duty on health and adult social care providers to share information about a person's care with other health and care professionals. It also makes provision about the safety of social care services in England, particularly with respect to the integration of information relating to users of social care services in England.
NHS Long Term Plan 2019	This made a commitment to give more power to individuals to manage their own care and support to make their own informed decisions.

References

Accounting Solutions Ltd (2020) 'The four quadrants of time management'. https://asl.co.nz/timemanagement/

Adair, J. (2000) *Effective Teambuilding: How to make a winning team*. London: Pan Macmillan.

Barnes, C. and Mercer, G. (eds) (2004) *Disability Policy and Practice: Applying the Social Model*. Leeds: The Disability Press.

Bonham, P. (2004) *Communication as a Mental Health Carer*. Cheltenham: Nelson Thornes.

Burnard, P. (2005) *Counselling Skills for Health Professions*. Cheltenham: Nelson Thornes.

Care Quality Commission (2022) 'Promoting partnership working to drive experiences and outcomes for people'. www.cqc.org.uk/news/stories/promoting-partnership-working-drive-better-experiences-outcomes-people

Covey, S.R. (2004) *The 7 Habits of Highly Effective People*. New York: Simon & Schuster.

Department of Health and Social Care (2022) 'Guidance: Expected ways of working between integrated care partnerships and adult social care providers'. www.gov.uk/government/publications/adult-social-care-principles-for-integrated-care-partnerships/expected-ways-of-working-between-integrated-care-providers-and-adult-social-care-providers

Department of Health and Social Care and Social Partnership Forum (2022) 'Social Partnership Forum – partnership agreement'. www.socialpartnershipforum.org/system/files/2022-07/Social-Partnership-Forum-Partnership-Agreement-2022.pdf

George, B. (2003) *Authentic Leadership: Rediscovering the secrets to creating lasting value*. San Francisco, CA: Jossey-Bass.

GOV.UK (2022) 'Policy paper: Health and social care integration: Joining up care for people, places and populations'. www.gov.uk/government/publications/health-and-social-care-integration-joining-up-care-for-people-places-and-populations

Health Foundation, The (2014) 'Person-centred care made simple'. www.health.org.uk/sites/health/files/PersonCentredCareMadeSimple.pdf

Helen Sanderson Associates (2015) 'All about outcomes'. http://helensandersonassociates.co.uk/outcomes/

King's Fund, The (2013) 'Volunteering in health and care: Securing a sustainable future'. www.kingsfund.org.uk/sites/default/files/field/field_publication_file/volunteering-in-health-and-social-care-kingsfund-mar13.pdf

LaFasto, F.M.J. and Larson, C.E. (2001) *When Teams Work Best: 6,000 team members and leaders tell what it takes to succeed*. Thousand Oaks, CA: Sage Publications.

Larson, C.E. and LaFasto, F.M.J. (1989) *Teamwork: What must go right/what can go wrong*. London: Sage Publications.

McKibbon, J., Walton, A. and Mason, L. (2008) *Leadership and Management in Health and Social Care*. London: Heinemann.

Mumford, M.D., Zaccharo, S.J., Connolly, M.S. and Marks, M.A. (2000) 'Leadership skill: Conclusions and future directions', *Leadership Quarterly*, 11(1): 155–70.

NHS England (2016) 'Joint review of investment in voluntary, community and social enterprise organisations in the health and care sector'. https://assets.publishing.service.gov.uk/government/uploads/system/uploads/attachment_data/file/524243/VCSE_Investment_Review_A.pdf

Nolan, M.R., Brown, J., Davies, S., Nolan, J. and Keady, J. (2006) 'The senses framework: Improving care for older people through a relationship-centred approach. Getting Research into Practice (GRiP) Report No 2'. Available from Sheffield Hallam University Research Archive (SHURA): http://shura.shu.ac.uk/280/

Primacare Living Solutions (n.d.) 'Innovations in care'. www.primacareliving.com/butterfly-model-of-care

Qureshi, H., Bamford, C., Nicholas, E., Patmore, C. and Harris, J. (2000) *Outcomes in Social Care Practice: Developing an outcome focus in care management and user surveys*. York: Social Policy Research Unit, University of York.

Rogers, C. (2002) *Client Centred Therapy*. London: Constable.

Social Care Institute for Excellence (2012) *The Research Briefing 41: Factors that promote and hinder joint and integrated working between health and social care services*. London: TSO.

Social Care Institute for Excellence (2015) 'Co-production in social care: What it is and how to do it, Guide 51'. www.scie.org.uk/co-production/what-how

Social Care Institute for Excellence (2020) 'Risk identification and virtual interventions for social workers'. www.scie.org.uk/care-providers/coronavirus-covid-19/social-workers/risk-identification

Social Care Institute for Excellence (2022) 'Co-production: What it is and how to do it'. www.scie.org.uk/co-production/what-how#whatis

Thompson, N. (2006) *People Problems*. Basingstoke: Palgrave Macmillan.

Tilmouth, T., Davies-Ward, E. and Williams, B. (2011) *Foundation Degree in Health and Social Care*. London: Hodder Education.

Timmins, N. (2015) *The Practice of System Leadership. Being comfortable with chaos.* London: The King's Fund. www.kingsfund.org.uk/publications/practice-system-leadership

West, M. (1994) *Effective Teamwork: Personal and professional development*. London: Blackwell.

West, M. (2004) *Effective Teamwork: Practical lessons from organizational research*. London: Wiley and Sons.

Yoder-Wise, P.S. (2007) *Leading and Managing in Nursing*. St. Louis: Mosby/Elsevier.

Useful resources and further reading

Griffith, R. (2015) 'Understanding the Code: Working in partnership', *British Journal of Community Nursing*, 20(5): 250–2.

Hunter, D. and Perkins, N. (2014) *Partnership Working in Public Health*. Bristol: Policy Press.

Innes, A., Macpherson, S. and McCabe, I. (2006) *Promoting Person-Centred Care at the Front Line*. York: Joseph Rowntree Foundation/SCIE.

Johns, C. (2000) *Becoming a Reflective Practitioner*. Oxford: Blackwell.

Nursing and Midwifery Council (2015) 'The Code: Professional standards of practice and behaviour for nurses and midwives'. www.nmc-uk.org/code

Reed, J., MacFarlane, A. and Clarke, C. (2011) *Nursing Older Adults: Partnership working*. Maidenhead: McGraw-Hill.

Rolfe, G., Jasper, M. and Freshwater, D. (2011) *Critical Reflection in Practice: Generating knowledge for care* (2e). London: Palgrave Macmillan.

Skills for Care (n.d.) 'Practical approaches to working in partnership: Practical examples of partnerships with adult social care providers'. www.skillsforcare.org.uk/resources/documents/Support-for-leaders-and-managers/Support-for-Registered-managers/Webinars/Leading-your-service/Practical-examples-of-partnerships-with-adult-social-care-providers.pdf

Social Care Institute for Excellence. www.scie.org.uk

Unit 510

Leading practice to manage comments and complaints

GLH 20

About this unit

As an adult social care provider you will, from time to time, have to deal with complaints from individuals using your service and perhaps from other providers or staff. While any mistakes that may have been made cannot be changed, people need to know that they will not happen again and assurances given that improvements will be made.

As a manager you must be aware of the requirements of the Health and Social Care Act 2008 (Regulated Activities) Regulations 2014. Regulation 16 specifies that you must have an effective and accessible system in place to identify, handle and respond to any received complaints from people using the service, or those people acting for them.

This unit will cover how to manage and deal with comments and complaints and how to lead good practice.

Learning outcomes

By the end of this unit, you will:

1 Understand the management of comments and complaints.

2 Be able to lead practice in acknowledging and responding to comments and complaints.

Getting started

Before you study the unit, think about the following:

- What comments and complaints have you received about the setting over the last year?
- Did you use the positive comments and deal with the complaints in a timely and efficient manner?
- How might you change the process of dealing with comments and complaints to ensure that you have a robust system in place?

LO1 Understand the management of comments and complaints

It is important that concerns and complaints procedures are not only visible in the workplace, but that staff and visitors are using the systems to manage situations that may involve safeguarding and risk management issues. Systems and processes that function poorly, or are not used, make it difficult for people to deliver high-quality care and this may be because staff do not use the information or, more simply, cannot find it. As the manager, you need to ensure not only that staff and visitors are aware of the policies, but that safeguarding is part of the cultural ethos of the setting and is embedded into the ways of working.

AC 1.1 Describe regulatory requirements, codes of practice and guidance for managing comments and complaints

Here, you will be required to describe that you know and understand current regulatory requirements, codes of practice and guidance for managing concerns and complaints.

Health and Social Care Act 2008 (Regulated Activities) Regulations 2014

Regulation 16 of this Act ensures that people can make a complaint about their care and treatment, and to do this you, as the manager, must ensure that the setting has effective systems for handling and responding to complaints from the individuals using your service. Complaints to regulated services must be investigated effectively and action taken rapidly. When a complaint is made, the care provider must provide the CQC with a summary of complaints and their response. Failure to do so may result in prosecution.

The Fundamental Standards state that a person in care must be able to complain about their care and treatment through the care provider's systems and that there will be a response to the complaint, which will be investigated.

Care Act 2014

The Care Act introduced a general duty on local authorities to promote an individual's wellbeing, and to have this in mind when planning and making decisions about them or their care.

Any individual who is not happy with their treatment or assessments is eligible to make a claim to social services, which should have a complaints procedure. If, after following the complaints process, the individual is unhappy with the outcome, a complaint can be made to the Local Government and Social Care Ombudsman (LGSCO).

Any safeguarding issue needs to be raised through organisational procedures.

Data Protection Act 2018

The Data Protection Act 2018, which is the UK's implementation of the General Data Protection Regulation (GDPR), enables people to raise complaints about misuse of data through the courts.

Public Interest Disclosure Act 1998

The Public Interest Disclosure Act 1998 describes the meaning of whistle blowing and ensures that protected disclosure is afforded to all who make a complaint. Section 19 of the Act introduces protection for whistle blowers from bullying or harassment by co-workers.

Health and Care Act 2022

This Act states that all services must adhere to national quality standards, and that there need to be procedures in place to assure quality and safeguarding and to consider complaints and commendations.

AC 1.2 Analyse the relationship between the management of comments and complaints and risk management and safeguarding

Here, you will analyse responses to comments and complaints and the processes of risk assessments and safeguarding.

Comments and complaints

Feedback in the form of positive comments and complaints should be dealt with in a positive way. You may have a system to receive suggestions from individuals using the service and using these to improve the service may prevent complaints from being made in the future.

Any complaints that are made need to be dealt with immediately to prevent issues escalating. Individuals, their carers and staff in the setting must feel comfortable raising issues and be assured of a prompt response and action taken. A badly handled complaint will affect the setting's reputation.

A positive acceptance of complaints as a way to improve service shows a responsive and open way of influencing change in the service.

Risk management

As a manager you will be familiar with the need to conduct risk assessments, and it is important that they are conducted with the individual and their family in attendance, if this is the wish of the individual. A situational approach needs to be taken here as not all individuals will have family to help or will want them to be involved. Adopting a person-centred approach requires that the choices and preferences of the individual are weighed against the anticipated risk and discussed with all concerned. When you enter into a contract of care with an individual you assume duties and obligations, which include respect for dignity and diversity and the promotion of equality and fairness. A risk assessment and subsequent action plan to which all involved agree does not mean that all risks are eliminated but that they are managed according to safe guidelines to which all agree.

Safeguarding

Individuals and their families need to be clear about how they can make a complaint without fear of recrimination. They also need to be reassured that any issue they raise will be dealt with rapidly. They must be advised that a whistle-blowing policy is in place and how they might use it should they wish to raise a concern.

Staff and partners from other agencies must be informed of the information that individuals and their families are given and should take responsibility for ensuring that they are well informed of the processes involved in safeguarding.

The Code of Conduct for Healthcare Support Workers and Adult Social Care Workers in England (Skills for Care and Skills for Health, 2013) outlines the duty of care to all those receiving care and support. As a legal requirement, staff are required to promote wellbeing and make sure that people are kept safe from harm, abuse and injury.

Reflect on it

1.2 Receiving complaints

Think about how you view the receipt of a complaint about the service. Do you see it as a failure or a way to make a change? Canvas staff and ask how they view receiving complaints. Is there a mindset change needed?

Is there a link between risk assessments carried out and the receipt of complaints? Might a change be required to ensure that risk assessments are carried out in a more efficient manner to remove the risk of a future complaint happening?

AC 1.3 Explain why those using services and others may be reluctant to comment or complain

Here, you will explain the reasons why an individual might feel unable or unwilling to comment or complain.

All individuals, their families, friends, carers and other practitioners involved in their care need to feel able to raise concerns if they are unhappy with aspects of the care.

Raising a complaint is difficult at any time, but in care the individuals, their families and friends may feel they will be treated differently if they do so. They may fear recrimination and therefore be reluctant to divulge cases of poor care and ill treatment at the hands of staff. They need to be sure that a complaint will be dealt with fairly and confidentially. If there is not a culture of trust in the setting this becomes even more problematic, so complaints to an external agency may be necessary.

Evidence opportunity

1.3 and 1.4 Developing a culture of trust in which to raise complaints

Explain why people may be reluctant to raise concerns. How can you develop a culture of trust in which individuals using your service feel safe to raise complaints or concerns?

AC 1.4 Describe attitudes and approaches that ensure comments and complaints inform continuous improvement of the setting/service

Here, you will describe your comments and complaints procedure and identify methods of ensuring that these are continually improved.

All people who enter your setting, whether they are team members, family/carers, visitors, volunteers, partners or other internal/external stakeholders, must be aware of the setting's culture and ethos. They need to be assured that feedback they give about practice will be received well and acted upon and that a culture of trust and openness is practiced throughout. They must be confident that no recrimination will occur if they need to complain.

When things go wrong, complaints will be made, and this will provide evidence of areas where your setting needs to improve. When you see areas that need improvement in your practices you can adjust the policies and procedures to address this. Handling complaints well can provide constructive opportunities for improvement. It might be that the team require extra training or closer supervision, and this can be monitored through complaints.

Complaints must be a priority for you, as failure to address them can lead to failure of the setting as people may start to lose faith in the care delivery and the staff. They must be dealt with as a matter of urgency and recorded accurately according to the processes outlined by the organisation. Confidentiality must be maintained throughout the process. Records need to be logged and reports made to the CQC.

It is also good practice to use information about concerns or complaints as a regular agenda item at team meetings, as this helps to keep staff mindful of the quality of their work and the need to address issues responsibly and honestly. Rather than apportioning blame to those involved in a complaint, lessons need to be learned and addressed. Any trends that emerge need to be risk assessed and reviewed to determine whether changes to work patterns and ways of working need to be made. Your annual service review should address what happened and what changes were made to address the complaints.

Making explicit use of lessons learned from concerns or complaints in service improvement plans, setting SMART targets and monitoring their achievement is a good way of developing the team and the setting. By setting specific and achievable goals about what needs to be done and putting into place tools to measure achievement and timeframes, improvements can be more effectively monitored.

Evidence opportunity

1.4 Improve handling of complaints

Identify your complaints procedure and describe how improvement plans are put into place.

AC 1.5 Describe ways of managing complaints which can be unreasonably persistent and abusive

Here, you will identify types of complaints that are persistent or abusive and describe how these can be effectively managed.

Persistent complaints

Repeat complaints may include those about issues that have already been dealt with or complaining about an issue without justified evidence. Sometimes the complainant will change the basis of the complaint, just to be heard. This can be frustrating to handle because emotions often run high, and you may start to feel angry and be unable to handle the situation effectively. The first step is to consider what the person is complaining about and why they are continuing to make the same complaint. A person who repeatedly complains may do so out of frustration or anger and feel unheard. By actively listening to them and asking questions you may be able to get to the bottom of their concerns.

When complaining, the person may also become very agitated, making it more difficult to reason with them. Remaining calm and professional is essential as you need to take control of the situation before it escalates.

Details of the complaint should be made available, so the complainant can be confident you are aware of the situation and can see what action has been taken already. A consistent approach will ensure that the complainant feels that their case is being taken seriously. Your team must adopt the same approach as you when dealing with persistent complainers, so make sure they know how to handle such people.

Abusive or unreasonable behaviour

If the situation is not being controlled then the complainant may resort to unacceptable behaviour, which has the potential to cause harm, injury or negatively impact the health and safety of you and your staff. The person may start to become abusive towards colleagues and make unfounded allegations. You need to be able to distinguish between persistent, but reasonable comments and complaints and those which are unreasonable or abusive. Even if a complaint has some truth in it a complainant's behaviour can still become unacceptable and even abusive.

Unreasonable behaviour is anything that might impact your staff and their work. Persistent emails or telephone calls about a complaint that do not provide new information may not appear to be severe, but they impact staff time and resources. Repeatedly demanding responses and insisting on speaking to the person in charge may also impact time.

Appointing a named point of contact in the setting to deal with the complainant may help. The member of staff who is going to deal with the complaint needs to be clear about how they would like the complainant's behaviour to change and should inform them why their behaviour is unacceptable or unreasonable. When dealing with violent and abusive outbursts, staff must remind the complainant such behaviour will not be tolerated. If the complainant informs staff of health concerns or disabilities they have, then staff need to adjust to this and be aware of their legal responsibilities under the terms of the Equality Act 2010. However, verbal abuse or violent behaviour of any kind should not be tolerated by staff under any circumstances.

The LGSCO makes decisions on complaints about councils or adult care providers in England and it is able to investigate individual complaints about councils, adult social care providers (including care homes and home care agencies) and other public service organisations.

Evidence opportunity

1.5 De-escalating conflict

Describe how you would deal with a person who is complaining and becoming increasingly angry. How could you de-escalate the situation?

LO2 Be able to lead practice in acknowledging and responding to comments and complaints

AC 2.1 Support team members to understand systems and procedures that ensure comments and complaints are actioned appropriately

Here, you will be required to show you can support team members to understand systems and processes relating to concerns and complaints, as well as to ensure that information and support are in place to enable individuals using services and their carers to raise concerns and make complaints when they wish to do so.

What is a complaint?

A complaint is the expression of dissatisfaction about an act, omission, decision or a service and may arise from the actions of a member of staff or an individual using the service.

When a complaint is made, a situational approach needs to be taken to determine what can be fixed immediately and what requires more in-depth investigation. Staff also need to be aware of individuals who have communication difficulties and may not be able to verbalise how they are feeling.

The type of complaint may be about:

- poor-quality care or the way the fees and charges are being handled
- poor complaint handling and delay in response
- assessments of need and safety and safeguarding.

Informing staff and others about procedures for complaints and concerns

Staff members and other professional and external agencies must be informed about the current procedures for complaints and concerns. Regular meetings addressing complaints and concerns, and discussions about how information is used, recorded and monitored should be a transparent process within the organisation. In this way staff will be more willing to take responsibility for the process.

Monitoring training

Staff training in relation to handling complaints and concerns should be recorded on the member of staff's individual personal development plan and on the plan in the setting's training record. Any training undertaken needs to be accurately recorded and audited.

Acknowledging anxiety about receiving concerns and complaints

Nobody likes to have complaints lodged against them and should this happen, a culture of no blame must be adopted. As a manager you should discuss the complaint with the member of staff and check that they are supported to make changes. You might find it helpful to use an improvement performance tool in such a situation. This begins by evaluating the employee's current performance to try to find out what might have gone wrong in this instance. Goals for improvement can then be set and performance monitored to see if their practice has changed. It is important that the member of staff takes responsibility for the complaint and the need to improve and for you to provide any necessary support to foster and facilitate this.

Acknowledging anxiety about raising concerns and the importance of whistle blowing

Staff may be anxious about repercussions when making a whistle-blowing claim, particularly when it involves a member of the team. Developing a climate of trust will mean staff are open and honest about their dealings with each other. If they notice poor practice, they should be encouraged to talk to each other in the first instance and then take concerns to the manager if they feel no change has happened. Team meetings can instil in staff the need to be vigilant about noticing when staff are struggling in their work and when they require support. If poor practice is noticed it should be challenged and further support provided.

Demonstrating a non-judgemental approach to those who raise a concern or make a complaint

If staff want to talk further about their concerns, they need to know that as the manager you will listen impartially and not judge them. An open-door policy means you are available at all times to discuss such issues and will do so confidentially. Individuals and their families must also clearly understand that they can approach you when they feel the need to and that they are welcome to discuss any issues with you.

As a manager you should discuss the complaint with the member of staff and check that they are supported to make changes. Again, an improvement performance tool may be useful.

Stretch and challenge

2.1 Creating a SMART target to respond to complaints

Create a SMART target to address a recent issue in your workplace that requires action to respond to a complaint or concern.

AC 2.2 Ensure accessible information and support is in place to enable, empower and encourage individuals and others

Here, you will be required to show how information is disseminated to team members and individuals in order for them to be able to raise comments and complaints and understand the complaints process.

Raising comments and complaints

Comments and complaints can arise from various sources. For example, you may receive positive comments or complaints through social media and via surveys of individuals using the service. You may also receive comments from regulatory bodies and partners that require actions.

You need to consider how you deliver comments and complaints to others in the setting. Sharing positive comments with the team is a powerful way of developing trust and an open culture. The way you deliver a complaint will need to be handled sensitively and in a fair and open way, without any display of anger or recrimination.

If the culture in your setting advocates fairness, openness and honesty, then feedback and complaints will be viewed in a positive way. Rather than viewing a complaint as a threat, it should be seen as an opportunity to improve things. Staff need to feel that problems picked up at an early stage will highlight poor practice which can then be put right. Staff and visitors should feel confident that their complaint or comment will be acted upon and their views heard.

Regulation 16 of the Health and Social Care Act 2008 (Regulated Activities) Regulations 2014 states that settings 'must establish and operate effectively an accessible system for identifying, receiving, recording, handling and responding to complaints by service users and other persons in relation to the carrying on of the regulated activity.' All staff need to know how to raise issues and understand how any feedback they give will be used and by whom.

SCIE offers guidance about how to deal with complaints. Staff must be briefed on the complaints procedure and short response timescales should be in place. The person complaining should be kept informed of the progress of the actions being taken and a clear report of the outcome of the complaint must be made. See SCIE (2020).

Follow-up on comments and complaints

Complaints made about things that have happened cannot be changed but you can take steps to ensure that they do not happen again. By recognising that a mistake has been made, and an authentic apology issued, the complainant can be assured that improvements will be put in place. This sort of response given verbally at first and then followed up in writing can give details of how the complaint was investigated, what the findings were and what further actions have been taken. Timescales for monitoring progress can be set and a next steps comment about what to do if they are not happy with the way the complaint has been handled can be put in place.

A follow-up meeting with the complainant at a later date to ensure that they are happy with the outcome is good practice.

Reflect on it

2.2 Deal effectively with comments and complaints

Think about how you deal with comments and complaints. Could there be a more efficient way in which you do this?

How do you ensure that the comments and complaints received are dealt with effectively and in a timely manner?

AC 2.3 Implement open and transparent systems and procedures

Here, you will demonstrate how to implement systems that ensure that team members feel that their complaints are dealt with in an open and transparent way.

Compassionately acknowledge comments and complaints

A feedback form that enables a complaint to be set out clearly, has space for the complainant's details and which gives an approximate timescale during which the complaint will be dealt with is a useful document to have in the setting. If the complainant wishes to escalate their complaint to a higher level, they can find out more on the Department of Health and Social Care website.

If you receive a complaint, your role is to listen well to what is being said. Remember that any comment or complaint is valuable feedback for your setting and gives you an opportunity to improve. Your team should also be encouraged to view the feedback positively.

Active listening

Active listening shows that you are concerned about what the person is saying to you and using skills such as repeating and paraphrasing their words demonstrates this. They need to know that you understand the problem. Using phrases such as 'I understand' and 'I see' can also help to build trust and rapport.

Respectful questioning

Respectful questioning is a useful skill to develop when dealing with complaints or comments. Such questions are non-judgemental, non-threatening and non-accusatory. It is easy to listen, but if the questions you ask are not respectful you will not achieve a good outcome from the discussion. In dealing respectfully with a complaint, avoid questions that start with 'why', as this word is often judgemental. Think about the question, 'Why did you do that?' There is an accusatory tone to it and the person answering is likely to feel defensive when trying to answer it. Instead, ask questions such as 'What went wrong?' and 'What can we do better?' An apology and respectful questions to elicit information about what the person needs you to do is more likely to be received well.

Respond to comments and complaints within agreed time frames

A complaint should be acknowledged immediately. This is the protocol adopted by local authorities. A full response should be issued within 10 working days. As some complaints take longer to resolve, it is good practice to let the complainant know why it will take longer.

AC 2.4 Implement learning from comments and complaints to drive improvements to the setting/service

Here, you will show how your setting can improve through learning from complaints and comments.

Complaints can provide feedback to elicit a change so, rather than viewing them negatively, try to view them as opportunities for practice to change and improve. Failure to adopt this attitude may result in further complaints being made to regulatory agencies and your setting having to deal with additional inspections and further worry.

Evidence opportunity

2.4 Improving your service

Explain how you have used comments and complaints to improve your service.

Legislation

Legislation	Key points
Data Protection Act 2018	The Data Protection Act 2018 replaced the Data Protection Act 1998. The Act enables people to raise complaints about misuse of data through the courts.
Health and Social Care Act 2008 (Regulated Activities) Regulations 2014	Regulation 16 specifies that settings must have an effective and accessible system in place to identify, handle and respond to any received complaints from people using the service, or those people acting for them.

References

Skills for Care and Skills for Health (2013) 'Code of Conduct for Healthcare Support Workers and Adult Social Care Workers in England'. www.skillsforcare.org.uk/resources/documents/Support-for-leaders-and-managers/Managing-people/Code-of-conduct/Code-of-Conduct.pdf

Social Care Institute for Excellence (2020) 'Dealing with concerns from people who use care services'. www.scie.org.uk/care-providers/concerns/dealing-with

Useful resources and further reading

Care Quality Commission (2022) 'Regulations for service providers and managers: Related guidance'. www.cqc.org.uk/guidance-providers/regulations-enforcement/regulations-service-providers-managers-related-guidance

Francis, R (2013) *Report of the Mid Staffordshire NHS Foundation Trust Public Inquiry*. London: TSO. https://assets.publishing.service.gov.uk/government/uploads/system/uploads/attachment_data/file/279124/0947.pdf

GOV.UK (2016) *Joint Review of Partnerships and Investment in Voluntary, Community and Social Enterprise Organisations*. London: TSO.

Local Government and Social Care Ombudsman www.lgo.org.uk/

Peters, S. (2012) The *Chimp Paradox: The mind management programme to help you achieve success, confidence and happiness*. London: Vermilion.

Public Health England (2017) *Reducing Health Inequalities: System, scale and sustainability*. London: PHE Publications.

Roberts, G.W. and Machon, A. (2015) *Appreciative Healthcare Practice: A guide to compassionate, person-centred care*. Keswick: M&K Publishing.

Skills for Care (2014) *The Care Certificate Standard 7: Privacy and dignity. What you need to know.* www.skillsforcare.org.uk/Documents/Learning-and-development/Care-Certificate/Standard-7.pdf

Social Care Institute for Excellence (2016) *Dignity in Care, Social Care Institute for Excellence Practice Guide 9*. London: SCIE.

Social Care Institute for Excellence (2017) 'DoLS: Best interests assessment'. www.scie.org.uk/mca/dols/practice/assessments/best-interests

Unit 511

Leading the vision of an adult care setting/service

GLH 22

About this unit

In this unit you will learn why compelling mission and vision statements for your organisation, together with clear methods of managing change, are important.

Your organisation's mission statement shows the purpose and direction the organisation is heading in. The vision statement clearly shows where the organisation wants to be in the future and should be accompanied by strategies for realising that vision. It communicates your organisation's values and its commitment to achieving its goals.

You will learn how to construct and communicate your vision for the setting and how to manage change using various models.

Learning outcomes

By the end of this unit, you will:

1 Understand how to develop a vision for the setting/service.

2 Be able to lead commitment and implementation of the vision and future direction of the setting/service.

Getting started

Before you study the unit, think about the following:

- How do you currently manage change in your setting?
- What is the mission and vision of your setting?
- How do you see the future of the setting developing and what changes might need to be made?
- How you currently develop plans for change and share these with staff.

LO1 Understand how to develop a vision for the setting/service

AC 1.1 Explain the meaning of 'leading a vision' for a setting/ service

Here, you will explain what a vision is and why it is required in a setting.

Part of leadership is the ability to scan the horizon and come up with a vision of where you would like the organisation to be in the future and what you would like to accomplish. If it is to be successful, the vision must be communicated to those who work in the setting and should inspire and focus their work.

As a manager, you need to generate a commitment to the organisation's vision, so it must be communicated in an appropriate way to staff. You want the team to buy into the vision and to keep the message going.

Having a clear vision can give your team direction and develop a forum for goal setting, whereas creating the vision yourself with little input from staff may mean you will spend a lot of time persuading others to buy in to the idea. You want commitment not compliance, so getting others involved in developing the vision will ensure that it becomes the team's vision.

Reflect on it

1.1 Having an organisational vision

What vision do you have for your setting? Ask yourself:

- How will the setting's daily goals and tasks align with the vision?
- How will I motivate staff when times get difficult?
- Who will support me?

Kotter's eight steps to successful change

Change can be frightening, so you need to help staff to feel comfortable with it.

John Kotter (1996) devised 'eight steps to successful change', which provides a useful starting point. Each stage recognises how individuals respond to and approach change, and Kotter identifies this through how we see, feel and then act towards change.

Kotter's model shows how managers can motivate people to buy into the change by 'owning' it. This is the important element of any successful change.

The eight-steps model can be reduced to four major factors:

- **The urgency factor**: The pressure to change is on the organisation. You need to get the team behind you to ensure successful outcomes.
- **The vision factor**: A clear shared vision is an imperative and, as manager, it is necessary to ensure that team members are with you and not against you. Motivation is the key here and you need to be aware of what motivates your team.
- **The resource factor**: The resources you need to implement change have to be identified before you proceed, and you need to ensure that these are provided. Without the necessary tools, your team cannot be expected to do the job.
- **The action factor**: When all else is in place, the next part of any change is to act. Having planned for change and implemented it, you need to check that it is working and act if it is not.

If the change is working, then maintaining the effectiveness and appropriateness of the change is good practice. By monitoring and analysing data produced you are able to evaluate its success or otherwise and to keep the team informed of progress.

Schein's levels of organisational culture

An organisations culture is made up of shared traditions, values and beliefs. These values influence staff in the organisation and determine how the organisation appears to others. Edgar Schein developed a model of organisational culture (1980) in which he identified three distinct levels as explained below.

Artifacts and behaviours

These are the visible elements which make the first impression on outsiders. They reflect the way the organisation runs. For example, a particular uniform or dress code is an artifact. Some companies may have activities that are undertaken by staff such as a breakfast club or an exercise class that all are encouraged to attend. There may also be an unusual layout of furniture or choice of style that is clearly connected to an organisation. Some Japanese companies, for example, believe that exercise will make their employees healthier and more productive and so they schedule exercise programmes during work hours. Honda was one of the first companies to take this on.

Espoused values

These affect how staff interact with and represent the organisation. Think about catchphrases of companies that indicate their culture and ways of working. Values of honesty, care and trust may be a strong part of your culture and you can communicate this via your mission statement, company or employee charters, and newsletters to the individuals using the service and their families.

Assumptions

According to Schein, the underlying beliefs of a group reflect the true way that the organisation works. They have developed as a result of the beliefs and behaviours embedded in the way the business runs and they manifest themselves in the values of the organisation. The values become embedded assumptions as they are repeated. A good example of an embedded assumption is the adherence to rules and policies that the organisation is governed by, but which are not discussed.

Johnson and Scholes' Cultural Web

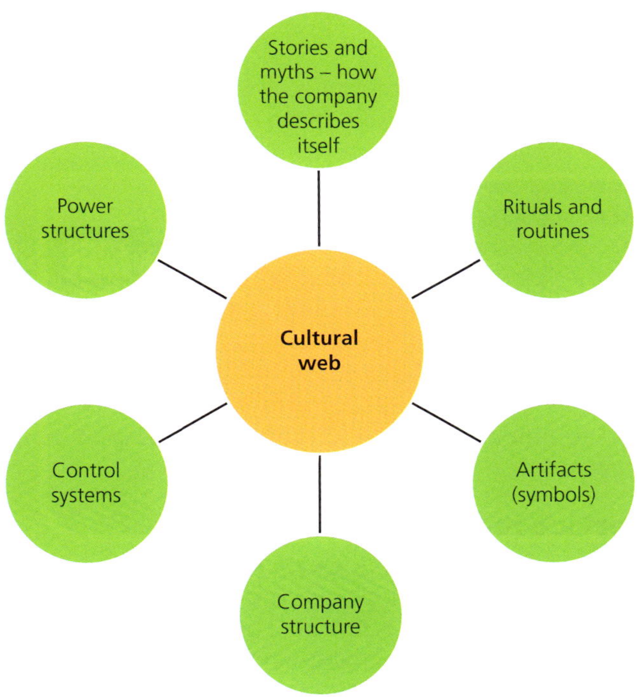

▲ **Figure 20** Johnson and Scholes' Cultural Web

During periods of organisational change, culture becomes a focus of attention. When there is growth in a company or partnerships with other companies are developed, the existing culture may be inappropriate. Changes that occur when two cultures collide can lead to low morale and absenteeism among staff.

The Cultural Web was developed in 1992 by Gerry Johnson and Kevan Scholes and is an approach for changing an organisation's culture. Six elements make up the 'paradigm' or model of the work environment and by looking at these factors, the bigger picture of the organisation's culture and what works and doesn't work can be realised.

The six elements are described below.

1. **Stories and myths**: How the company describes itself sheds light on its values and the behaviours it encourages. These include the words that the company uses to describe itself and its history, for example how the company was founded, how the people that work there describe the company and how it works.
2. **Rituals and routines**: This describes the behaviour of staff and the actions they carry out that the organisation values and wants from its employees.
3. **Symbols**: These are the visual representations of the organisation, including logos and dress codes. This is similar to the artifacts in Schein's model.
4. **Organisation structure**: This is the company structure as defined by the organisational chart, and the lines of power and influence within that structure.
5. **Control systems**: The ways that the organisation is controlled, such as the financial systems, the way in which quality and standards are maintained, and the ways in which staff are rewarded.
6. **Power structures**: These are the people with real power in the organisation and involve perhaps one or two key executives, or a particular department. These people are the most influential on operations and strategic direction.

Source: Adapted from Think Insights (2022)

Using the cultural web to make changes in an organisation requires a review of its current culture, and then a look at the six elements to see how they align with current operations. By looking at the differences between the two you can determine what you need to change.

McKinsey's 7S framework

McKinsey's 7S framework provides a useful decision-making tool. It was developed in the late 1970s by former McKinsey consultants Tom Peters and Robert Waterman (2004). The framework identifies seven internal elements of an organisation that need to align for it to be successful. These elements can either be hard or soft.

The hard elements are:

- Strategy – these are the organisation's plan for building and maintaining a competitive edge over its competitors.
- Structure, or how the company is organised.
- Systems, such as the daily activities and procedures to get the job done, including formal processes and IT systems.

The soft elements are:

- Shared values – these reflect the organisation's general work ethic.
- Style of leadership used.
- Staff – the employees and their general ability.
- Skills and competencies of the staff.

Shared values are at the centre of the model and are essential for the development of all the other elements. These need to balance and reinforce each other to ensure that an organisation performs well.

The model is a useful change management tool as it enables you to identify which of the 7S elements need to be realigned in the organisation to improve its performance, or which need to remain aligned during other changes that the organisation is undergoing. Examples of such changes include the development and introduction of new processes and systems, restructuring, organisational mergers, the development of new partnerships or a change in the organisation's leadership.

Evidence opportunity

1.1 Using a model to explain leading a vision

Using one of the models described above, explain the meaning of 'leading a vision' for your setting/service.

AC 1.2 Evaluate own role in developing a vision for a setting/service

Here, you will be required to evaluate the aims and objectives of your vision for your service area, with consideration of the areas discussed in this section.

The business planning process – maintenance and potential growth

In developing your business plan and vision for your setting, you will have answered two questions:

- What is the current state of play or where are you now?
- Where do you want to be in one, three or five years' time?

You can then define what needs to be done and by when to accomplish the goals of the organisation. It is important that you are aware of the changes that may be happening to the setting as new guidelines are developed and as the competition around you changes. Without such knowledge, your organisation will not grow and could even fail.

Competition/market competitors – national and local – and risks – actual and potential

Like any retail or customer care service, a care home or other care provision needs to be sustainable and provide the best quality of care. A potential risk of not doing so may be the closure of the service. For example, if a care service is not providing good care that the people using the service are happy with, it may find that it loses them to other services. A failing domiciliary service may ultimately lose the contract for providing care and support in that area. A residential care provision that is continually rated 'needs improvement' or 'inadequate' by CQC during inspections may share a similar fate, with individuals moving elsewhere. So, you need to be aware of the competition and what is referred to as the 'market economy' in the national and local areas and understand the strengths and weaknesses of each competitor. A market economy describes an exchange of goods between buyers and sellers. In adult care this means that individuals have more choice about who provides their care. You should also be aware of the risk that competitors pose for your service and you may need to act to diminish this.

Aside from the risk posed by competitors in the field, adult care managers also need to acknowledge the risk of other factors that can damage a business if they are not considered or prevented. For example, cyber-attacks when computer systems are targeted resulting in data breaches. There has also been an increase in telemedicine and other innovative ways in which people can access care, as well as new forms of technological support for people with different communication needs. Infection risk is another area of concern. As a manager there is a growing need for you to be aware of these risks to your business and so you will need to think about ways in which these can be managed.

Service redesign

Having assessed the competition and what they offer, you may decide to redesign your services to improve the way in which care is provided or to move ahead of the competition. For example, it may not simply be a case of redesigning the care space but perhaps the way in which the care is delivered. You may also consider redesigning how the workforce is used and could look at developing new roles. If staff training has been an issue, you might consider developing a mentor system to ensure that new staff are trained while working. However you plan to develop the area, it is the aims and objectives of the service area and the wider organisation together with the mission and vision statement that need to be prioritised.

Research it

1.2 Business planning

Look at a variety of articles dealing with business planning. Think about what your role is in this process and make notes.

Local and national data that informs your service area

In Unit 503 AC3.2 you looked at factors and drivers likely to have an impact on service provision and determined that these are often driven by national data and legislation as well as local need. The demographics of your local area will inform how your service runs. For example, there may be a greater number of older adults or young people, and this will mean a different approach to the services you offer.

Needs of individuals requiring care and support services and needs of local communities

Integrated Care Boards (ICBs) collect data on the types of people in a population, their age demographic and needs. These needs then need to be met with the development of appropriate services. As mentioned previously, a high number of older adults with complex needs will require different services and support than those in an area where there is a significant mental health need.

As a manager, it is important that your aims and objectives for the future are aligned with the vision of the organisation. The business planning process should clearly address needs for the future to ensure that your setting is sustainable. You should be aware of the market economy, potential competition and changes to service delivery, all of which will affect the individuals using your service.

New trends in digital technologies and innovations

In social care, the introduction of online meeting platforms and message apps such as WhatsApp has provided platforms for people to communicate with loved ones using voice and video, thereby maintaining a connection to their family and wider communities. Your role as a manager may be to embrace such technology within your own service.

During the pandemic lockdown, visiting individuals in care homes, residential homes and hospitals was stopped completely, so the use of video calls to maintain communication between families increased.

Remote ways of working are now accepted as standard and we are now realising the benefits that digital technologies can bring to care provision.

Engaging in change and growth

Change will either bring about growth or it can contribute to its failure. In moving your service forward, you must not only be aware of the changes that are happening, but also the need to move with them. You can have real influence if you engage in change and growth. This may mean you require more staff to grow as a business and to rival competitors if you are working in a private business, or you may need to retrain staff to fulfil the needs of the service. Perhaps your staff are unfamiliar with the use of new digital technologies and therefore require upskilling.

Evidence opportunity

1.2 Your personal role in developing a vision for services

Reflect on the areas covered above and the changes that have happened to your own service and role.

Define your personal role in relation to developing a vision for services.

AC 1.3 Describe how factors may affect the vision and future of the setting or service

Here, you will be required to describe the internal and external factors that may affect the vision.

A vision for the setting/service

A number of factors can affect the vision for the setting or service. Financially, your service may have been affected negatively by changes in funding or by other unforeseen events. For example, in the aftermath of the COVID-19 pandemic you may struggle to ensure that funds are available for staffing and the general running costs of the setting. In addition, the adult social care sector also struggles with staffing and this may impact how you set your vision for future care and support.

Legislation changes and the need to update policy and procedure will also affect the way you see the setting developing. Additional partnership working and integration of other services may not have been in your original vision but may now have to be factored in.

Co-production is a further factor that needs to be taken into account. It describes new ways of partnership working to develop preventative services for people who need care. For more on co-production, see Unit 509 AC2.2. By strengthening services and supporting assessment, your setting can help to further plan and shape the local care facilities.

Future of the setting/service

Factors affecting the future of the setting that need to be considered include environmental changes and new digital technologies. Health and wellbeing of staff and the individuals using the service is now at the forefront of policy, while the NHS vision statement 'enabling people to live healthier and more independent lives through high-quality seamless care' is a useful guide to inform the vision for your setting.

> **Reflect on it**
>
> **1.3 Factors affecting the future of your setting**
>
> Consider how the following factors affect the future of your setting:
>
> - finance
> - staffing
> - legislation
> - policy and procedures
> - partnership working
> - integration of other services
> - co-production
> - digital technologies
> - health and wellbeing of staff and individuals.

AC 1.4 Explain how to ensure the vision and future direction of the service remains compatible with the service

Here, you will be required to explain how the vision is relevant to the future aspirations of the setting and the continuing care of individuals and making sure the service is going in the right direction.

Internal aspirations of the service

As a manager, you will be responsible for identifying and recognising the areas within your own service that require improvement, so you can continually offer enhanced person-centred care that meets the needs of those who use adult care services. You will need to future proof the setting and ensure that it remains compatible with your aspirations for service.

Service delivery: Your current services may still be using some outdated models of service delivery. This may be due to the way funding is allocated to a service and so you have sought to provide a cheaper option to deliver care. As the manager, you need to take a critical look at how your service is delivering care and then think about ways in which improvements can be made to meet person-centred ideals.

Internal policy and procedures: As change occurs and as more research and government reports are published, policies and procedures will need to be updated to accommodate change.

Stakeholder opinions: Staff, those in receipt of support and care services and other stakeholders will also have opinions as to the future of the setting and should be involved in decision making. They may have excellent suggestions as to how the setting may be enhanced and by involving them, you can gain a wealth of knowledge about improvements that can be made. Autonomous and empowered staff are likely to be innovative and bold in their thinking and unafraid to voice their opinions.

Complaints and compliments system: This can also provide valuable insight into how well or poorly a service is being delivered. By analysing these things, you will be able to see clearly where improvements can be made. For example, a persistent complaint may be a sign for you as a manager that a change needs to be made. But if you are getting compliments about either a care practice or a member of staff, then you can also learn valuable lessons from this, as this is something that you can use to offer even better care. Again, as a manager, you will play a key role in recognising the improvements that need to be made and capitalising on good practice to offer even better service.

Quality monitoring: Without monitoring quality, you cannot be sure you are delivering the best and most efficient care required by individuals. This activity of monitoring and scrutinising must become a major part of the daily work you undertake.

Recruitment and workforce training and development: The way in which staff are recruited will be done according to the changes that have been identified in the strategy design and operational delivery. Training and development will also be revised as a result of newer, more innovative ways of working.

Involvement of individuals using the service: The involvement of individuals in their own care has already undergone great change but must move forward even more to enhance the care individuals receive. Enabling individuals to be part of team meetings and to engage more in the running of the care setting may be a way forward. By undertaking surveys of individuals' opinions, you can gain a wealth of information about how you function and whether you can improve.

External adult care system

A wealth of policy and guidance has been published and this has influenced how health and adult care is delivered in the UK. It is important to keep up to date with this in order to strengthen your edge in care service.

Government policy reforms and reports have significant impacts on adult social care, so managers need to review these to determine how they affect their own service areas. Public inquiries and the outcomes of reviews held in cases of failures in care practice give further guidance into how you need to work to safeguard and promote the welfare of the individuals using care services.

CQC reports and inspections may point out the need to change practice in order to effect improvement and give guidance on how to ensure that safe and high-quality care is given. Additionally, your own internal inspections and quality audits are a useful way to ensure that service delivery is of a high quality.

Staff development forms an important part of the future plans for your setting. The Care Certificate is an agreed set of 15 minimum standards that all health and social care workers must adhere to, developed by Skills for Care, Health Education England and Skills for Health. Although it is not a mandatory qualification, workers in care have the opportunity to complete this qualification, which has directly influenced the way in which care is improving.

Information technology changes rapidly but is essential to advance your business and to check on quality.

Communities change over time, so you need to keep track of local changes so you can determine how your organisation needs to adapt. Are you living in an area where life expectancy is particularly high or low?

Your role is to keep ahead of the changes that occur. Failure to do so may result in missing vital clues as to how your service needs to improve in order to stay viable and safe. There is no doubt that social care service design and strategy will continue to change in the future to meet the growing needs of an increasing older population, for example.

You will also be required to ensure that the options you formulate are bold, innovative and embody the core values of adult care. You may also need to think about different ways in which support can be delivered to meet not only local needs but also the needs of those who may move to the area for a specific service and to offset rising costs.

Stretch and challenge

1.4 Areas that require improvement to ensure the vision and future direction of the service remains safe

Several internal and external factors have been identified that impact your service. Explain how you can ensure that your service is compatible with these in the future.

LO2 Be able to lead commitment and implementation of the vision and future direction of the setting/service

AC 2.1 Build support for those implementing and communicating the vision and future direction of the setting/service

Here, you will understand how to communicate forward thinking vision and strategy confidently and engagingly and inspire others to follow.

Sharing the vision

> *If I really want to improve my situation, I can work on the one thing over which I have control – myself.*
>
> Source: Covey (2004)

In order to engage others and build support for the future of the setting, you must be able to communicate the way forward for them and be a force for change yourself. A lot of the time this requires you to work on yourself initially. You need to develop a sense of self and an awareness of how you conduct yourself and respond to others. For example, you need to know what your strengths and weaknesses are and have an understanding of your own beliefs, attitudes and emotions. By having this level of self-awareness you can start to understand other people.

Leading a group requires the ability to motivate them, so where do you start?

Think back to some of the leadership models you looked at in Unit 500, and in particular Maslow's hierarchy of needs, which demanded that certain needs must be met before somebody may be able to undertake a task. For example, if someone is hungry, they may not be at their best to undertake the task you want them to do. So send them for lunch first! This is a simple way of making a difference to somebody, but what else might you need to do to motivate them further?

When staff are being requested to buy into something new, communication and transparency of purpose are crucial to success.

Team meetings with agendas giving team members opportunities to contribute should be set up and other forms of communication such as email or using a mobile phone. WhatsApp, Instagram or other instant messaging apps may also be useful to communicate care changes or other practice enquiries. Team meetings are a good vehicle to communicate how the organisation is moving towards its vision.

Suggestions from staff should be encouraged and considered.

You also need to ensure that the people in your care and their families are well informed about how the organisation is striving to meet their needs. Meetings will be an opportunity to communicate this.

In communicating an organisational vision to your team and those in receipt of care, you first need to target your message to your audience and inform the staff about what they are working towards. Talking to staff about where the organisation is heading helps to create a shared vision and purpose.

Many teams and organisations arrange events to keep people informed of what is happening and link these in with awards evenings and socials. In smaller settings you might consider other methods to ensure that staff feel part of the organisation and feel that any contribution they make is valued and respected. Team meetings and supervision provide an opportunity to update staff on strategic changes and the organisational vision.

As a manager you need to be confident about the work of your organisation and its vision in order to inspire others. This requires you to have a good understanding of the strategies of the organisation and how it intends to move forwards.

Reflect on it

2.1 What motivates you?

List the things that enhance your job for you and give some examples about what makes you want to do them.

You may have put down things like being treated with kindness and fairness and being listened to. Being praised is also highly motivating. Showing an interest in your staff and encouraging them by giving them additional responsibility is also a way to motivate people.

What strengths do you have in motivational thinking/speaking, and how do you inspire others to follow?

Evidence opportunity

2.1 Communicating forward thinking vision and strategy

Communicate to your assessor forward thinking vision and strategy with consideration of the topics discussed in this section.

Invite them to observe a team meeting or training session where you are informing staff of changes.

Encouraging ownership of the vision

What does it mean to take ownership of the vision and to buy into it? When staff take ownership of their work, they make thoughtful decisions and take responsibility for what they do. They feel accountable for their actions and so will be more motivated. Feeling accountable for what happens in the workplace and caring about what we do means we will be more invested in future developments and plans.

Encouraging staff to move with you and to own the new vision will mean demonstrating what success will look like. It is important that staff realise that change is necessary to ensure success and how that will affect them and the work they do. Communicate to staff the reasons for the change and why their work is important. Individuals will be more engaged in change if they believe it to be important.

Trust is also important here because if staff do not feel trusted, they are less likely to take the initiative in their work as they will expect to be criticised if they do so. Communication and a shared understanding of the objectives the whole team are working towards is crucial.

AC 2.2 Support stakeholders to be aware of the vision of the setting/service and understand the impact this may have on them

Here, you will be required to demonstrate the aims and objectives of the vision to other stakeholders and manage their expectations of the service.

Partnership working refers to the relationships between individuals, their carers, service providers and care professionals.

Stakeholders need to be part of the decision making with respect to the vision in the setting and any changes that are to be made because they have a vested interest in how the service works. By effectively communicating with them you can ensure that they receive information that is relevant to their needs so that they can continue to support the individuals using the service.

One method of communicating is to involve stakeholders in community meetings. These may be a regular way of ensuring that the community is kept up to date with change, innovation and the way in which the organisation is moving forward. Regular staff meetings are also part of the communication strategy in care organisations.

Stakeholders, such as commissioning agencies or the local authority, families and individuals who commission their own services, need to engage with the work of the setting to be fully informed of the vision and the way forward with respect to the service. They have an interest and an investment in the business and, as such, require to be fully aware of ways in which the service is developing. They must have clarity about how change will affect them and how it might impact their own businesses.

Your organisation is part of a much wider community and groups of professionals, and you will be liaising with and calling on the services of those who work in social work, community nursing staff, infection control teams, the justice system and education staff. You will also come into contact with carers, the individuals receiving the care and their family and friends.

Your communication with groups may be via individual meetings in which you liaise with and meet with one person from a group, or as part of regular group meetings.

Additionally, there may be shared marketing and other ways in which you communicate. You need to ensure that stakeholders are made aware of how the organisation is moving forward and what the expectations for the service are. Conference calls using Teams, Zoom and Webex, for example, are all valuable digital methods by which you can link with stakeholders.

Evidence opportunity

2.2 Support stakeholders to be aware of the vision of the setting/service and understand the impact this may have on them

Provide evidence for your assessor that all stakeholders (internal and external) are aware of service expectations, using appropriate communication strategies such as the ones discussed in this section.

Reflect on it

2.2 Creating awareness of forward thinking

Draw a spider diagram which shows the internal and external stakeholders you work with. Write an account of how you engage with these stakeholders to create awareness of forward thinking.

AC 2.3 Create a plan to implement the vision and future direction of the setting/service

AC 2.4 Review stages of the plan

Here, you will be required to create service development plans, including management meetings, staff supervision, strategic planning and research and development activities.

Service development planning is concerned with change. The way in which individuals in the service and stakeholders external to it are involved in this is crucial to its successful implementation.

A service development plan includes an analysis of the needs of a population and identifies how these needs can be met using the resources available.

Your own service development plan will feed into a much larger document but may just be about your own setting. For example, you will be asked to develop a plan of how your service will meet the objectives of the organisation as a whole and this will then be linked into the wider organisation plan.

Management meetings and staff supervision

Planning inevitably involves a cycle of events and it is crucial that staff are kept aware of change through meetings and supervision sessions.

The first step in any planning process is to assess the current situation and then demonstrate reasons why a change is needed. Staff need to be sure that the decision to change is necessary to support the organisation in moving forward. Your service development plan will be useful here to communicate the vision of the service, both in terms of your own setting and how partners and stakeholders fit into that vision.

Strategic planning

A strategic plan starts with a vision at the top of the pyramid (see Figure 21) and this is then cascaded throughout the organisation. Strategic planning may involve changes to job roles, processes, policy changes and structural reorganisation, so staff must be aware of the impact this is likely to have on them.

Research and development

There may be an opportunity for staff to be involved in research and development activities, such as surveys or fact-finding projects, to identify how change will be effective or how it might impact current work.

The service development plan is likely to include evidence you have collected from various aspects of your work. For example, there may be data collected from staff surveys and surveys of the individuals using the service that can be used to argue for more resources in certain areas. Staff may have undertaken research in the form of projects or literature reviews which again may support requests for changes to practice or simply show how the service is working to move the wider organisation forward.

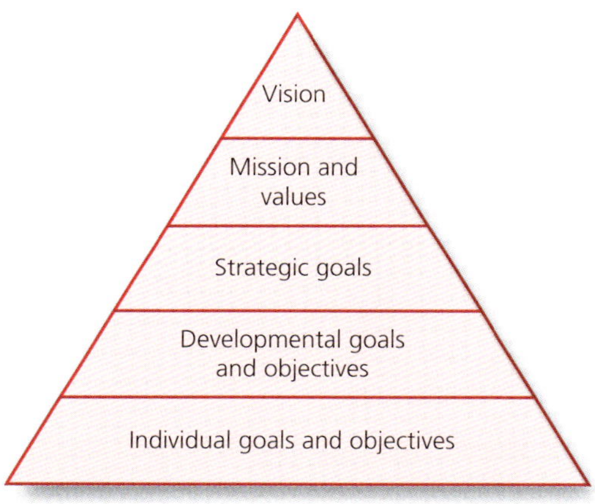
Vision
Mission and values
Strategic goals
Developmental goals and objectives
Individual goals and objectives

▲ **Figure 21** Strategic planning

Once evidence and data has been gathered, budgets can be assessed and a programme of how a change can be implemented and monitored can be drawn up.

One way to ensure that you plan and monitor changes in the setting is to use a Gantt chart (see Figure 22). This simple planning method shows the tasks that need to be undertaken, when they should take place and how long each task will take to complete. You can colour code each task as red, amber or green to show its progression. The sequence of each task can also be shown.

> **Evidence opportunity**
>
> **2.3 and 2.4 Create service development plans to support the vision**
>
> Show your assessor service development plans you have created. How do you ensure that they support the vision and that the vision is both shared and owned by those implementing and communicating it, such as your staff?

AC 2.5 Monitor stages of the plan

Here, you will be required to demonstrate the impact of the plan in relation to your expectations.

At various points you will need to review and monitor the plan, undertaking checks on whether objectives have been met. You can start to review the data collected in the last action and determine if changes need to be made. Your target date for a piece of work may not have been met so adjustment can be made here. You might also see obvious strengths or weaknesses emerging that can be dealt with as they arise.

Your plan needs to be adaptive so that it can survive changing circumstances. The organisation's mission and vision may remain the same, but your objectives and goals may require changing or updating.

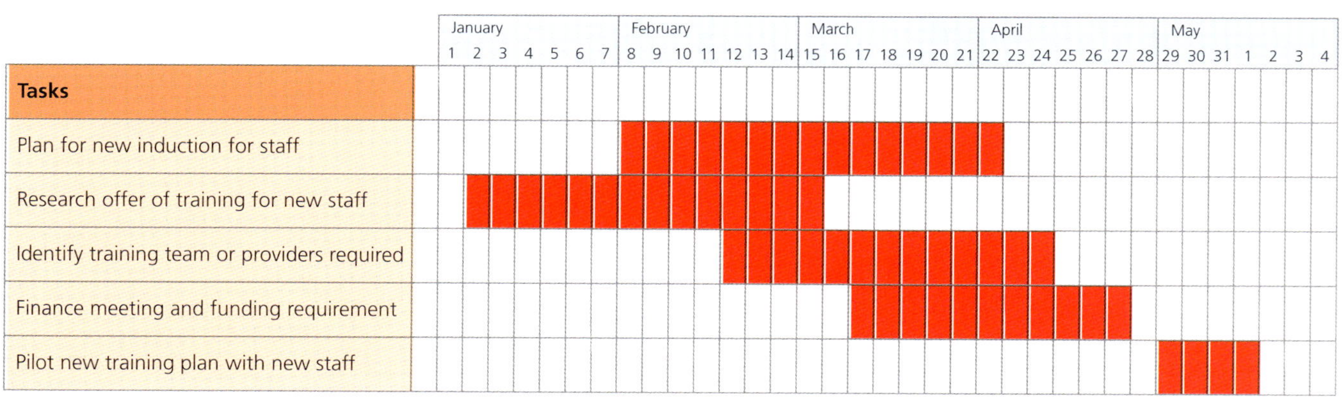

▲ **Figure 22** Gantt chart

AC 2.6 Revise stages of the plan, adapting implementation if required

Here, you will demonstrate how the plan can be updated and adapted as necessary to fit the aims of the service.

Once the plan is implemented you need to check that it covers all the required areas for change. It should show the strategic goals and how success against these will be measured, the team responsible for change and who will oversee the implementation of change.

During the implementation process, managers should focus on staff and enable them to achieve the goals of the plan. There may be challenges that result in adjustments being needed, so it is essential to keep the lines of communication open and the organisation's vision constantly in mind.

Positive change management and future vision for the service

By having a positive change management plan in place, everyone in your setting will have a vision of what the change looks like and how it will be reached. This means you can check how successful your project is at various stages and motivate your staff along the way.

Evidence opportunity

2.5 and 2.6 Monitor service development plans against measurable goals

Using service development plans that you have created, together with your organisation's strategic plan if there is one, show how you have monitored the plans against measurable goals and comment on how you have adapted the plans when obvious weaknesses occur.

References

Covey, S.R. (2004) *The 7 Habits of Highly Effective People*. London: Simon & Schuster.

Kotter, J.P. (1996) *Leading Change*. Brighton, MA: Harvard Business School Press.

Think Insights (2022) 'Cultural web – A model to align culture with strategy'. https://thinkinsights.net/strategy/cultural-web-model/

Waterman, R.H. and Peters, T. (2004) *In Search Of Excellence: Lessons from America's Best-Run Companies*. USA: Collins Business Classics.

Useful resources and further reading

Care Quality Commission (2015) 'Guidance for providers on meeting the regulations'. www.cqc.org.uk/sites/default/files/20150324_guidance_providers_meeting_regulations_01.pdf

Care Quality Commission (2021) 'How CQC monitors, inspects and regulates adult social care services'. www.cqc.org.uk/sites/default/files/How_CQC_regulates_adult_social_care_November_2021.pdf

Department of Health, Skills for Care and Skills for Health (2013), 'Code of Conduct for Healthcare Support Workers and Adult Social Care Workers in England'. www.skillsforcare.org.uk/resources/documents/Support-for-leaders-and-managers/Managing-people/Code-of-conduct/Code-of-Conduct.pdf

Goleman, D. (1998) *Working with Emotional Intelligence*. New York: Bantam Books.

Gopee, N. and Galloway, J. (2009) *Leadership and Management in Health Care*. London: Sage.

GOV.UK (2021) 'A guide to good practice for digital and data-driven health technologies'. www.gov.uk/government/publications/code-of-conduct-for-data-driven-health-and-care-technology

Maslow, A. (1987) *Motivation and Personality*, New York: Harper & Row.

McClean, S. (2012) *Power and Empowerment in Health and Social Care*. London: City & Guilds.

McGrath, J. and Bates, B. (2017) *The Little Book of Big Management Theories and How to Use Them*. London: Pearson.

Owen, J. (2015) *The Mindset of Success: From good management to great leadership*. London: Kogan Page.

Peters, S. (2012) *The Chimp Paradox: The mind management programme to help you achieve success, confidence and happiness*. London: Vermilion.

Residential Forum (1997) *Managing a 'Skills for Health home from Home': A companion to 'Creating a home from home', a guide to standards. London:* The Residential Forum.

Reynolds, M. and Holwell, S. (eds) *Systems Approaches to Managing Change: A practical guide*. London: Springer.

Skills for Care (2013) 'Leadership starts with me'. www.skillsforcare.org.uk/Developing-your-workforce/Care-topics/Leadership-skills/Leadership-starts-with-me.aspx

Skills for Care (2016) 'Manager Induction Standards'. www.skillsforcare.org.uk/Support-for-leaders-and-managers/Developing-leaders-and-managers/Manager-induction-standards.aspx

Unit 512

Continuous improvement within adult care

GLH 25

About this unit

Continuous improvement is about creating organisational and process change to enhance service. In this unit you will learn about the ways in which this is carried out and how it can streamline care services, reduce waste and costs and improve the quality of care overall.

You will learn how to lead continuous improvement and create a culture that supports innovative change. You will also look at change management and change models.

Learning outcomes

By the end of this unit, you will:

1. Understand continuous quality improvement in adult care.
2. Be able to lead continuous improvement in practice.
3. Be able to lead a culture that supports innovation and change to improve outcomes for individuals.
4. Understand how to implement effective change in adult care.

Getting started

Before you study the unit, think about the following:

- What does continuous quality improvement mean to you?
- How do you lead on good practice in this area in your setting?
- What innovations and change programmes have you been involved in or would like to implement in the setting?

LO1 Understand continuous quality improvement in adult care

AC 1.1 Explain the meaning of quality improvement

Here, you are required to explain the term continuous improvement and its role in maintaining quality in care. As a key driver for your service it is part of the fundamental standards for inspection

Quality improvement in adult care

Quality improvement is a co-ordinated approach to problem solving using specific methods and tools to bring about improvements that can be measured. Using this approach, those experiencing issues that affect their care quality are given the 'time, permission, skills and resources they need to solve them' (Jones et al., 2021).

A key driver for any service should be to maintain and improve the quality of care delivered. The CQC's fundamental standards are in place to ensure that adult social care services provide high quality, person-centred care. If the service is not regulated the standards are still useful guidelines.

Inspections may highlight areas of concern to which attention must be paid. In 2019, 17 per cent of regulated adult social care services in England were delivering care that was not achieving CQC standards (CQC, 2019).

The updated CQC report 'The state of health care and adult social care in England 2021/22' (CQC, 2022) reports that for the years 2020–22 there has been a 'small increase' in this number, although the report does not specify what that increase is. It does, however, comment that 83 per cent of adult social care services were rated as 'good or outstanding', which suggests that the change is insignificant but still requires improvement.

Failing to address areas for improvement will impact quality of care and the reputation and sustainability of the service.

If you have a service that is already achieving the CQC's fundamental standards, making continuous improvements or achieving a 'good' or 'outstanding' rating will ensure that your setting remains stable and meets the changing expectations of the adult social care service.

Continuous quality improvement in adult care

Change happens with great frequency and often comes from external factors such as changes in the economy, technology, society or environmental issues. This means that we need to continually evaluate whether our services have room for improvement and whether they are still fit for purpose.

Continuous quality improvement involves making incremental improvements over time. In an adult social care setting it requires an organisational approach that involves all team members in planning and implementing ongoing improvement strategies. This will be a gradual process, since change can lead to a 'fear factor' for staff and destabilise the team. Significant change can feel threatening to staff so small improvements that gradually encourage change and can be implemented quickly has its advantages. For example, some change simply requires eliminating a single step in a process, which results in savings in time and costs as well as improving the process.

For continuous improvement to work, the team need to feel safe in order to challenge practices and share new ideas to aid development.

> **KEY TERM**
>
> **Continuous quality improvement**: Continual actions to improve the outcomes for individuals and to develop the workforce.

Quality improvement tools and techniques

The NHS and Department of Health and Social Care (DHSC) definition of quality is that the delivery of care is 'effective, safe and provides as positive an experience as possible by being caring, responsive and person-centred'. This definition further states that care should also be 'well-led, sustainable and equitable, achieved through providers and commissioners working together and in partnership' (Jones et al., 2021).

In 2017, the DHSC and partners across adult social care sectors published the paper 'Quality Matters', an initiative to improve the quality of adult social care. To make a difference to people who use adult social care services, the document sets out a clear vision of shared commitment to high-quality person-centred adult care and support. It highlights quality as being everybody's business and sets out clear action plans supporting the priorities for improving quality, working alongside the quality strategy for the NHS, building on partnerships and co-ordinated care.

Quality improvement tools and techniques are processes and strategies that can help you to better understand, analyse and communicate how you are managing quality improvement efforts. You will look at some of these in AC1.2.

Reflect on it

1.1 Upholding quality of care

What are the ways in which you currently ensure that quality of care is upheld in your setting?

What evidence do you have to show that the CQC's fundamental standards are in place in your setting and ensure that the services you provide are of a high quality and meet person-centred care needs?

AC 1.2 Explain how to meet regulatory and best practice guidance requirements using continuous quality improvement tools and techniques

Here, you will explain how to meet best practice guidance using different models for quality improvement.

Quality improvement is the systematic use of methods and tools to continuously improve quality of care and outcomes. There are several methods and techniques that might be used. Regulatory and guidance changes demand that adult social care settings continually address change and look for ways to improve the quality of their care offer.

The model for improvement, six sigma and lean six sigma are supported in NHS literature as useful tools and methods. While there is no favoured method, it is the process of having a systematic approach to quality improvement that is deemed important.

The 'Quality matters' document sets out seven steps to maintain and improve the quality of care that people experience:

1 Set clear directions and priorities.
2 Set standards for what high quality care looks like by bringing clarity to quality.
3 Use information to improve the quality of care through performance and quality reporting systems so that quality can be measured and published.
4 Celebrate and share good and outstanding care to recognise and reward quality.
5 Maintain and safeguard quality by working together to reduce risk and protect people from harm.
6 Improve leadership, management, professional and institutional culture, skills and behaviours to build capability to assure quality and sustain improvement.
7 Stay ahead, by developing research, innovation and planning.

Based on work by the Health Foundation: A Clear Road Ahead (2016), this modified version was developed by the National Quality Board in their Shared Commitment to Quality.

The commitment is to help everyone improve the quality of adult social care by adapting these seven steps to their care setting.

Model for improvement

The model for improvement was developed by Associates in Process Improvement in the USA and is a framework to support continuous improvement. It is made up of two key parts:

- three questions that drive all improvement
- the plan-do-study-act or PDSA cycle (also known as the PDCA or plan-do-check-act cycle).

The three key questions

Using the framework, the team would ask three key questions:

1 What are we trying to accomplish?

   This identifies what needs to be improved. It is important that this is a statement which is specific, has an end point that can be achieved, matches the goals of the organisation and is measurable.

2 How will we know that a change is an improvement?

   This question requires teams to identify outcome measures, i.e. how the aim of the project is measured, and process measures that track the steps or changes that occur during the process to see how they influence the outcome.

   There are three types of measures that can be used at this stage: outcome, process and balancing measures.

   - Outcome measures show the impact on the individuals using the service of what has been implemented and the end result of the improvement work. For example, you might measure the impact of how independence is promoted with individuals.
   - Process measures look at the way the systems and processes work to deliver the outcome required. For example, you can measure the arrival and departure times for domiciliary care visits or look at the number of support plans that are in place and are being used and reviewed within a time frame. It is also possible to check that support plans have been completed according to agreed policy .
   - Balancing measures reflect how the change may be affecting other parts of the system and look at the unintended consequences of the improvement effort. Unintended consequences can be both positive and negative. For example, in promoting independence there may need to be an increase in the number of staff or training may have to change.

These measures will track the progress against the original improvement statement.

3 What changes can we make that will result in improvement?

This can be a team effort in which ideas are generated and theories are put forward for discussion.

The three questions enable the team to explore what they want to achieve and what ideas for change might make a difference. Having identified these, think about how the change can be measured to demonstrate improvement.

The PDSA cycle

The second part of the model is the PDSA cycle. This is where the steps of planning, doing, studying and acting (PDSA) are undertaken. The cycle then returns to planning for the next stage of continuous improvement.

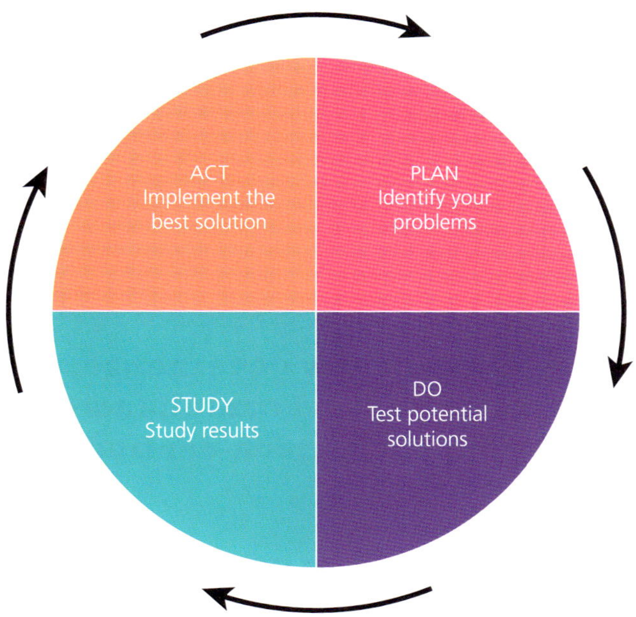

▲ **Figure 23** The PDSA cycle

Six sigma

Six sigma is a management technique that focuses on statistical improvements to a process using qualitative measurements. Users of six sigma follow the DMAIC approach:

- **Define**: Focus on a faulty process in the workplace, outline the problem and identify goals for the project.
- **Measure**: Make a statistical measure of the problem to understand the process and to provide a benchmark measure.
- **Analyse**: The process is analysed by isolating each part or input and the potential reason for the failure is identified. The root causes of the problem are defined.
- **Improve**: The team work to improve the system performance.
- **Control**: Controls are added to the process to ensure that it does not fail again.

The use of six sigma has evolved and has been applied in more general management with a focus on meeting consumer requirements, improving staff retention and improving and sustaining products and services. For adult social care, six sigma might be applied to intensively analyse care and support processes to assess if the needs and expectations of individuals are being met. By identifying what is critical to the quality of the service for individuals, measurements can then be applied to see whether their needs are actually being met. For example, we might apply six sigma to Positive Behaviour Support (PBS) for people with behaviours that challenge. PBS helps staff to understand the reason for the behaviour they are seeing so that people's needs can be met more readily.

A recurring incident of behaviour that challenges might be due to a lack of understanding of how to promote positive behaviour. By applying the six sigma steps to focus on the problem and measure the incidents, it might be possible to analyse the root cause of a particular issue, which can then be improved.

Six sigma has also been applied with lean principles (see below) to produce a more useful approach.

Lean six sigma

The 'lean approach' originated in Japan's car industry, but the principles can be used in care settings as a quality management method.

Lean emphasises the individual's position as central to all activities and aims to eliminate or reduce activities that do not add value to the individual. To do this, lean six sigma's operational principles involve five steps for continuous improvement. These are:

- Defining what adds value to individuals.
- Identifying the mapping value streams, which are the pathways that deliver care.
- Making these value streams or pathways flow by removing waste, delay and duplication.
- Enabling individuals to 'pull' value towards them, so that their care meets their needs. These might involve a different use of resources or staff.
- Aiming for perfection as an ongoing goal.

Evidence opportunity

1.2 Comparing models

Explain to your assessor how you might use the tools and techniques for continuous improvement, meet regulatory requirements and embed best practice guidance. Refer to PDSA and the lean six sigma tools.

AC 1.3 Outline the potential signs or indicators of poor practices in relation to quality improvement

Here, you will outline the ways in which poor practices may be identified during quality improvement.

An unintended outcome of applying a quality improvement plan may be the uncovering of unsatisfactory practices and performance. Your drive to improve quality of care may reveal poor standards of work, with frequent mistakes being made and staff unable to follow a job through due to a lack of resources. You might also discover that staff are not working to a satisfactory standard, lacking commitment and drive. It might also reveal a lack of skill and poor attitudes to the individuals using the service.

Evidence opportunity

1.3 Indicators of poor quality care

Outline to your assessor potential signs of poor quality care emerging in your setting. What will you notice?

AC 1.4 Explain how quality assurance practices inform quality improvement activities

Here, you will explain quality assurance and the ways in which it can help in managing quality improvement.

Quality assurance and quality improvement are two concepts which help you to manage quality, but they are different and require definition.

- Quality improvement involves systematic approaches which analyse the current performance of the setting and identifies actions to take to improve care.
- Quality assurance refers to how you monitor procedures or processes to ensure that they are meeting the expected levels of quality standards.

There are several ways in which you as the manager can monitor procedures and processes. Satisfaction surveys of individuals using the service will be one way to measure how care is being given. The supervision cycle, appraisals and one-to-ones with staff members are also good indicators of whether staff are achieving their objectives. Ad hoc spot checks can reveal work practice anomalies, or indeed good practice.

By monitoring a particular procedure or a process you can determine the competency of a member of staff to ensure that they are working to the expected quality standards. For example, a quick check on hand-washing technique might reveal that a staff member has not been diligent, which might then have consequences for the individuals in their care. For domiciliary staff working in people's homes, checks may be made in supervision sessions. You might wish to address moving and handling techniques to determine that this regular practice is being carried out safely in the person's home.

Evidence opportunity

1.4 Meeting quality assurance practices

Explain how quality assurance practice supports improvement. How has this led to improved care in your setting?

AC 1.5 Explain how governance, adult processes and compliance activity support person-centred practice

AC 1.6 Explain how governance and audit processes can support outcome-based practices

Here, you will explain how governance, audit processes and compliance activities can support person-centred and outcome-based practices.

Person-centred practice

Person-centred practice puts the person at the centre of everything you do, recognising the uniqueness of every person as a complex individual. It respects the individual's needs and preferences and the knowledge they bring about their care and support needs. By applying a person-centred care approach, you can tailor the care to the needs of the individual, supporting them to develop the knowledge, skills and confidence to manage and make informed decisions about their own support needs.

KEY TERM

Person-centred practice: A way of working that recognises the complexity and unique nature of individuals and places them at the centre of the care given, respecting their needs, preferences and knowledge.

Outcome-based practice

Outcome-based practice is a method used in adult social care services designed to have a direct effect on an individual and is similar to person-centred practice. An outcome is the end result of planned care and the impact it has on the individual after an activity or service. Outcomes-focused services, like person-centred ones, are those that aim to achieve the priorities that the individuals themselves identify as important. It is a way of planning, designing and monitoring services to work together to maximise an individual's independence and quality of life.

Governance

Governance is a system by which care organisations are held accountable for continuously improving the quality of their services. The system ensures that all individuals using a service are safeguarded and that high standards of care are delivered. Governance will ensure that monitoring systems for all care processes are in place and there is an assurance of a person's safety and quality of care throughout the setting.

Adult processes

Person-centred care and outcomes-based care, in which the individual is at the centre of the care process, require that key principles are applied to the adults who require support in the process. A person-centred approach to safeguarding adults is a dynamic process that must be undertaken *with* people rather than done *to* people.

The Department of Health and Social Care (2022) highlighted the following key principles that must be followed as part of the safeguarding adults process:

- **Empowerment**: Person-centred care presumes that person-led decisions and informed consent is part of the process. Adults need to be consulted about their desired outcomes.
- **Protection**: Adults must be safe and have support and representation during the process.
- **Prevention**: The likelihood of repeated abuse must be eliminated and the person's contribution to this should be recorded in safeguarding plans.
- **Proportionality**: Safeguarding procedures must be proportionate and as unintrusive as possible, appropriate to the risk presented.
- **Partnership**: Agencies must work constructively to make adults feel safe.
- **Accountability**: Safeguarding processes should be conducted in transparent and consistent ways and all practice must be subject to external scrutiny (e.g. through the courts).

Compliance

Compliance refers to following rules and laws. It is about doing the right thing in accordance with regulations and government legislation. Failure to do so can lead to legal action being taken.

There are four types of compliance.

- Regulatory compliance means following local and national laws and regulations that are relevant to adult social care. This means that trust is established both internally and externally to the setting.
- HR compliance covers topics such as the maintenance of employee documentation, recruitment procedures, pay and employee benefits. Being compliant ensures that complaints or legal issues are kept to a minimum. HR compliance ensures that the setting is operating lawfully.
- Data compliance ensures that the information you need to collect is correctly organised and stored and managed legally and safely. If your setting is data compliant, data will be safeguarded against loss, theft and misuse.
- Health and safety compliance is about providing a safe working environment as well as a safe environment for individuals. This ensures that staff and individuals are not being put in danger or at risk of injury.

Evidence opportunity

1.5 and 1.6 Comparing outcome-based and person-centred practice

Explain how governance, audit processes and compliance activities support outcome-based and person-centred practice in your setting.

LO2 Be able to lead continuous improvement in practice

AC 2.1 Monitor progress towards the implementation of person-centred practice

AC 2.2 Evaluate progress towards the implementation of person-centred practice

Here, you will monitor and evaluate systems and processes that your setting uses in order to implement person-centred practice.

Evaluate systems and processes

The appropriateness and usability of systems and processes within an organisation determine whether those systems and processes help to promote positive outcomes in person-centred care. The first step is to ensure that they are clear and well-understood and set the standards of the behaviours expected of all employees in the workplace. When designing policies there are three requirements:

1. The policy must be clear about person-centred practice and positive outcomes.
2. There should be no possibility of misinterpretation of what is intended.
3. The policy must address the issue directly and must reflect current legal requirements.

Policies provide a framework for promoting positive outcomes, but if they are not monitored or staff are unclear about how they should be practising, then your service may not be offering person-centred care.

You must ensure that there have been no amendments, extensions or changes to relevant laws. A well-designed policy is essential in promoting a positive culture that celebrates diversity in the workplace and how this is linked to person-centred practices. All new policies should be agreed or designed in consultation with unions or employee representatives.

Policies should:

- give clear examples of what person-centred practice and diversity is and how it can affect positive outcomes
- give examples of what constitutes discrimination, harassment, bullying and intimidating behaviour, including cyber-bullying, work-related events and harassment by third parties
- state that if discriminatory behaviour has occurred it will be treated as a disciplinary offence.

Every policy should be monitored and regularly reviewed for effectiveness, including:

- records of complaints including why and how they occurred and who was involved – an analysis of trends will help you to identify if the policy is working or if there are any systemic problems
- individual complaints to ensure that action plans were implemented as intended, to identify resolution and to identify whether there was any evidence of victimisation for those involved.

Evidence of feedback from those in receipt of care and support

The individuals using your service can provide you with first-hand knowledge about their care and how they perceive it, and this can be facilitated by arranging meetings where they are given an opportunity to speak out. Anonymous surveys can also be used. The 'complaints, compliments and comments' systems are also a good way to audit practice. For those individuals with limited verbal or written communication, the use of visual sheets and questioning may be helpful. Sign language and reading the body language of the person can be invaluable in determining how individuals are feeling about their care and support.

Colleagues

Your colleagues need to have a safe way to comment upon care and practice and this may be achieved through appraisal and supervision but also staff meetings. As a manager you may want to stress that you have an open-door policy that enables people to come and express concerns at any time.

Contributions from others involved in supporting those in receipt of care and support

Carers and others who support the individuals using the service should be able to meet with the manager. Although this might be time consuming, you may want to set aside a fortnightly meeting slot for all to come in to discuss needs. They may also be able to access the complaints, compliments and comments system and user surveys.

> **Evidence opportunity**
>
> **2.1 and 2.2 Implementation and evaluation**
>
> Collect evidence to demonstrate how you monitor, review and evaluate the implementation of person-centred practices and the achievement of positive outcomes for individuals within your setting. This should include robust feedback from those referred to in this section.

AC 2.3 Monitor progress towards the achievement of positive outcomes

AC 2.4 Evaluate progress towards the achievement of positive outcomes

Here, you will monitor the effectiveness of interventions to ensure a continuous cycle of improvements.

To lead a sustained, continuous cycle of improvement in social care, you need to monitor and evaluate the achievement of outcomes to ensure success. Research published by the American Psychological Association says that the chances of success are even more likely if the outcomes are reported on and if progress is publicly or physically recorded (Science Daily, 2015).

Harkin et al. (2016) looked at the effectiveness of interventions or treatments which prompted the participants to monitor their goal progress. Focusing mainly on personal health goals, such as losing weight or changing diet, the study showed that if participants monitored their progress towards a goal there was an increased likelihood they would achieve that goal. Publicly recording results also led to improvements. Best practice can then be adopted for the future.

The adoption of a person-centred approach to care means that discussions and engagement among individuals, their families and care professionals can highlight the risks and benefits to the individuals and the outcomes they desire. This has enabled care outcomes to be more explicitly expressed, which in turn ensures that monitoring those outcomes is easier. Asking the individuals in your setting to self-report whether outcomes have been achieved is one way that you can monitor progress. Staff and individuals can evaluate achievements against goals identified in the care/support plan.

The use of satisfaction surveys and meetings are all ways in which the progress against a plan of care can be monitored. For those with limited communication, the use of stories with pictures may be useful to gain feedback. Using real-time interviews with individuals and their families will provide good insight into the individuals' needs

AC 2.5 Create opportunities for individuals and others to provide feedback on their experiences of the setting/service

Here, you will ensure that individuals using the service and other relevant stakeholders have opportunities to provide feedback and that this feedback is acted upon effectively.

An important function as a leader and manager is to be able to deliver feedback, yet it is often a skill that is ignored, neglected or done badly.

The only way to drive change and help teams to develop is to create a culture in which feedback is not only effective but also welcomed, whether it challenges practice or celebrates it.

Giving feedback can impact morale and must therefore be carried out sensitively and truthfully. One of the things that is difficult about constructive feedback is that informing somebody that they need to change a certain behaviour or practice is uncomfortable. Telling the truth about something you know may not be received well is very challenging, so there is a tendency to avoid it or try to soften the blow.

You may have heard of the 'praise sandwich' technique where negative feedback is sandwiched between two positive statements. For example, 'I can see that you are excellent at communicating with the individuals in our care and you are always friendly and approachable. I do have some concerns about your tone with staff. You can be quite abrupt and this may be seen as rude. As an important part of the team your work is good and working on this aspect of your communication would make it even better.'

The criticism here is flanked by two pieces of praise so the recipient can feel positive. Unfortunately, it has been shown that the critical information, that of poor communication with staff, is lost amidst the praise and the person may therefore not respond to how important this is. It is also possible that the praise might be seen as insincere.

Feedback must therefore be specific, honest and clear. It is guidance about what to keep doing and what needs to be changed or improved upon.

Sustained and lasting success as a leader comes only when people can effectively lead themselves and are able to influence, engage and collaborate with others. These elements are at the heart of personal, team and organisational effectiveness and feedback.

Development is at the heart of staff feedback and is an important part of staff appraisal. This should provide an opportunity for staff to celebrate their achievements and to set targets for the future. There should be a clear action plan in place for any targets to be achieved.

Creating a feedback culture requires you, as the leader, to seek and respond to feedback yourself. This is a hard thing to do as you are opening yourself up to criticism that may be difficult to receive. However, in doing so you will highlight the importance of feedback to staff, and it will give you the opportunity to learn from the feedback you receive.

Evidence opportunity

2.5 Seek feedback about yourself as a leader

Undertake interviews with individuals and their families and ask them for feedback on their experiences.

AC 2.6 Use the views of individuals once they have been acknowledged

Here, you will show how you receive feedback and undertake respectful questioning in order to better acknowledge feedback received.

When you ask for feedback from others it is important to acknowledge the feedback that they give you and then to act upon it, as this can make them feel their efforts have been recognised and they are valued. Receiving praise can motivate an individual and enhance their performance. Positive acknowledgement of what a member of staff has to say to us recognises their skills and dedication.

Negative feedback can often feel threatening, so it is important to be respectful. You might get complaints from individuals using the service or from staff and these need to be managed well.

Listening and paying attention to what someone is saying shows that you are receptive. However, active listening is much more than simply listening. It involves paying full attention to the speaker to demonstrate that you are fully involved in the conversation and are able to respond in a more fulfilling way. Effective communication in this way can enhance relationships at work and staff are more likely to feel better understood and valued.

Asking respectful questions will enable you to gain more information about the complaint or feedback. It will also give you the opportunity to say how you will act on what you have been told. A respectful question is not judgemental or accusatory in its tone and will encourage the person to open up more. You will need to plan your questions carefully as a disrespectful one will close the conversation down and could even lead to conflict. Questions that start with 'Why' are unhelpful as this word sounds accusatory. For example, 'Why did you do that' sounds like an accusation whereas 'What led to that action?' will be better received.

Techniques for active listening include:

- focusing on the conversation and being mindful of what is being said, with no interruptions
- paying attention to non-verbal cues which may say more than words. Mehrabian (1972) concluded that in face-to-face conversation, communication is 55 per cent non-verbal, 38 per cent vocal and 7 per cent words
- giving encouraging verbal cues to elicit a response. Saying 'Yes, I see' or 'I understand' together with smiling or nodding will enable the speaker to feel they are being heard
- clarifying and paraphrasing information will help you understand and determine whether you have gained full knowledge of what the person is saying
- leaving judgement behind and remaining neutral. Approach each conversation with an open mind and do not criticise.

Evidence opportunity

2.6 Use feedback from individuals

What changes might you make as a result of the feedback gained from individuals using the service and their families?

AC 2.7 Evaluate evidence-based research in best practice for person-centred and outcomes based practice

Here, you will be required to research and evaluate up-to-date, reliable literature and/or other publications relevant to your area of study to establish best practice that supports the above.

Evidence-based practice is about incorporating evidence from research and making professional judgements as a result of the new knowledge and applying it to formulate care decisions.

As a care practitioner you are duty bound to perform care in a safe way and to be accountable for what you do. To 'do no harm' is the essential premise of evidence-based practice and the need to be able to demonstrate that the care you provide is safe and effective is a reasonable expectation.

As an effective practitioner accountable for your own safe practice, you need to have access to and be up to date with the research related to your own area and be able to critically appraise such work. As a manager of staff in your setting, you are accountable when it comes to ensuring that the staff have embraced the notion of evidence-based practice.

In making a decision about how and what care is to be given, it is important to have an accurate picture of the research available and to construct sufficient evidence from it to support your actions. In supervising staff you need to ensure that their practice is based on good, sound evidence and that they are informed as to how they might be able to improve their practice consistent with new initiatives in care.

KEY TERM

Evidence-based practice: Refers to using information from high-quality research and applying it within practice to make informed decisions about an individual's care.

Research it

2.7 Best practice guidelines

The following publications are useful for best practice guidelines about person-centred care and positive outcomes.

Take some time to read a couple and to make short notes for your portfolio.

- The Health Foundation (2014) 'Person-centred care made simple'.
- Care Quality Commission (2022) 'Adult social care: Information for providers'.
- Skills for Care and Skills for Health (2013) 'Code of Conduct for Healthcare Support Workers and Adult Social Care Workers in England'.
- NHS Confederation (2012) 'Delivering dignity: Securing dignity in care for older people in hospitals and care homes'.
- Social Care Institute for Excellence (n.d.) 'Dignity in care'.

Evidence opportunity

2.7 Evaluate evidence-based research to identify best practice

Show your assessor that you have researched up-to-date, reliable literature and/or other publications relevant to your area of study that supports best practice. Evaluate the use of person-centred and outcome care practice by highlighting the strengths and the weakness of each.

AC 2.8 Identify areas where digital technology could enhance person-centred outcomes based practice

Here, you will identify the ways in which digital technology can be used in a setting to reduce health inequalities.

The agenda to provide better digital technology to transform services provides adult social care with a huge opportunity. The Skills for Care website contains excellent resources to help adult social care staff to develop digital leadership and to grow and develop as confident and skilled digital leaders.

Digital technologies have the potential to improve social care and in 2019 the government brought together information technology teams from the Department of Health and Social Care, NHS England and NHS Improvement to form NHSX.

NHSX commissioned reviews of the current extent of digital technologies and skills in the adult social care sector and Skills for Care are a key partner in this work.

The reviews explored the current use and effectiveness of digital technology in adult social care and also identified the barriers to accessing and supplying digital technology.

The review also looked at how future use of digital technology would look, together with the required skills and digital capabilities of the adult social care workforce.

Research it

2.8 Digital inclusion

Look at 'Digital technology in social care' on the Skills for Care website (Skills for Care, n.d.).

One example of digital inclusion is Liam House, a residential home for ten adults with learning disabilities. The team were looking for a way to reduce paper use and move their care management online. Using 'Log my Care', a free care home software tool, staff were able to easily plan, record and co-ordinate care on an app. With all care notes logged through the app, carers were able to read the latest information on the residents and view any handovers.

The benefits of using an online system include a reduction in paperwork and improved consistency. A small care home has limited storage space for files, so moving paperwork online can make things easier.

How might your setting use digital technology to enhance the care you provide?

Skills for Care supports developing digital leadership and growing the wider sector's skills and offers training for leaders. The benefits of being more digitally aware include extension of the services on offer, greater independence and control over individuals' care and freeing up the time care workers spend on administration tasks, leaving space for more face-to-face care.

AC 2.9 Identify lessons learned

Here, you will be required to show evidence of how any incidents that can or may have occurred inform your leadership and management of service practice in respect of person-centred care.

Lessons learned from national incidents and events

Identifying mistakes or near mistakes and assessing whether these could have been avoided is an important activity. It is important that this is seen as a productive activity and not a punitive or disciplinary one. Its primary focus is about learning from an incident or set of behaviours in order that changes can be made to improve things.

In 2001, Margaret Panting, a 78-year-old woman, died after suffering 'unbelievable cruelty' while living with relatives. Following her move from sheltered housing to her relatives' home, her death five weeks later revealed 49 injuries on her body, including cuts made by a razor blade and cigarette burns. This case became the catalyst for introducing the Section 4 offence of 'causing or allowing the death of a child or vulnerable adult' into the Domestic Violence Crimes and Victims Act 2005.

Lessons learned from internal incidents and events

On a smaller scale, investigations into minor mistakes and accidents are designed to enable learning from reflection on the circumstances that allowed an accident or mistake to happen. Importantly, getting the balance between investigation, reflection and assigning blame is crucial. If staff feel they are going to be unfairly blamed or punished for mistakes, it may prevent them from reporting them or coming forward with concerns. An organisation that supports its staff to raise concerns, to acknowledge deficits and to report mistakes is much more likely to be a learning organisation than one where this is not the primary culture. An open organisation provides the conditions for someone to acknowledge and investigate and to reflect on how things can be improved or done differently.

Untoward incidents that occur in care work need to be fully investigated and reviewed. In recommending proposals for improvements to systems and procedures, you could begin by looking at how you process complaints, what happens with incident and accident reports and how care/support plans are used. You need to first ensure that they are up to date and are useful for determining how well your safeguarding procedures are working.

Identified poor practice

Unsatisfactory work performance and poor practice might manifest in a number of ways. As a manager you may observe staff making frequent mistakes, not following a job through, or being unable to cope with instructions or tasks.

Managing poor performance may require you to invoke formal procedures whereby you undertake an investigation of the reasons for poor performance, discuss this with the member of staff and then give them time to improve. Clear advice on how improvement can be made and the provision of training and supervision must be offered and staff must also be aware of the consequences of failing to improve.

Accidents, errors and 'near misses'

Protecting people in our care requires that accidents and errors must be identified and investigated in order to provide learning from each incident. The CQC requires all regulated social care settings to provide audits of the accident records, which might reveal whether anything connects to poor practice. Reflective practice, including incident analysis (where you analyse an incident by considering what happened, how and why it happened, what might reduce the risk of it happening again and what you learned), enables you and your team to reflect on behaviours, interactions and incidents and to identify ways of enhancing or improving practice.

Errors and 'near misses' may also be recorded.

Concerns and complaints – informal and/or formal

Any complaint or concern that is brought to your attention needs to be dealt with in a structured way and you must document how the issue has been handled. You must not be complacent about the effectiveness of policies and procedures that have been designed to support a culture that promotes and assures equality and respect for person-centred practice. An annual audit of how effective such policies are and how complaints have been handled is a good way of checking whether this issue remains at the forefront of people's minds and practice.

There is a great deal of emphasis on evidence-based practice and best practice. This is another means of reflection. It has involved somebody identifying an issue and researching it in order to generate evidence. Best practice means analysing different ways of doing things in order to identify whether there is a preferred way of undertaking the activity. Access to up-to-date learning resources is important in supporting staff to keep abreast of new evidence and best practice.

AC 2.10 Act on lessons learned from national incidents and events and internal incidents and events

Here, you will show how you have acted on lessons learned from nationally reported events and those that occur within the setting.

Evidence opportunity

2.9 and 2.10 Acting on lessons learned

How are incidents or near-misses dealt with in your setting? How did the death of Margaret Panting impact the law and social care? Show your assessor evidence of how such events can inform leadership and management practice in respect of person-centred care. Include, for example, the topics discussed in section 2.9.

Reflect on it

2.9 and 2.10 Lessons learned

Ensuring that you maintain confidentiality, draw on a real example of a failure, mistake of a standard practice or a practice that required change and write a report that answers the following questions:

- What happened?
- Was the incident reported to senior staff?
- If the incident was reported to senior staff, who did they (senior staff) report it to and why that individual (or agency)?
- How was the individual causing the incident perceived?
- What actions resulted from the incident?
- Are policies and protocols fit for purpose?
- If a similar thing occurred again, are you confident that employees feel sufficiently well supported to report the issue?
- What changes could you make to make it easier for staff to raise issues that can improve service and manage risks?

AC 2.11 Evaluate how positive outcomes for individuals are facilitated

Here, you will evaluate the ways in which collaboration within the setting can improve outcomes for individuals.

Internal systems and processes

The way you lead and manage your team directly impacts the culture of the setting and this, together with the organisation's mission, values and vision statements, will affect positive outcomes for both staff and the individuals using the service.

The internal systems and processes that are in place can affect how the workplace functions and how staff work together. In an open culture, staff are encouraged to collaborate on ideas and solutions. The internal systems in place will be staff orientated and processes will value the staff. Collaboration will be part of the process of leadership, including mentorship and facilitation. Systems that are hierarchical with an emphasis on rules and regulations are likely to govern behaviour of staff in a more controlling manner.

Both of these types of internal systems can affect the outcomes of individuals in a positive or negative way.

Agreed ways of working

An agreed way of working is a policy or procedure in your setting that you need to abide by. For example, you may have a regular practice in which a handover session for staff coming on to a shift are given information from those who have finished their shift.

With person-centred care it may be that you are all using the 6Cs – values that are integrated into adult care which shape the way your work is carried out:

- **Care**: Having an individual's best interests at heart and doing whatever you can to maintain or improve their wellbeing.
- **Compassion**: Expressing empathy and concern for the individual and understanding them and their situation.
- **Competence**: Possessing the knowledge and skills to provide what is required and showing that you have the ability to understand the individual.
- **Communication**: Speaking and acting in a way that the individual can understand and listening actively.
- **Courage**: Being able to express concerns without fear of reprisal and being able to try something new.
- **Commitment**: Being dedicated to providing care and support for the individual while understanding the responsibilities you have as a social care worker.

Individuals and others being involved in the decision-making process

Decision making happens every day in the life of a manager and those decisions affect the care and day-to-day running of the setting. Decisions are made a little easier when others are involved in the decision-making process, so families, friends and the individuals themselves will give a more diverse approach to the decision being made. By bringing others into the conversation with different disciplinary and cultural backgrounds, a fresh perspective on the task or problem is gained. Further benefits of including others in the decision-making process include increased engagement of staff and the families and friends of the individual, increasing trust as you show how much you value their opinions. It can also help you to see your own blind spots about certain issues as new ideas are articulated.

Collaboration is fostered by involving others and creates opportunities to share ideas, learn from each other and work towards organisational and personal goals.

> **Evidence opportunity**
>
> **2.11 Ensuring positive outcomes**
>
> Provide an evaluation of the following four areas, showing the strengths and weaknesses of each and how they facilitate and lead to positive outcomes for individuals:
>
> - ✔ internal systems
> - ✔ processes
> - ✔ agreed ways of working
> - ✔ individuals and others being involved in the decision-making process.

AC 2.12 Plan for improvements to internal systems and processes and agreed ways of working

Here, you will develop a plan for improvements in the setting that will have benefits for person-centred care.

As a manager, you must review and update systems, processes and practices to ensure that they continue to contribute positive practice.

It is only by doing this that an organisation can grow and improvements can be made. In your own setting, for example, you might start by making a simple change to encourage everyone to invest in person-centred care. By putting up posters and giving out details via leaflets, individuals in your care and their families can be encouraged to ask questions and play a more active role.

Additionally, you might encourage the team to identify what can be changed in the service to improve outcomes for individuals and then discuss the ways in which those changes can be made. It is important to have explicit aims, which means being clear about what the setting is trying to achieve in improving its approach to person-centred care. In this way, the outcomes from the changes can be measured more readily.

> **Evidence opportunity**
>
> **2.12 Review the extent to which systems, processes and practice facilitate positive outcomes**
>
> Undertake a review and update of the systems, policies and practices you have in place to ensure that they facilitate improvements to agreed ways of working. Show evidence of this to your assessor.

AC 2.13 Lead implementation for improvements to internal systems, processes and agreed ways of working

Here, you will be required to show you can actively identify improvements and plan and implement changes to systems, processes and agreed ways of working.

> **Reflect on it**
>
> **2.13 Change management**
>
> Think of a change you have had to make in your care setting and critically analyse the way in which you led the team in each of the following areas. Examine each heading to determine how effective your change was. Give one example for each heading.
>
> - Driving changes in service strategy and operational delivery, e.g. what was the change?
> - Business development and related opportunities. How did the change affect the business?
> - Overcoming resistance and barriers to change. What resistance did you get and how did you handle it?
> - Leading by example – setting best practice. How did you lead by example?
> - Incorporating, inspiring and encouraging others to recommend changes in care service provision, e.g. teams and those in receipt of care services. How did you inspire your team?

Any improvement made to systems, processes and ways of working requires a change management approach to be taken for it to be wholly successful.

Lewin's change management model

Kurt Lewin's change management model is a three-stage theory of change, commonly referred to as 'Unfreeze – Change – Freeze (or Refreeze)', but it also includes something you may be familiar with in today's adult social care setting – the use of force field analysis.

Unfreezing

This stage is about preparing for the change and making sure there is shared understanding about the nature and rationale for the change. Deadlines need to be created because this motivates you towards the change. If there is no deadline there will be no action. Force field analysis comes into play in this stage: this is the time to weigh up the pros and cons of change before any action is taken. If there are more positive factors for the change then staff are more likely to move with it and be motivated. Think about the last major change you made at work. Maybe you decided to change a process of working or a method of delivering care. These big decisions involve listing the advantages (pros) or disadvantages (cons) of such a change and staff need to be on board with these developments. This is where force field analysis and the unfreezing take place.

Change

The change or transition is the process of making the change or moving towards the change. As you start to implement the change there is a steep learning curve, so staff need to be given some time to understand what is happening.

Freezing

Once the first two stages have been successfully negotiated, freezing or refreezing, as it is sometimes referred to, happens. In this stage, the change becomes the norm and staff start to feel comfortable in new routines. This has been criticised by some writers as being a little simplistic because change is happening so rapidly, particularly in care settings, that we are not given the luxury of becoming comfortable in new routines. What you can do is support staff and reinforce the change whenever you can.

Evidence opportunity

2.13 Change and improvement

How do you actively identify improvements and plan and implement changes to systems, processes and agreed ways of working? Show your assessor the process of improvement you favour to demonstrate your understanding.

The advantages of the Lewin model are its simplicity and the number of steps involved. It is easy to plan for and implement. The disadvantages are the time it takes to 'unfreeze' current thinking and practice. Some critics also point to the lack of instructions as to how to accomplish each step. Your role as manager will be to engage staff in this activity by training them in the use of force field analysis. They will need support to ensure that they have a clear picture of what the end result following an implemented change is likely to look like. This will require clear communication and explanation during each stage.

The manager's role is to lead on improvements within the setting and you also need to be able to plan for and implement any changes required. The use of SMART objectives for staff, and ensuring that team objectives are set, will be a useful tool to develop improvements in the delivery of adult care.

Evidence opportunity

2.13 Plan and lead the implementation of improvements

Show your assessor how you actively identify improvements, plan and implement changes to systems and processes.

LO3 Be able to lead a culture that supports innovation and change to improve outcomes for individuals

AC 3.1 Outline the meaning of culture, innovation, change and transformation in relation to adult care

Here, you will outline key terms relating to the culture of a setting.

Culture

The culture of an organisation influences the staff members and the operation of the work environment each day. Culture is the way things are done in the setting and the way in which people behave and perform. The practices and behaviours that have been identified as important to an organisation set the standard for how staff should conduct themselves.

Innovation

Innovation means building or producing something new. This might be a system or process or a product. It can also be a new way of doing something or a new way of thinking. Innovation can be a powerful tool for change and for improving social care practice.

Change

There are three types of change that all managers should be aware of:

- **Developmental change**: This happens when a need arises and improvements have to be made to the current process.
- **Transitional change**: This involves recognising that a new course of action must be taken and it requires a plan to make the change happen.
- **Transformational change**: This happens when a process fails and a new process emerges. It is usually unplanned and may need to be refined.

Source: Adapted from Management Training Specialists (2009)

> **Evidence opportunity**
>
> **3.1 Identifying change**
>
> Outline your understanding of culture, innovation, change and transformation. Provide a definition for each term.

AC 3.2 Evaluate the achievement of outcomes for individuals to identify where improvements could be made

Here, you will evaluate ways in which improvements can be measured in order to improve outcomes for individuals.

Measuring outcomes is essential to show that changes to care or services have resulted in an improvement. You looked at the model for improvement and PDSA improvement cycle in AC1.2 and this is a good place to start. If the achievement of outcomes is not shown then there has been no improvement, and there will be a need to try something new.

By setting and using quality measures you can calculate how well your service aligns with a quality statement. This in turn helps to highlight changes to your service that you could make. The three measures you can look at are:

- the environment or setting
- the activity carried out
- the end result or impact.

The individuals using your service will have set personal outcomes or goals that describe what they need to support their wellbeing and these can be measured by returning to the three questions of the PDSA model. What did you want to achieve? Was there an improvement? If not, what will the next step be?

> **Evidence opportunity**
>
> **3.2 Evaluating outcomes to identify possible improvements**
>
> Evaluate the achievement of outcomes for individuals to identify where improvements could be made. Engage with individuals and assess outcomes against their care/support plans. What improvements have you noticed? What further improvements to their care might be made?

AC 3.3 Work with others to identify the transformation and innovation opportunities for service improvement

Here, you will demonstrate ways in which the service can be transformed and how innovation can be introduced in a setting.

Transformation

Transformation means 'a change of form' and to do this in your setting you will need to completely change how you do and see things and how care is structured and delivered. By engaging the individuals using your service, their carers, family and friends, your colleagues, peers and team members, you can access a diverse range of views and ideas that may be innovative and new.

Transformation starts with the recognition that change needs to happen. It is about doing things differently for better outcomes for those who use your service. The response to change is often not well received because change can be scary and unpredictable. It often requires risks to be taken and attitudes, beliefs and behaviours to change.

Innovation

Innovation includes the development of ideas and concepts to solve problems in a more creative way. Developing innovative and creative skills involves taking risks and engaging in independent and sometimes unconventional thinking. Innovation requires a different sort of mindset to explore new ways of working.

Reflect on it

3.3 Change and innovation

How do you feel about change and innovation? Write an honest reflection on how you manage enforced changes to your setting.

AC 3.4 Utilise the expertise of individuals and/or others

Here, you will explain the Social Care Innovation Network and how this can be utilised to improve service and develop new innovations and manage change to the service.

Driving innovation and improvement

The Social Care Innovation Network is funded by the Department of Health and Social Care and is a partnership between SCIE, Think Local Act Personal (TLAP) and Shared Lives Plus. It was set up to support innovative approaches to social care Also, local authority services have experts by experience in their strategy groups and these individuals can supply valuable input into the types of service they would like to see delivered. The white paper 'People at the heart of care' (DHSC, 2022b) provides a ten-year strategy to address all aspects of social care, which includes involving people and organisations across the sector working in partnership with stakeholders and people who draw on care to support the implementation of the measures set out.

In 2018, Phase 1 of the Social Care Innovation project revealed that while there were many good examples of innovative approaches to care, they failed to take root and survive beyond short-term funding. Since the definition of innovation is subjective, some ideas will be seen as radical by some groups whereas others may view them as old and outdated. The Network views innovation as approaches to care that see people as citizens first and promote wellbeing. The first question to consider is 'What does a good life look like?' rather than 'What changes are needed to services?' If you undertake to support individuals in this way, a different picture of a good care and support system emerges, and this has been defined as an Asset-Based Area.

An asset-based approach is one in which rather than looking solely at problems and what the service cannot provide or do, the attention is turned to what the organisations and people of each area can do. By bringing together the expertise of people, time, creativity and resources of everybody in a given area, a more positive approach to care is developed.

It may be that your own area already engages with services in this way but to have more of an impact, it will require whole systems and areas to align with this approach. The Network argues that change can only be led when practitioners act as local citizens, working as partners, not 'providers', and taking the share of responsibility for the best use of resources.

Asset-based areas respond to needs but look for potential, recognising that their own service has limitations, and empowers citizens by redefining the role of providers as working with, not for, people.

Source: Adapted from Social Care Innovation Network (2019)

Research it

3.4 Social Care Innovation Network

Research the report by the Social Care Innovation Network, 'Getting under the skin of it' (2019). The report is based on the principle that people want a life and not a service and highlights how change might be encouraged by the development of asset based areas.

Read section 5 'What can be done locally to support the growth and spread of innovation?' and prepare a short report to show how your local area might benefit from this development.

Driving change

Service strategy differs from operational delivery and, as a manager, you need to be clear about each of these terms.

A setting might have a strategic plan in place, together with key performance indicators for staff and services offered. These goals will provide a three- to five-year plan to help the organisation to meet individuals' needs both now and in the future. The strategic plan will look closely at what is done at operational levels and try to plan for change, which will ensure that the service remains sustainable and competitive in the future. It will also give an indication of how the setting will develop and evolve over the years to ensure that it remains fit for purpose in the future. You should be mindful of the political and legislative drivers that will change the service provision, the market trends as well as demographic changes happening, so that in the five-year span you will be evolving the setting to meet all those needs you may want to serve.

It is most important in driving change that we do not become overly concerned with the everyday activities and work that move the service forward on a daily basis. There is a tendency to focus more on getting through the day and providing the care that's needed, so you may be forgiven sometimes if you forget the bigger picture that is the strategic strategy.

You need to have both streams working together and your staff must be aware of where the setting is heading and how what they do links into that. Focusing just on what you do now to get through the day is foolhardy and a number of adult social care provisions have fallen into this trap. For example, when mandatory training for care staff was cited in legislation, some managers/owners of homes buried their heads in the sand and decided it was not for them. They failed to see the bigger picture, which meant that inspection strategy was also changing. At the next inspection, many found they did not meet the requirements for trained staff, and they did not receive a favourable inspection grading.

It is imperative that staff are fully aware of the threats and opportunities that exist and can offer their solutions to everyday problems, in order to be part of shaping the future.

In managing change, leaders have to ensure that employees buy into the vision for the service, and this requires good communication, with clear and consistent information. You must also show understanding if there is resistance to change. People need to feel included in decisions and, as a manager, your role will be to help staff to overcome any resistance.

In a leadership role, others will look to your behaviour and be guided by it. Take a moment to reflect upon somebody you have worked with whom you admired. What characteristics did they have that you liked and would like to copy? For example, you may have worked with people who under pressure managed to keep a perspective that meant everybody around them felt calm and in control. They dealt with challenging situations in a rational way and managed to keep a sense of humour in the process. You may, therefore, take that example and try hard to emulate that in your daily work. You may have also worked with people who under stress would snap at staff and become completely unapproachable until the situation was under control. This is a behaviour that you certainly do not want to copy as it can completely change the team spirit. When managing change, a positive attitude towards it can be inspiring for others who may otherwise feel anxious.

As a manager you need to set examples that drive the vision and strategy forward and at the same time inspire and encourage staff to do the same. You can go a step further in this and ask and encourage staff, as well as those who use such services, to recommend changes for developing an entrepreneurial spirit and innovation.

Reflect on it

3.4 Impact of personal behaviour

Take time to think about the behaviour you display in your role and how this impacts others. How do you ensure that you remain positive in times of change and challenge?

LO4 Understand how to implement effective change in adult care

AC 4.1 Explain the term 'change management' in adult care

Here, you will explain what change management is and how it may be needed in the setting.

Change management is a process of planning, implementing and monitoring changes in an organisation. To ensure the smooth implementation of a change process, staff and the individuals using the service need to be prepared for the change. Change can be difficult, so it is good to have a plan to help them through the transition. A simple plan, prepare, implement, monitor and evaluation cycle will ensure that change is carefully managed (see AC4.3).

KEY TERM

Change management: A systematic approach to dealing with the transition or transformation of an organisation's goals, processes or technologies. The purpose of change management is to implement strategies for effecting change, controlling change and helping people to adapt to change.

AC 4.2 Explain models of best practice in 'change management'

Here, you will explain different models in how to approach change.

Any change you make in your life brings about uncertainty and the tendency to ask yourself 'what if' questions: What if I am wrong to do this? What if everything goes wrong? You can get into a cycle of negative thinking about your own intentions. Even if the source of change is your own choice, it can still be scary. Self-created change may cause you anxiety but the motivation to make the change was entirely your own. This is different from changes imposed from external sources.

Change management theories and models identify ways that change can be managed well. Lewin's change management model was discussed in AC2.13 and Covey's '7 Habits' in Unit 509 LO2. In Unit 511 AC1.1 you looked at Kotter's eight steps to successful change model and you can refer to these now. Additionally, some models from other disciplines are also worth looking at.

Kolb's learning cycle

Kolb (1984) developed a cycle of experiential learning, and this has led to the development of models of reflective practice. Kolb recommends that we need to recall our observation of an event, reflect on the observations, develop and research some theories about what we saw and then decide on some action as a result of the process (Jasper, 2003). With respect to change, similar processes are utilised and Kolb's model, written with Frohman, is a lengthier version of Lewin's and is shown in Figure 24.

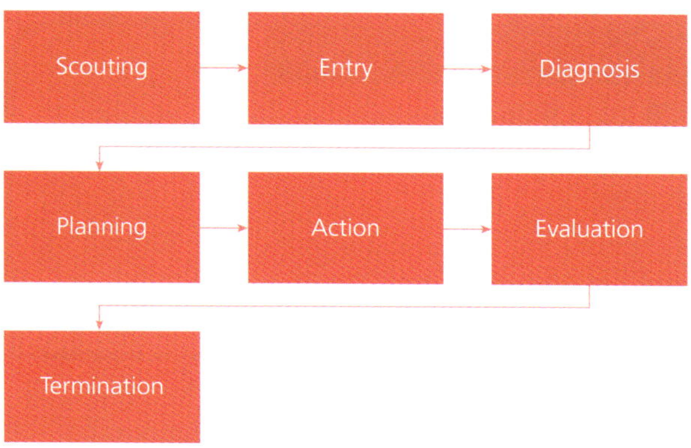

▲ **Figure 24** Kolb and Frohman's change model

This model looks at the stages of organisational change as a relationship between an organisational consultant (designer) and their client (user).

- **Scouting**: The consultant and client look at each other's needs in order to decide if there is a fit.
- **Entry**: A starting point for the project is selected, with initial goals and objectives set. Commitment to the project is also declared. The two parties build a trust relationship and a 'contract' for who will lead the project.
- **Diagnosis**: Data gathering begins and the problem is clearly defined. The consultant and client look at the available resources (including commitment) to see if it is feasible to continue.
- **Planning**: Planning begins with the consultant and client clearly defining the specific objectives and examining alternative ways to accomplish these. Any proposed solutions are judged as to the impact they will have, and an action plan is then put into place.
- **Action**: The consultant and client put into practice the best solution.
- **Evaluation**: The action plan is assessed as to its level of achievement of the goals set and the consultant and client decide whether more work is needed or to terminate the plan.
- **Termination**: The consultant and client make sure that all involved with the change have mastered new ways of working and have control of the new systems in place.

Source: Adapted from Buse et al. (2013)

The advantage of using Kolb's learning cycle lies in its effectiveness in improving performance in experiential learning, but a disadvantage of it is that the **experiential learning** model does not always fit with all situations. Staff may already be aware of this model as an experiential learning cycle and a way of reflection and in managing change in your setting. Your role as manager will be to show how it can be used as a way to introduce change in practice.

> **KEY TERM**
>
> **Experiential learning**: The process of learning through experience.

Herzberg's Two-factor theory (motivation–hygiene)

Frederick Herzberg's theory of motivation identified that the motivators or factors that brought high morale to staff are achievement, recognition, responsibility and promotion prospects within the role and the nature of the job. These factors can motivate staff if they are present and can increase job satisfaction. Alternatively, hygiene factors such as pay, company policy, type of management, benefits and relationship with colleagues are, according to Herzberg, likely to lead to job dissatisfaction if they are ignored or absent. They were not considered to be 'true' motivators but rather were expected conditions of normal working life.

Herzberg found that to increase motivation in workers, dissatisfaction had to be avoided and this was accomplished by addressing the hygiene factors, meaning workers were not negative about their jobs. This led to people who were calmer in their workplace and happier. He determined that by addressing the motivators, job satisfaction could be increased. When managing a team this is worth investing in. For example, you may have no control over the pay somebody gets but you can address the way in which they are perceived and valued in their role.

The advantage of Herzberg's theory lies with the factors that motivate and demotivate groups of employees and, as a manager, you will have some control over these. A disadvantage of Herzberg's theory is that factors that motivate can change; they may also be different for some people. Employees may have very different views as to dissatisfaction and satisfaction at work and, as a manager, you need to work towards achieving no dissatisfaction at work. This means, for example, addressing the hygiene factors in the workplace and ensuring that working conditions, pay relationships and company policy all benefit the employees. As a result, staff are likely to be more positive at work and job satisfaction can then be worked upon by introducing the motivators such as responsibility, recognition and achievement.

Kubler-Ross Five-stage model – the change curve

You might be familiar with Elizabeth Kubler-Ross' five stages of grief in her book *On Death and Dying*, which were said to represent the normal range of feelings people experience when dealing with bereavement.

You can appreciate that change often involves some sort of loss, so the five-stage model has been adapted and applied to managing change.

Kubler-Ross' five stages of grief (Figure 25) are:

- denial
- anger
- bargaining
- depression
- acceptance.

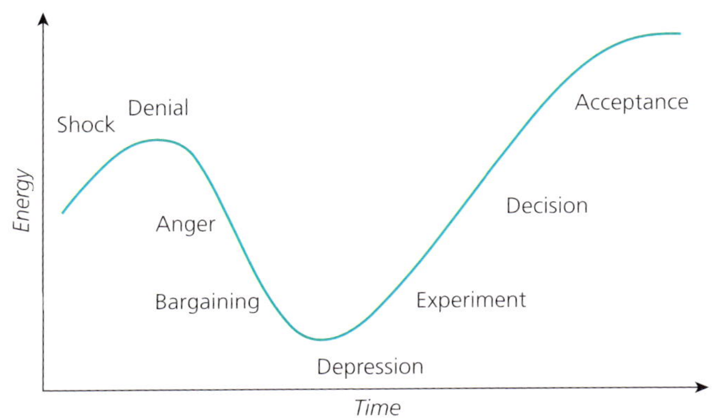

▲ **Figure 25** Kubler-Ross change curve

Kubler-Ross explained that these are normal reactions we have to tragic news and called them defence or coping mechanisms that we need to move through in order to manage change. Any change in the workplace may see staff going through similar stages.

Since the model was created, two further stages have been added, which are:

- experiment (after depression)
- decision (after experiment).

These stages evolved into what Kubler-Ross terms the change curve, which shows the levels of emotion or energy experienced by people as they deal with change. Even though it depicts a linear process, individuals move in and out of stages and it does not follow that we can expect somebody in shock and denial to move straight into anger. They may well do, but they may also simply move straight on to acceptance.

When you use this model, you can identify and understand how your staff are dealing with change and also have a better understanding of the reactions you are seeing and why staff are behaving in a particular way.

As a change model, one advantage is that it identifies how others are dealing with and reacting to change and, in this way, you can see why your colleagues may be behaving in a particular way. A disadvantage is that it does not describe the wide range of emotions that people may feel. It assumes that we all react similarly, but cultural differences may bring about different emotional reactions.

Evidence opportunity

4.1 and 4.2 Change management models

Explain the change management theories and models in terms of their relevance and how you apply them or would apply them in your current leadership and management practice.

AC 4.3 Describe the processes of 'change management'

Here, you will describe how change management can be implemented within the setting.

When undertaking change management in your organisation, it is helpful to view this as a series of steps.

Step 1: Prepare the staff in your organisation

The first step in any change is to prepare your staff, the individuals using your service, their families and commissioning agencies. At this stage you will need to focus on helping staff to understand why the change needs to happen. It may be that a new government directive requires you to address systems in the setting that will impact ways of working. By making your staff aware of the challenges facing the organisation you can start to show them how this is affecting the setting and how it will affect them. This should lead to an initial buy-in, removing any resistance.

Step 2: Plan for change

Having prepared staff for the change, a robust plan must developed. The plan must have a set goal to work towards, with key performance indicators that show how success will be measured. Project stakeholders and a team must be chosen to oversee the task of implementing the change and the actual steps and actions that will be taken.

A risk assessment will be needed to identify what challenges might be faced along the way. Implement the changes by following the steps in the plan. During that time, staff need to be encouraged to do their best to achieve the goals and to anticipate and deal with risks that may arise. Communication is key at this stage.

Step 3: Embed changes into culture and practices

When the change has been accomplished you need to prevent a return to the previous way of working by embedding the changes into the company's culture and practices.

Review progress and analyse results

The effects of the change must be reviewed and analysed as it may or may not have been successful. Conducting analysis and review can offer insights as to how the change was handled and what lessons can be learned from the process as a whole.

> **Evidence opportunity**
>
> **4.3 Identify and plan a change**
>
> Describe how you would implement and manage a change within your setting.

AC 4.4 Describe tools and skills needed to inspire change, development and innovation across the setting/service

Here, you will describe the skills needed to ensure that change can be implemented in the setting.

Your setting will be changing every day and the most important skills you need to manage change are communication skills. Change can be difficult for staff, so they need to be aware of every part of the change process. You therefore need to clarify what is happening and be honest about the change. Resistance happens when people do not understand why a change is needed. Ensuring that staff and those using the service understand what the change is for and giving them support to help them play their part means they are more likely to buy into the process.

Part of communication is the need to listen. Listening is a two-way process and by gaining feedback from staff about how the change is working and taking ideas on board, the process will be easier to manage. Staff who are invested in the change and who feel their opinions matter will make sure the change sticks.

Developing trust through effective leadership ensures that people feel motivated to make change happen. Being part of the change and being listened to is crucial for success. Staff must feel that they are valuable and that they are contributing to the change in some way. By building trust you can show that you care about what your staff think and feel, and they will be more likely to engage with the project.

Projects fail when they are not measured correctly so you need to be able to identify the key performance indicators (KPIs) that measure success. Staff need to know that their efforts have not been in vain and that the change has led to an improvement.

> **Evidence opportunity**
>
> **4.4 Tools and skills needed for change**
>
> Describe the tools and skills you will need to undertake a developmental change in your setting or service.

AC 4.5 Outline the range of external drivers for change in adult care

Here, you will outline the way in which external aspects such as the law and demographic changes might impact the need for change in the setting.

Changes that might be imposed upon you from the government and other external drivers will include those due to legislative changes, and service providers are duty bound to amend their ways of working as a result of these.

Impact of legislative changes

Legislative changes to the Mental Capacity Act 2005, together with the introduction of the Down Syndrome Act 2022 and the Autism Act 2009, impact the care provisions in these areas.

For example, with two million people in England and Wales lacking capacity to make decisions for themselves those working with these individuals require a knowledge of how best to help the process.

The Autism Act 2009 committed the government to publishing an adult autism strategy to transform services for adults with autism. The strategy set out key actions and recommendations for central government and local authorities to meet. These included the need to increase awareness and understanding of autism, to develop a clear pathway for diagnosis, to improve access to services and to support people to live independently. Employment and the need to involve local partners to develop relevant services was also an area for change.

The Down Syndrome Act 2022 aims to improve access to services and to improve the quality of life for people with Down syndrome. It calls for all service provisions, including local authority and commissioning services together with health, social care and education, to recognise that people with Down syndrome have specific needs that must be met.

The impact and benefit of changes in the law may be that cost savings can be made if ways of working are altered. For example, involving people in their own health and care by offering the information and support they need to manage their independence means they may be less likely to need more complex support. A disadvantage of legislative changes is that there is usually no choice but to implement them. You may also not be privy to the reason behind a change, which can make it more difficult, particularly if you believe it is unnecessary or you cannot see any benefit to it, even though there is obviously a benefit and clear rationale for it. In these circumstances you have not had the time to process what is going on and to reflect upon the change and it is then you may start to feel anxious and try to resist the change. However, it is important to embrace the positives and focus on how such legislation can bring about positive change.

Reflect on it

4.5 External drivers for change

Outline the external drivers for change affecting your setting.

AC 4.6 Describe how external drivers for change impact on adult care settings/services

Here, you will describe how commissioning agencies, legislation, public opinion, finances, etc. mean that settings have to change their ways of working.

CQC inspection process

'Change' is also part of the CQC inspection experience and can be a process that causes anxiety among staff. Before an inspection, staff may make changes to how they are working (i.e. 'self-created' change) but inspection may also bring about (or 'impose') changes to the way in which care is being delivered in order to meet standards. This can lead to improved ways of working.

Revenue/funding changes and staffing/workforce changes

Changes to the way in which care is funded and budgetary cuts will impact both staff and the individuals using the service and may lead to workforce changes. This can, of course, impact staff negatively causing anxiety and concern about job losses and reduced salaries. The benefits may result in a more streamlined workforce that is working more efficiently, but such change requires careful handling and sensitivity.

Managerial strategy, operational objectives, changes in service/business ownership and mergers

New policies can occur as a result of:

- legislative changes
- regulatory/inspection changes
- revenue/funding changes
- staffing/workforce changes
- managerial strategy and operational objectives
- changes in service/business ownership, mergers.

All of these points may create feelings of anxiety among your staff and, as the manager, you need to appreciate why this is so. Any change, whether it is self-created or imposed, is likely to cause stress. If you choose to move to a new house, you may be excited about the prospect, but you may also fear the unknown that comes with such a big life decision. With imposed change, we may try to ignore it or actively resist it by not buying into that change. What is the emotion behind resisting change? Think back to your self-imposed change and the thinking that went on. What if it's the wrong decision? The emotion that is foremost is one of fear and any change that your staff have to deal with will invariably expose their fear in a variety of ways. They may fear being unable to adapt to the change or that they lack the ability to undertake new work. For example, the implementation of a new IT system may mean that staff have to learn how to use a new system and change their way of working. An example of this sort of change was described earlier when we highlighted how staff in an adult social care setting changed the way they reported care via an app rather than on paper. Had the change not been introduced in a sympathetic manner by including staff in the decisions, it may have been met with anger, frustration and disapproval for the way in which they were being treated. The underlying fear may also have been due to the loss of a system they felt worked well but may also have been due to concern about potential job losses.

Fredrickson (1998) argued that negative emotions result in a fight or flight type of response which limits our thoughts and actions. We become overly concerned with the threat and want to run away. Change in organisations is inevitable and by establishing positive ways of dealing with it you can help staff to embrace it rather than fear it. If you feel good about something you take more interest in it and are curious about what might happen. By taking a more positive view of change and recognising how it can bring about better working conditions, you can help staff to embrace it.

Reflect on it

4.6 Changes in the setting

What was the last major change you had to deal with in your setting?

How did you feel about it and how did it impact your thinking?

Evidence opportunity

4.6 Imposed changes

Look at the following list and describe how these imposed or self-created changes have impacted your service. Consider the impact on your staff.

- ✔ Commissioning agencies.
- ✔ Legislative changes.
- ✔ Regulatory/inspection changes.
- ✔ Revenue/funding changes.
- ✔ Staffing/workforce changes.
- ✔ Managerial strategy and operational objectives.
- ✔ Changes in service/business ownership, mergers.

AC 4.7 Explain success factors and barriers in respect of implementing effective change

Here, you will explain ways in which a setting can implement change.

Success factors

If a business is to remain viable and competitive it needs to develop new products and processes and in care work this may mean looking at new ways of working. This requires changing the way you do things and, as already noted, this might be unsettling.

Service vision and service strategy

The vision of a service sets out its direction and broad aims and distinguishes it from other organisations. For example, your vision might be 'to improve outcomes for individuals'. The service strategy determines how the organisation intends to reach that vision. There are a number of ways in which you can reach the vision, but innovation and entrepreneurial strategies are likely to give you the edge over other similar providers. As the manager, you need to develop a culture of curiosity and openness within the team to encourage new ways of thinking about providing care.

Operational planning and delivery

With a strategic plan in place it is a managerial task to develop an operational plan that details the day-to-day tasks needed for the smooth and efficient running of the organisation or setting and for the people who work there. It will outline staff roles, responsibilities and duties so that everyone is aware of what is expected of them. These will be in keeping with the overall objectives of the organisation or setting. The operational plan will focus on 'what', 'who', 'when' and 'how much' to ensure that everyone is aware of their role.

An operational plan changes over time and managers need to be able to manage those changes. For example, in a competitive field of work, change may be required because of new updates and guidance from government or there may be changes to finances. As the manager, you need to be able to manage the change and to help others to see the advantages of it. High levels of competition require organisations to move forward by embracing change and adapting new technology and methods.

Service quality

Within the operational plan there will be reference to how the quality of the service is to be monitored and maintained. Audit tools will be available and quality measures need to be adhered to. Changes may need to be made because of surveys and audits to improve the delivery of quality care.

Integration and integrated services/the wider adult care system

With the inclusion of wider care services you must ensure that other services are made fully aware of any changes. Changes may come about because of working with external stakeholders where operations become more complex. Managing such changes may involve transitioning staff, groups and projects from one way of working to another.

Change management theories and models, when correctly implemented, can support innovation and business development by empowering staff to improve their practice. Staff who are informed and supported throughout the change are likely to offer less resistance.

Evidence opportunity

4.7 Innovation and business development

Explain success factors and barriers to implementing effective change in your setting. Use your setting's vision statement to support your explanation.

	Define (say what each of these terms means to your setting)	Change theory utilised for each of these concepts (what is the change theory utilised for service vision, service strategy, etc.?)	Comment on how it supported your work
Service vision	e.g. what is your service vision or mission?	e.g. how has it been developed or changed over time and how was it delivered to staff?	e.g. what areas did it support?
Service strategy			
Operational planning and delivery			
Service quality			
Integration and integrated services/the wider adult care system			

Barriers

You have looked at why people dislike the idea of change, and it is suggested that fear is at the heart of this. Think of the last time a change occurred in your workplace in which you had no say and had been given no information about why it was needed. How did you feel?

Resistance to change and a lack of understanding about why change is necessary can be a real barrier to people committing to change. Also, the structures put in place by the commissioning agencies may be difficult to input and be a barrier to change. If there is no leadership to help you through the change it will be difficult to be inspired to make it work. If staff issues about the change are not defined and addressed, staff will not engage with the change and morale will plummet.

SCIE has supplied guidance on dealing with barriers to change in various areas of care, including participation and co-production. There is guidance for individuals using care services on how they can be supported in overcoming some of the barriers to individual participation by having systems that are flexible and that take into account the way in which their individual circumstances influence the ability to participate.

Also, for adult social care managers, SCIE have introduced a new digital resource to support managers to deal with change within their settings. The resource features change management tools to help support change. The new interactive digital format means that people will be able to quickly use and apply the tool to real-life issues. (See Social Care Institute for Excellence, n.d.)

Communication is a vital aspect in effectively managing change. Sometimes it can help to present your team with a problem that needs to be solved, rather than simply telling them about a solution that is already going to be implemented. Giving people an opportunity to work together to find a solution makes it more likely that they will understand the reason for change and be ready to adopt the change with less resistance.

Staff engaged in adult social care are, on the whole, committed to delivering quality of care. If, as a manager, you can demonstrate how a change will improve that delivery and be better for the individuals using the service, staff are more likely to accept it.

Another crucial factor in eliciting commitment to change is to keep channels of communication open and to ensure that the team understands the vision and strategic direction. Team meetings with agendas giving team members opportunities to offer their ideas should be set up and other forms of communication, such as email, WhatsApp and other forms of instant messaging may also be useful, but you should consider the advantages and disadvantages of these. Communicating through discussions and appraisals is a good way to ensure that all are aware of the changes and how they might be affected. Suggestions from staff should be encouraged and considered.

In working with others, you need to promote a shared vision by ensuring that everyone is involved in decision making and is aware of the need for the change.

Stretch and challenge

4.7 Change management

Explain your role in change management.

References

Buse, F., Mangu, S.I., Buse, G.F. and Slusariuc, G.C. (2013) 'The strategy of implementation and integration of the Decision Support Systems having in view achievement of a performant management at SC Energetic Complex, Oltenia, SA'. *Journal of Engineering Studies and Research*, 19(2).

Care Quality Commission (2019) 'The state of health care and adult social care in England 2018/19'. www.cqc.org.uk/sites/default/files/20191015b_stateofcare1819_fullreport.pdf

Care Quality Commission (2022) 'The state of health care and adult social care in England 2021/22'. www.cqc.org.uk/publication/state-care-202122/concern#ratings

Department of Health and Social Care (2017) 'Adult social care quality matters'. https://assets.publishing.service.gov.uk/government/uploads/system/uploads/attachment_data/file/795351/Adult_Social_Care_-_Quality_Matters.pdf

Department of Health and Social Care (2022a) 'Care and support statutory guidance'. www.gov.uk/government/publications/care-act-statutory-guidance/care-and-support-statutory-guidance

Department of Health and Social Care (2022b) Policy paper 'People at the heart of care: Adult social care reform'. www.gov.uk/government/publications/people-at-the-heart-of-care-adult-social-care-reform-white-paper/people-at-the-heart-of-care-adult-social-care-reform

Fredrickson, B. (1998) 'What good are positive emotions?' *Review of General Psychology*, 2(3): 300–19.

Harkin, B., Webb, T.L., Chang, B.P.I., Prestwich, A., Conner, M., Kellar, I., Benn, Y. and Sheeran, P. (2016) 'Does monitoring goal progress promote goal attainment? A meta-analysis of the experimental evidence'. *Psychological Bulletin*, 142(2), 198–299. https://doi.org/10.1037/bul0000025

Jasper, M. (2003) *Beginning Reflective Practice*. Oxford: Nelson Thorne.

Management Training Specialists (2009) 'The three types of change'. www.mtdtraining.com/blog/three-types-of-change.htm

Mehrabian, A. (1972). *Nonverbal Communication*. New Brunswick: Aldine Transaction.

Science Daily (2015) 'Frequently monitoring progress toward goals increases chance of success'. www.sciencedaily.com/releases/2015/10/151029101349.htm

Skills for Care (n.d.) 'Digital technology in social care', www.skillsforcare.org.uk/Support-for-leaders-and-managers/Managing-a-service/Digital-technology-and-social-care/Digital-technology-in-social-care.aspx

Social Care Innovation Network (2019) 'Getting under the skin of it'. www.thinklocalactpersonal.org.uk/_assets/Social-Care-Innovation-Network-Phase-1.pdf

Social Care Institute for Excellence (n.d.) 'SCIE media releases'. www.scie.org.uk/news/mediareleases/

Useful resources and further reading

Care Quality Commission (2022) 'Adult social care: Information for providers'. www.cqc.org.uk/guidance-providers/adult-social-care

Health Foundation, The (2014) 'Person-centred care made simple: What everyone should know about person-centred care'. www.health.org.uk/publications/person-centred-care-made-simple

Hunter, D.J., Perkins, N., Visram, S., Adams, L., Finn, R., Forrest, A. and Gosling, J. (2018) *Evaluating the Leadership Role of Health and Wellbeing Boards as Drivers of Health Improvement and Integrated Care across England*. Durham: National Institute for Health Research.

NHS Confederation (2012) 'Delivering dignity: Securing dignity in care for older people in hospitals and care homes'. www.nhsconfed.org/publications/delivering-dignity

Public Health England (2017) *Reducing Health Inequalities: System, scale and sustainability*. London: PHE Publications.

Roberts, G.W. and Machon, A. (2015) *Appreciative Healthcare Practice: A guide to compassionate, person-centred care*. Keswick: M&K Publishing.

Sanderson, H. and Lewis, J. (2003) *A Practical Guide to Delivering Personalisation: Person-centred practice in health and social care*. London: Jessica Kingsley Publishers.

Skills for Care and Skills for Health (2013) 'Code of Conduct for Healthcare Support Workers and Adult Social Care Workers in England'. www.skillsforcare.org.uk/resources/documents/Support-for-leaders-and-managers/Managing-people/Code-of-conduct/Code-of-Conduct.pdf

Social Care Institute for Excellence (n.d.) 'Dignity in care: Privacy and dignity in care'. www.scie.org.uk/dignity/care/privacy

Zambrano-Monserrate, M.A., Ruano, M.A. and Sanchez-Alcalde, L. (2020) 'Indirect effects of COVID-19 on the environment'. *The Science of the Total Environment*, 728, 138813. https://doi.org/10.1016/j.scitotenv.2020.138813

Unit 513

Effective communication in leadership and management in adult care

GLH 20

About this unit

Effective communication and information management demands that you know yourself well, are aware of what you bring to your communication, and how you might impact those you communicate with.

The purpose of this unit is to revisit the systems of communication used in care work and in particular when managing information in a care setting. In any relationship, be it personal or working, effective communication skills play an essential part, and being able to communicate well is one of the most important aspects of your role as a leader and manager.

Misunderstanding and misinterpreting the message can lead to team conflict and disrupt the smooth running of the organisation. It can also lead to ineffective delivery of services and unproductive teamwork. Being an effective communicator is therefore key to successful working.

In this unit, you will explore the different models of communication, how to develop communication systems and practices which will support positive outcomes, understand how you can implement systems for effective information management and support others to communicate effectively.

Learning outcomes

By the end of this unit, you will:

1. Know how to use communication skills to achieve positive interactions.
2. Know how to manage and resolve conflict.
3. Be able to communicate effectively with others.
4. Be able to develop communication practices.

Getting started

Before you study the unit, think about the following:

- What different models of communication are there in your setting, and how might they apply to your management practice?
- What systems do you have in place to ensure that all staff fully understand the policies and procedures that apply to their practice and how is this monitored?
- What are the barriers to effective communication within **service delivery teams**?
- Why is it important to lead others in maintaining accuracy in record keeping?

KEY TERMS

Service delivery teams: Teams within **multidisciplinary groups** such as the primary care team, social care team, hospital, housing and other services used within your own setting.

Multidisciplinary groups: Groups of people with different specialist skills. For example, the group may have people with medical and care expertise and others with specialist knowledge of housing and other services.

LO1 Know how to use communication skills to achieve positive interactions

AC 1.1 Explain how to achieve positive interactions within an adult care setting/service

Here, you will explain different types of communication and communication models.

Communication skills

To be skilled in communication requires you to use a variety of interpersonal techniques and to be able to adapt the way in which you communicate according to a variety of factors. As a manager, your skills lie in listening actively to staff and other people you meet in your work in order to make decisions and to negotiate issues that may arise. Your role requires you to deliver information and provide feedback. You will use several methods to do this, including attending meetings, training staff, assessing the individuals using your service and writing reports.

Crawford et al. (2006) suggest that:

> *Communication is something we do in our internal world of thoughts and in our external world by speaking, writing, gestures, drawing, making images and symbols or receiving messages from others.*

Effective communication is the means by which you deliver and receive a message and both need to be consistent in order for the communication to work. Communication is the basis of interaction, so skills in speaking, writing and especially listening are essential in social care. As a manager, you will interact and communicate with a range of people within social care settings, including the individuals using your service (who may be vulnerable), their families, staff, visitors and other professionals. You may sometimes communicate with individuals who are going through a personal crisis or are upset, and this requires skill to make sure they feel supported and valued.

The effectiveness of your communication skills as a manager and leader within the care setting will undoubtedly lead to the success of the organisation and the team with which you work.

Methods of communication

You will use verbal and non-verbal methods of communication to meet different needs. For more information on methods of communication, see Unit 509 AC1.8.

Reflect on it

1.1 Methods of communication

Which different methods of communication do you use in your role? Provide a reflective account and list the types of communication you use at work and comment on how effective each type is. You might address when and how you use verbal, non-verbal, sign, pictorial, written, electronic and assisted methods. These may be personal, organisational, formal, informal or public (information/promotional).

Models of communication

Linear models

The Shannon and Weaver model of communication (1949) is one of the earliest linear models of communication (see Figure 26). In a linear model the communication process and the transfer of information are in one direction.

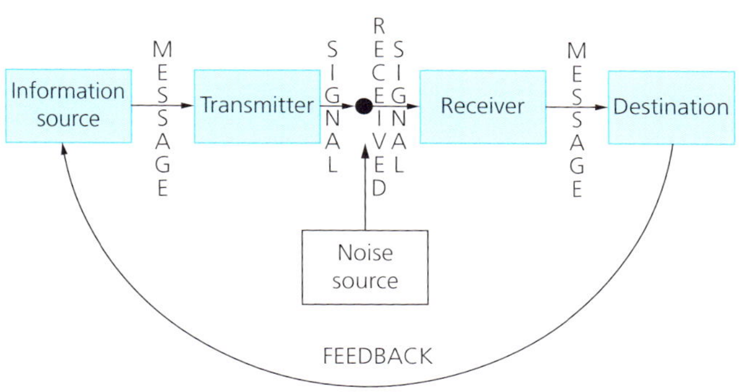

Figure 26 Shannon and Weaver's model of communication (Businesstopia, 2018a)

In the Shannon and Weaver model:

- the information source or the sender has a message to deliver
- the transmitter is the sender who transmits the message by the method (channel) they have chosen, e.g. voice, machine, text, email
- the receiver or decoder receives or hears the message as a series of signals and translates it
- the destination is the means by which the message is received, e.g. ears during face-to-face communication, phone, computer, etc.
- noise refers to any physical disturbances in the environment that may prevent the message from getting through. Noise can occur at any stage in the transmission.

An example of linear communication being used in service provision is when a manager issues instructions in an emergency. The transmitter asks the receiver to phone for an ambulance. The receiver is not expected to offer their own ideas. The feedback from the receiver may be agreement and then making the phone call.

Transactional models

Transactional models of communication describe the exchange of messages between sender and receiver. Both take turns to send or receive messages, so that every part of the communication process (such as the transmitter, receiver, environment and medium) is constantly changing. This model requires the receiver to listen to the sender for successful communication, and both sender and receiver are regarded as communicators.

Wood's (2004) transactional model (see Figure 27) offers a more complex communication process than Shannon and Weaver's linear model. In this model, messages are sent back and forth with a focus on interpretation of their meaning. As language develops, we notice that different meanings may be assigned to the same word. From a cultural point of view, this may result in miscommunication because we cannot always be sure that a word has the same meaning for two people. For example, words such as 'wicked', 'bad' and 'sick' mean something very different to young people than to older generations. There are many more examples of how words change. The words we use alter depending on the situation and the people involved and, because of this, we can never be sure that a word has the same meaning for two people (Porritt, 1990). This is particularly important when communicating feelings, as the strength of the word may differ between people.

This model recognises the differences in social, cultural and relational contexts and that understanding communication depends upon a shared response. Communication depends upon various physical, cultural, environmental, social, psychological and emotional factors, so we cannot always predict the response of another person.

An example of transactional communication in service provision may be talking to an individual about their food preferences face-to-face. The sender (staff member) asks the receiver (the individual) what they like to eat. The receiver feeds back by telling them (so becomes the sender, while the staff member becomes the receiver). The original sender may then clarify by asking more questions and taking into account non-verbal communication. It is very much a two-way process. In a managerial position, you may speak to the person that you manage about training needs in an appraisal meeting or receive feedback on your own performance.

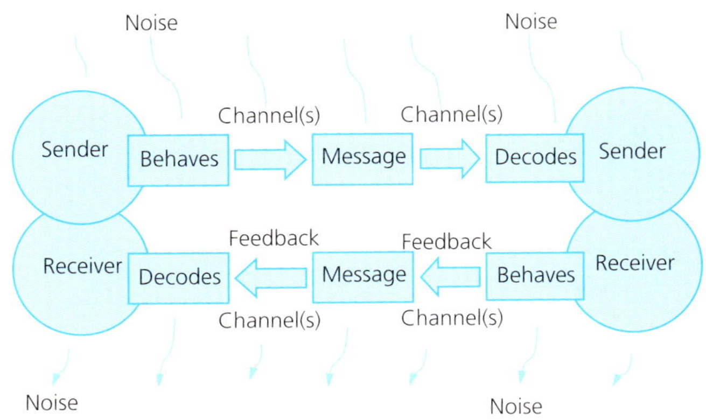

Figure 27 Wood's transactional model of communication (Businesstopia, 2018b)

Interactive models

Schramm's interactive model (1954) is similar to the transactional model in that there is a two-way process of communication and it includes an 'interpreter' to address the problem of meaning (see Figure 28). This model recognises the psychological frame in which interaction occurs.

For example, our attitude towards the sender may influence our understanding of the message. As a manager, you may react differently to a complaint from a service provider you know well, because you are more familiar with the way they communicate, than to a complaint from an individual who has recently started using your service. The context in which the message is sent is also important. Shouting the word 'fire' in a crowded area will receive a very different response than if it is shouted on a firing range.

The difference in meanings between cultures is also addressed in this model. When we come into contact with people from different cultures we are often confronted with new meanings for familiar words, and also different behaviours and gestures. This can quickly become a barrier to communication due to misunderstanding.

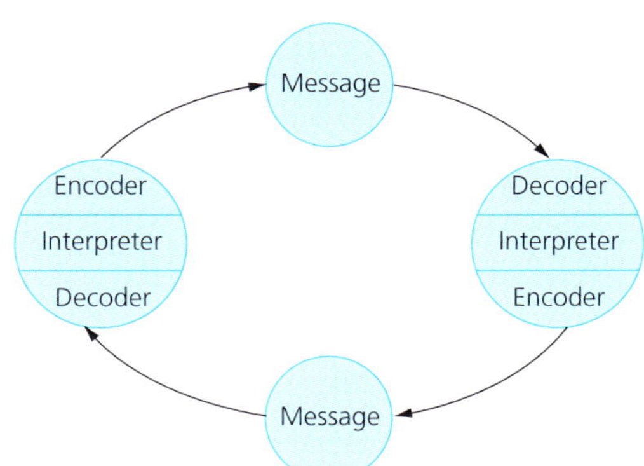

Figure 28 Schramm's model of communication

For example, staff members who have grown up in the UK may be put off by the direct way of speaking that some cultures favour and others may find the lack of eye contact, which is a sign of respect in some cultures, misleading and even believe it to be disrespectful. As a service provider and as a manager, you should be aware of, and make allowances for, changes to communication due to cultural differences.

Schramm's model of communication suggests that messages need to be decoded and interpreted before they can be understood. Decoding and interpreting may result in a different understanding from that intended by the encoder (sender of the message).

Reflect on it

1.1 How do you communicate?

Think about the ways in which you communicate with different people in your setting. Write a short reflective account about how your communication may change according to the people you meet who may have a different outlook on life or different values to yours. Consider how this might hinder the response and the meaning you get from the interaction.

SOLER/SURETY models

SOLER was a model first developed by Egan in 1975 and is used widely in a variety of settings (Egan, 2002). It is an acronym that can be used to aid non-verbal communication, for example between a therapist and their client. Table 6 shows how wordless messages can be given and received. This can be applied equally well to the roles of manager and team member.

Stickley (2011) developed the acronym SURETY. It adds to the SOLER model by including touch and the importance of individual intuition, encouraging us to think about therapeutic space.

S: Sit at an angle

U: Uncross legs and arms

R: Relax

E: Eye contact

T: Touch

Y: Your intuition

In a management role, you communicate with people who may be in a subordinate position to you, as well as those in more senior roles, peers and others such as visitors or other service providers. The way you communicate may differ based on the different people you communicate with, but it will be useful to apply the principles of SOLER and SURETY as these will help you to be an effective communicator.

Research it

1.1 SOLER and SURETY

Give three examples of when SOLER or SURETY could be useful models to use in your own setting and practice.

Evidence opportunity

1.1 Theoretical models of communication and their relevance to practice

Provide an explanation of how a–d below can help you to achieve positive interactions with the individuals in your care setting/service:

a. communication skills

b. methods of communication

c. models of communication

d. leadership and management responsibilities.

Table 6 Explanation of Egan's SOLER model

S	**Sit squarely**	Sit at an angle to the other person so that you are at either sides of an imaginary corner. This enables you to see all aspects of their non-verbal communication, which you might not see if you were sitting side by side. This position is less threatening than sitting face on.
O	**Open position**	Sit with uncrossed arms and legs to convey to the client that you are open and not defensive.
L	**Lean slightly towards the client**	Leaning towards the client shows that you are interested and want to understand their problem.
E	**Eye contact**	It is important to get the balance right. The client will feel uncomfortable if you stare and will think that you are not interested if you do not look at them at all.
R	**Relax**	If you are relaxed, you can concentrate on listening rather than worrying about how to respond to individuals.

Source: Tilmouth and Quallington (2015)

The role of phatic communication

This is simply 'small talk' or the type of speech that you use to be sociable. So, for example, you might say to somebody 'take care', 'have a nice day' or simply mention the weather. You are not necessarily stating a fact or passing on information; you are just moving the conversation along.

Burgess (1964) defined phatic communication as speech to promote human warmth and in care work this certainly has a place. Although it is sometimes thought to be trivial, it helps to establish a human touch to your communication. For example, you might ask a team member how they are or ask how their daughter got on in her football match at the weekend. Think about the last time somebody remembered a personal fact about you and how it made you feel. As a manager, you need to take an interest in your workers.

Also bear in mind that people who struggle with phatic communication often come across as very direct, so it's useful to be prepared, and not to use small talk if they become impatient with what they regard as 'unnecessary' communication.

Formal communication vs informal communication

Formal communication is official communication that passes through a setting, whereas informal communication is usually on a smaller scale and is not official, such as telling a colleague about an immediate issue when you pass them in the corridor. We see formal communication happening when there are hierarchies in place and there is a chain of command. It comes generally in written form, such as via email, and provides evidence that communication has happened. It might also be in the form of a PowerPoint presentation or a safety talk to staff. Informal communication is generally oral in nature and tends to happen in an ad hoc manner. There may be little to support what has been said. You may, for example, tell a colleague where they can find an individual they're looking for. It might also be a general conversation between team members and individuals.

The type of communication you use in your personal communication with members of staff and friends will be different to the type you might use in an organisational context. For example, your language may be more formal when you speak to individuals or members of the multidisciplinary team and less formal in your everyday life.

Self-awareness and perception awareness in communication

One of the things that we often do not pay enough attention to is our body language. Argyle (1994) pointed out that non-verbal communication can have as much as five times the impact on a person's understanding compared with the words spoken, so if you are displaying negative non-verbal signals this can prove problematic. Communication can be broken down as follows:

- 7 per cent is what you say in words.
- 38 per cent is contributed by how you say it (volume, pitch, tone, rhythm, etc.).
- 55 per cent reflects your body language (facial expressions, gestures, posture, etc.).

It is also useful to remember that individuals in a social care setting may have communication difficulties and may not pick up the non-verbal cues communicated (Crawford et al., 2006).

The way in which you present yourself can have as much if not more impact on whether your message is listened to and understood. When communicating:

> *Our attention is focused on words rather than body language. But our judgement includes both. An audience is simultaneously processing both verbal and non-verbal cues. Body movements are not usually positive or negative in and of themselves; rather, the situation and the message will determine the appraisal.'*

Source: Givens (2006)

It is vital to ensure that your behaviour and bodily actions match your speech. Awareness of the way in which you conduct your non-verbal communication is just as important as what you say in some cases.

Leadership and management responsibilities

Not everyone who works in your setting will have knowledge of methods or models of communication so it is your responsibility to ensure that they develop these skills. At the simplest level staff must be able to use any communication methods employed by the individuals in their care, so training is essential.

Responses to individuals must be appropriate, so it is important that staff understand the basics of communication and adapt to the ways in which individuals wish to communicate. A good place to start would be to organise some training in which staff address **self-awareness**.

KEY TERM

Self-awareness: The ability to notice the self and to be able to recognise our behaviour and personality.

Self-awareness is to be aware of your own character and feelings and sometimes this can be difficult. Being self-aware means knowing your own emotions and recognising the feelings arising from those emotions when they happen. Self-aware staff can be more in control of what is going on during interactions with others and within themselves and will be able to regulate their emotions appropriately. You may feel angry or sad at times, but it might be inappropriate to show those feelings at work. **Perception awareness** is the ability to understand what you are conveying to others via your non-verbal communication. How you present yourself to others can communicate much about you.

KEY TERM

Perception awareness: The ability to recognise how and what we are communicating to others through our non-verbal communication.

Reflect on it

1.1 Non-verbal communication

How do you use non-verbal communication? Take a few minutes to look at the people around you. Even if they are unaware of you watching them, they are still communicating with you. Can you, for example, tell how somebody is feeling by the way they are standing? Are they smiling? How are they dressed? What is their walk like? All of these things are communicating something.

Now apply this exercise to yourself. How do you communicate with your staff when you are not speaking to them? What are you conveying? Do you always feel like a professional? How do you convey that to your staff? What actions show this? Write a short reflective account and think about how models of communication apply to this.

Reflect on it

1.1 Communication models and practice

How do you present yourself to your staff and what do they actually see? Write a short reflective piece about your own body language.

Compile a table that explains the models of communication described above and give new examples of how they might be applied in your service provision. How might you use the Shannon and Weaver model of communication, Wood's (2004) transactional model and the SOLER/SURETY model?

AC 1.2 Explain the circumstances in which a leader/manager may use communication skills, including methods and models of communication to achieve maximum impact

Here, you will explain how different communication skills and communication models can be used in the setting.

Communication skills and methods

Every day you will communicate with a wide range of people. Figure 29 shows the different types of people you will deal with as part of your role. You may need to use particular skills to get your message across to some of these people. Recognising this is paramount since many barriers to communication arise from inappropriate language and terminology, which effectively means the message is lost. For example, the delivery of factual information can be quite impersonal and may be inappropriate when dealing with a vulnerable child or adult with complex needs or learning disabilities, or someone who is depressed or autistic and therefore requires a more empathetic response. However, a medical professional may require a factual response.

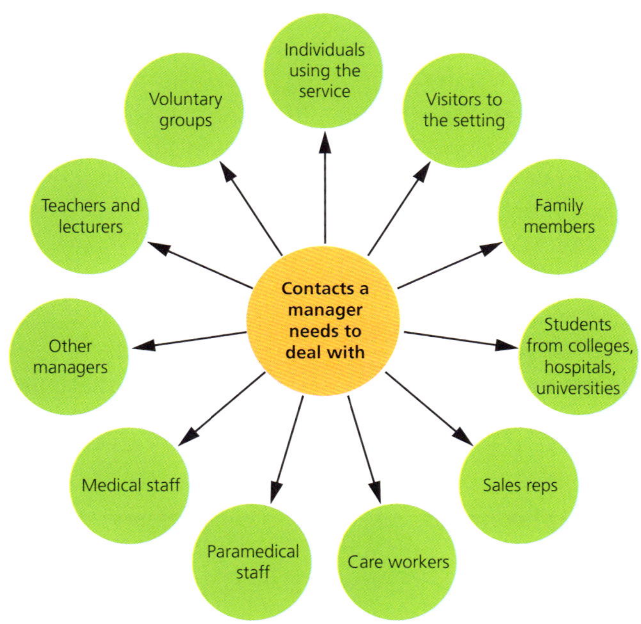
Contacts a manager needs to deal with
Individuals using the service
Visitors to the setting
Family members
Students from colleges, hospitals, universities
Sales reps
Care workers
Paramedical staff
Medical staff
Other managers
Teachers and lecturers
Voluntary groups

Figure 29 As a manager, you will need to deal with a range of people

Therefore, for the message to be received and understood, you must match your communication with the individual you are speaking to and the circumstances in which the interaction takes place. For example, a person you manage may be distressed after dealing with a stressful situation, so they may not be listening to what you are trying to say. In this situation, it might be better to write the information down or to have another conversation at a better time.

Davis and Fallowfield (1991) reported on failure of communication and lack of empathy, and Graham (1991) described how a breakdown in respectful relationships leads to poor communication. Hewison (1995) highlighted power relationships and barriers to communications.

How to communicate with individuals with different care needs

Recognising individual ways of communicating is the first step to understanding and using suitable communication to meet specific needs. You will need to tailor your communication to meet the individual needs and preferences of the person you are communicating with. Skills for Care offers guidance on different communication methods (see Skills for Care, 2016).

It is important to remember that every person will have individual and unique ways of communicating, so active listening should always be applied to ensure that a person's needs are understood. Below are some examples of the type of communication that may be required, but remember that communication is complex and should be tailored to individual preferences and needs.

- **Depression**: A person with depression needs to be spoken to in a clear and concise way as they may be slower to respond.
- **Dysarthria**: (Difficulty in articulating due to a brain condition.) This type of condition can be very frustrating for a person as they try to communicate but often fail to find words. The use of electronic aids, picture cards or symbols may help.
- **Language difficulties**: Again, this is frustrating and if an interpreter is unavailable then pictures and drawings can be used.
- **Dementia**: Speak clearly and slowly and use short sentences. Maintain eye contact and give the person time to respond. They must not feel patronised or a nuisance, so patience is needed here.
- **Complex needs**: The form of communication that is best depends on the person's needs. For example, multiple sensory loss may require electronic forms of communication.
- **Sensory loss**: If the person has lost hearing ability or is partially sighted you can use a hearing loop, Braille or other forms of communication the person is familiar with.
- **Autism needs**: Too much information can be a barrier to communication, so any extraneous information needs to be filtered out. It is best to use the person's name and to ask for their attention before talking to them and giving instructions. Saying less and speaking slowly will aid communication. The use of symbols and pictures may help.
- **Learning disabilities**: People with a learning disability usually feel that the best way to communicate with them is face to face and one to one, using easily understandable words. Mencap has a useful guide, 'Communicating with people with a learning disability' (Mencap, n.d.).

Research it

1.2 Communication and interpersonal skills

It would be useful to research further and explore more recent texts dealing with communication and interpersonal skills, for example Moss (2020), and/or watch relevant TED talks on the internet. TED talks are usually 20-minute instructive talks from leaders in their field and often cover communication, among other topics.

Evidence opportunity

1.2 Communication for maximum impact

Explain to your assessor how a–c can be used for maximum impact. Give an example for each one.

a. the communication skills you use
b. the methods of communication you have employed
c. the models of communication.

You might like to consider what was successful and what you would do differently next time.

Models of communication

The transactional models discussed in AC1.1 will be appropriate to use in most circumstances as feedback is useful in many situations. As you want to know how others are feeling, using a model that requires open questions, such as the linear model proposed by Shannon and Weaver, might be appropriate for giving factual information to staff.

AC 1.3 Explain how communication skills underpin achievement of positive outcomes for individuals, leadership and management of teams and sustainable relationships and partnerships

Here, you will explain how communication skills can help individuals to reach positive outcomes, benefit you in the leadership role and build relationships.

Achievement of positive outcomes for individuals

It is important to develop communication systems and practices that support positive outcomes. Positive outcomes are any beneficial outcomes for adults that lead to improved health, emotional wellbeing and quality of life. As a manager you will ensure that your service provides safe care, free from discrimination and harassment, where individuals and staff have choice and control, dignity and respect.

The goal is for individuals, their families and friends to experience the best care possible and yet there are constant reminders of how communication fails in health and social care.

The white paper 'People at the Heart of Care' (DHSC, 2022) is the government's ten-year vision for the reform of social care. Social care and support affects over 10 million adults of all ages and individuals draw on support at different stages of their lives. The need for care can develop suddenly or gradually, and can also be needed for a temporary period.

The vision covers areas such as:

- housing, technology and innovation
- empowering individuals, unpaid carers and families
- a strategy for the social care workforce.

There is to be an injection of £5.4 billion over the next three years to support the reforms.

The NHS Long Term Plan pledges to keep all that is good about the health and social care services but to tackle head-on the concern about future proofing the service and ensuring that with improved funding and better communication between health and social care services.

The challenge in both health and adult social care has been to reduce the barriers between the sectors of primary care, secondary care, social care, voluntary, independent and housing providers and an important part of the new way of working has been the identification of the responsibilities of local authorities and how they need to be involved in areas where social work can make a difference.

Good communication enables you to make decisions, promote rights and enable choice for individuals. This means promoting a person-centred service. Good communication also ensures that staff and individuals are empowered and can support each other well in their work.

An area where communication is likely to break down is an inappropriate environment. Have a look around the room in which you are sitting. How does it make you feel? Think about it for a moment. Is it welcoming? Or is it untidy, busy, crammed, too large? Are the chairs too far apart?

Also take a good look at where and when you conduct important communications with staff. The initial impact of a room or building can have a huge effect on how people feel and can influence the success of an interaction. In a domiciliary setting you may have little control over the actual physical environment, but you may be able to reduce the volume on radios or TVs in order to ensure that communication is not hindered in this manner.

As a manager, you will need to be aware of the environments in which you hold meetings such as appraisals. You should also be aware of the environments in which the individuals using your service are spending most of their day. A noisy environment may mean your message is not heard, impacting the outcomes you may have expected. A room that is poorly lit may mean that you are unable to clearly read the other person's body language or make eye contact. Where furniture is placed can impact communication: in meeting rooms or living spaces in the setting even the position of the chairs can affect the interactions.

The way that our environment communicates with us is extremely important. How cold or warm the room is and even the colour on the walls can affect how comfortable we feel, and how and what we choose to communicate.

You will be aware of the need for privacy when carrying out sensitive types of communication, such as breaking bad news or reprimanding someone. But have you thought about the impact your own setting will have on others? Thinking about these things will enable you to create, choose and work in environments well suited to the needs of the people you work with and manage, and ultimately those for whom you provide care and support. The important point for individuals who are being cared for in their own homes is that they have the time to express their needs and preferences and that you have a good understanding about the person being supported and how they wish to communicate.

Staff attitudes and stigma and how this might affect positive outcomes

Staff have their own beliefs, attitudes and **prejudices** and, as a manager, you need to be aware of this in order to encourage cultural awareness and non-judgemental communication. Staff who demonstrate **stigma** and discrimination towards individuals using the service will be providing a poor standard of care and communicating in an unfair way. Staff need to accept and value the people with whom they interact and display a non-judgemental attitude in order to demonstrate good communication skills.

Have you ever felt judged or that the other person was not listening to you? In this situation it is very difficult to be open and honest about your feelings and needs. If you judge the people with whom you are interacting, whether they are staff or the individuals using the service, they may feel they are unable to open up to you, which might be detrimental to the organisation's aims and objectives. In other words, your failure to communicate effectively or to ingrain this principle in your staff will lead to lack of success.

You will regularly come into contact with people whose feelings, values and attitudes are different to yours. Although you may not share a person's views or particularly like the stance they take, as managers and leaders of a setting you have to show tolerance of these views (providing they are not contravening any anti-discrimination policy). You need to be fully aware of how you come across to those you are communicating with. It is possible that you may communicate your dislike of somebody through your body language or the way you speak to them; this will have a negative effect on the interaction and may lead to conflict in the workplace.

Evidence opportunity

1.3 Impact of communication

The achievement of positive outcomes for individuals, leading and managing teams and maintaining sustainable relationships and partnerships all require good communication skills.

Explain, by giving examples, how each of these is met by using good communication skills.

KEY TERMS

Prejudice: An unreasonable, preconceived judgement or opinion that is not based on knowledge, evidence or experience.

Stigma: This implies that a characteristic held by some people or groups deviates from social expectations. For example, some people will not admit to being depressed because of the stigma of mental illness in society.

Partnership working: The use of inclusive and mutually beneficial relationships in care work that improve the quality and experience of care. It refers to the relationships between individuals, their carers, service providers and care professionals.

Leadership and management of teams

There are a number of reasons for communicating as a manager and leader, including:

- delegation of work
- conducting meetings
- presentations
- supervision and appraisal
- report writing
- building the team
- negotiation
- interviewing.

All of these tasks in themselves are detailed and can be further broken down to reveal more complex levels. For example, before undertaking a supervisory role, you need to be aware of what it entails. Your list might include:

- function of supervision
- who requires it
- mechanics of how it is carried out
- record-keeping policies
- conduct of the interview
- evaluating the process.

Meeting communication needs

Whatever the communication need, a good working relationship is essential and this demands trust and the ability to talk openly and honestly. The other person may need to feed back to you, to report a complaint of abuse, for example, and as a manager you should ensure that you equip them with the skills to do so. During your daily work you will undertake a variety of roles and will need to adjust your communication to each circumstance. Effective communicators make appropriate choices when it comes to deciding how they interact and they are clear about the purpose of the interaction. The different people to which you will have access will require different types of communication and you may find yourself advising, instructing, welcoming, assessing, observing, informing and counselling.

Sustainable relationships and partnerships

Effective adult social care is provided in collaboration and partnership with others, either in the same team (internally) or across a range of agencies and disciplines within the care sector (externally).

You will spend time building personal and organisational or partnership relationships and trust within those relationships matters. The success of your setting or team depends upon the ability to collaborate and build effective working partnerships with both internal staff and those outside the organisation. Building sustainable relationships is also a useful indicator of how successful you are as a leader because good relationships will motivate staff and others to do their best.

All **partnership working** depends on effective communication and good working relationships. As part of a care team that goes beyond the boundaries of your own organisation, you need to be aware of the need to build team links with external bodies.

Partnership working is an important means of making improvements in adult social care. It depends on effective partnerships between the different professions and organisations involved in commissioning and delivering services and interventions. It requires shared communication systems, including shared databases, records and files, to ensure that consistency in care is maintained and decision-making processes are clear. This may not be something that is currently available to adult social care settings, but with the digitalisation agenda could be a future goal.

The Care Act 2014 simplified and improved the existing legislation in care and these changes mean that more people are now able to access care and support from local councils or other organisations in the community. They also have more choice about the type of support and care they need. In addition, different ways to pay for care and support are now available. This means that communication between partners must be firmly established to ensure that all parties are talking to each other and have the individual at the heart of the care.

Evidence opportunity

1.3 Poor communication and its impact on relationships

Explain how poor communication could affect the relationships and partnerships you have at work and in your personal life. Give examples to support your work.

LO2 Know how to manage and resolve conflict

AC 2.1 Describe approaches for conflict management and conflict resolution

Here, you will be able to describe different ways of managing and resolving conflicts.

As individuals we all have different values and personalities, as well as unique preferences and certain unconscious biases. Being self-aware means recognising how our behaviour affects others as well as how others' behaviour affects us. Because of these differences, conflict will arise from time to time. Changes in the organisation can also lead to conflict.

As a manager, it is your responsibility to try to resolve conflicts. Conflict resolution means finding a solution to a disagreement that everyone is happy with. The danger of ignoring conflict is that it can lead to resentment and a lack of trust in the team. By developing skills to manage conflict fairly you will be able to support your teams.

Ignoring conflict

This is a tempting way forward but will lead to the situation getting worse. Conflicts that are ignored reappear later as resentment continues to increase. As soon as you are aware of a conflict situation, deal with it.

What is the issue?

You first need to establish the facts. By taking the time to talk to each individual involved you can find out exactly what the issue is and how each person perceives the problem. You can also ask what they see as an appropriate solution.

Bring the parties together to talk

When you have the facts you can become a mediator in a conversation between those involved in the dispute. In a neutral environment they can be encouraged to brainstorm solutions to the issue and encouraged to actively listen to each other's point of view. The ideal outcome is for all parties to understand the issue from each side and to identify possible solutions.

Continue to monitor the situation

When a solution has been identified, checks need to be put in place to see that it is working. As a manager, you should check in from time to time with all those concerned to determine that all is well. If not, then be proactive in working with both parties to identify alternative solutions.

Managing conflict implies managing negative emotions and disagreement. If this can be reframed as incompatible ways of dealing with a situation, it can be helpful to use a model to manage conflict.

Thomas Kilmann conflict model

This model was developed by Kenneth Thomas and Ralph Kilmann in the 1970s. It describes behaviour in terms of two axes – assertiveness vertically and co-operation horizontally – with the following types of behaviour at the extreme ends of the axes.

- **Co-operative**: This type of behaviour is supportive and open, being positive, empathetic and warm. It is constructive and engaging.
- **Un-cooperative**: A cold, suspicious, detached way of being, which takes the focus away from people and relationships.
- **Assertive**: This type of behaviour, although dominant and challenging, is also in control and shows confidence and strength. It is authoritative and direct.
- **Unassertive**: This type of behaviour is passive and submissive.

Within these dimensions are five types of conflict resolution that use these approaches to different degrees:

- **Competing**: This is an assertive (dominant) approach with un-cooperative behaviour (top left on the diagram) and may be experienced as aggressive. In this sort of conflict situation it is best to increase your own assertiveness but to show you are co-operative rather that competitive. By using open questions you will gain more understanding about how a person is feeling and you can confront their behaviour in a more meaningful way as you try to understand their point of view.
- **Avoiding**: This is unassertive (submissive) and un-cooperative behaviour (bottom left of the diagram). This may be the sort of behaviour you use when experiencing conflict but by recognising it in others you can deal with it by trying to engage with them positively. By reducing your assertiveness (dominance) and becoming more co-operative and warm you can help somebody feel more secure. Adjusting your body language to something that is not perceived as threatening and lowering your tone of voice and smiling will help.
- **Accommodating**: This type of behaviour is unassertive and co-operative and may be considered to be the preferred behaviour but it is not good to always act this way all the time. The tendency to simply agree or be over talkative without really listening may happen here. In dealing with this behaviour you need to keep on track and summarise what the person is saying to you to maintain focus.
- **Collaborating**: This is the best way to deal with conflict as it requires you to be both assertive and co-operative. Most people wish to avoid conflict if possible, so it is easier to adopt a warmer and more co-operative way of being than it is to be challenging and aggressive.
- **Compromising**: This is the middle ground in the model, as it sits at the centre of both axes. It is a useful way to deal with conflict when the other ways are not appropriate. A solution can be negotiated that both parties are happy with.

Reflect on it

2.1 Kilmann model

Using the Thomas Kilmann model, describe how you would deal with a conflict in your setting

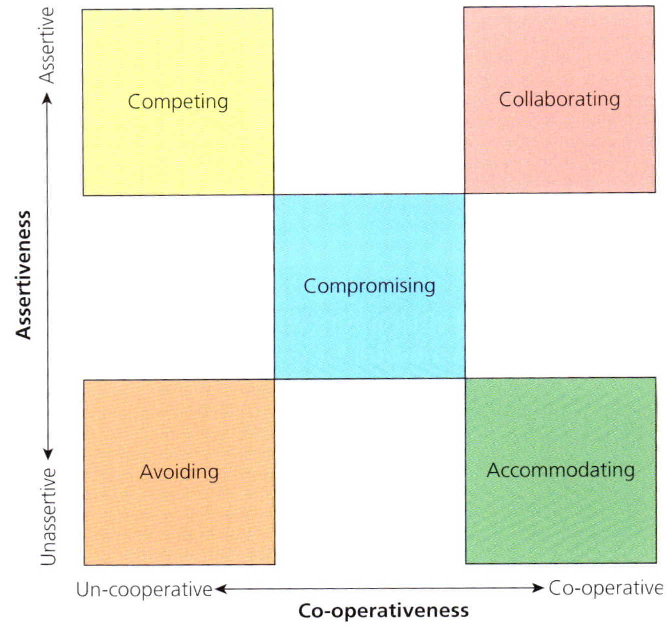

Figure 30 The Thomas Kilmann conflict model

AC 2.2 Outline factors within workplace that may cause friction and conflict

Here, you will outline the causes of friction and conflict in a setting.

You will not get along with every person you meet and it is the same at work. With so many different personalities operating in one space, conflict and friction can occur. However, the behaviours that some people exhibit can have a toxic effect on the rest of the team. Setting the right tone for the development of healthy relationships is part of the leader's role.

Three types of behaviour affect how the workplace operates.

Passive behaviour

Passive behaviour is practiced to avoid conflict or rejection. Someone who is passive often lets others take control and they invariably are disappointed because their needs are not being met, which can lead to resentment. Examples of passive behaviour include remaining quiet when being criticised even if it is unjust and going along with someone else's plans even though you had plans to do something else. Passive body language can include avoiding eye contact and fiddling with hair, clothing, etc., as well as shrinking down to avoid being noticed.

Passive-aggressive behaviour

Being passive-aggressive is an indirectly aggressive way to behave. Expressing anger is not an acceptable emotion, so a person who is showing passive aggression will mask that anger by adopting other hostile behaviours. Asking somebody who is subordinate to you to do something they do not particularly want to do may result in this type of behaviour. The person wishes to avoid the request but does not openly say this and so may seek to exert control over the situation in a less direct or recognisable way, one that seems innocuous on the surface, but which has an underlying aggressive streak. In the workplace this can have negative effects on the staff. For example, staff who are aggrieved in some way at a decision you have made may respond by not communicating with you, disengaging from work or just being sulky or obstructive. They may accept a task but then take a long time to complete it or fail to complete it. Procrastination or being stubborn may also be forms of this behaviour.

Examples of passive-aggressive behaviour include:

- the use of backhanded compliments such as 'I saw you did the stock take yesterday … that was a surprise'
- indirectly refusing a request by not saying no, but also not doing the task
- being sarcastic with other staff
- 'keeping score' about how often others are supposedly treated more kindly or leniently than they are
- not finishing their work on time and or even withholding important information in order to punish the team.

Communication is difficult when this behaviour is displayed as the person will tell you they are okay even when they are obviously angry. They deny what they feel and simply shut down communication. This sort of behaviour negatively affects relationships as by not openly voicing their feelings, others will struggle to understand why their requests are being ignored.

Microaggression

A **microaggression** is an unintentional or unconscious form of discrimination and the person making the comment may think they are complimenting the person. For example, commenting on the appearance of a female colleague, saying that a person who belongs to an ethnic minority 'speaks English so well', jokes about being 'blond' in reference to someone's intelligence. Microinvalidations occur when we undermine the struggles of target groups. Discrimination is present in our daily lives, and we negate its reality if we insist it does not exist.

KEY TERM

Microaggressions: Subtle and indirect statements or incidences of discrimination against a particular group.

Aggressive behaviour

Aggressive behaviour is any act that might cause damage or harm to people or property. Sometimes aggression can lead to abuse when there is a desire to take power and control. Recognising the potential for aggressive behaviour in others can help to control the triggers that might be causing it.

Aggression can also be seen in coercive or manipulative behaviour. You might observe the following types of aggressive action:

- Physical aggression includes hurting somebody by hitting, kicking or punching.
- Verbal aggression is shouting and swearing, or hurling insults to cause pain.
- Relational aggression is actions taken to damage another person's reputation or relationships, for example bullying and gossiping.
- Hostile aggression happens when emotional or reactive acts specifically target another person to harm them, resulting in a fight that causes physical harm.

Evidence opportunity

2.2 Behaviour within the setting

Outline the factors you may have observed in your setting that might cause friction or conflict. You might like to reflect on how you dealt with it.

AC 2.3 Evaluate personal skills that underpin conflict management and conflict resolution techniques

Here, you will evaluate your own approach to managing conflict.

The range of emotions you experience in the workplace will manifest themselves in a positive or negative way and you need to be aware of these feelings and the impact your emotions have on the people around you. Displaying positivity in the face of conflict will help the workforce to overcome the issues and this impact will be shown in a more productive and upbeat workplace.

Conflict can often lead you to view an individual in a negative way and you may therefore avoid communicating with them. This will affect your work and may also change your behaviour in the workplace. John Adair (2000) draws on the Thomas Kilmann model of five strategies for dealing with conflict and highlights how you may deal with this. You can force your ideas through in a competitive manner, or confront the individual, bringing all the issues to the fore. This could lead to a compromise or some sort of collaboration. You might also avoid the whole situation by opting out of any discussion. A more positive method might be to accommodate the issue so that feelings are not hurt.

Stress

When you feel stressed, you may feel under threat from many sources. Stress is a response to overwhelming situations, and this will undoubtedly affect your emotions. As a manager, you need to be able to deal with the stress you may be feeling in a productive manner. It is useful to have some strategies you can use to help you to respond appropriately to staff.

Negative emotions

These are unhelpful and, as a manager, although you may experience such emotions from time to time, you need to try to develop your emotional intelligence to ensure that your emotions are not affecting your workforce.

As a manager, you will need to adapt the way you communicate to suit your audience. This requires a professional response to all situations. You must always be respectful, no matter how negative the situation is and whatever the emotions being exhibited by the person you are communicating with. By being open, honest and clear in your communication, you can show empathy for the feelings of others.

Passive-aggressive behaviour

Passive-aggressive behaviour may have been learned in childhood and needs to be addressed for harmony in the workplace to be restored. As a manager, you can resolve this issue by avoiding passive-aggressive behaviour yourself and instead ask the staff member to identify what it is they are aggrieved about and then discuss possible solutions. Using active listening and being impartial and patient with them will help them to improve their behaviour.

Passive behaviour

Being passive or acting like a victim is also a destructive form of behaviour and is another way in which people may show emotions. It may be unintentional and can occur as a result of being unable to express one's emotions. The victim will fail to take responsibility for their work and will endeavour to get you to pity them. It is always somebody else's fault that they have been unable to do the job you asked them to do, or they may be persistently late coming in or ask to leave early every day. In dealing with this behaviour you will need to ensure that limits are set that are non-negotiable and be firm about the impact of the person's behaviour on others.

People may react in this way simply because they have gained sympathy for their behaviour in the past. It may be that they have legitimate reasons for such behaviour, and there may be issues outside work troubling them. Changing this behaviour can be accomplished by building the person's self-confidence and helping them to take responsibility for their own actions.

Open communication in all types of conflict situation can help others to become aware of the behaviours they are adopting and to elicit change.

Evidence opportunity

2.3 Personal skills in managing and resolving conflict

Evaluate the personal skills that underpin conflict management and conflict resolution techniques.

Case study

A member of your staff, Mary, has recently undergone a traumatic separation from her husband. She has three small children and is struggling to make ends meet. She finds it difficult to get to work on time and has been late several times recently. You know she does not have family in the area to help her get the children to school.

When you ask to see her to try to resolve some of her issues, Mary is aggressive and quite rude. This makes you feel angry, particularly as you are trying to come up with a solution to her problems. However, fighting anger with anger does not work and you need to consider how you might approach this problem in a different manner.

How might you deal with this situation?

Perhaps you will empathise with Mary's plight and ask her how she might see a way forward. It is likely that she has been unable to take time out to note the decline in her work or her lateness. You might suggest a change in hours to help her to get to work on time, or a reduction in her hours of work until she can settle her children into a more favourable routine. Perhaps Mary might work the same number of hours but at times when the children are at school.

The way you deal with the situation will affect the whole workforce, as they will be aware of the situation. The trust and rapport you have with the team can be strengthened or weakened depending upon the way in which you deal with Mary.

Evidence opportunity

2.3 Resolving conflict

Having read the case study, what skills would you use to manage and resolve this sort of conflict?

Make an evaluation of your own personal skills that shows your strengths and weaknesses with respect to conflict management and conflict resolution techniques.

LO3 Be able to communicate effectively with others

AC 3.1 Demonstrate a range of effective communication styles, methods and skills expected of leaders and managers in adult care

Here, you will show how you can communicate in a range of different styles when relevant.

Becoming an effective communicator

To gain trust and to develop a team who are inspired to work for the good of the setting there must be effective communication in place. Without it, information can be misinterpreted or lost, and this will result in barriers being set up, leading to a lack of trust and progress.

An essential skill is the ability to adapt your communication style. You must understand your audience and adapt to a style that suits them. Each member of staff will have different motivations, so you will need to tailor your communication to influence them. Not all will respond in the same way so the way you communicate will need to change to get your message across. Some people want a direct style and need to be told exactly what to do, whereas others respond badly to this, preferring to have some autonomy over their tasks.

The skill of active listening will ensure that staff know you care about what they say as your focus is truly on them. By asking for opinions and ideas and then actively engaging in the conversation they will feel valued and nurtured.

Being transparent in your dealing with staff is also essential. Openly sharing the organisation's goals, aspirations and challenges and owning your mistakes will empower staff to do the same.

It is important to be very clear about goals, particularly if they are not being met. If this is the case, communication needs to change and a simpler message sent out. Encouraging staff to actively problem solve and be creative will help to develop a safe environment in which there is transparency and trust.

In a survey by Businessolver (2018), **empathy** was ranked as the top leadership skill for a successful business. Ninety-six per cent of respondents said it was important for their employers to demonstrate empathy. Building a stronger, more productive culture requires that you acknowledge and understand how your staff feel.

> **KEY TERM**
>
> **Empathy**: Being able to understand and share the feelings of another person or having the ability to experience another person's condition from their perspective.

Effective communicators adapt their communication style to the situation and respond in sensitive and empathetic ways to the needs of those they are communicating with. In supporting others to become effective communicators, you must be an effective role model and reflect on how you are communicating your messages.

Effective communicators are those who are not only aware of the different ways of communicating but also the need to affirm the self-worth of the person with whom they are interacting with. What do we mean by this?

Be empathetic

Rogers (1980) referred to the need for empathy, which is the ability to 'put yourself in the shoes of others' or to understand a person's frame of reference. Active listening skills are the best way to show empathy. This is different from showing sympathy, which might make a person feel pitied.

For more on emotional intelligence, self-awareness, social awareness and relationship management, see Goleman's leadership styles and emotional intelligence in Unit 500 AC1.2.

Take a non-judgemental approach and listen

Have you ever felt judged in a conversation or that the other person was not listening to you? In this situation, it is very difficult to be open and honest about your feelings and needs. If you judge the people with whom you are interacting, whether they are staff or the individuals using the service, they may feel they are unable to open up to you, which might be detrimental to the organisation's aims and objectives. In other words, your failure to communicate effectively or ingrain this principle in your staff will lead to a lack of success.

Help staff to communicate with individuals using the service

As a manager and leader, you can support effective communication by ensuring that your staff are aware of the need to be flexible in how they communicate within different contexts and to engage in communication that is empathetic and values the people they are interacting with. It is also useful if members of staff understand any communication plans that are developed in partnership with speech and language therapists to enable continuity of care. Individuals will have different communication needs and it is important that staff can address these needs by having a firm understanding of different communication methods such as sign language. They may need to have specialist training in these.

Staff need to be mindful of how to communicate verbally with certain individuals in ways which show a respect for their differences and needs. Non-verbal communication may also pose barriers to effective communication so staff need to be sure they are aware of how this may affect their interactions. For example, when communicating with somebody who is angry, it is important to approach the conversation in a way that will not escalate the situation. Staff may need advice on how to do this and may also require training in dealing with this sort of situation. Also see LO1 for more information about communication skills that both you and staff you manage will need.

Reflect on it

3.1 Developing empathy

Look at the Businessolver 'State of workplace empathy' report and make notes on how you might increase your own empathy skills (Businessolver, 2018).

AC 3.2 Apply communication skills appropriately for maximum impact

Here, you will demonstrate the appropriate method of communication for different situations.

Communicating the message

The message you are sending and the way it is received is important to ensure that you gain understanding.

You will use both written and verbal communication to provide instructions and feedback and to discuss issues with the people you manage. However, just because you and your colleagues are speaking the same language, it does not follow that you each clearly understand what is being said, or that you each understand the other. How many times have you said to somebody, 'But that is not what I meant!' Perhaps your written communication has been taken out of context and somebody has felt angry about what you have proposed.

When you are face-to-face with a person there are other senses at play. It is easier to see that you might have been misunderstood if you assess the other person's body language. The values and beliefs that a person brings to the communication may also affect the way in which they receive the message.

Written communication is even more likely to be misunderstood or misinterpreted because it is not supported by body language and often you are not present with the reader to explain exactly what you mean. Writing loses some of the nuances of verbal conversation and this can lead to the message being misinterpreted. It is therefore useful after the message has been read to ask for clarification that what has been communicated has been understood.

Communicating to an audience

You need to be aware of the audience with whom you are communicating in order to get your messages across well. Adapting your message to fit with their communication style and understanding is important because it will be more effective. For example, speaking to a visitor in the same way that you speak to your staff may mean the information given is lost on them, as they may have a limited understanding of the technical jargon you use.

Emotional context of self and others

The role that emotional intelligence and feelings play in communication is discussed in AC2.3 of this unit and Unit 500 AC1.2. Being aware of your emotions and feelings will help when communicating with other people. By noticing the emotions of other people, you will better understand what they are communicating to you and why. Communication is as much about how something is communicated as it is about what is being said.

Communication and emotion are closely linked. Emotions experienced while communicating with others can affect the message being sent, whether verbal or non-verbal. Emotions being experienced by the listener may be so strong that they are unable to understand what is being said to them and the message is lost.

Communication style of others

Understanding how others communicate is key to getting your message across to them. You looked at passive-aggressive behaviour in AC2.2 and AC2.3 of this unit. Aggression can affect communication and you need to be aware of this when communicating with others. Rather than adopting an aggressive stance to put your point of view across, you should aim to develop and use an assertive communication style, which includes the use of 'I' statements and maintaining eye contact.

Reflect on it

3.2 Improving own communication style

What aspect of your communication would you like to improve? Do you, for example, express passive-aggressive behaviours at times? Perhaps your written communication is less than clear. Think about the changes you need to make to communicate appropriately for maximum impact.

AC 3.3 Manage barriers to communication

Here, you will demonstrate barriers to communication and how to overcome them.

There are a number of things that can interrupt effective communication. Physical barriers such as poor sound during a telephone or conference call can make a message hard to hear. Technical issues can also mean messages get lost and we have all experienced the dropping of the internet in meetings! There are other barriers to consider, too:

- An individual who does not enjoy their work will often be poor at both giving and receiving information. Unfortunately, this is a difficult barrier to mend because the mindset of the person experiencing disaffection needs to change.
- Not engaging in active listening leads to assumptions being made about others' needs based on your own perceptions.
- Another barrier is that of a lack of transparency and trust. For example, if your staff do not believe the message you are giving them, they will find it difficult to communicate with you and you them.
- As mentioned previously, your style of communication may also present a barrier. Perhaps you employ a very direct style which some staff members find difficult to handle and may even lead to conflict. They may prefer a softer, more empathetic approach.
- Cultural differences in communication may also present barriers. Strong accents and the use of idioms may be difficult for both individuals and staff to understand.

Evidence opportunity

3.3 Barriers to communication in the setting

What are the barriers to communication in your setting and how will you manage these?

LO4 Be able to develop communication practices

AC 4.1 Monitor communication systems and practices for effectiveness in the work setting

Here, you will show how to evaluate the communication system in your setting.

Information sharing

The way you work with others demands that you are open about what you do and effective in sharing information. Local strategic partnerships are an integral way of working that enable settings to share information and sometimes services to enable individuals to be cared for more effectively. You need to be aware of the policy in place for partnership working. This will detail how information is to be shared and stored to protect the confidentiality of individuals, as well as detailing referral processes and recording procedures.

For effective partnership, communication systems must be robust, confidential and standardised so that all staff who need to access records understand how they can do this without compromising confidentiality. All partners need to be involved in improvements to the ways in which this is done. Clear protocols as to who is responsible for updating information and who has access to data need to be in place to ensure effective use.

Working environments

Issues associated with different communication systems used within the workplace are covered in Unit 509 AC1.8 in the section 'Communication limitations'.

Stretch and challenge

4.1 Ways in which communication underpins effective service operation

Demonstrate to your assessor how communication impacts effective service operation in relation to the topics discussed in this section. For example, what are some of the communication difficulties you have with partnership working? How do you share information and is the process robust and safe?

Research it

4.1 Communication in your setting and partnerships

Design a questionnaire to obtain feedback from the following groups of people about the communication systems currently used in your setting:

- individuals using the service
- family and carers
- staff
- visitors
- other professionals you deal with.

The following questions may be helpful:

- How is information shared within your organisation and among your team and partners?
- Where does communication break down?
- What is good about your communication?
- What needs to be changed?
- Is there anything missing?

When you believe you have the information you need, set down some proposals to improve the communication systems.

Evidence opportunity

4.1 Monitoring systems for communication

Review and monitor existing communication/information delivery systems. Consider some of the changes you might make to ensure that they are safe and fit for purpose.

AC 4.2 Evaluate the effectiveness of communication systems and practices that promote positive outcomes

Here, you will evaluate the effectiveness of communication systems in your setting.

Good communication has a positive effect on service-user outcomes. The individuals you support, and those close to them, want to be able to participate in their own care and be part of any decision making, so staff need to be able to communicate sensitively and in a clear and compassionate manner. Positive outcomes mean people are encouraged to share information and are also given clear information that they understand.

It is important to evaluate the internal communication systems and practices within your workplace, identifying potential issues and barriers that relate to the specific needs of people providing and using adult care services.

Internal communication refers to the way in which staff communicate, for example via one-to-one discussions with managers or informal discussions with each other. Emails, memos, texting, social media, annual reports and printed materials such as newsletters also convey messages throughout an organisation.

External communication is for organisations and people operating outside the organisation and focuses on spreading news and information to the public, to individuals using the service and to other stakeholders to reflect the ethos and values of the organisation.

Evaluating

In evaluating a communication system, you look at its pros and cons to determine whether there are any deficiencies you need to address and whether changes need to be made to address new initiatives. You can do this in two ways:

- Search for information to support the current level of function with respect to communication.
- Analyse and interpret that information to decide on a plan of action.

In determining the effectiveness of a system or practice it is essential to monitor its use and review it regularly. For example, the policy on daily record keeping may state how staff should record support and care needs, but this needs to be monitored to see whether the process being used is, in fact, efficient and maintains good continuity of care and communication. Once you have collected the information, you need to analyse it. To do this you should examine all the data from the daily records and then determine its positive and negative aspects. One way this can be carried out is to obtain casual feedback from individuals as to how well they feel the system works. However, it is far better to collect information that may be used in auditing your service and can provide evidence to external bodies of continual progress and quality assurance in the organisation.

There are several useful ways in which you can formally ask for feedback. For example, you may use forums (groups of individuals who meet to discuss the quality of the service) and meetings when the quality of services can be discussed and recorded in the minutes. This provides valuable information on how individuals feel about the service and how the care is being delivered. Recording is central to good, person-centred support, so you might wish to investigate whether the individuals feel it is working with respect to continuity of care and whether the records kept are truly identifying the changing needs of the individual.

The care you give and the way you deliver that care have a significant impact, not only on the users of the service but also on staff morale, and as such, any feedback is essential in measuring the quality of the care you provide.

Evidence opportunity

4.2 Evaluate efficiency

Show your assessor how you monitor and evaluate the efficiency of internal and external communication systems and practices. How do you identify potential issues and barriers in relation to the specific needs of people providing and using adult care services?

AC 4.3 Propose improvements to communication systems and practices

Here, you will demonstrate which methods of communication would be most effective in your setting.

Improving communication can be done through meetings and reports for staff and for the individuals using the service. For example, if a member of staff suggests a change to current practice, it is important that the idea is considered and discussed at a team meeting. The change may be useful but may require some refinement before full implementation.

Any proposed change will require you, as the manager, to ensure that all staff are aware of what needs to be done and that a plan of action is in place. Any revised working practice must be discussed and fully understood by staff and others involved in the setting. New responsibilities may arise that may require training and time. By communicating all the information to staff and having guidelines in place, the changes can be presented in a clear and efficient way to ensure success.

Research it

4.3 Improving communication systems

Safeguarding adults reviews often comment upon poor communication as one area requiring improvement to care. Undertake a small-scale study to monitor the communication practice within your own setting and evaluate how effective it is. Identify any improvements that could be made to the practices and make recommendations for revised systems.

Reflect on it

4.3 Revised communication systems and practice

Reflect on the way in which you led the implementation of a revised practice of your communication systems in your setting.

Which communication practice in your setting did you change and why? How did you recommend this change to your team? Make notes to document your thoughts.

AC 4.4 Lead the implementation of improvement to communication systems and practices

Here, you will show how you as a leader can ensure improvements in communication within your setting.

Improving communication practice

It is an important part of the leadership role to ensure that communication practice is implemented and improved upon over time. Effective communication can help an individual feel safe and secure and you need to take time to ensure that the individuals using your service are able to express their needs clearly.

Improving your own effort in this can be helped by:

- communicating with the individual when they are alert and able to respond
- enabling sufficient time for the conversation and allowing for breaks so the individual can take stock of what is being said
- ensuring that the environment is conducive to communication and communication isn't being conducted in a noisy or poorly lit area
- ensuring that you face the person, maintain eye contact and speak clearly
- using suitable language and regularly checking understanding.

Good communication is not only important for the individuals using your service. You will need to ensure that your members of staff are also aware of the different forms of communication and are supported to be effective communicators in order to deliver the best possible outcomes for individuals.

SCIE provides useful information about good communication, including a communication skills e-learning course (see SCIE, 2008). It has not been updated since 2008, but it remains relevant, although policy and laws may have changed.

Evidence opportunity

4.4 Implementing improved communication systems

How will you lead the implementation of improvement to communication systems and practices in your setting? What do you think requires improvement and how will you lead the change on this?

Reflect on it

4.4 Evaluating effectiveness of communication systems and practices

How do you evaluate the effectiveness, quality and performance of communication systems in your setting? What standards do you use? Why is it important to ensure accurate communication?

Choose one of the communication systems in your setting (the complaints procedure, for example) and write an account reflecting on and evaluating the quality of the organisation's performance relating to that system.

Review communication policies in line with legislative and regulatory requirements.

The Gov.uk website provides details of the relevant legislation relating to information and communication and how to keep them secure. This legislation includes:

- Data Protection Act 2018
- Freedom of Information Act 2000
- Human Rights Act 1998
- Equality Act 2010
- Terrorism Act 2006
- Official Secrets Act 1989
- Malicious Communications Act 1988
- Privacy and Electronic Communications (EC Directive)
- (Amendment) Regulations 2011
- Police and Justice Act 2006.

In September 2021, the Department for Digital, Culture, Media and Sport launched its consultation 'Data: a new direction' to inform development of proposals to reform the UK's data protection laws, as part of the UK's National Data Strategy (GOV.UK, 2022). During the COVID-19 pandemic, the government, businesses, organisations and public services were able to share vital information quickly. This sharing of data use saved many lives, enabled new ways of working and kept the economy running. The National Data Strategy aims to build on this and improve data use in all walks of life.

You need to establish that systems are in place to ensure that significant changes to the law are identified, and processes implemented to cover them. Your staff should be aware of changes to legislation that will affect their practice, for example the ways in which the Data Protection Act 2018, which is the UK's implementation of the General Data Protection Regulation (GDPR), is different to the Data Protection Act 1998. One way of keeping up to date with legislative and regulatory requirements is to read sector news, blogs and websites, and to undertake regular training. If you model this and encourage it as good practice, your team will do the same.

It is important to be critical of the way in which you communicate in your setting as poor communication is often held up to be the cause of inadequate care being delivered and/or staff being unhappy in their work.

Legislation

Legislation	Key points
Data Protection Act 2018	This Act deals with the processing and protection of data on individuals. It applies to the processing UK residents' personal data.
General Data Protection Regulation (GDPR)	This Regulation provides detailed guidance to organisations on how to govern and manage people's personal information. It also applies to the processing of EU residents' personal data.
Care Act 2014	Sets out the key responsibilities of local authorities in meeting the needs of individuals who require help and support to promote their wellbeing. Its main aim was to provide integrated care and to introduce the right to an assessment for all.

References

Adair, J. (2000) *Effective Teambuilding: How to make a winning team*. London: Pan Macmillan.

Argyle, M. (1994) *The Psychology of Interpersonal Behaviour*. London: Penguin.

Burgess, A. (1964) *Language Made Plain*. London: English Universities Press.

Businessolver.com (2018), 'State of workplace empathy: Executive summary'. **https://info.businessolver.com/hubfs/empathy-2018/businessolver-empathy-executive-summary.pdf**

Businesstopia (2018a) 'Shannon and Weaver model of communication', *Businesstopia*, January 6, 2018. **www.businesstopia.net/communication/shannon-and-weaver-model-communication**

Businesstopia (2018b) 'Transactional Model of Communication', *Businesstopia*, January 6, 2018. **www.businesstopia.net/communication/transactional-model-communication**

Crawford P., Brown, B. and Bonham, P. (2006) *Communication in Clinical Settings*. Cheltenham: Nelson Thornes.

Davis, H. and Fallowfield, L. (eds.) (1991) *Counselling and Communication in Health Care*. Cirencester: Wiley.

Department of Health and Social Care (2022) Policy paper 'People at the heart of care: Adult social care reform'. **www.gov.uk/government/publications/people-at-the-heart-of-care-adult-social-care-reform-white-paper/people-at-the-heart-of-care-adult-social-care-reform**

Egan, G.E. (2002) *The Skilled Helper*. Belmont, CA: Brooks/Cole.

Givens, D.B. (2006) *The Nonverbal Dictionary of Gestures, Signs and Body Language Cues*. Washington: Center for Nonverbal Studies Press.

GOV.UK (2022) Department of Digital, Culture, Media and Sport, 'Data: A new direction – government response to consultation'. **www.gov.uk/government/consultations/data-a-new-direction/outcome/data-a-new-direction-government-response-to-consultation**

Graham, R.J. (1991) 'Understanding the beliefs of poor communication,' *Interface*, 11, pp. 80–2.

Mencap (n.d.) 'Communicating with people with a learning disability'. **www.mencap.org.uk/learning-disability-explained/communicating-people-learning-disability**

Porritt, L. (1990) *Interaction Strategies: An introduction for health professionals*. London: Churchill Livingstone.

Rogers, C. (1980) *A Way of Being*. New York: Houghton Mifflin.

Schramm, W. (1954) 'How Communication Works', in W. Schramm (ed.) *The Process and Effects of Communication*. Urbana, IL: University of Illinois Press, pp. 3–26.

Shannon, C. and Weaver, W. (1949) *The Mathematical Theory of Communication*. Urbana, IL: University of Illinois Press.

Skills for Care (2016) 'Communication skills in social care'. **www.skillsforcare.org.uk/resources/documents/Developing-your-workforce/Care-topics/Core-Skills/Communication-skills-in-social-care.pdf**

Social Care Institute for Excellence (2008) 'Communication skills e-learning course'. **www.scie.org.uk/e-learning/communication-skills**

Stickley, T. (2011) 'From SOLER to SURETY for effective non-verbal communication', *Nurse Education in Practice*, 11: 395–8.

Tilmouth, T. and Quallington, J. (2015) *Diploma in Leadership for Health and Social Care*. London: Hodder Education.

Wood, J. (2004) *Communication Theories in Action: An introduction*. Belmont, CA: Wadsworth/Thomson Learning.

Unit 514

Managing the effective handling of information in adult care

GLH 20

About this unit

You collect huge amounts of information on a daily basis, including both electronic and physical information. Managing this information requires that the organisational structure is capable of collecting, storing and distributing that information to various audiences including the individuals using the service, families, partners and staff.

In this unit you will learn about your role and responsibilities relating to the effective handling of information and how to respond to data breaches. You will learn how to lead on the implementation of policies, procedures and systems for effective information handling to meet legal and ethical requirements and will be able to explain how your own service or setting's business continuity plan informs the management of a data/cyber security breach following agreed ways of working.

Learning outcomes

By the end of this unit, you will:

1. Understand effective information management.
2. Be able to implement systems for effective information management.

Getting started

Before you study the unit, think about the following:

- What information are you privy to on a daily basis?
- How is information stored and used in your setting?
- How do you ensure that confidentiality is maintained and that your systems of storage are secure?

LO1 Understand effective information management

AC 1.1 Outline own role and responsibilities in effective information handling management

Here, you will be required to outline your role and responsibilities with respect to handling data and information.

Care settings handle and process a great deal of information, much of which is sensitive and confidential. Looking after information properly and ensuring confidentiality is a crucial role for you as a manager, as the repercussions of data loss or unauthorised data use will be significant.

Every care setting must have in place a policy that clearly shows the responsibilities and processes for information handling, to ensure that confidentiality is maintained by all staff. The legal duty on care settings is to protect the information and to follow data protection principles.

As the manager, you need to ensure that the standards for handling information are documented clearly in your setting's policies and procedures. Secure data storage systems for all information must be in place. You may have physical storage such as filing cabinets that need to be kept locked, as well as electronic storage on computers, USB drives or external hard drives that must be password encrypted.

AC 1.2 Describe how to support others to effectively handle information

Here, you will describe how you support others in handling information.

As a manager, you must support individuals to handle their own personal data wisely and safely. Online fraud is an increasing threat to our safety and staff should be aware that they can advise and assist individuals to understand the dangers of passing on personal information, and help them to devise ways of protecting themselves.

All staff handling information should have been trained to do so safely. Staff training on data protection and information handling must be undertaken and you should ensure that compliance with training is monitored and documented. Training should be updated on an annual basis.

In larger settings a Data Protection Officer who is responsible for monitoring compliance with GDPR might be appointed.

Staff need to be aware of the security risks involved with information handling. For example, they need to understand that their passwords must be unique to them and should never be shared. They should be encouraged to have several different passwords so that should one password become compromised, other accounts are not put at risk.

The practice of locking computers when they are left unattended should become a habit and staff must be made aware of how screen content can be viewed if this is not done. The confidential nature of the information staff are able to access in a care setting must be clearly covered in all induction and subsequent training.

The same data protection rules apply to the data on people who are cared for in their own homes. There are advantages to keeping care records in people's homes to ensure continuity of care should a different carer take over. The records will document the support that has been provided in accordance with the support plan. However, there may be reasons why individuals do not wish to keep records in their own homes. For example, they may think that this is inappropriate in the informal setting and, if detailed records are being written, these take time and encroach upon the time allocated for support.

Moving from paper-based to digital recording is certainly a wise move as data can be protected more easily when it is password protected.

The CQC supports the Health and Social Care Act 2008 (Regulated Activities) Regulations 2014: Regulation 17, which ensures that providers have systems and processes in place for effective governance, to assess, monitor and mitigate any risks relating to the health, safety and welfare of people using services and others.

With respect to record keeping, providers must securely maintain accurate, complete and detailed records for each person using the service.

> **Research it**
>
> **1.1 and 1.2 Safety of information held**
>
> Conduct a survey of your setting to check the safety of the information you hold. Are staff diligent about locking computers? Is there sharing of email passwords?
>
> Look at your policy and determine how you might ensure the safety of information in your setting.

AC 1.3 Explain how own setting/service business continuity plan informs the management of a data/cyber security breach following agreed ways of working

Here, you will explain your setting's planning for dealing with potential security breaches.

The main sources of guidance that inform your setting about how to handle information will come from your own organisation's policies and procedures relating to:

- information handling
- GDPR and data protection
- confidentiality
- codes of practice.

Your codes of practice and policies will reflect the legal requirements for data protection. Since Brexit, UK organisations must comply with the:

- Data Protection Act 2018, which is the UK's implementation of the GDPR and applies to processing UK residents' personal data.
- General Data Protection Regulation (GDPR), which also applies to the processing of EU residents' personal data.

Your policy must also include guidance on what to do in the event of a data breach or a cyber security alert and how to prevent this from happening.

No organisation can be immune to data breaches but you can take steps to minimise this risk. There are a number of common breaches you need to guard against. These include the following:

Information stolen due to human error can occur if a computer is left unlocked or if a laptop is accidentally left somewhere outside the organisation and is stolen. This can result in a large amount of data being stolen.

The NHS in Wales became a victim of computer hackers in March 2017 when personal information of thousands of medical staff was stolen (BBC, 2017). This included their names, dates of birth, national insurance numbers and data relating to radiation exposure of staff who worked with X-ray equipment. The data had been stored and processed by a private IT contractor until its security was compromised. Encrypted systems and not sharing codes or passwords increase data security.

Ransomware is the act of your computer being hacked and a message being sent telling you that the hacker is holding your information to ransom.

A very simple hack happens when passwords are stolen. Writing passwords down and sharing them with others as well as having passwords that are easily guessed can lead to information being stolen.

Phishing attacks come from third parties who create genuine looking sites, for example mirroring online banking websites. When a bank customer logs onto their site and inputs a password, criminals then have the user's bank details and their password and are able to access their bank account.

Staff should be told not to open emails from anyone they do not know or a source that they do not trust. The message must be reported as spam using your setting's method for this. Sensitive information such as passwords or bank account numbers should never be sent via email.

Opening an attachment from a company or person you do not know may lead to a virus being introduced into the computer system. Staff and the individuals using the service should know not to reply to or click on links inside spam emails. All computers should have antivirus software installed which scans email attachments.

Malware, such as viruses, is harmful to any setting, especially those in which personal data is accessed on a daily basis. A virus in a care setting's computer system could wipe the data of the individuals using the service, leading to serious and injurious results.

Completely protecting your organisation from data breaches is not possible, but you can train your employees to understand the consequences of data breaches and how it is possible for someone to hack into your system in order to ensure that everyone takes all steps possible to minimise the risks.

Staff should be required to change their passwords regularly by setting timers on them. They must also be aware that any sensitive information they carry with them outside work must be kept as safely as possible.

Evidence opportunity

1.3 Protecting information and data

How does your setting protect its information and computer data? What antivirus software is in place and what are the guidelines for staff with respect to emails and breaches of security?

AC 1.4 Explain how to respond to a data breach

Here, you will explain your setting's plan when dealing with a security breach.

A data breach occurs when there is accidental or deliberate loss of information without permission. Your setting's policies should detail how a data breach will be dealt with should one occur. For example, a member of staff may accidentally send an email to the wrong person, leaking information about another. Staff need to know what they should do to rectify the situation. You must immediately set up an enquiry to obtain the facts that led to the breach. This involves writing down the facts about the incident, for example what happened and why, how many people were involved and when it happened. You should also record the actions you took following discovery of the data breach.

You then need to find out what has happened to the personal data affected. It should be recovered if this is possible. If information is sent to someone by mistake, they should be asked to delete it.

In the case of a stolen laptop or tablet, appropriate systems should be installed so that the device can be wiped remotely to minimise the risk of personal data being retrieved and used. Changing all passwords after a cyber incident will help too.

You need to assess the risk of potential harm the breach may cause, for example, safeguarding issues, identity theft or significant distress.

If a simple mix up has occurred, then there may be little or no risk involved, but a serious breach might cause significant harm. If the risk is small you may not have to do anything but if the risk of harm is greater you will need to inform those affected about what has happened and then give clear advice as to the steps they can take to protect themselves, and what you will do to help.

The Information Commissioner's Office (ICO) is the regulator responsible for ensuring that all organisations comply with the Data Protection Act 1998 and for promoting good practice in information handling. Your breach may require you to report to the ICO to provide details about what happened and when, as well as a risk assessment of the situation and what you have done to contain the breach.

Research it

1.4 Information Commissioner's Office

See ICO (n.d.) for information on how to handle a data breach. See also the government white paper on 'A cyber resilient health and adult social care system in England: Cyber security strategy to 2030' (DHSC, 2023). The government's strategy looks at the functions of health and social care services and the importance of protecting them from the disruptive impact of a cyber-attack. Ensuring that individuals' data is protected is a challenge in sectors that are complex and where interdependent systems with different risks and needs co-exist. The strategy sets out an approach that will apply across health and social care systems, adult social care, primary care and secondary care.

LO2 Be able to implement systems for effective information management

AC 2.1 Lead the implementation of policies, procedures and systems for effective information handling to meet legal and ethical requirements

Here, you will be required to show the legal and ethical requirements for handling information and be able to implement the policies and procedures for effective information handling.

Any system of information management must be legally sound. Information shared in organisations must be kept confidential and staff need to be aware of their role in this. Beauchamp and Childress (1994) define confidentiality as 'keeping secret' information given to a person by another. It is infringed when that information is disclosed to someone else without the giver's consent.

Adult social care staff are required to fulfil their duty of care and maintain confidences obtained via their work so you, as a manager, need to respect this requirement. However, if a public interest issue is at stake, then a confidence may be broken. For example:

- if a crime has been committed or you believe it is about to be
- if malpractice has occurred
- if abuse is suspected
- to prevent harm to self or to others
- if professional misconduct has occurred.

If there is a breach of confidentiality within your workplace, then you as the manager are obliged to take disciplinary action and/or legal action. From a legal point of view, you are obliged to follow the laws associated with maintaining confidentiality, including:

- Care Act 2014
- The Health and Social Care (Safety and Quality) Act 2015
- Data Protection Acts 1998 and 2018
- Human Rights Act 1998
- Freedom of Information Act 2000
- Equality Act 2010
- Public Interest Disclosure Act 1999 (often referred to as the 'Whistle Blowing Act').

Other guidelines are:

- setting-specific guidelines, drawn up for a setting's unique circumstances
- clinical governance requirements
- CQC essential standards for quality and safety
- Caldicott Report recommendations 1997
- Skills for Care guidelines.

From an ethical point of view, care professionals explicitly or implicitly make a promise to the individuals using their service to keep their information confidential, thus respecting the autonomy of the individual. But problems arise when decisions need to be made that require certain personal information to be shared. For example, Article 10 of the Convention on Human Rights and Biomedicine states that: 'Everyone has the right to respect for private life in relation to information about his/her health care' (European Parliament and Council of the European Union, 1995). Any information you gain must be ethically sourced and accurate, and care must be taken to not mislead or distort what you have been told. For example, if you use direct quotations from an individual, these must not be changed as this could distort the meaning. Any inaccuracies or misleading statements that are brought to your attention should be corrected immediately. The use of pejorative or emotive language must be avoided at all costs and a courteous and respectful approach should always be your aim.

As a manager you need to ensure that you have implemented effective information management systems that meet all legal and ethical requirements and are safe with respect to confidentiality and data protection.

Evidence opportunity

2.1 Effective information management systems

Show how you support your staff to understand and adhere to the legal and ethical requirements of information management systems in relation to the services you provide, and how you implement such systems. What evidence do you have?

AC 2.2 Lead practice to address legal and/or ethical conflicts that arise between maintaining confidentiality and information sharing

Here, you will be required to show that you lead practice which considers both legal and ethical conflicts relating to the area of service, and consider the areas covered in this section.

One of the tensions with respect to confidentiality lies in the use of information and its safekeeping. This is an important issue on a national scale. SCIE clearly sets out some key messages. Adults have a general right to independence, choice and self-determination including control over any information about themselves that is held. This can be overridden in certain circumstances, such as emergency or life-threatening situations when sharing relevant information with emergency services must be carried out without consent.

Legally, sharing sensitive, personal information is not prevented within organisations within the parameters of the Data Protection Act 2018 and the General Data Protection Regulation (GDPR). If there is a safeguarding concern, then sharing confidential information may be justified and staff should inform the individual if they need to share their information without consent. Individuals can choose whether or not their data is used for planning and research and there are different types of data sharing that can be opted out of. For example, an individual can stop their providers from sharing their data in certain circumstances.

As a manager of a setting, you and the individuals that you manage may come across various obstacles when trying to ensure confidentiality and keeping information safe. There will be legal and ethical conflicts that may arise, some of which are explored below. It is your duty to ensure that the people you manage are aware of the actions to follow and that these are clearly outlined in the policies and procedures for your setting.

Relatives expecting information without consent

Occasionally a relative will call and ask for information about an individual in your care. Your first duty is always to the individual. If the individual has not given **consent**, then you will not be able to discuss their care with the relative unless they have power of attorney.

Information may be shared with the consent of the individual. Some residential care organisations will write in the individual's notes the details of those who may have access to information. If it is kept digitally, this information may be password protected and the person asking about the individual may be asked to declare the password before information can be shared. When the people you manage come across an issue like this, they will approach you for advice about the best course of action. You should be able to advise them of best practice and also advise them of any occasions when confidentiality may be breached.

Capacity issues

The Mental Capacity Act (MCA) 2005 was designed to empower individuals who may lack the mental capacity to make their own decisions about their care and treatment. Capacity refers to having sufficient understanding and memory to understand the situation that a person finds themselves in, but this is specific to the decisions being made and a situational approach must be taken here. Those who may lack capacity are individuals such as those who have dementia, a severe learning disability, a brain injury or a mental health condition, or who may be affected by a stroke or unconsciousness caused by an anaesthetic or accident.

The MCA contends that care professionals must assume that somebody has mental capacity unless a capacity assessment proves otherwise and also that individuals must be given help to make decisions based on information that they understand.

There is also provision within this law for an **advocate** to make a decision on behalf of the person if they lack capacity at a future date and this is done through a power of attorney document. A decision made by an advocate must always be in the individual's best interests. Confidentiality must always be maintained, and a person needs to give consent before information about them is shared.

> **KEY TERMS**
>
> **Consent:** To give permission for something to happen. It may be verbal, written or implied but always needs to be obtained.
>
> **Advocate:** An individual who acts for or on behalf of another, particularly if the person lacks capacity in some way or simply requires help to speak out.

Consent issues

As a manager, you will also need to ensure that the people you manage are aware of consent issues when working with the individuals that they care for. They must be aware that before any support can be given to an individual, their consent must be obtained. This may simply mean asking them if what you are planning to do is OK to go ahead with. For example, if you are going to help an individual with their personal needs, consent is gained by explaining what you are going to help them with and then asking them if they agree to this.

Consent has to be a voluntary action agreed by the individual and not one which has been influenced by another person. It also has to be 'informed' – all information, including benefits and risks, must be explained and any alternative support described. The person also has to have capacity. This is decision-specific and we should never assume that if someone is not able to make a particular decision this means they can't make other decisions.

Whilst it is good practice to gain the individual's consent to share information, staff must not guarantee confidentiality, but should inform the person if they need to share their information without consent.

Daily records need to be shared with colleagues as they contain important information about the support given. Local escalation policies and protocols need to be in place so that any concerns with respect to safeguarding can be forwarded to the relevant authority straight away. Staff and volunteers should always report safeguarding concerns to their line manager except in emergency situations. (See SCIE, 2015 for further details.)

Power of attorney – lasting versus enduring

The role of the **Lasting Power of Attorney (LPA)** replaced Enduring Power of Attorney (EPA) in 2007. An EPA made before then is still valid. The difference is that an LPA, which is a legal document, enables an individual with capacity to appoint a person or persons to make decisions about their health and welfare, property and financial affairs should they become unable to do so themselves, without being subjected to pressure or fraud. There are two types of LPAs:

- a Financial LPA, which allows decisions about an individual's money and property to be made by the attorney
- a Health and Care LPA, which allows the attorney to make decisions about an individual's medical treatment and day-to-day care.

Additionally, the individual can give power to the attorney to make decisions regarding the receipt of life-sustaining treatment if needed. Each of these decisions is made with legal documentation to support them. An **Ordinary Power of Attorney (OPA)** allows one or more people to act as attorneys and to make financial decisions. It is a temporary arrangement used when a person is unavailable for a while due to being away or in hospital, is finding it difficult to access their bank account or wants somebody to supervise their funds for a while. The OPA is only valid while the individual still has mental capacity to make decisions and can be limited in its use.

> **KEY TERMS**
>
> **Lasting Power of Attorney (LPA):** A legal document that allows anybody over the age of 18 to appoint one or more people to support the decision-making process should the individual become unable to do so. The person must have the mental capacity to undertake this step.
>
> **Ordinary Power of Attorney (OPA):** A temporary arrangement that allows a person to nominate an attorney to undertake financial decisions while they are temporarily incapacitated.

Reflect on it

2.2 Breaching confidentiality

Think about when you might have to breach an individual's confidentiality. Under what circumstances would you be prepared to do this and how would you go about it?

Evidence opportunity

2.2 Legal and ethical conflicts between maintaining confidentiality and sharing information

What are the legal and ethical conflicts relating to your own area of service? Show your assessor how you lead practice that considers both legal and ethical conflicts relating to your area of service. Consider the areas discussed in this section.

Alternatively, use the headings above and tell your assessor how you deal with them and how you help those you manage with ethical conflicts and issues with respect to confidentiality and information sharing.

AC 2.3 Identify team's training needs in relation to handling information

AC 2.4 Implement a plan that addresses team's training needs in relation to handling information

Here, you will identify the training requirements for the setting to ensure that data is handled correctly and then implement a plan to address those requirements.

Data protection is a legal requirement so your staff must be trained to comply and understand the importance of it. Failure to do so could result in, at best, a complaint and, at worst, a fine.

The law does not specify which training your staff should undertake, but it should be relevant to their role in the organisation. The training should provide data protection basics and details about what information can be given to individuals using the service, their families and others.

Data protection is everyone's responsibility, so you'll need to provide training to everyone who works for you, including temporary staff and volunteers.

Evidence opportunity

2.3 and 2.4 Assess staff training needs

Undertake a skills analysis of your staff and complete a training plan for handling information. Show which staff are qualified in this area and those who require training.

Construct a simple questionnaire detailing some of the areas you believe staff should understand about data protection and confidentiality. Survey your staff to get an idea of their current knowledge.

What training will you supply as a result of completing Q2?

Legislation

Legislation	Key points
Data Protection Act 2018	This Act deals with the processing and protection of data on individuals. It applies to the processing UK residents' personal data.
General Data Protection Regulation (GDPR)	This Regulation provides detailed guidance to organisations on how to govern and manage people's personal information. It also applies to the processing of EU residents' personal data.
Mental Capacity Act 2005	This Act informs individuals about what they can do to plan and ensure that someone else can make decisions for them if they ever lack capacity to do so for themselves.
Health and Social Care (Safety and Quality) Act 2015	This Act aims to improve safety and quality of care and places a duty on health and adult social care providers to share information about a person's care with other health and care professionals.

References

BBC News (2017) 'Thousands of Welsh NHS staff's data stolen in hack'. 13 March. www.bbc.co.uk/news/uk-wales-39249975

Beauchamp, T.L. and Childress, J.F. (1994) *Principles of Biomedical Ethics*. Oxford: Oxford University Press.

European Parliament and Council of the European Union (1995) 'Directive 95/46/EC of the European Parliament and of the Council of 24 October 1995 on the protection of individuals with regard to the processing of personal data and on the free movement of such data'. *Official Journal*, L281, pp. 31–50.

Social Care Institute for Excellence (2015) 'Safeguarding adults: Sharing information'. www.scie.org.uk/safeguarding/adults/practice/sharing-information

Useful resources and further reading

Department of Health and Social Care (2023) Policy paper 'A cyber resilient health and adult social care system in England: Cyber security strategy to 2030'. www.gov.uk/government/publications/cyber-security-strategy-for-health-and-social-care-2023-to-2030/a-cyber-resilient-health-and-adult-social-care-system-in-england-cyber-security-strategy-to-2030

Information Commissioner's Office (n.d.) '72 hours - how to respond to a personal data breach'. https://ico.org.uk/for-organisations/sme-web-hub/72-hours-how-to-respond-to-a-personal-data-breach

Rethink Mental Illness (n.d.) 'Nearest relative under the Mental Health Act 1983'. www.rethink.org/carers-family-friends/what-you-need-to-know/nearest-relative

Social Care Institute for Excellence (2020) 'Privacy and dignity in care'. www.scie.org.uk/dignity/care/privacy

Unit 515

Leading person-centred practice

GLH 40

About this unit

The purpose of this unit is to enhance the manager's knowledge of the theory, principles, understanding and skills required to promote and implement person-centred practice and to lead the implementation of active participation of individuals.

You will look at how the development of the personalisation agenda from a service-led provision has changed the face of care in the UK.

You will also deal with consent in practice and what this means for individuals. This addresses the issue of active participation as a way of working that recognises an individual's right to participate in the activities and relationships of everyday life as independently as possible. The individual as an active partner in their own care or support is given a voice in adult care service provisions and is no longer regarded as a passive recipient. You will be introduced to various models of person-centred practice to enable you to lead and encourage the active participation of the individuals using your service.

Learning outcomes

By the end of this unit, you will:

1. Understand person-centred, outcomes-based practice.
2. Understand the value of person-centred practice in partnership working to enable individuals to achieve their desired outcomes.
3. Be able to lead person-centred practice to facilitate positive outcomes for individuals.
4. Understand the relevance of relationships when promoting health and wellbeing.
5. Be able to lead practice in recognising individuals' relationships.
6. Understand positive risk taking in the context of supporting individuals.
7. Be able to lead the implementation of practices, policies, procedures to manage risk and positive risk.

Getting started

Before you study the unit, think about the following:

- How do you think services can be managed to meet best practice guidelines and benchmarks for person-centred practice?
- What training and support do staff need to ensure that services achieve positive outcomes for individuals who use the services?
- What kinds of integrated services are currently provided to facilitate the achievement of positive outcomes for individuals who use the services?
- How can services be improved to ensure that individuals receive a person-centred approach to their care package?
- How can person-centred practices enhance relationships?
- Why is positive risk taking part of person-centred care?

These are some of the things you should start to think about; you will find out more about them throughout the unit. It would also be useful to come back to these questions as you study the unit.

LO1 Understand person-centred, outcomes-based practice

AC 1.1 Evaluate ways of working

Here, you will evaluate ways of working in a person-centred way using strength-based approaches.

Strength-based approaches

Strength-based (or asset-based) approaches look first at the individual's skills and resources and at the support they receive from the people around them and the community. The term 'strength' refers to the things that meet the individual's needs, enabling them to deal with the challenges they face in life and to achieve their goals. These strengths include their personal resources such as knowledge, skills and abilities, their social network and resources and community resources, also known as 'social capital' and/or 'universal resources'.

Adopting a strength-based approach involves a collaborative process between the individual and the people supporting them, so the quality of the relationship that develops between them is crucial to the process. Working in such a collaborative way enables the individual to be a co-producer of the services and support rather than just a consumer of them.

Person-centred practice

Person-centred practice is a care approach in which individuals access social care services as an equal partner in their care and support. They are at the centre of all decisions relevant to them.

SCIE's definition of person-centred care places the person at the centre and as the expert of their own experience. Rather than adult social care workers making decisions about what is best for an individual using the service, the individual, and their family where appropriate, become equal partners, planning their care and support to meet their needs, goals and outcomes.

The emphasis of support moves to 'doing with' the individual rather than 'doing to', enabling a more active approach to designing the care and support that the individual needs and wants.

> **KEY TERM**
>
> **Person-centred practice:** A way of working that recognises the complexity and unique nature of individuals and places them at the centre of the care given, respecting their needs, preferences and knowledge.

The Care Act 2014 further moved this agenda on by making it a main focus in care and identifying the outcomes that matter to the individual. 'Outcomes' are defined as the end-results of services for individuals, so an outcomes-focused service is one that prioritises the care that the individual identifies as most important to them. This means they can specify the care that will have a greater impact on their wellbeing. For example, a positive outcome for somebody might be that they are able to stay in their own home with carers and professionals coming in to deliver personal and medical care rather than them being taken into hospital or long-term social care.

Person-centred care or personalised care is, therefore, about making the individual requiring the care the central figure in the process. 'People at the heart of care' (DHSC, 2022) is the government's response to the reform of social care and sets out a ten-year vision for adult social care. For many people, care begins at home and this vision for adult social care puts people and families as a central focus at the 'heart' of care . The vison offers choice and control to individuals and promotes their independence so that they can live well as part of a community. It further recognises unpaid carers and treats them fairly.

Personalisation enables individuals to build a system of care and support tailored to meet their needs and designed with their full involvement. It is about ensuring that the individual has their choices taken into account and their culture and ethnicity respected. Historically, a 'one size fits all' approach to care was used and this meant the individual had to fit into and access already existing care services, whether those services were appropriate or not.

The term 'person-centred care' is now used to describe care that is user-focused, promoting independence and autonomy. Collaborative and partnership approaches to care often use the term 'person-centred' to describe their ethos (Innes et al., 2006).

Positive practice is about treating people in a compassionate manner, with dignity and kindness. It is a means of truly embedding person-centred care, with its focus on the individual and their specific needs, and not just undertaking a tick-box exercise. Person-centred thinking is about the values, skills and tools staff can use to get to know an individual to find out what is truly important to them to be able to support them properly. By adopting this mindset, care workers can focus entirely on what matters to the individual and ensure that they are listened to and supported every step of the way in the decisions that are made. Helen Sanderson Associates offer a set of templates for person-centred thinking tools that enable individuals to think and plan for their life (Helen Sanderson Associates, n.d.)

The templates can be used to structure conversations with individuals to gain as much information as possible from them, helping to improve understanding and communication. The information gathered then informs the care and support the individuals require.

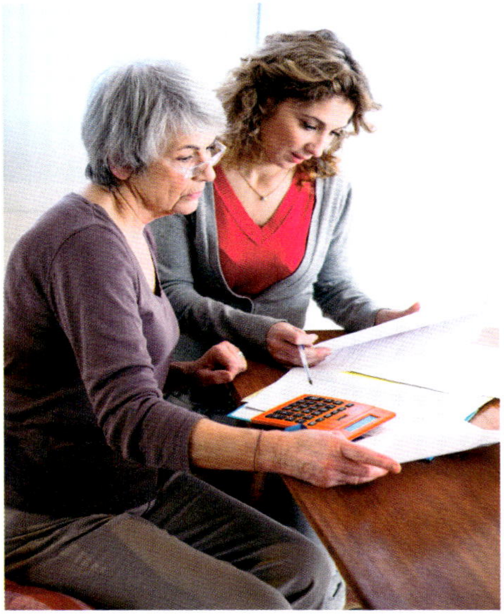

Figure 31 A care/support plan is user-focused, taking into account individual needs and wishes

> **Reflect on it**
>
> **1.1 Person-centred practice as positive practice**
>
> What do you think person-centred practice is? Describe its benefits. How is this positive practice? How is this used in your setting?

Active participation

Active participation refers to an individual's right to be an active partner in their own care or support, rather than a passive recipient. Person-centred practice adopts an inclusive and collaborative approach and the language you use is important. For example, the words you choose need to enable and facilitate the individual. Using an encouraging tone is far better than adopting a stance that might limit the individual's actions. You should not 'allow' a choice but rather enable or facilitate it. This way of working encourages the individual to participate in the activities and relationships of everyday life as independently as possible. This in turn will give them confidence and belief in their abilities, which brings with it a sense of pride and success.

Consider for a moment how you might feel if you were never consulted about the support you need. You merely had to accept the decisions made about you and do as you were told. It would not be very long before you were completely switched off and passive in whatever was being done to you. You might even feel that you were being undervalued with respect to your wishes. It could also have a detrimental effect on your personal and professional relationships, affecting your overall wellbeing.

By being an active partner in care, the individual is able to build relationships that will enhance their wellbeing and independence.

Active participation is mentioned in the 'Code of Conduct for Healthcare Support Workers and Adult Social Care Workers in England (Skills for Care and Skills for Health, 2013), which outlines the behaviour and attitudes expected of those who work in the sector. Although the code is voluntary, it is suggested as best practice.

Standard 7 in the Skills for Care 'Care certificate' defines active participation as a way of supporting an individual's right to be an active partner in their own care and support. It is about privacy and dignity and references active participation as a way of ensuring that individuals have a right to participate in activities and relationships as independently as possible (Skills for Care, 2014). As the expert in their own care, indviduals know exactly what they need and want, and will want to participate in activities and relationships as independently as they can. As care workers, we can never assume what a person will want.

To evaluate how active participation has enhanced the wellbeing and quality of life of the individuals using your service, you could ask for feedback via questionnaires or interviews. You might also encourage individuals to discuss their experiences as a group in a forum. Any information gained can then be acted upon, with individuals kept informed of how this will be done.

Outcomes-based practice

Outcomes-based practice refers to individuals' aims or objectives; things individuals want to achieve or need to happen. This approach focuses on supporting individuals to achieve the outcomes that are important to them and offers innovative approaches to enable this.

Outcomes-based practice specifies what the person at the centre of the care process needs to do to achieve their care and support aims. This has created a results-based accountability culture that relies on data-driven decision-making processes to help to improve the lives of citizens and the community as a whole. Being accountable in this way means evidence is provided for the outcomes achieved and services can be judged on whether individuals are better off as a result of the services' input.

The key benefits of such care are:

- individuals can choose the care they prefer and need to improve their quality of life
- individuals can have more choice and any changes to their needs can be responded to more quickly
- care workers can work closely with individuals to enable them to become more independent

- partnership working is strengthened
- evaluating the effectiveness of services is easier because outcomes measures are set out.

Several approaches to outcomes-based practice have been identified. These include the following:

- **Results-based accountability**: Also known as outcomes-based accountability. It uses data-driven decision-making processes to help solve problems and is a way of thinking and acting that improves the lives of people in the community. It has been developed to improve the performance of an organisation's services.
- **Outcomes management**: Helping individuals and providers make care-related choices based on knowledge of the effects those choices may have on the individual's life.
- **Outcomes into practice**: Focuses on the outcomes people value.
- **Logic model**: A logical framework and theory of change used by funders, managers and evaluators of programmes to assess effectiveness.

Whichever model is used, the basic premise is that outcomes-based practice is a new way of working that replaces the needs-led approach that tended to focus on the immediate situation and support requirements that would be provided by the care professional.

Evidence opportunity

1.1 Person-centred practice

Evaluate the strengths and weaknesses of each of the following four ways of working using examples from your own setting:

- ✔ strength-based approaches
- ✔ person-centred practice
- ✔ active participation
- ✔ outcomes-based practice.

AC 1.2 Describe how strength-based approaches and person-centred practice influence outcomes-based practices

Here, you will describe different influences on outcomes-based practices, including different approaches and practices.

Strength-based approaches

The strength-based approach identifies and assesses the individual's strengths and capacity and examines how they currently interact with the community. In this way, the individual's outcomes and aspirations are identified at the care and support planning stage. The assessor, along with the individual, identifies strengths and then together they set the outcomes needed to achieve positive change and build supportive relationships.

Person-centred practice

Person-centred approaches ensure that the individual is able to identify and prioritise the outcomes they want from the care provision, whether that is their immediate care needs or future goals.

The link between the two

Helen Sanderson Associates (2015) demonstrates the link between the two terms by describing person-centred outcomes as:

- being a personal and not a service perspective
- controlled and influenced by the person
- specific to the person and able to be measured (HSA, 2015).

In an attempt to ensure that all individuals requiring care have their needs met holistically, the 'personalisation' agenda was introduced.

It is clear that to support positive change for individuals, outcomes-based practice and person-centred practice need to be interlinked. It is possible to have an outcomes-based service that is purely service-led and not person-centred at all. In other words, it meets the needs of the setting rather than the individual. However, by linking the two, the individual is able to choose the care required to fit their own lifestyle and needs. Your role is to ensure that staff are fully open to enabling choice and autonomy so that the individuals they care for can become more independent and empowered in their own care setting. This will require staff training and supervision to ensure that they have the individuals at the heart of everything they do.

Reflect on it

1.2 Person-centred care and strength-based approach

Person-centred care reflects the values of empowerment and personalisation that underlie contemporary approaches to social care in the UK. The strength-based approach is similar in that it requires practitioners to work in collaboration with the individuals using the service, supporting them to do things for themselves, having first established their capacity and skills, and the support they have in the local community.

Write a reflective account of your own views on these two models and describe how you meet these needs in your organisation.

Evidence opportunity

1.2 Approaches to person-centred and strength-based practice

Describe how strength-based approaches and person-centred practice influence outcomes-based practices.

AC 1.3 Analyse how outcomes-based practices impact on individuals

Here, you will analyse how outcomes-based practice can impact an individual's wellbeing and control over their environment.

Health and wellbeing

An outcomes-based approach to care is driven by aspirations which are unique to the individuals using the services. Outcomes are the impact of services on a person's life, therefore outcomes-based services aim to achieve the priorities that the individuals themselves identify as important. Any goals set are those they have set for themselves and describe what they want to achieve.

These need to be goals that have been assessed and discussed so that the individual and those supporting their care can work towards them together. The aim is to ensure that people who need care and support are enabled to live their best lives possible, building on their own strengths and capabilities. In this way, wellbeing is enhanced.

Independence and choice and control

Having the independence to make our own choices is part of what makes us human and yet we take this for granted until we become unable to engage in certain activities. Anybody who has suffered a debilitating illness will know how losing independence and control of our lives can happen slowly without us even realising it.

A commitment to maintaining a person's independence, choice and control begins with a personalised care/support plan with outcomes clearly detailed. The person involved, together with their family and an adult social care professional, will create outcomes that show how they will be supported, enabling as much independence, choice and control as possible.

Being free to make our own decisions and choices is a liberating feeling. A person with a learning disability, such as Down syndrome, may have choice removed from them by family who feel this is the right thing to do, and well-meaning care workers may think this is fine. As unique people with our own identity, values and goals in life, we need to be able to maintain the ability to think and act for ourselves. As a care worker you must empower the individuals you care for to do the same.

Autonomy is about making decisions for ourselves and keeping control of our lives. Being masters of our own environment and adapting to and modifying our situations in order to progress and achieve what we need is a vital part of this. When an individual requires support and care, this may seem to be difficult to achieve, but it is imperative to keep the lines of communication open and to access the individual's desires about how they wish to live and how they can remain in control of their circumstances as much as possible.

Evidence opportunity

1.3 Ensuring independence, choice and control

Give a detailed account describing how outcomes-based practices impact an individual's health and wellbeing, independence and choice and control.

Use an example from each heading to support your answer and explain how strength-based approaches and person-centred practice influence outcomes-based practice for the individual.

LO2 Understand the value of person-centred practice in partnership working to enable individuals to achieve their desired outcomes

AC 2.1 Evaluate the role of partnerships, collaboration and co-production with individuals and others in enabling individuals to achieve their desired outcomes

Here, you will be introduced to the various aspects of partnership working. Collaboration and co-production will be required to evaluate these types of working.

Partnerships, **collaboration** and **co-production** are all terms that identify ways of working with individuals, networks, communities and other professionals and organisations.

KEY TERMS

Collaboration: The practice of care professionals working in partnership with individuals and members of the public to improve outcomes.

Co-production: Working in partnership and sharing power between people who require care and support. It includes carers, families and citizens.

Partnerships

You will be aware of how working in partnership with other local services has improved care for people. For example, the local GP service will offer primary care but will also be able to link in with physiotherapy, chiropody or leisure services should people need such care. Care homes or other provisions may link in with local hairdressers or health clubs to provide services for the wellbeing of the individuals in their care. Private care companies may be engaged as partners to provide services the statutory sector cannot provide and this all enhances the individuals' experience.

Collaboration

Collaboration describes how working with partners, and gaining an understanding of their needs, can establish mutually beneficial and respectful relationships without losing focus of the outcomes or the needs of either party.

Co-production

Co-production was first mentioned in the Care Act 2014, when it was suggested that it be a key part of implementing the Act. It was to be used to develop preventative, strength-based services, and to support assessment.

Co-production describes an equal relationship between the individuals using a service and the people responsible for the service working together to decide the best way to design and deliver services. It recognises that individuals, their families and friends have knowledge and experiences that can be used to help make services better, not only for themselves but for other people who access care. They are, after all, experts in their own care and support because of their lived experience.

Provider collaboratives

In August 2022, the Care Provider Alliance published its guidance on 'Adult social care provider partnerships in Integrated Care Systems.' This guide recognises the role adult social care providers play in the Integrated Care Systems (ICSs) and the need for collaborative working to face the challenges in the system.

The Care Provider Alliance represents the national voice of adult social care and, following the Health and Care Act 2022 with the further development of ICSs, it supports integration in the provision of health and social care. It recognises that some adult social care providers are still at the early stages of understanding and engaging with ICSs, but there is strong support for local systems to make opportunities for adult social care providers to be an active part in these new arrangements to better support individuals using adult care services.

NHS England launched provider collaboratives or partnerships as a way of bringing two or more NHS trusts together for the benefit of the individuals using the services in each trust. This move is part of a shift in the way the health and care system is organised. The aim is to put greater emphasis on partnerships as a way of dealing with increasing demand for services and a lack of funding, which has been made more acute by the COVID-19 pandemic.

Historically, provider organisations have worked together to address challenges. There have been documents and reviews aimed at making these collaborations more effective, with the goal of bringing together the different types of organisations involved in partnership working:

- The NHS Five Year Forward View (2014) aimed to deliver integrated care by breaking down barriers between services.
- The Dalton Review (GOV.UK, 2014) explored organisational models to underpin this. It identified five themes:
  1. One size does not fit all – recognising that care should be delivered which best suits local circumstances.
  2. Quicker transformational and transactional change is required, so simplifying the processes of changes should be addressed
  3. Ambitious organisations with a proven track record are encouraged to expand their reach and have greater impact.
  4. Overall sustainability for the provider sector is a priority.
  5. A dedicated implementation programme to make change happen.
- The Carter Review on productivity in NHS hospitals (GOV.UK, 2015) showed that improvements could be made, leading to the Five Year Forward View for Mental Health which brought together commissioning and service providers. The NHS Long Term Plan (2019) emphasised the development of collaborative working, which in turn has led to:

- NHS-led provider collaboratives, where providers of specialised mental health, learning disability and autism services agreed to work together to improve care in their areas, and
- formal provider collaboratives and integrated care systems which are described in 'Integrating care: next steps to building strong and effective integrated care systems across England' (NHS England, 2020), and NHS guidance on 'Working together at scale: guidance on provider collaboratives' (NHS England and NHS Improvement, 2021).

Research it

2.1 Provider collaboratives

Read 'Provider collaboratives: Explaining their role in system working' on The King's Fund website (The Kings Fund, 2022).

What is the rationale for provider collaboratives and how do you think they can enhance care?

Evidence opportunity

2.1 Evaluating the role of partnerships, collaboration and co-production

Evaluate the role of partnerships, collaboration and co-production with individuals in your own setting and say how this achieves their desired outcomes.

AC 2.2 Describe own setting/service's role in enabling individuals to build and maintain relationships and connections with their community

Here, you will describe how involvement in the community can assist individuals in developing relationships.

What is a community? Various definitions describe it as a group of people with different characteristics who are linked by social ties or relationships and who share common perspectives. We all live in communities, which describes the location part of the definition, but there are other communities based on shared interests, such as a sport community or an art community.

Communities provide support to individuals and the individuals in your setting may already engage with their local community, participating in social and recreational activities, leisure services, spiritual and cultural services.

A number of relationships are built in communities and individuals will be part of a range of relationships that are important to them that go beyond family.

As the population ages and more people live longer, it is likely that more support will take place within people's homes and the community rather than in hospital. Support will also be needed for people with learning disabilities and those with long-term conditions. Your setting may have a role in the delivery of that care or may provide a service that helps people in the local community. How you market and promote your service to the local community is important in developing a sustainable service for the future.

In line with government policy on person-centred practice, services must respond to individuals' wishes and choices to ensure positive outcomes. The Department of Health's 'Transforming Community services' programme (Department of Health, 2011) showed that integrated care improves quality outcomes and efficiency through better use of resources. Individuals using your service and those of your partners, stakeholders and others in the community with whom you work will benefit from better resources and more positive health outcomes.

Evidence opportunity

2.2 Community involvement

Describe how your own setting/service enables individuals to build and maintain relationships and connections with their community.

- ✔ How do you promote your service within local communities?
- ✔ How do the individuals using your service and your staff engage and integrate with the wider community?
- ✔ How does working with other community and outreach services support the development of care provision within the community, for example retail or charity outlets, community cafes, hairdressers and chiropodists?

AC 2.3 Analyse how integrated service provision that crosses traditional boundaries may achieve better outcomes for individuals

Here, you will analyse how traditional boundaries compared to integrated service provision can provide better outcomes for people.

Traditionally, delivery of care in the UK was fragmented and based in various settings. A move to a multidisciplinary approach to care in the 1960s saw the sharing of facilities and later partnership working was encouraged. The focus on disease and care management and the use of the medical model changed in the 1990s and, driven largely by finance, the move to integrated care was seen to be the way forward.

The social model was adopted by most disability organisations, having been created by people with disabilities themselves, and in 2014 it was endorsed by the Government Equalities Office. This model looks at the barriers that prevent people with disabilities from being able to participate fully in day-to-day life and further seeks to remove these barriers to enable greater access to work and independent living. It recognises that attitudes towards people with disabilities also create barriers to inclusion.

Integrated service provision is joined up, co-ordinated care planned around the desires, needs and preferences of the individual and has been developed through the personalisation agenda and person-centred care.

The benefits of the philosophy behind person-centred care are clear, but despite extensive support by government, policy makers, practitioners, individuals and their families, there remain difficulties with implementation. Traditional boundaries still exist and there are still funding and training issues in addition to the occasional communication failures and lack of information. Organisational barriers, where policies are different and staff incentives and structures don't fit well with other organisations, can also be a problem.

As individuals experience more complex health issues, their care may be provided by several different health providers and this can result in care services that are fragmented, difficult to access and not based around the individual's needs.

Good integrated care can reduce this problem by reducing the gaps and inefficiencies in care and also provides opportunities for financial savings between services. The joined-up approach reduces confusion for both the individual and the health professional and prevents care from being repeated. In the past, it was relatively easy for individuals to get lost in a system where health professionals located in different areas did not engage with professionals from different disciplines. It should be mentioned, however, that not all people who require support in the community also require healthcare.

The Local Government and Public Involvement in Health Act (2007) set out the government's plans to promote public and community influence in health and social care. The intention was to make NHS organisations more accountable to their local populations and to strengthen the voice of individuals using care services.

The Act states that the local involvement networks were developed for:

- promoting and supporting the involvement of people in the commissioning, provision and scrutiny of local care services
- reviewing and monitoring the commissioning and provision of local care services.

Person-centred care is about enabling people to have choice and control in their care and lives, and as wellbeing has been shown to link to social inclusion and active participation, it requires integration with local communities. As a manager and a leader, your focus will be on how you might improve the quality of the service and transform the current ways of working to ensure that a more person-centred agenda is followed. This will require you to understand the role of local government and the wider community of health services such as the NHS, GPs, the private/independent sector, the voluntary sector and the local community.

One of the biggest challenges you may face is enabling individuals with diverse needs to access employment. Employers must consider how to make adaptions to enable those with neurodiverse needs, such as autism, Down syndrome and other learning disabilities, to fully participate in employment. The National Autistic Society supplies a guide to employing people with autism (National Autistic Society, 2020).

The Down's Syndrome Association also provides a tailored employment programme called Workfit, which brings together employers, training them about the learning profile of people who have Down syndrome and how they can be supported in the workplace. (See their website for more details: Down's Syndrome Association, n.d.)

Evidence opportunity

2.3 Analyse integrated service provision

Analyse how an integrated service provision that crosses traditional boundaries may achieve better outcomes for individuals. Identify the strengths and weaknesses in your answer.

LO3 Be able to lead person-centred practice to facilitate positive outcomes for individuals

AC 3.1 Facilitate the development and implementation of a plan to ensure team members have the training and development needed to support individuals in person-centred ways to achieve desired outcomes

Here, you will show how you can plan for training and development for team members in person-centred practice.

The training programme you offer new staff and refresher training for experienced staff must be underpinned with knowledge about person-centred care. Skills for Health, Skills for Care and Health Education England (2017) have published a framework called 'Person-centred approaches' that provides advice, training and development and includes a number of underpinning principles to guide an organisation's approach to training and development on the topic.

One such principle is that of behaviour change. Although the concept of using a person-centred approach for care is not new, it is not always seen in some settings, so a reminder of the sort of behaviours you need staff to exhibit to encourage a person-centred approach must be included in training.

In line with co-production methodology, the framework also recommends that training is co-produced, with the individual contributing reflections and stories of their experience. You may have started on this process in the evidence opportunity for AC1.3.

Research it

3.1 Person-centred approaches

Look at the 'Person-centred approaches' framework published by Skills for Health, Skills for Care and Health Education England (2017). This focuses on healthcare but aspects of it are useful for all adult care services.

How could you incorporate some of the material into a short training session to encourage staff to adopt a more person-centred way of thinking?

AC 3.2 Support team members to work in partnership with individuals and others to recognise and respond to individuals' changing strengths, needs and preferences

Here, you will be required to provide evidence of how you manage others to work with those in receipt of care and support, ensuring that you adapt your approaches to meet an individual's changing needs.

The person who is at the centre of decision making must feel like they are actively involved. Too often an individual can feel like they are merely a passive attendant at a meeting, with little say in what goes on. It is easy to take for granted the work you do, with all its related administration, meetings and bureaucracy. For individuals using a service, this may be overwhelming, and it would take a lot of confidence on the individual's part to question anything put forward. You need to enable your staff to ensure that individuals are happy to participate in their care. This may require managing them in following a set process that ensures that needs are consistently met. This is covered in Unit 509 AC4.8.

Reflect on it

3.2 Changing needs

Reflect on an incident in which you and the team needed to adapt the care approach in response to an individual's changing needs or preferences. How did this affect the person-centred approach?

Evidence opportunity

3.2 Managing others to adapt approaches

Provide evidence of how you manage staff to work with those in receipt of care and support, ensuring that they adapt their approaches to meet an individual's changing needs.

For example, during supervision you might set an action plan for staff to provide examples of how they react to an individual's changing needs. You may ask them what strategies they use to give individuals the confidence to speak up. Perhaps they could provide a sample care/support plan with annotations to show where each step has been accomplished.

AC 3.3 Support others to apply person-centred approaches to ensure positive outcomes for individuals and those important to them in complex situations

Here, you will be required to show how you support your team to adopt person-centred approaches when working with individuals during complex situations.

Support can be psychological, physical, social, financial, environmental or emotional, or a mix of any of these. An individual with complex needs may present with two or more needs affecting their mental or physical health, for example financial and social needs. What makes this complex is that such needs interact with and exacerbate one another, leading to individuals experiencing several problems at the same time. For example, somebody who has made choices about their wishes that clash with those of their family may feel depressed and isolated. This can affect all aspects of their life, which might exacerbate issues with poverty and relationships.

All care settings need to support and guide family, friends, advocates, carers and other professional disciplines in obtaining information from individuals to ensure that their wishes and choices are taken into account. This requires shared systems of working across traditional boundaries. For example, occupational therapists who visit a setting to help with independence issues may need access to records and care/support plans. Carers and significant others may also require such information to support the person in their own home. When developing ways of working that involve different teams and other people linked to the individual receiving the care, the following points should be considered:

- The individual is always at the centre of the process.
- Family and friends are partners in the care process.
- The care/support plan is a guide to what is important to the individual and shows what support they need.
- A care/support plan helps the individual to be part of their community and is not merely a description of the services they need.

The plan is a continuous process and does not stop once it has been written. Those involved should continue to evaluate and act within the plan to help the individual to achieve the best quality care.

In reviewing care, you need feedback about how the needs and preferences of the individual have been met and whether changes may be required. The supervision process for staff is a good way to gain feedback and time can be given to review which approaches worked well and which did not. For family members, friends, advocates and other professionals, reviews of care need to be planned and there should be regular meetings or forums to enable this.

The manager's role is to ensure that guidelines for practice that highlight the support needed for individuals are available for staff and the wider team to ensure that seamless care is provided. Decisions about support are made during the assessment process and are then translated into outcome-focused plans, which detail 'important to' and 'important for' sections. These support plans ensure that care given is standardised to reduce the risk of variation throughout the day. For example, a staff member who may not have been involved in the initial assessment needs to be aware of how an individual is supported and how they wish to be treated so that the same care can be continued. Practice protocols will provide guidance and as a manager you are responsible for ensuring that they are upheld and implemented. Sometimes it may be necessary to involve other members of the wider disciplinary team to provide a different area of expertise so staff need to know how a referral to other professionals can be made.

Evidence opportunity

3.3 Person-centred approaches to ensure positive outcomes for individual

Demonstrate to your assessor how your team adopts person-centred approaches when working with individuals in complex situations and how you support them in this endeavour.

AC 3.4 Facilitate the development and review of individuals' care and support

Here, you will demonstrate your involvement in ensuring that individuals are involved and that their preferences are met.

Ensuring that individuals and others are actively involved

Recognising that the individual is an expert in their own care, the Health Foundation has highlighted four principles for person-centred care (Health Foundation, 2014). These are:

1. Treat people with dignity, compassion and respect.
2. Provide co-ordinated care, support and treatment.
3. Offer personalised care, support and treatment.
4. Enable individuals to recognise and develop their strengths and abilities, so that they can live an independent and fulfilling life.

By adopting a person-centred mindset and using the tools developed by Helen Sanderson Associates, person-centred reviews explore what is happening from the individual's and others' perspectives. This means that adult care providers can offer better support to individuals by ensuring that the experiences of the person, their family and those supporting them are taken into account. Additionally, these reviews can create psychologically safe environments where individuals feel comfortable expressing themselves honestly. People living with long-term conditions often know more about managing their condition than care professionals and are able to communicate their needs and the support they require.

Co-production, as mentioned earlier, is the concept of sharing power within the care relationship. Individuals work with personal support networks and professional services to help organisations become agents for change rather than just service providers.

Ensuring that plans and activities reflect individuals' preferences, wishes, strengths and needs

Wilcox et al. (1994) identified key ideas in the form of a five-rung ladder of participation relating to the stance an organisation promoting participation may take, as shown below.

- **Information**: Telling people what is planned.
- **Consultation**: Offering options, listening to feedback, but not allowing new ideas.
- **Deciding together**: Encouraging additional options and ideas and providing opportunities for joint decision making.
- **Acting together**: Not only do different interests decide together on what is best, they form a partnership to carry it out.
- **Supporting independent community interests**: Local groups or organisations are offered funds, advice or other support to develop their own agendas within guidelines.

Your policies and procedures which are in place will support this.

Risk assessment needs to form part of the systems and processes that support individuals. You should also agree on how the care required is assessed in your workplace and how wishes, choices and preferences are agreed upon and met.

Participation in daily activities

In care, the term 'daily living activities' is used to refer to daily self-care activities such as:

- personal care
- shopping
- working
- education
- socialising.

As a professional, you must assess the individuals in your setting to determine their ability or inability to perform these daily living activities. By measuring in this way, you gain knowledge of their functional status and can determine how independent they are.

A managerial responsibility here is to determine the ways in which staff are enabling the individuals in their care to actively participate in their support and that their wishes, needs and desires are what lead the discussion and planning. This can be done by observing practice and through the appraisal system.

> **Evidence opportunity**
>
> **3.4 Personal care of individuals**
>
> Show your assessor how you ensure that the individuals using your service are involved in their support and that their preferences are met.

AC 3.5 Manage resources to ensure that individuals can make choices about their health and wellbeing to achieve positive outcomes and reasonable adjustments are provided to enable individuals to access care and support

Here, you will be required to manage resources to ensure that individuals are actively informed and supported to make healthy choices through a person-centred approach in maintaining their wellbeing.

As the manager, you are sometimes limited with regard to the resources you have at your disposal. Individual needs and wishes should, however, be a priority and you will need to look carefully at the resources you have to achieve this where possible. For example, it may simply require a redeployment of staff to ensure that an individual is able to engage with a hobby or a group meeting outside the setting.

> **Evidence opportunity**
>
> **3.5 Manage resources to ensure that reviews of individuals' preferences, wishes, needs and strengths are valued within the achievement of positive outcomes**
>
> Show your assessor how you manage resources to ensure that reviews of individuals' preferences, wishes, needs and strengths are valued within the achievement of positive outcomes.

Resources

Funding and services

To ensure that the individuals using your service experience positive outcomes, you need to be clear about the resources at your disposal and how they will be used. Care/support plans need to be financially resourced, taking into consideration the availability of services, which of course may change over time. Therefore there needs to be a continual check on what is happening with an individual's care. Your role is to ensure that the budget you are given is used wisely; you may have to identify where savings can be made elsewhere to ensure that the financial resources needed for an individual's care are available.

Funding may be reduced or demand for a particular service may increase, making it more difficult for individuals to access the service. Adjustments to the plan should be made in accordance with how it is progressing.

When you audit or monitor a provision, you make a judgement as to how the resources have been used and whether there has been a positive impact on the individual. For example, you may have decided that, by inputting more funding into a community outing, individuals will experience improved quality of life, resulting in a positive outcome. The resources here would be seen to be well-used and effective.

You should also monitor the ways in which the programme of activities you have planned for the individuals in your setting has improved their wellbeing. A simple evaluation questionnaire can provide feedback on whether they enjoyed a session and this will help you determine whether to repeat it. It is likely that you have in place an evaluation system to enable everyone involved in the setting to comment and document how such care is working.

Carers, the individuals receiving the care and service care providers all need to provide regular feedback about the care package and any need for adjustment. At the start of the whole care planning process, you will have put into place a means for providing feedback. You will also have identified the key people in the process:

- **Person receiving the care**: As the central figure in the care process, there needs to be a clear process for individuals to record how they experience the care received. This can be achieved using a checklist, perhaps on a weekly or monthly basis, regular contact via email, telephone or meetings with the care manager or the person facilitating the care, and recording the care given on a daily basis on the daily record.
- **Family and friends involved in the care**: Feedback from these individuals is valuable, but form filling can be laborious and time consuming. They may feel overwhelmed with having to provide a regular feedback form, so you need to be able to obtain their views in another way, perhaps via a weekly phone call or email.
- **Adult care professionals and service providers**: It is important that at meetings and in discussion with colleagues and service providers you can determine how the resources are being managed and how well the budget is being used. At these meetings you can also undertake a review of how an individual's support package is meeting their wishes and achieving a positive outcome for them. The individual and their family should be included in these review meetings if possible.

Staff

Your staff are your biggest resource. It is important that they are trained to promote good health and healthy choices to the individuals in their care. In planning, care staff must be aware that the promotion of good health and giving individuals information to help them to make healthier lifestyle choices are as important as managing long-term chronic conditions. Staff can advise individuals about healthy choices, but the decision to follow this advice, of course, lies with the individual.

Evidence opportunity

3.5 Support individuals to make healthy choices

Show how you manage resources to enable individuals to make choices about their health and wellbeing to achieve positive outcomes.

Give an example from your practice to show how you make adjustments to enable the individual. For example, somebody who is at the end of life may wish to eat food we might consider not particularly healthy. The positive outcome for this individual of eating something they really like far outweighs our attempt to help them to eat a more balanced diet.

Reflect on it

3.5 Health and healthy choices

Write a short reflective account of how you have promoted good health and healthy choices in one aspect of your provision and how you engaged your staff with it. For example, how did you promote the idea of nutrition?

Reflect on it

3.5 Managing resources

Give an example of how you have managed resources so that individuals can achieve positive outcomes in your setting.

How does your organisation monitor resources and evaluate progress towards the achievement of outcomes for the individuals using your service? Write a reflective account of the process undertaken and place copies of relevant documentation in your portfolio.

AC 3.6 Implement systems and processes for recording that identifies progress towards achievement of individual's desired outcomes and implementation of person-centred practice

Here, you will show how the setting implements systems that record an individual's preferences to ensure that person-centred practice is implemented.

The process of implementing systems and processes to record person-centred care is about recognising and documenting changes to circumstances. You will already have systems in place that record the care to be provided and to evaluate that care. As a service provider, you are required to regularly ask for feedback from the individuals using your service and their families about how well you deliver the service. Individuals need to be active participants in their care so their input might be part of the records.

An outcomes-based approach to care differs from a task-based approach. A task-based approach sets out in detail every task that a care worker must undertake with each individual, but an outcomes-based approach is much broader as it is set by the individual. For example, the individual may set an outcome of getting out of bed, washed, dressed and comfortable every morning. How that is achieved is entirely up to the individual and how they are feeling.

Outcomes tend to focus on wellbeing rather than achieving specific long-term goals. Records should monitor the progress of the individual towards their outcome, so that all staff are able to observe progress and gain information. In order to record progress, there must be a clear statement of the outcome, a plan of how the outcome will be achieved and regular feedback about progress.

Care assessment and care/support plans are useful systems for documenting care. Handwritten records and notes are still used but many settings and partners now use electronic formats for storing records. Electronic records may include:

- care/support plans
- daily records and Medication Administration Records (MARS)
- GP and primary healthcare team records
- outpatient records
- test results, including photographs of the individual, X-rays, pathology and other laboratory records.

You may also have letters to and from the individual, or their medical professional's or social worker's emails, texts and recordings.

All of these records describe the care the individual is receiving and are, of course, confidential. As a manager, you must ensure that the systems and processes in place conform to the requirements of GDPR.

It is most important that you do not underestimate the input from carers, family and others in the care of an individual. Should a carer become too ill to continue in the caring role for a while, there must be a procedure in place to ensure that care for the individual can be continued as planned.

As a manager, you need to engage with families to ensure that they feel included in the care-planning process and that they have somebody they can access if they need to. Families and other carers can sometimes feel socially isolated, so it is useful to have systems in place to inform them about support groups and help that is available.

Another system could be for carers to have a monthly meeting to discuss the progress of the care being given to the individual and to suggest any changes if necessary. There might also be a system in place whereby a carer can telephone a direct number to speak to a staff member about the care where appropriate.

Evidence opportunity

3.6 Implementing systems, processes, procedures and practices

Review the systems you have in place by commenting upon the strengths and the weaknesses of the processes.

You may find it useful to collect the documentation you use to show how you go about recording progress in care and the achievement of outcomes. Do you think the process and the system you use are useful? Give reasons for your answer.

What systems and practices are in place to address the needs of family and other carers?

LO4 Understand the relevance of relationships when promoting health and wellbeing

AC 4.1 Explain why it is important to follow a proactive approach when supporting individuals to build and maintain relationships

Here, you will explain the importance of positive relationships for individuals within a setting.

Our health and wellbeing are affected by the people we have around us and the strength of those relationships. Enabling and helping the individuals using your service to build positive relationships is a crucial part of your role.

Positive relationships with others result in feelings of happiness and a sense of wellbeing and give us purpose and belonging. Research has shown that the benefits of social connections are linked to good mental health.

For young adults in care and older people, care and support needs may change and become complex. It is possible that some of their relationships will become difficult to maintain or even come to an end. This can result in individuals becoming lonely and isolated, which is bad for both their physical and mental health.

Loneliness and isolation remain the key predictors for poor mental and physical health. Having a lack of good relationships and long-term feelings of loneliness have been shown by a range of studies to be associated with higher rates of mortality, poor physical health outcomes and lower life satisfaction.

According to the Campaign to End Loneliness, there are 1.2 million chronically lonely older people in the UK and 9 million lonely people. Find out more on the Campaign to End Loneliness website.

AC 4.2 Describe how having an open, proactive culture, which supports individuals' rights to have the relationships they choose, can support health and wellbeing

Here, you will describe your role as a leader in developing a positive culture within a setting and its impact on health and wellbeing.

One of the CQC's 5 Key Lines of Enquiry (KLOEs) is 'Are they well-led?', which refers to the leadership, management and governance of an organisation (CQC, 2022). To ensure that high-quality care is being provided and that individual needs are met, the CQC assesses the culture and ethos of the organisation and asks, 'How does the service promote a positive culture that is person-centred, open, inclusive and empowering?'

Take a moment to remind yourself what culture actually means. A useful definition is that all staff in the setting think, behave and work in a way that complies with the ethos and values of the service. Culture covers all aspects of organisational life and is about how things are done on a daily basis. It involves how staff interact with each other and how they go about their work. It determines how decisions are made and draws people together. An organisation that is cohesive and value-led improves the workplace for the staff and the quality of life of the individuals using the service. Culture is covered in more detail in Unit 511 AC1.1 and Unit 512 AC3.1.

Everyone has the right to personal relationships, but the need to protect individuals in a care settings from harm and from sexual abuse has been a focus and in the past may have led to the discouragement of relationships.

CQC have reported incidents of a sexual nature arising in homes with providers notifying them about a sexual incident. These incidents included those observed by staff, allegations of abuse, and the effects on people. These notifications revealed lack of awareness of good practice in sexual safety and sexuality and supported further recommendations for change.

One of the CQC recommendations led to the Skills for Care guidance on 'Supporting personal relationships' to be updated so that staff know how to protect the individuals in their care from sexual abuse and how to support them to develop and maintain relationships and friendships. Individuals should be able to express their sexuality and settings should aim to develop a culture where people and staff feel empowered to talk about sexuality and raise concerns around safety (Skills for Care, n.d.). This can only be achieved in a culture that is open and proactive and supports the development of individuals' relationships and friendships.

Evidence opportunity

4.1 and 4.2 Promoting a person-centred culture

Refer back to your last CQC report and look at the 'Are they well-led?' section and the question 'How does the service promote a positive culture that is person-centred, open, inclusive and empowering?'

How did you score and what will you do to improve this?

If you are not a regulated service, explain the importance of following a proactive approach when supporting individuals to build and maintain relationships and describe how such an open, proactive culture supports individuals' rights to have the relationships they choose.

AC 4.3 Analyse the support an individual may need to maintain and build relationships

Here, you will analyse the methods by which team members can create a supportive environment for individuals when building relationships.

The Care Act (2014) promotes the principle of 'wellbeing', and this recognises the importance of relationships in physical health and emotional wellbeing.

Staff should work towards reducing isolation for individuals, helping them to develop and maintain relationships and friendships. This is an important part of their role in promoting wellbeing.

Everyone who uses care services must be protected from becoming isolated and potentially inactive. Friendships, hobbies and interests should be actively encouraged.

Recognising the benefits of a friendship to the individual and the value this can bring to their life should be supported through shared decision making. Staff who are informed and trained can support the individual by having discussions about relationships and the types of friendships the individual has in order to minimise risk and increase positive experiences. By developing a proactive approach to support relationships, individuals can be supported to have the relationships they choose, with minimal risk of harm.

If it is evident that a friendship is developing into a more intimate relationship, staff should be able to create an environment in which individuals are free to discuss it and this means addressing the values and beliefs of the organisation and acknowledging sexual intimacy as a fundamental human need.

As a manager, you will need to engage with staff and develop an open, blameless culture that positively supports sexuality and relationships and is truly person centred. Staff may find relationships easier to discuss if they have a set of local guidelines and policies to give structure to conversations and to capture information from the individual about their intimate needs.

Evidence opportunity

4.3 Support individuals to build relationships

Analyse how you can support an individual to maintain and build relationships.

AC 4.4 Outline when external services may be required to enable an individual to maintain or build relationships

Here, you will outline how multi-agency working can support the individual when building relationships.

The decision to support individuals in the maintenance of relationships must be shared with the wider multidisciplinary team, if this is appropriate. As a manager you might need help from other external services to help individuals maintain or build relationships, such as the individuals' work colleagues, faith leaders or club members. Community or educational facilities may also be useful sources of support. This means that all staff must be aware of the protocols and plans that are in place to support the individual in maintaining relationships.

Evidence opportunity

4.4 Using external services to enable an individual to maintain or build relationships

Outline when external services, such as faith groups, friends and social activities, may be required to enable an individual to maintain or build relationships.

LO5 Be able to lead practice in recognising individuals' relationships

AC 5.1 Lead a culture which fosters approaches that recognise and value an individual's gender identity, sexuality and relationship needs

Here, you will identify an individual's needs in relation to their sexual identity, sexuality and relationship needs.

Individuals who receive care and support in their own home or who are moving into a care home may feel this marks an end to friendships, relationships or sexual activity. Care settings, therefore, need to consider the practical implications of maintaining privacy and understanding what the individual needs.

Young people reaching adulthood may develop needs of a sexual nature and may also have questions about their own identity, which may be confusing for them. Friendships are also very important at this time and there may be a concern that transitioning from school to work or college may disrupt these.

As sexual expression is a natural human need, care providers must assess individuals' relationship and sexuality needs. You also need to ensure that staff understand what is meant by sexuality and sexual orientation.

Sexuality describes sexual feelings, thoughts and what attracts a person to others. It is diverse and personal, and it is an important part of the individual. It includes a person's gender identity – their internal, personal sense of being a man or a woman or somebody who does not identify themselves as either. It also includes personal body image and sexual desires and experiences, regardless of age. Gender identity is about a person's own sense of self.

Sexual orientation describes a person's physical and/or emotional attraction to another person.

Personal pronouns refer to the set of words that a person uses to represent their gender identity accurately. These might include 'he' and 'she' or gender neutral expressions, such as 'they' and 'ze'.

The language we use can sometimes unconsciously make assumptions about people. We also need to be aware that derogatory language can reinforce stereotypes and labels, and may exclude certain groups of people. Generally, descriptors that refer to personal attributes, such as race, gender, sexual orientation, disability and age, should be avoided unless they are relevant.

It is important that your organisation understands the definition **LGBTQIA+** and promotes and supports LGBTQIA+ inclusive practices so that individuals' equality, diversity and human rights are respected.

KEY TERM

LGBTQIA+: Stands for lesbian, gay, bisexual, transgender, queer/questioning, intersex, asexual and other terms (such as non-binary and pansexual).

Research it

5.1 LGBTQIA+

Research the sexualities included in LGBTQIA+ and check your understanding of each.

AC 5.2 Promote an open, proactive culture where individuals and others feel confident to discuss gender identity, sexuality and safe relationships

Here, you will demonstrate how you establish a culture within a setting that enables individuals to freely express their sexuality.

Staff should be trained in gender identity and sexuality to enable confident discussions to be had. At induction and subsequent ongoing training on sexuality and relationships, staff should be enabled to respond to situations that may arise with the individuals in their care, so they can have open conversations with them. Having a template for opening up such discussions may be helpful. Individuals should be asked to feed back on how approachable the staff are with regard to this.

Training and awareness of equality, diversity and human rights issues will help staff to be self-aware and can also help them explore any unconscious bias they have about the sexuality needs of older people or those living with disabilities.

The CQC has published guidance for CQC inspection staff and registered adult social care providers on relationships and sexuality in adult social care services – see Care Quality Commission (n.d.).

This CQC guidance provides much needed support to help individuals express their sexuality and to have their needs met, recognising that experiencing sexual feelings and desires is healthy, but when personal care and support is needed there is a loss of privacy.

The guidance helps providers to understand that enabling the individuals using their service to manage their sexuality needs and giving them access to information to help them develop and maintain relationships and express their sexuality is important.

As a manager and a registered provider you need to be able to demonstrate how your service supports people to meet their sexuality needs. During an inspection you will be asked questions about people's sexuality needs, such as the following:

- Does the organisation have a relationship and sexuality policy?
- Does the organisation recognise that people have different ways of experiencing and expressing sexuality?
- Are staff trained to support people with their personal relationship needs?
- Are there examples that demonstrate positive support for relationships?
- Is there accessible information about, and links with, sexual health services?
- What is the policy for enabling people to have guests staying overnight?
- How does the setting accommodate people who are in existing friendships and relationships?
- How are people encouraged and supported to develop friendships and relationships?
- Are people using the service given information and support about relationships and sexual health?
- Can people be signposted to a local organisation that provides this service?
- Are staff aware of what action to take if they have concerns that someone is at risk of harm or abuse?

Source: Care Quality Commission (n.d.)

Evidence opportunity

5.2 Sexuality and sexual orientation of individuals

Using the questions above, provide evidence that shows you are actively addressing sexuality, gender identity and sexual orientation with the individuals using your service.

AC 5.3 Ensure individuals and others have access to support, information and advice about relationships and sexuality

Here, you will demonstrate how information on relationships and sexuality is provided to individuals in the setting.

During a care assessment and the discussions that ensue, you will determine the care and support needs that an individual has and the support and information they require about relationships and sexuality. You need to ensure that the relatives and friends of the individual are involved in care-planning processes and assessments and are aware of the decisions made. Others who have contact with the individual also need to be aware of decisions made, for example colleagues and peers, team members, visitors to the work setting who have a connection to the individual, and volunteers.

Research it

5.3 Meeting the needs of individuals' relationships and sexuality

How well does your setting meet the needs of individuals with respect to giving advice and support about relationships and sexuality?

Does a change in culture need to be made?

LO6 Understand positive risk taking in context of supporting individuals

AC 6.1 Explain how positive risk taking can contribute to the achievement of positive outcomes for individuals

Here, you will explain the benefits and possible concerns of positive risk taking for individuals.

The benefits and drawbacks of positive risk taking are covered in Unit 508 AC1.5. You should, however, ensure that you take the time to check what the benefits of risk-taking in your own setting might be and also the concerns you and your staff might have.

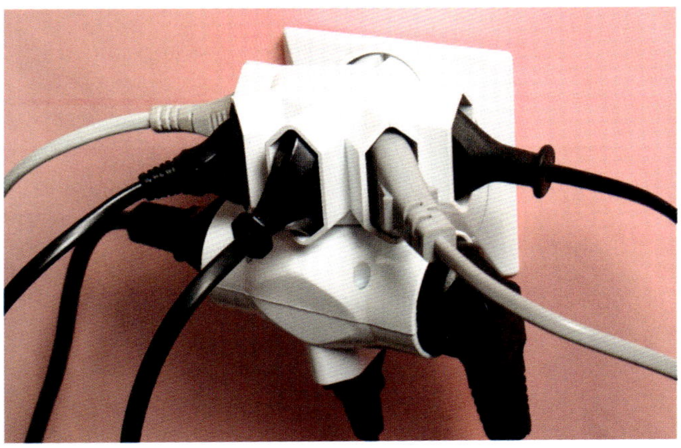

▲ **Figure 32** It is important to assess the environment for risks to individuals

Reflect on it

6.1 Positive risk taking

Positive risk taking is about identifying the potential risk in a situation or activity and then developing a plan to overcome it.

How do your staff enable the individuals in your setting to take risks in a safe and considered manner to enhance their quality of life?

AC 6.2 Describe the potential impact of a risk-averse culture on person-centred practice and the wellbeing of individuals

Here, you will describe how risk aversion can affect the way in which staff work with individuals.

Attitudes to risk are discussed in Unit 508 AC1.5.

Reflect on it

6.2 How do you view risk?

Think about how you view risk. Are you risk-averse in your personal life and does this extend to your work life?

Undertake a risk assessment for an individual who wishes to take an evening class, then ask a member of staff to do the same activity and make a comparison. What does it show you?

AC 6.3 Analyse the considerations which need to be applied in the management of positive risk taking

Here, you will analyse the management of positive risk taking.

Positive risk taking involves comparing the pros and cons of one choice of action against another. Being able to take carefully thought-out risks is empowering for individuals and is vital for them to feel they have control over their lives. Supporting individuals who use your service to plan and monitor activities that they wish to take part in that may involve some risk is essential in order to provide care that also provides choice and control for individuals.

Positive risk taking is covered in detail in Unit 508 AC1.5.

Evidence opportunity

6.3 Enabling increased choice and control to ensure positive risk taking

Using your findings from AC6.2, analyse the considerations that need to be applied in the management of positive risk taking.

AC 6.4 Explain how supporting others to balance risks and rights promotes person-centred practices

Here, you will explain the ways in which staff can be supported to assess the appropriate level of risk taking for an individual.

Staff must be supported to incorporate risk enablement and safeguarding into their work but they may require guidance and reassurance. An overwhelming desire to protect the individual from harm may take away the individual's choice and limit their activity. By adopting a risk-enablement approach, staff can be assured that carefully considered risks can actually be a good thing and will empower the individual. Staff need to feel confident that in supporting individuals to take more control over their lives, they will improve their wellbeing. By operating in a person-centred way, safeguarding is more personal.

Family and friends can be involved in important decisions, and this can also reassure them that their loved one is having their specific needs met. Families need to be supported to understand how to balance risk against the individual's rights as these can sometimes conflict.

Evidence opportunity

6.4 Assessment and balance of risk

Provide an explanation of how supporting others to balance risks and rights promotes person-centred practices.

LO7 Be able to lead the implementation of practices, policies, procedures to manage risk and positive risk

AC 7.1 Lead a culture which promotes the benefits of positive risk taking in person-centred practice where the wellbeing of individuals is recognised

Here, you will show how the benefits of positive risk taking can be shared with staff in the setting.

As the registered manager in a setting you need to ensure that clear policies outlining the organisational approach to positive risk taking are in place. These policies and procedures should weigh up the potential benefits and harms and identify the potential risks.

You are responsible for ensuring that staff receive training, including updates and refresher courses, and that the policies include guidance on safe and positive risk taking. Staff should also be able to access support when a decision regarding an individual is being made.

The deputy manager needs to support the manager in the above practices and deputise when necessary. The deputy manager also requires knowledge of the methods to manage risk positively and should support the manager in developing plans and arranging for available resources and support to minimise risk in the workplace.

There must be a collective understanding by all involved that positive risk taking is part of person-centred practice. The risk policies and procedures should be available to all people who come into the service and they should be encouraged to adhere to them.

Evidence opportunity

7.1 Ensuring team members are aware of policies and procedures relating to positive risk taking

Show your assessor evidence of how you lead a culture that promotes the benefits of positive risk taking in person-centred practice.

How do you measure the wellbeing of individuals?

AC 7.2 Facilitate a person-centred approach in the management of risks

Here, you will show how positive risk taking fits in with the process of person-centred care.

Promoting a culture of risk enablement and positive risk taking requires the individual using the service to be at the centre of the planning process so that they and the people important to them can understand the risks involved in the activity they wish to undertake. They can then make an informed decision whether they are willing to positively take risks to achieve their goal.

All risk taking activities should focus on the individual's strengths so that any activity undertaken is within their abilities. This will lead to an increase in confidence. However, anyone with capacity to make decisions cannot be stopped from undertaking a risk that you might consider to be dangerous.

Evidence opportunity

7.2 Seek the views of an individual regarding risk taking

Show how your management of risks uses a person-centred approach.

AC 7.3 Evaluate own and others practice in leading a balanced approach to risk taking

Here, you will evaluate how to plan for the appropriate level of risk suitable for an individual.

A balance must be struck between people's choice to do everyday activities and the duty of care owed by settings to their staff and to the individuals using their service.

The dangers associated with a risk and the potential benefits of risk taking must be identified.

By encouraging staff to adopt a positive approach to risk that ensures positive outcomes for individuals in receipt of services, a better service can be offered in line with personalised adult social care.

A positive approach to risk taking means involving everybody working together to achieve positive outcomes for the individuals in the setting. Identifying and managing risk should promote their independence and social inclusion.

In undertaking an evaluation of risk, it is important not to lose sight of person-centred approaches to care and choice. In this approach, risk is identified and assessed to establish the possibility of danger, harm or accident. A risk assessment in social care is used to protect individuals and staff from harm. Care providers are required to undertake assessments for each person for whom care is being provided. The Health and Safety Executive define 'sensible risk assessment in care settings' as balancing decisions to prevent risk with helping the person to live a full life and move towards their goals.

Methods to control or mitigate against risks should also be in place. For example, wherever possible it is best to eliminate a risk. Removing a trip hazard is an easy way to mitigate against a fall.

When mitigating against risks to individuals, you must be mindful of the choices they have made and prioritise a person-centred approach when selecting control methods.

Evidence opportunity

7.3 Managing risk in the setting

Look at the strengths and weaknesses of the way you and others practice a balanced approach to risk taking.

Legislation

Legislation	Key points
Care Act 2014	Sets out the key responsibilities of local authorities in meeting the needs of individuals who require help and support to promote their wellbeing. Its main aim was to provide integrated care and to introduce the right to an assessment for all.
Local Government and Public Involvement in Health Act (2007) incorporated	Incorporated the recommendations of 'A Stronger Local Voice' (Department of Health, 2006) and set out the government's plans to promote public and community influence in health and social care.

References

Care Provider Alliance (2022) 'Adult social care provider partnerships in Integrated Care Systems'. **https://careprovideralliance.org.uk/assets/pdfs/asc-provider-partnerships-in-integrated-care-systems.pdf**

Care Quality Commission (2022) 'The five key questions we ask'. **www.cqc.org.uk/what-we-do/how-we-do-our-job/five-key-questions-we-ask**

Care Quality Commission (n.d.) 'Relationships and sexuality in adult social care services: Guidance for CQC inspection staff and registered adult social care'. **www.cqc.org.uk/sites/default/files/20190221-Relationships-and-sexuality-in-social-care-PUBLICATION.pdf**

Department of Health (2007) *Putting People First: A shared vision and commitment to the transformation of adult social care*. London: TSO.

Department of Health and Social Care (2022) Policy paper 'People at the heart of care: Adult social care reform'. **www.gov.uk/government/publications/people-at-the-heart-of-care-adult-social-care-reform-white-paper/people-at-the-heart-of-care-adult-social-care-reform**

GOV.UK (2014) 'Dalton Review: Options for providers of NHS care'. **www.gov.uk/government/publications/dalton-review-options-for-providers-of-nhs-care**

GOV.UK (2015) 'Productivity in NHS hospitals: Lord Carter's review of efficiency in hospitals shows how large savings can be made by the NHS'. **www.gov.uk/government/publications/productivity-in-nhs-hospitals**

Health Foundation, The (2014) 'Person-centred care made simple: What everyone should know about person-centred care'. **www.health.org.uk/publications/person-centred-care-made-simple**

Helen Sanderson Associates (2015) 'All about outcomes'. **http://helensandersonassociates.co.uk/outcomes/**

Innes, A., Macpherson, S. and McCabe, I. (2006) *Promoting Person-Centred Care at the Front Line*. York: Joseph Rowntree Foundation/SCIE.

NHS (2014) 'Five year forward view'. **www.england.nhs.uk/wp-content/uploads/2014/10/5yfv-web.pdf**

NHS (2019) 'The NHS long term plan'. www.longtermplan.nhs.uk/publication/nhs-long-term-plan/

Skills for Care (2014) 'The Care Certificate Standard 7. Privacy and dignity: What you need to know'. www.skillsforcare.org.uk/Documents/Learning-and-development/Care-Certificate/Standard-7.pdf

Skills for Care (n.d.) 'Supporting personal relationships'. www.skillsforcare.org.uk/Developing-your-workforce/Care-topics/Supporting-personal-relationships/Supporting-personal-relationships.aspx

Skills for Health and Skills for Care (2013) 'Code of Conduct for Healthcare Support Workers and Adult Social Care Workers in England'. www.skillsforcare.org.uk/resources/documents/Support-for-leaders-and-managers/Managing-people/Code-of-conduct/Code-of-Conduct.pdf

Skills for Health, Skills for Care and Health Education England (2017) 'Person-centred approaches'. www.skillsforhealth.org.uk/wp-content/uploads/2021/01/Person-Centred-Approaches-Framework.pdf

Wilcox, D., Holmes, A., Kean, J., Ritchie, C. and Smith, J. (1994) *The Guide to Effective Participation*. York: Joseph Rowntree Foundation.

Useful resources and further reading

Campaign to End Loneliness. www.campaigntoendloneliness.org

Care Quality Commission (2020) 'Promoting sexual safety through empowerment: A review of sexual safety and the support of people's sexuality in adult social care'. www.cqc.org.uk/publications/major-report/promoting-sexual-safety-through-empowerment

Department of Health (2011) 'Transforming community services. Demonstrating and measuring achievement: Community indicators for quality improvement'. https://assets.publishing.service.gov.uk/government/uploads/system/uploads/attachment_data/file/215624/dh_126111.pdf

Down's Syndrome Association (n.d.) 'Workfit'. www.downs-syndrome.org.uk/our-work/services-projects/workfit/

Francis, R (2013) *Report of the Mid Staffordshire NHS Foundation Trust Public Inquiry*. London: TSO. https://assets.publishing.service.gov.uk/government/uploads/system/uploads/attachment_data/file/279124/0947.pdf

Helen Sanderson Associates (n.d.) 'Person-centred thinking tools'. http://helensandersonassociates.co.uk/person-centred-practice/person-centred-thinking-tools/

Kim, D. A., Benjamin, E. J., Fowler, J.H. and Christakis, N.A. (2016) 'Social connectedness is associated with fibrinogen level in a human social network', *Proceedings of the Royal Society B*. https://doi.org/10.1098/rspb.2016.0958

Kings Fund, The (2022) 'Provider collaborations: Explaining their role in system working'. www.kingsfund.org.uk/publications/provider-collaboratives

National Autistic Society (2020) 'Employing autistic people – a guide for employers'. www.autism.org.uk/advice-and-guidance/topics/employment/employing-autistic-people/employers

Parliamentary and Health Service Ombudsman (n.d.) 'Introduction to the social and medical models of disability' www.ombudsman.org.uk/sites/default/files/FDN-218144_Introduction_to_the_Social_and_Medical_Models_of_Disability.pdf

Social Care Institute for Excellence (2015) 'Care Act guidance on strengths-based approaches'. www.scie.org.uk/strengths-based-approaches/guidance#whatis

Unit 516

Leading a service that promotes health and wellbeing in adult care

GLH 18

About this unit

This unit is about health and wellbeing and how you can lead and develop a culture that promotes individuals' wellbeing and independence. All individuals in your care should be able to enjoy full and meaningful lives and be connected to those important to them as well as to their communities.

To do so they need to be involved in co-designing how their care and support services look and are provided. It is important that they and their loved ones are able to influence the care they have as this supports their health and wellbeing. You will also be introduced to the factors that influences health and wellbeing and will learn about your role in providing sufficient training, support and supervision to enable team members to monitor individuals' health and wellbeing.

Learning outcomes

By the end of this unit, you will:

1. Be able to lead a culture that promotes individuals' wellbeing and independence.
2. Understand the importance of promoting individuals' health and wellbeing.
3. Be able to lead practice in promoting individuals' health and wellbeing.

Getting started

Before you study the unit, think about the following:

- How will you promote the wellbeing and independence of yourself, staff and individuals in your setting?
- Why do you think this is an important consideration?
- How might you ensure that your setting provides a culture where individuals are able to enjoy full and meaningful lives and be connected to those important to them?

LO1 Be able to lead a culture that promotes individuals' wellbeing and independence

AC 1.1 Lead a culture where an individual's preferences, wishes, needs and strengths are prioritised and responded to

Here, you will learn about how the culture in which you work can have both positive and negative effects on the preferences, wishes, needs and strengths of the individuals within it.

Changes to sections of the Care Act in 2022 updating the government guidance on wellbeing have required local authorities to promote wellbeing when carrying out their care responsibilities and to apply 'the wellbeing principle', which puts wellbeing at the heart of care and support. The wellbeing principle applies where a local authority is carrying out a care and support function, or making a decision, in relation to a person.

Wellbeing is fundamental to the overall health of an individual, enabling them to successfully navigate and overcome difficulties and helping them to achieve their goals. Research has shown that a greater sense of wellbeing relates to increased physical benefits, such as lower incidences of cardiovascular disease, stroke and sleeping difficulties, as well as the psychological effects of increased self-esteem, optimism and happiness (Kubzansky et al., 2001, Ostir et al., 2001, Ryff et al., 2004 and Lyubomirsky et al., 2005).

Wellbeing is about feeling good and being able to function well as we go through life. Being older brings with it the challenge of ageing. As a care professional, you need to understand what these challenges are, how the individual experiences them and how they affect the individual.

Wellbeing exists in two domains:

- **Subjective wellbeing** (or personal wellbeing) is how the individual feels about themselves – how satisfied they are with life and whether it is meaningful. It engages with the person's positive emotions.
- **Objective wellbeing** is based on assumptions about human needs and rights and includes aspects such as adequate food, physical health, education and safety. You can gain this information by asking people whether they have a specific health condition or by looking at reports showing mortality rates and life expectancy.

KEY TERMS

Subjective wellbeing: This relates to how an individual feels and how satisfied with life they are. Levels of subjective wellbeing are influenced by internal factors, such as personality and outlook on life but also external factors, such as the society in which an individual lives. Also referred to as personal wellbeing.

Objective wellbeing: This is based on material, quantitative indicators and is measured by what people have in society. Educational opportunity, housing and the built environment in which a person lives, being part of a community and having enough money are all indicators of objective wellbeing.

Some individuals will find that certain aspects of wellbeing will be more relevant to them than others. For example, the ability to engage in work or education will be an important outcome for some, so this may require a more flexible approach.

A care setting can promote a person's wellbeing in a number of ways, but it requires a personalised approach to care and a culture of putting the individual at the heart of the care process. An important assumption is that the individual is best placed to judge their own wellbeing.

In promoting wellbeing, no single set approach can be possible as each individual case must be considered on its own merits. Individuals will have different needs, wishes, strengths and preferences that need to be taken into account. Your service must consider how to meet each person's specific needs and not simply try to fit them into a particular service or way of working.

Evidence opportunity

1.1 Promotion of wellbeing

Provide evidence to show how you lead a culture that promotes the wellbeing and independence of individuals in your setting.

AC 1.2 Lead a culture which enables individuals to enjoy full and meaningful lives connected to those important to them and their communities

Here, you will demonstrate ways in which individuals in your setting can participate in activities.

Wellbeing, as described in the government guidance and as set out in the Care Act 2014, relates to:

- personal dignity (including treating the individual with respect)

- physical and mental health and emotional wellbeing
- protection from abuse and neglect
- control by the individual over their day-to-day life (including in relation to the care and support provided and the way it is provided)
- participation in work, education, training or recreation
- social and economic wellbeing
- domestic, family and personal relationships
- suitability of living accommodation
- the individual's contribution to society.

Friends, relatives and support networks who are involved in caring for the individual need to be considered in planning care as they are a significant part of the individual's lives.

During the assessment process, settings must consider the individual's needs but also the most relevant aspects of wellbeing to them. For example, the individual may wish to be closer to their families, so location may be important to them. By ensuring that this is taken into account, the care professional is able to identify how care and support from family and friends and other services or resources in the local community could help the individual to achieve their outcomes.

When assessing individuals, care professionals should look holistically at how the individual wishes to live their life. This will mean considering that any support needed takes into account the person's skills and ambitions for a fulfilled life. This includes the role the individual's family and friends play in helping them and also the role of the local community and the various activities offered via clubs, groups and activities. Sometimes particular feelings or beliefs (including religious beliefs) impact the choices that a person makes about their care, and these should be taken into account. This is especially important where a person has expressed such views in the past, but no longer has capacity to make specific decisions for themselves. The overall goal is to support the person to live as independently as possible for as long as possible.

Evidence opportunity

1.2 Helping individuals to participate in social and educational opportunities

Describe the types of activities, clubs, support groups and educational classes that the individuals in your setting are supported or encouraged to pursue. How do they maintain contact with those people who are important to them?

Could you do better to enable them to enjoy full and meaningful lives?

AC 1.3 Lead a culture which enables individuals and those important to them to influence and co-design how care and support services are provided

Here, you will demonstrate co-design and how it can be effective in developing services within the setting.

A care culture that enables individuals and those important to them to influence and co-design their care is one in which co-production (working in partnership and sharing power) is practiced. See Unit 509 for more on co-production.

The Care Act 2014 included the concept of co-production, defining it as partnership working between people who draw on care and support, carers and citizens to improve public services. SCIE have also produced guidance about the concept of co-production. For more information, see SCIE (2022).

Co-production should be used to develop 'preventative, strength-based services, support assessment, shape the local care market, and plan information and advice services' (SCIE, 2022).

The key features of successful co-production initiatives include a redefinition of those who access care and support as people with skills rather than just needs, so building on people's existing capabilities.

There needs to be a breakdown of the barriers between people who draw on care and support and professionals, with a more reciprocal arrangement being made where people get something back for putting something in. A mutual way of working with people working together to achieve shared objectives needs to be developed. It also involves work with peers and personal support networks alongside professional networks in order to help organisations to become agents for change rather than just being service providers.

Evidence opportunity

1.3 Co-design

Demonstrate how you lead a culture that enables co-design.

LO2 Understand the importance of promoting individuals' health and wellbeing

AC 2.1 Describe factors that influence individuals' health and wellbeing

Here, you will describe social, economic and physical factors that might affect health and wellbeing and assess how a person's characteristics may affect their care.

The World Health Organization (2017) describes the factors that influence our health as determinants of health and these include:

- the social and economic environment
- the physical environment
- the person's individual characteristics and behaviours.

Included within these determinants of health are environmental, physical, social, financial and psychological factors.

Social and economic environment

Where we live, work, are educated and even where we were born all impact our health and wellbeing. These social, physical and environmental determinants impact a wide range of health, functioning and quality-of-life outcomes. For example, the availability of healthy food, clean water, a living wage and safe living environments affect our physical and psychological health. If these needs are not met, we are at risk of developing health issues.

Additionally, discrimination, living with exposure to violence and crime, a lack of social support and social disorder can lead to impoverished living conditions and an increase in risk of disease.

Income and social status remains a factor affecting health with higher income and social status linked to better health. The greater the gap between the richest and poorest people, the greater the differences in health.

Physical environment

Our physical environment is something that we tend to take for granted. Access to safe water and clean air, healthy workplaces, housing, communities, education and even roads all contribute to good health. People who have jobs are generally healthier while access to social support networks and good health facilities all impact the quality of our health.

The context in which people live their lives determines their health, so it is important not to judge individuals with poor health, as often the factors that contribute to their situation are beyond their control.

Person's individual characteristics and behaviours

Individual behaviour plays an important role in health outcomes. For example, a non-smoker is likely to have a reduced risk of developing heart disease. Someone who chooses a diet based upon processed food and takeaways may be risking obesity and the health conditions linked to this. Many public healthcare interventions focus on trying to change individual behaviours, for example tackling substance abuse, encouraging a healthy diet and increasing physical activity, as these can reduce the rates of chronic disease. However, such measures often fail when an individual's income is an issue.

Genetics and inheritance also have a role in determining an individual's lifespan, healthiness and the likelihood of developing certain illnesses.

> **Reflect on it**
>
> **2.1 Impact of life experiences**
>
> Think about how your life experiences have impacted your own health and wellbeing. What might you have changed and what was beyond your control?

AC 2.2 Explain own role and role of others in monitoring, assessing and promoting individuals' wellbeing

Here, you will explain the objective and subjective measures that can be taken to promote wellbeing.

Wellbeing can be monitored and assessed using a range of approaches, including **objective measures** and **subjective measures**.

You may already be collecting data on objective measurements. For example, if you work with adults you might be measuring the number of individuals who engage with external support groups to enhance their quality of life. You might also collect information about food preferences in order to plan menus or you might explore how assistive technology is being accessed and used.

Subjective measures ask people directly how they are doing and feeling. Individuals can then articulate how they are feeling and whether their needs are being met. It is up to them to decide what makes a difference to them in their daily lives and whether they feel their needs are being met.

KEY TERMS

Objective measures: Examine the factors that affect someone's life; they include measures of education, employment, health, housing, income and environmental quality, which can be used to monitor how people feel and function.

Subjective measures: Measure what people say about how they are feeling. Standardised daily self-reports on symptoms and feelings can be used to measure how individuals are feeling at any given time.

The Measuring National Wellbeing programme was introduced by the government in 2010 with the aim of providing an indication of the progress and wellbeing of people in the UK (Office for National Statistics, 2018). The Office for National Statistics (ONS) asks questions to evaluate how satisfied people are with their life overall, whether they feel they have meaning and purpose in their life, and also what emotions they experience during a particular period, such as how happy or anxious they feel.

Evidence opportunity

2.2 Personal wellbeing

Provide an explanation of how your role promotes an individual's wellbeing. In your setting how do you and others monitor wellbeing? What assessment do you make and how do you promote it?

AC 2.3 Explain own role in providing sufficient training, support and supervision to enable team members to monitor individuals' health and wellbeing

Here, you will explain the training needs for team members to be able to accurately assess an individual's wellbeing.

Staff may require some additional training to enable them to help the people in their care with wellbeing goals, so providing an update on the Care Act 2014 is a good place to start. Staff need to be familiar with the requirements of this Act, as they need to uphold its principles when working in a model of continuous improvement.

The Department of Health and Social Care has produced guidance on the Act, which states that 'promoting well-being involves actively seeking improvements in the aspects of wellbeing ... when carrying out a care and support function in relation to an individual at any stage of the process from the provision of information and advice to reviewing a care and support plan' (GOV.UK, 2022).

Wellbeing is a broad concept and will mean different things to each individual using your service. As such, staff need to be able to identify what is important to each individual in order to promote their wellbeing. Providing holistic care encompassing more than just the individual's physical health may require a change in your setting's perspective of care.

For example, working with people with dementia can be challenging, but a change to ways of working over the last 20 years has shown significant benefits. Dementia Care Matters (now Meaningful Care Matters) launched the Butterfly Model of Care as an antidote to the 'impersonal, unstimulating' environments of many care homes' 'dementia units'. David Sheard's work focused on the detached way in which people were being treated and, together with care professionals, he started work to reshape the environment. Creating an approach where feelings matter most, he began training staff to challenge old ways of working and to embrace new approaches.

His first step was to remove anything that was part of an institutional approach to create an environment in which there was no 'them and us', removing uniforms, nursing stations and drug trolleys and the usual ways in which staff monitored individuals. The recruitment of staff also changed and people with emotional intelligence from any walk of life, not just those with care backgrounds, were employed. Finally, the whole environment was changed and a more family-orientated place without former hospital-like spaces was adopted. See McAlees (2018) for more information.

Evidence opportunity

2.3 Promote wellbeing for individuals

Explain how you provide training, support and supervision to enable team members to monitor individuals' health and wellbeing.

AC 2.4 Evaluate how lines of accountability and responsibility are understood when delegating healthcare tasks

Here, you will evaluate how delegation takes place within the setting.

What is the difference between being responsible for something and being accountable? Often the terms are used synonymously but they are different.

- Responsibility is task-oriented and can be divided up among several people so that your staff may be responsible for completing part of a task or project.
- Accountability must be accepted by someone for them to take ownership of the task. That might be you. So, if you have accountability for a project or a task then you are willing to accept responsibility for your actions and outcomes.

Delegating healthcare tasks to others in your team requires that certain protocols are in place. As a care professional you will remain accountable for the appropriateness of the delegation, and you will need to be sure that the person can do the task.

Your responsibility is to make sure that delegation does not harm any person in your care and that the member of staff is competent and understands what is being asked of them.

If you are delegating tasks, you must ensure that training and supervision is provided so that the staff member will feel confident in what they are doing. Any delegated healthcare task is a shared responsibility requiring clear guidelines, protocols and escalation plans to be in place.

Clear procedures for the care worker to follow in an individual's care/support plan must be in place, together with management of risks and advice on what to do and who to contact if there are any concerns.

Keeping full records of training given, including dates and when refresher training is required, is also good practice.

What should be clear to everybody is that the responsibility and accountability for the individual remains with the care professional who delegated the task.

Evidence opportunity

2.4 Delegating tasks

Evaluate your understanding of accountability and responsibility when delegating tasks. Consider healthcare tasks, such as the completion of MAR sheets, administration of medication, receiving, recording and the disposal of medication, and also simple first aid. What are you accountable and responsible for with respect to these actions? What healthcare tasks are you not responsible or accountable for?

LO3 Be able to lead practice in promoting individuals' health and wellbeing

AC 3.1 Lead practices which support others to meet an individual's identified health and wellbeing needs

Here, you will show how you support team members to meet an individual's identified health and wellbeing needs.

As a care professional you need to encourage individuals and their support network to be involved in the design and delivery of the services they are accessing so that what is important to them is understood by all.

As a manager you may need to educate family and friends about the principles of person-centred planning and encourage them to respect the fact that their loved one is the best person to decide what care they need. For example, an individual may wish to make choices about the types of mobility aids they use but their family may feel that a wheelchair is the best option. By ascertaining the strengths and abilities of the individual, a decision can be made. The individual can also own their decision by having the care/support plan written in the first person. For example, 'I would like to use a walking frame rather than always using my wheelchair.'

By getting involved in their own needs, individuals have more control over their lives and will have better health and wellbeing as a result.

Evidence opportunity

3.1 Supporting others to meet an individual's needs

Demonstrate how your leadership supports others to meet an individual's identified health and wellbeing needs.

AC 3.2 Lead practice which supports others to monitor, and assess changes to, individuals' health and wellbeing using agreed ways of working

Here, you will show how you lead team members in assessing the individual' health and wellbeing.

All members of the support team around the person using the service need to be aware of how they can assess changes to health and wellbeing and work with the individual to ensure that they are at the heart of choices made. As the manager you need to lead on this and ensure that the agreed ways of working are monitored and any changes in an individual's health and wellbeing are picked up early. You will need to provide support for carers and family, loved ones and friends in addition to the professionals from other services and team members who all need to understand the ethos of person-centred care and work under your leadership.

The changing needs of the individual will require changes to the care/support plans that are in place. These are dynamic records that must be reviewed constantly to maintain a safe and healthy life for the individual. Any changes in the individual's health need to be documented in the care/support plan or reported to a person in charge to ensure that all those working with the individual have access to the new information. It may be that the individual is having trouble sleeping and various actions have been taken to help. The care/support plan will show what has worked and what hasn't and how the change has been received by the individual.

A care/support plan provides evidence of the care that has been given. Staff change shifts or go on holiday and temporary workers come to the setting who will need to have access to a well-informed, up-to-date care/support plan.

Evidence opportunity

3.2 Support others to monitor and asses change

Undertake a review of how you support your staff to monitor and assess the health and wellbeing of individuals, using agreed ways of working. What training do staff receive to show how they monitor change and how it should be reported?

AC 3.3 Lead practice which supports others to understand the importance of early identification of deterioration in an individual's health and wellbeing

Here, you will show the possible signs of deterioration in an individuals' condition and the steps to be taken in these circumstances.

The health of individual in a care setting can change at any time, and it is good practice to ensure that there are systems in place that can identify these changes early so that treatment and care can be given. Using a system by which staff can easily check someone's current health status will enable them to escalate their concerns more quickly.

The rates of emergency admissions in England for people aged 65 years or over rapidly declined in the period March–June 2020. In 2016/17, there were approximately 192,000 emergency admissions from care homes in England of people aged 65 years and over. Between March and May 2020, this fell to 6255 admissions for suspected or confirmed COVID-19, while rates for other emergency admissions also fell (Grimm et al., 2020).

There are a number of programmes in place to proactively assess care needs so that deterioration in the health of individuals is picked up at an early stage.

Enhanced Health in Care Homes (EHCH)

The Enhanced Health in Care Homes (EHCH) framework aims to reduce emergency admissions from care homes by using a more proactive approach so that the number of emergency admissions from care homes is reduced. The framework aims to deliver care with the support of multi-disciplinary teams including primary care, specialists, community-based care services and care home staff. The NHS Long Term Plan contains a commitment to roll out EHCH between 2020 and 2024.

For more information, see Care Provider Alliance (2021).

National Patient Safety Improvement Programme

NHS England has introduced a number of National Patient Safety Improvement Programmes (SIPs) to support safety, continuous learning and improvement across the healthcare system (NHS England, 2021). One of these SIPs is the Managing Deterioration Safety Improvement Programme (ManDetSIP). Staff should be clear on the aims of ManDetSIP so they can recognise and reduce deterioration-associated harm.

One of the key aims of ManDetSIP is to increase the adoption of deterioration management tools, such as the National Early Warning Score (NEWS) 2, developed by the Royal College of Physicians as a system for scoring the physiological measurements that are routinely recorded at the individual's bedside. The NEWS2 scoring system measures six physiological parameters:

1 respiration rate
2 oxygen saturation
3 systolic blood pressure
4 pulse rate
5 level of consciousness or new-onset confusion
6 temperature.

A score of 0, 1, 2 or 3 is allocated to each parameter. The higher the score, the further it is from the normal range. The scores for each parameter are then totalled to get a final score.

Physiological parameter	Score						
	3	2	1	0	1	2	3
Respiration rate (per minute)	≤8		9–11	12–20		21–24	≥25
SpO_2 Scale 1 (%)	≤91	92–93	94–95	≥96			
SpO_2 Scale 2 (%)	≤83	84–85	86–87	88–92 ≥93 on air	93–94 on oxygen	95–96 on oxygen	≥97 on oxygen
Air or oxygen?		Oxygen		Air			
Systolic blood pressure (mmHg)	≤90	91–100	101–110	111–219			≥220
Pulse (per minute)	≤40		41–50	51–90	91–110	111–130	≥131
Consciousness				Alert			CVPU
Temperature (°C)	≤35.0		35.1–36.0	36.1–38.0	38.1–39.0	≥39.1	

▲ **Figure 33** The NEWS2 Scoring system. Reproduced from: Royal College of Physicians. *National Early Warning Score (NEWS) 2: Standardising the assessment of acute-illness severity in the NHS*. Updated report of a working party. London: RCP, 2017.

As you can see from the table in Figure 33, the normal range is shown in the 0 column so anything outside that requires assessment as it could indicate a deterioration in the individual's health. This is more information than you will require in your role, but may be of interest to care managers.

- A low-risk score of 1 to 4 requires prompt assessment by a qualified member of staff to decide on whether there needs to be a change in the frequency of monitoring or an escalation of clinical care.
- A low-to-medium-risk score of 3 in any single parameter requires an urgent review by a doctor to determine the cause and to decide on changes to be made.
- A medium-risk score of 5 to 6 requires an urgent review by a doctor to decide whether to escalate to a critical care team.
- A high-risk score of 7 or over will require emergency assessment by a critical care team, and transfer to high-dependency care.

In order for the NEWS2 system to work, staff must be trained to understand the normal parameters of these physiological signs and the indications that there is a deterioration in an individual's condition. Examples of these for the NEWS2 parameters are as follows.

Respiration rate

This is one of the first signs of deterioration. The normal respiration rate should be between 12 and 20 breaths measured over one minute. An individual may be seen to be having a laboured breathing pattern with increased effort being made to breathe and breathing potentially affecting their speech. Their colour may also change, with a pallor and blueness around the lips.

Oxygen saturation

Oxygen saturation measures how much haemoglobin is currently bound to oxygen compared with how much remains unbound. The tissues extract more oxygen from the haemoglobin in blood cells, causing the saturation of blood to fall. Levels below 95–99 per cent saturated are an indicator of deterioration and indicate that the individual is not getting enough oxygen into their body. Some individuals, however, may be stable at low levels due to other health conditions, so you need to ensure that staff are aware of this.

Pulse rate

A normal heart rate is 60–100 bpm. However, individuals may present with a different baseline and some people with heart conditions such as an irregular heartbeat or a low heart rate still function well. Medication, sepsis and low oxygen levels may also affect the heart rate.

Systolic blood pressure

A late sign of deterioration relates to blood pressure (BP). Adequate BP is essential for the delivery of oxygen and nutrients to the body.

Temperature

Temperature is a significant measure of deterioration. A high or low temperature can be a sign of sepsis so staff must recheck the individual's temperature and perhaps the thermometer being used, increase fluid intake and, if the temperature is high, remove clothing or bedding. A temperature of less than 35°C or greater than 38°C must be referred to an appropriate clinician.

Fluid balance, although not part of the NEWS2 parameters, is also an indicator of deteriorating health and a good indicator of hydration status. Urine output should be 0.5 ml/kg/hour.

Level of consciousness

Neurological assessment must always include an assessment of the individual's level of consciousness. There are a number of scales in use, but the AVPU scale is a simple and effective method to assess consciousness. When faced with an unwell individual, the following should be assessed:

- New confusion: Are they confused or disorientated?
- Voice: Can the person respond when you talk to them?
- Pain: If unresponsive to voice, do they respond to a pain stimulus?
- Unresponsive: If none of the above applies then the person is unconscious.

Evidence opportunity

3.3 Early identification of deterioration in individuals

Develop a short training course that will support others to understand the importance of early identification of deterioration in an individual's health and wellbeing.

AC 3.4 Lead practice which ensures others record and respond to assessments and observations of an individual's health and wellbeing

Here, you will show the need for record keeping to track an individuals' health and wellbeing.

Observation involves using all your senses to monitor any changes in the individual. Care professionals who work in certain settings have access to objective measures to monitor and record changes in health. They are trained to undertake measurements of vital signs, such as breathing, blood pressure, pulse and temperature. They will also monitor how much the person eats and drinks and their fluid input and output. Accurate recording of these readings will provide a comparison if anything changes.

You would not expect an individual's family, friends or visitors to undertake physiological measures, but they can help to monitor change in other ways. Subjective observations are the signs you might see or the symptoms the individual may complain of. They may also report changes for the good. A visitor to a person's home may notice the individual looks pale or complains to them of having a headache or feeling sick. Visitors and family should be encouraged to report these changes to the care professional for further investigation.

Evidence opportunity

3.4 Recording and assessing individual's health and wellbeing

Show the assessor how you record and assess an individual's health and wellbeing in your own setting. How do you ensure that everybody in the setting is aware of how to respond appropriately to a change in an individual's health? Complete a short piece of work that shows the process of recording.

AC 3.5 Implement procedures which involve others in responding to any changes in an individual's health and wellbeing

Here, you will demonstrate the setting's policies when an individual's health needs change.

In developing and implementing a policy or procedure, you should include all those involved so that they understand the need for the procedure.

Having in place an effective policy or procedure at the setting means you can ensure that others will be clear about how they should respond to changes in an individual's health and wellbeing. Bear in mind that changes are not always negative, and a positive change should also be reported, as a change to the care/support plan will still be needed.

Make sure the steps a person needs to take to report a change are clear and in plain English and that they specifically state what actions should be taken.

Put your policy and procedure in writing and make sure everybody has access to it.

Provide information and instructions to those who need to implement the procedure.

Follow up to ensure that the policy or procedure is working, and that staff are 'leading by example' in implementing it.

AC 3.6 Work in partnership with individuals and others to agree roles and responsibilities in achieving individuals' health and wellbeing outcomes

Here, you will explain and demonstrate the 6Cs and how to work in partnership with other care professionals to achieve them for individuals.

All those involved with individuals using adult care services, whether as a care professional or as a family member or friend, have a moral responsibility to ensure that the individual receives care that is based on the 6Cs – six values that apply to social care:

- **Care**: Have the individual's best interests at heart to maintain and improve their wellbeing.
- **Compassion**: Feel empathy for someone and understand what they are going through.
- **Competence**: Understand what the person needs and have the knowledge and skills to provide it.
- **Communication**: Actively listen and speak and act in a way that the person can understand.
- **Courage**: Try out new things or speak out if you are concerned about something.
- **Commitment**: Be dedicated to providing care and support but also understand the responsibility you have as a worker.

Each individual in a care setting must be placed at the centre of their care and support, which should be designed to fit the individual, rather than the individual being made to fit existing routines.

Evidence opportunity

3.5 Managing changes to individuals' health and wellbeing

Consult with individuals, their families and others to determine how best the setting can manage changes to their health and wellbeing.

What procedures might be implemented to involve others in responding to any changes in an individual's health and wellbeing?

References

Care Provider Alliance (2021) 'Enhanced health in care homes: A guide for care homes' https://careprovideralliance.org.uk/enhanced-health-in-care-homes-cpa-guide

GOV.UK (2022) 'Care and support statutory guidance'. www.gov.uk/government/publications/care-act-statutory-guidance/care-and-support-statutory-guidance

Grimm, F., Hodgson, K., Brine, R. and Deeny, S.R. (2020) 'Hospital admissions from care homes in England during the COVID-19 pandemic: A retrospective, cross-sectional analysis using linked administrative data.' *International Journal of Population Data Science*, 5(4): 1663. https://ijpds.org/article/view/1663

Kubzansky, L.D., Sparrow, D., Vokonas, P. and Kawachi, I. (2001) 'Is the glass half empty or half full? A prospective study of optimism and coronary heart disease in the normative aging study'. *Psychosomatic Medicine*, 63(6), 910–16.

Lyubomirsky, S., King, L. and Diener, E. (2005) 'The benefits of frequent positive affect: Does happiness lead to success?' *Psychological Bulletin*, 131(6): 803–55.

McAlees, M. (2018) 'Butterfly Care Homes bring humanity to those living with dementia'. www.carehome.co.uk/news/article.cfm/id/1602499/Butterfly-care-homes-bring-humanity-to-those-living-with-dementia

NHS England (2021) 'The National Patient Safety Improvement Programmes'. www.england.nhs.uk/patient-safety/patient-safety-improvement-programmes/#ManDet

Office for National Statistics (2018) 'Personal well-being frequently asked questions'. www.ons.gov.uk/peoplepopulationandcommunity/wellbeing/methodologies/personalwellbeingfrequentlyaskedquestions

Ostir, G.V., Markides, K.S., Peek, M.K. and Goodwin, J.S. (2001) 'The association between emotional well-being and the incidence of stroke in older adults'. *Psychosomatic Medicine*, 63(2): 210–15.

Royal College of Physicians (2017) 'National Early Warning Score (NEWS) 2: Standardising the assessment of acute-illness severity in the NHS. Updated report of a working party'. London: RCP.

Ryff, C.D., Singer, B.H. and Dienberg Love, G. (2004) 'Positive health: Connecting well-being with biology'. *Philosophical Transactions of the Royal Society of London B: Biological Sciences*, 359(1449):1383–94.

Social Care Institute for Excellence (2022) 'Co-production: What it is and how to do it'. www.scie.org.uk/co-production/what-how

World Health Organization (2017) 'Determinants of health'. www.who.int/news-room/questions-and-answers/item/determinants-of-health

Useful resources and further reading list

Young Minds (2021) 'The impact of Covid-19 on young people with mental health needs'. www.youngminds.org.uk/about-us/reports-and-impact/coronavirus-impact-on-young-people-with-mental-health-needs/

Unit 517

Leading and promoting equality, diversity, inclusion and human rights in adult care

GLH 30

About this unit

Equality, diversity and inclusion are key principles in the delivery of a quality care service and your role as a manager will be to ensure that you encourage and promote these values. In this unit you will look at how all individuals can access support and care regardless of their circumstances, and how you need to provide a fair, personalised and diverse service. You will learn more about the terms equality, diversity, inclusion and human rights and how you can develop a culture in your setting that promotes, values and celebrates these concepts within adult care.

Learning outcomes

By the end of this unit, you will:

1. Understand equality, diversity, inclusion and human rights in relation to adult care.
2. Be able to lead a culture that promotes, values and celebrates equality, diversity, inclusion and human rights within adult care.

Getting started

Before you study the unit, think about the following:

- What do you understand about equality, diversity, inclusion and human rights and how this affects the way you work?
- What is the current culture within your care setting and how does it promote equality, diversity, inclusion and human rights?
- What are the policies and practices you see on a daily basis that support this?

LO1 Understand equality, diversity, inclusion and human rights in relation to adult care

The importance of understanding **equality**, respect for **diversity** and **inclusion** in care work cannot be overestimated. It is important that practice in your setting is reinforced by these principles and it is your responsibility to ensure this through training and meetings.

KEY TERMS

Equality: Treating individuals or groups of individuals fairly and equally irrespective of race, gender, disability, religion or belief, sexual orientation and age.

Diversity: In this context, means equal respect for people who are from different backgrounds.

Inclusion: Exhibiting positive behaviour to ensure that all people have an opportunity to be included and not excluded because of their individual characteristics.

AC 1.1 Summarise current legislation underpinning equality, diversity, inclusion and human rights in relation to adult care

Here, you will understand the main legislation that covers equality, diversity, inclusion and human rights.

Legislation relating to equality and diversity

The equality and diversity laws that are especially relevant to social care are the Equality Act 2010, the Care Act 2014, the Human Rights Act 1998 and the Mental Capacity Act 2005. Details of other relevant legislation are also described.

Equality Act 2010

The Equality Act 2010 clearly identifies that if a social care organisation provides goods, facilities, services or functions to the public then it must make sure that it does so within the requirements of the law. The Act brought together a number of individual pieces of legislation into one law in order to make the law on equality, diversity and discrimination much clearer and simpler.

The nine main pieces of legislation that merged to form the Equality Act are:

- Equal Pay Act 1970
- Sex Discrimination Act 1975
- Race Relations Act 1976
- Disability Discrimination Act 1995
- Employment Equality (Religion or Belief) Regulations 2003
- Employment Equality (Sexual Orientation) Regulations 2003
- Employment Equality (Age) Regulations 2006
- Equality Act 2006, Part 2
- Equality Act (Sexual Orientation) Regulations 2007.

The Act applies to private, statutory and voluntary organisations, no matter their size. Equality law affects all those working and volunteering in an organisation.

Human Rights Act 1998

The Human Rights Act 1998 outlines the basic human rights and principles of equality and freedom that all those in the UK are entitled to. Its five main principles are: fairness, respect, equality, dignity and autonomy. Sometimes, however, human rights can be restricted if a person breaks the law or in the interests of national security. The Act supports individuals' rights to dignity and respect and to be treated fairly when accessing care or support services.

Care Act 2014

The Care Act 2014 underpins all work with vulnerable adults to ensure that adults give consent for support that is tailored to them and has been chosen by them. This legislation ensures that information and services for the provision of care and support are fair and clear to everyone involved.

Mental Capacity Act 2005

The Mental Capacity Act 2005 aims to help people who are unable to maintain their independence, dignity and the right to freedom. Deprivation of Liberty Safeguards (DoLS) were put in place to aid vulnerable individuals to maintain their right to dignity and equality. These are in the process of being replaced by Liberty Protection Safeguards (LPS).

The Mental Capacity Act 2005 (MCA) also empowers individuals who lack the mental capacity to make their own decisions. The impact of this Act for individuals using care services has been to liberate them from previous restrictive practices in which they had no say over their care or treatment. Forward planning can now be undertaken and advance statements about what will happen when an individual no longer has capacity to speak for themselves can be put in place.

Special Educational Needs and Disability Act 2001

All education settings are required to make reasonable adjustments for people with disabilities so that they can be offered the same opportunities and choices as people who do not have disabilities, for example a specialist support person for an individual with a learning disability or the provision of teaching and learning materials in alternative formats such as Braille for individuals with sight loss.

Evidence opportunity

1.1 Investigate the legal context underpinning equality, diversity and inclusion

Summarise the legislation underpinning equality, diversity and inclusion.

Reflect on it

1.1 Impact of legislation and policy

Which law has had the most impact on the care you provide to individuals? For example, you may comment on how the MCA has changed the way you undertake assessment for care.

Case study

In each of the following cases, identify whether you think discrimination has occurred and whether there is a case to appeal to the law through the Equality Act 2010.

1. Mary, 62, applies for a job as a care assistant. Despite having previous experience in this area of work, she is not offered an interview. She is told that she has not been shortlisted for the position because of her age.

   In this instance, discrimination due to age has occurred.
2. Parminder attends a day centre. She overhears another attendee making comments about her skin colour and dress to a member of staff.

   In this instance, we need more information to determine what is being said. It might be a case of unconscious bias, but still requires investigation.
3. Gemma has a long-standing disability and uses a wheelchair. She is required to attend meetings for the care service she works for, but these meetings are always held in an upstairs room in an old building with no lift. She finds being carried upstairs humiliating and has stopped attending the meetings. Her manager is adamant that she must attend.

   In this case, Gemma's employer has not made adjustments for her being a wheelchair user, so this is discriminatory.
4. Wendy, a white, middle-class woman aged 40, has applied for a post in a women's refuge set up specifically to cater for young Asian women. The refuge is funded by the local Asian community. The advertisement specifically identified being Asian as a necessary characteristic.

   In this case, the advertisement specially asks for an Asian candidate, so is acceptable and not discriminatory.
5. Andrew has been off sick with depression for five months. While on sick leave and a week before he is due to return to work, Andrew is invited for an interview with his manager, who suggests that he should hand in his resignation.

   This case requires investigation, but it seems to discriminate against mental health issues.

AC 1.2 Describe how current legislation underpins equality, diversity, inclusion and human rights in supporting own role that promotes a culture which values individuals and others

Here, you will describe how you, as a manager, will develop an inclusive and diverse culture within your setting.

As the manager of a care service you have a key role in ensuring that equality and anti-discriminatory practice are promoted as core organisational values and that the law is complied with. Public sector organisations and other organisations that carry out public functions, such as those in the social care sector, must have 'due regard' to eliminate conduct that is prohibited under the Equality Act.

The Equality Act 2010 provides for the protection of people and their different characteristics, with specific protections in respect of:

- age
- disability
- gender reassignment
- pregnancy and maternity/paternity
- race
- religion or belief
- sex/gender
- sexual orientation.

By creating an inclusive culture you involve everybody. Having a communications policy that encourages staff to identify any issues with inequality and to make suggestions for improvements is a step forward to creating an inclusive culture. Appointing **diversity champions** across the organisation to raise awareness and engage others is good practice too.

You might wish to review organisational policies, procedures and practices to determine how they support and demonstrate inclusion through fair operations. Staff training in equality, diversity and inclusion will not only raise awareness, but can also provide a vehicle to deal with sensitive and difficult subjects, such as unconscious bias.

KEY TERMS

Diversity champions: People in your organisation who drive inclusion and diversity objectives and make sure they are achieved. Champions are responsible for supporting and developing the equality, diversity and inclusion agenda.

Socialisation: The process through which we are taught the norms, customs, roles, values and beliefs of our society. We are socialised first into our own families and communities and this is termed primary socialisation. Secondary socialisation occurs when we enter the education system or have contact with religion and the media.

Tackling bias, whether conscious or unconscious, needs to start at induction and should be part of the continuing development of all staff. Your recruitment and selection policies must have diversity, equality and inclusion at the heart of the process. You should pay attention to the language used in adverts, job descriptions and application forms to try to ensure that you attract diverse applicants. There must be a clear statement showing the setting's commitment to equality, diversity and inclusion, as defined in the Equality Act 2010. Potential candidates must feel that they will be treated equally by the organisation and there should also be opportunity for marginalised members of society, for example people with disabilities, special needs or those from minority groups, to apply for jobs.

People need to feel that they are not only included but appreciated and valued too.

Evidence opportunity

1.2 Promoting an inclusive, diverse and equal culture

How does the current equality, diversity, inclusion and human rights legislation help to promote a culture that values individuals and others in your own setting? Supply an example.

AC 1.3 Explain other influences that impact leading a culture which values individuals and others

Here, you will explain external influences that may affect the culture within your setting.

Societal

The society we live in and the way we are raised influences our behaviour every day, even though we may be unaware of this. Social influences in organisations involve the particular behaviours, tactics and strategies that are used by individuals to shape outcomes. An individual's **socialisation** might affect the organisation's culture in both positive and negative ways.

To function well in a society we need to find our place within it. We are guided by family, teachers, our community and the media about norms, values, beliefs and how we are to live. We are also affected by workplace culture.

Our behaviour is a result of the personal values we hold, while the decisions we make are based on knowledge, morals and ethics. The values we have learned throughout our lives become part of our personality and make-up. When we are faced with a decision or have a choice to make, we will always consider what we value most in making that decision.

Being at the receiving end of care can be quite distressing and may be made all the more so if the person delivering the care is less than sympathetic and does not appear to value the person. The culture of the organisation must reflect the values of care and respect and not be influenced by any inappropriate beliefs, attitudes or behaviour of those who work there, as this can lead to the development of a toxic work culture.

Historical

People who use services that have closed cultures are more likely to be at risk of abuse, harm and breaches of their rights under the Human Rights Act 1998 and the Equality Act 2010. Such cultures were found at Whorlton Hall, an independent hospital that featured in a BBC Panorama programme in 2019 (CQC, 2020), Winterbourne View Hospital (Department of Health, 2012) and the Mid Staffordshire NHS Foundation Trust (Francis, 2013). These cases exposed the extremely damaging effects a service with a closed culture can have on the individuals using that service and highlighted the importance of an open culture within the care service.

The events at the Mid Staffordshire NHS Foundation Trust were tragic and resulted in loss of life and a loss of faith in the care system. The culture of the organisation had become toxic, with leadership that lacked control and staff who betrayed their professional values in order to survive. It was reported that a defensive culture had sprung up in which money and targets were more important than compassionate values. Following a public inquiry, the Francis report led to the introduction of robust safeguards being put in place to avoid a recurrence of what happened. With renewed policy and legislation, a new regime on inspection and a more robust return to individualised care and choice, this historical event serves now as a reminder that the development of a good culture in care is of vital importance. Safe, effective, respectful and compassionate care is the only expectation and standard for individuals using adult care services.

Additionally, the Orchid View safeguarding review highlights the need to strengthen the quality of care, governance and financial monitoring, with independent organisations.

The Orchid View nursing home, owned and managed by Southern Cross Healthcare, had a number of safeguarding alerts and investigations. Following an anonymous call to the police, five members of staff were arrested and questioned. Although there was insufficient evidence to pursue criminal charges, the inquest in 2013 found that five people had 'died from natural causes attributed to neglect' and that several other people 'died as a result of natural causes' with 'insufficient evidence to show that this suboptimal care was directly causative' of their deaths. (WSASB, 2014.)

Reflect on it

1.3 Socialisation

Think about how you have been socialised in society and how this has shaped your values, beliefs and behaviour.

Consider how you have changed as a result of education and the decisions you have made.

AC 1.4 Explain the impact discriminatory or closed cultures have on individuals and others within adult care

Here, you will explain the adjustments that may be needed within a setting to ensure that individuals are not subject to discriminatory practices.

Under the Equality Act 2010, individuals using adult care services have the right not to be discriminated against on the basis of protected characteristics. People with disabilities have a right to 'reasonable adjustments' to ensure that they can access an equal standard of care.

As a manager in a care setting, you need to ensure that the people in the care of your staff are protected from both direct and indirect discrimination.

A closed culture will include identifiable risk factors and warning signs. For example, you might be aware that staff are operating a 'no leave' policy for some individuals and that restrictive practices are being used. Without a DoLS in place this is not acceptable. These individuals could become highly dependent on staff for their basic needs, with staff undertaking basic care rather than giving the individuals a choice. You may notice a lack of understanding on the part of staff and/or a lack of warmth when dealing with individuals. Care/support plans may be written entirely by the staff rather than in partnership with the individual. In addition, they may be standardised rather than written to meet the needs of each individual and may not reflect what the individual wants.

Evidence opportunity

1.4 Discriminatory or closed cultures

Explain how discriminatory or closed cultures impact individuals and others within adult care. Can you supply an example of this?

AC 1.5 Evaluate how own values, beliefs and experience may impact practices and behaviours relating to equality, diversity, inclusion and human rights within adult care

Here, you will evaluate your values and explain how unconscious and confirmation biases can be confronted.

An individual's values, beliefs and experience are often deeply ingrained and acquired through learning and upbringing. The person may have been encouraged to believe that certain attitudes and behaviours are acceptable. It is only when these values, beliefs and attitudes are challenged, either by new information during training and education, or different experiences, that they may be seen to be flawed. Even when individuals' views can be shown to be discriminatory, deeply held beliefs may be resistant to change and this is termed prejudice. This can often impact how a person treats others.

You have already seen that unconscious bias can affect your thought processes and the decisions that you make. Other biases are explained below:

- Affinity bias is when you feel a connection with another person simply because you have shared life experiences. For example, someone may have attended the same university as you, or grown up in similar circumstances. Having these biases might lead to you favouring them because they are more like you. This can be problematic when deciding who to recruit or promote.

- Confirmation bias means drawing conclusions about others based on your own personal beliefs and biases. You look for behaviours/traits in others which 'confirm' your biases. For example, you may form an initial view about a job applicant based purely on attributes that are irrelevant to the role. You may know the school they went to and have a view that it was not a 'good' one. If this type of bias occurs at an interview, it could result in leading questions being asked and interpreting the answers as confirmation of the initial (biased) opinion.

It is clear that these types of bias can particularly impact minority groups and form a barrier to having a diverse workforce.

> **Evidence opportunity**
>
> **1.5 Your impact on quality, diversity, inclusion and human rights**
>
> How do your own values, beliefs and experience impact practices and behaviours relating to equality, diversity, inclusion and human rights within adult care? Give an example using the STAR framework to shape your answer:
>
> **S**ituation: What was the background?
>
> **T**ask: What did you do?
>
> **A**ction: What action did you take?
>
> **R**esult: What were the results?

AC 1.6 Evaluate how the values, beliefs and experience of others may impact practices and behaviours relating to equality, diversity, inclusion and human rights within adult care

Here, you will evaluate how biases of team members can be overcome to ensure that individuals receive the correct care.

To ensure that equality, diversity and inclusion are effectively embedded in an organisation, all staff in all roles and others who may enter the setting, such as families, visitors, volunteers and other care professionals, must embrace and implement these principles.

The values outlined for adult social care are safety, dignity, independence, privacy and communication and it is expected that all staff uphold these values. But what happens when they don't? Maybe you work with a carer who does not value independence as you do and the care they give is very hands on, taking away individuals' rights to be involved in their own care. This is likely to lead to some dissatisfaction on your part as you struggle to uphold the individuals' rights.

The role of the manager is crucial in identifying and removing barriers to the implementation of these values and principles. As a manager, you must lead and foster an environment where any discrimination or exclusion is actively challenged and addressed.

All organisations have their own culture or, as Thompson (2011) suggests, a 'symbolic universe' in which a shared set of meanings, beliefs, values, norms and practices is based. It is, more simply, 'the way we do things'.

A prejudice is an attitude or belief based on a faulty and inflexible generalisation that can lead to negative emotions and discriminatory actions. Prejudice can lead to unacceptable behaviours, including harassment, bullying and victimisation, as well as poor standards and abuse of power over others. Harassment, bullying and victimisation are all behaviours that individuals are protected against under the Equality Act 2010; remember, it is not just individuals and groups that can be prejudiced and discriminatory. Prejudice does not necessarily cause someone to discriminate unfairly, but examining such beliefs and values and questioning them is a first step in recognising and tackling prejudice.

Exclusion refers to barring somebody from a service or an activity or not allowing a group or an individual to join in due to a barrier of some sort. Whatever way it occurs, it is disabling and a form of discrimination. Discriminating against someone generally implies conferring disadvantage or oppression on that individual, which impacts negatively upon their self-concept, their dignity, their opportunities or their ability to get justice.

> **Evidence opportunity**
>
> **1.6 Others' impact on quality, diversity, inclusion and human rights**
>
> The values, beliefs and experience of others may impact practices and behaviours relating to equality, diversity, inclusion and human rights within adult care. Evaluate how this happens in your setting. Give an example.

LO2 Be able to lead a culture that promotes, values and celebrates equality, diversity, inclusion and human rights within adult care

AC 2.1 Evaluate own and others' inclusive practice

Here, you will evaluate your own and team members' approach to inclusive practices.

To practice care inclusively means that people in your care are included in all aspects of life and are not isolated in any way. To exclude an individual from something is to take away their control and limit their dignity. It is unsupportive and discriminatory.

The individuals using your service need to feel connected and involved with other people in the local community to support their independence, dignity and self-respect. To practice inclusivity, your setting must endeavour as far as possible to remove the barriers between the setting and the outside world and ensure that there are no barriers inside the setting that might hold individuals back.

Reflect on it

2.1 Promoting values and celebrating equality

What rationale would you give to explain why you promote values and celebrate equality, diversity, inclusion and human rights?

AC 2.2 Evaluate how the setting/service promotes, values and celebrates equality, diversity, inclusion and human rights

Here, you will evaluate how human rights are embedded within the service.

Organisational culture

According to Mullins (2009), the culture of an organisation has a powerful influence over the behaviour and practices of the people within it. Complex interactions occur between individuals within organisations and sometimes this can lead to conflicts of interest and abuse of power if safeguards in the form of policies and practices are not in place to help counteract this.

Formal power structures supported by policies and procedures that provide a framework to help everyone understand expectations and responsibilities is a requirement in most, if not all, organisations. Policies that show who's who in the organisation, lines of responsibility and lines of management give an idea of the power structure in a setting.

Power is exercised through management structures and is evident in an organisational hierarchy by role and position, and sometimes by virtue of specialist knowledge or experience. Within this system, each layer has some exercise of power over those below and this is acknowledged and understood by both those in leadership roles and those who are subordinates. When individuals step outside the responsibilities of their role, those in leadership positions are empowered to take appropriate sanctions to ensure the smooth and effective running of the organisation. This type of power is legitimate and provides a framework for keeping the organisation running effectively. However, power also operates on an informal level.

Informal power is more difficult to understand because it is insidious, operates beneath the surface and is not formally acknowledged. Such power is not related to role or position – some people are natural leaders and have an innate ability to influence others, and this may be entirely independent of their position within the organisation. Where this is a positive, value-based influence it can be invaluable to the manager in spreading good practice.

As manager, you might use your position to encourage your staff to adopt anti-discriminatory and non-judgemental attitudes in their work by challenging discrimination. This can be accomplished by being a good role model and demonstrating fairness and anti-discriminatory practice to all individuals using your service and to staff. Discrimination should be challenged at all levels of the staff structure and staff need to feel that they are able to report practices they believe to be wrong. Through training sessions and supervision, as well as clear job descriptions, staff will understand their role in relation to equality, diversity and inclusion.

Powerful personalities on the team may influence others negatively, encouraging them to cut corners, bend rules or manipulate situations for their own advantage. The impact of this may mean that individuals and other members of staff are treated in an unfair manner, and this will compromise the equality, diversity and inclusion of the service. As the manager you must then take steps to minimise their influence.

Training and supervision

You may need to remind your staff about issues surrounding equality, diversity and inclusion at team meetings and update them on the policies and procedures. You can also recommend training to remind them of their duty with respect to this.

Communication

When creating or updating a policy, it is important that a strategy for communicating the policy is designed at the same time. A policy that nobody knows about is of no value. It should be tailored to the different networks within the organisation to ensure that all staff are aware of it. It also needs to be clear who the policy is aimed at – staff in general, individuals using the service or visitors.

Many organisations have staff intranet sites, so a pop-up alert is a good way of raising awareness. This allows you to add a link to the policy and to highlight changes to existing policies. You could also add a frequently asked questions page or examples of cases to illustrate how the policy can be applied in practice. You can also check out the effectiveness of your communication by doing informal and random checks to see whether staff are aware of the policy.

Training

Raising awareness, although crucial, is not enough. Equality, diversity and anti-discrimination policies need to be supported by staff training. This helps people to really think about their responses to different situations and how these can be improved. It also ensures that staff are up to date with the latest legislation and practice. Training can be provided as part of the staff development programme or via an online package.

Provide advice and support for staff when complaints are made

A reflective, learning organisation tries to identify issues before they become grievances or complaints. Consequently, a well-publicised opportunity to access advice, support and counselling should be a feature of how organisations engage with diversity and equality. One way is to recruit an adviser, trained to provide initial informal advice to any person who believes they are being discriminated against. They can talk through their situation and look at all the options before they take action. Often talking through an issue and being believed and supported is enough to enable the individual to draw on their own reserves and tackle the issue directly or change the situation in some way.

Having a diversity champion will help to keep equality at the forefront. Reflecting on best practice in your own and other organisations is valuable. It is not necessary for the manager to take on this role – it can be an opportunity for someone interested in this area to extend their skills and develop their role.

No matter how you decide to implement this type of awareness, your aim is to support compliance with equality legislation and to eliminate discriminatory behaviour.

Research it

2.2 Organisations that champion diversity, equality and inclusion

Research an organisation other than your own and comment upon how it has championed diversity, equality and inclusion.

AC 2.3 Revise practices, policy or procedures to improve how the service promotes, values and celebrates equality, diversity, inclusion and human rights

Here, you will assess the practices within the setting and see how they can be improved to be more effective.

It is important not to be complacent about the effectiveness of the policies and procedures you have in place to support a culture that promotes and assures equality and respect for diversity and inclusion. Occasionally, a policy may reinforce discrimination and exclusion inadvertently, perhaps because of the language used or because it refers to out-of-date practices. An annual audit of effectiveness is a good way to check whether equality and diversity remain at the forefront of people's minds and practice. The types of activities that can be used to monitor the effectiveness of your policies include:

- Surveys: A quick questionnaire will assess how well the individuals using your service feel their differences are respected and equality is promoted by your staff.
- Observation: When you work alongside others, you can observe how well staff promote equality and respect diversity.

Research it

2.3 Systems and processes that promote equality and inclusion or reinforce discrimination and exclusion

Look at the systems and processes that promote equality and inclusion or reinforce discrimination and exclusion in your workplace and comment on how effective they are.

Evidence opportunity

2.3 Policies, systems, processes and practices that promote equality, diversity and inclusion

Look at the policies in your own setting that relate to equality, diversity and inclusion. Show your assessor that you can lead practice with others in reviewing and evaluating current systems and processes. Explain how you make improvements where required. You might, for example, review and evaluate the policies with your staff in team meetings and make improvements to them.

What do you think the strengths of your policies are? Could they be improved and, if so, how?

Research it

2.3 Gaps, shortfalls and improvements

Undertake some research to identify the gaps or shortfalls in systems and processes in your own setting and propose improvements to address these.

Reflect on it

2.3 Systems and processes

Think about the systems and processes that promote diversity, equality and inclusion in place in your organisation and reflect on how attitudes to these things have changed during your practice as a care professional. Give some examples of the changes you have noted and how they now affect the individuals using your service. Are there any improvements that can be made?

AC 2.4 Monitor changes and improvements that lead to better outcomes for individuals and others in own setting/service

Here, you will review improvements to the setting's policies to ensure that they are effective.

Monitoring improvements enables you to see the effect that implemented changes have had on practice and ensures that mistakes are rectified. However, first you need to assess the current situation. For example, you may be aware of a change in an individual's wellbeing due to the support the staff have put into place.

By investigating the practice and having one-to-ones with staff you can see examples of change leading to good practice.

Once you have this knowledge you can look at your current procedures and identify areas where changes could be made to improve the situation for other individuals in the setting. The next step is to talk to your staff to ensure that they understand the reasons for the change and to discuss with them how they should implement this. Once you have drawn up new guidelines and staff are aware of them, you can set a deadline to check whether the policy has improved the situation for individuals and to obtain feedback from your staff as to how they feel the guidelines are working.

AC 2.5 Review changes and improvements that lead to better outcomes for individuals and others in own setting/service

Here, you will review the changes made to assess their effectiveness.

Evidence opportunity

2.4 and 2.5 Determine the effectiveness of a practice used within the setting

Undertake a review of a practice in your setting to determine its effectiveness. How have you monitored the practice in its development?

Discuss with staff changes they could make to enhance the outcomes for individuals. Document the changes to be made and monitor the new practice over a period of one month. Report back to staff on the outcomes.

AC 2.6 Challenge discrimination, harassment and exclusion in ways that are likely to achieve change and promote positive outcomes

Here, you will review methods of challenging discrimination, harassment and exclusion within a setting.

As a manager, you must ensure that equality, diversity and inclusion are effectively embedded within the organisation and that all staff in all roles embrace and implement these principles. You must lead and foster an environment where any discrimination or exclusion is actively challenged and addressed.

If it is communicated that equality and diversity are everybody's responsibility, it confers an obligation on employees to challenge or report discrimination when they encounter it. If a care worker has concerns about the individuals in their care, they must voice these concerns in a safe environment without fear of victimisation or losing their job. It can be daunting for employees who have to continue to work in an organisation in which an investigation, suspension or prosecution occurs as a result of their challenge. While the expectation is that individuals should raise challenges and concerns, it is imperative that they can do this in a supportive and protective environment. For more on disclosure and whistle blowing, see Unit 507.

If an employee loses their job as a result of disclosure and wants to claim compensation, an employment tribunal must be satisfied that the employee's actions to whistle blow and make the disclosure were reasonable.

Reflect on it

2.6 Challenge unacceptable behaviour

Think about a time when you have had to challenge discrimination, harassment or exclusion, for example maybe you had to challenge a member of staff's behaviour towards an individual or perhaps you challenged an individual for using discriminatory language.

How did such a challenge make you feel and how was the incident resolved? It might be good to get a witness testimony from somebody who observed the incident.

AC 2.7 Support others to challenge discrimination, harassment and exclusion in ways that are likely to achieve change and promote positive outcomes

Here, you will review the setting's policies on challenging discrimination, harassment and exclusion in order to support team members and individuals and provide active support.

Exclusion refers to barring somebody from a service or an activity or not allowing a group or an individual to join in due to a barrier of some sort. However it occurs, exclusion is disabling and a form of discrimination. Harassment is any physical or verbal behaviour directed at somebody that is unwanted and makes that person feel humiliated and uncomfortable. This is also discriminatory.

Discriminating against someone generally implies conferring disadvantage or oppression on that individual, which impacts negatively their self-worth, dignity, opportunities or ability to get justice.

Discrimination takes many forms:

- stereotyping
- marginalisation
- invisibilisation
- infantilisation
- medicalisation
- dehumanisation
- trivialisation.

Organisations must develop, implement and monitor policies and methods of working that support anti-discriminatory practice. These should raise awareness about unacceptable behaviours and provide a structure for individuals to challenge such behaviours. This includes the responsibility of management to ensure that all staff work within the policy and respect the difference of others. Most organisations will have equality and diversity policies that should also explicitly identify how staff seek to redress when they believe there is non-compliance with a policy or law. For example, this can be accomplished through staff meetings and in supervision.

Importance of challenging discrimination

Discrimination causes people to feel devalued, worthless, angry, hopeless and powerless, and undermines their confidence. From an organisational or managerial perspective, this can have a significant impact on the effectiveness of your workforce as well as the individuals being cared for. Discriminatory practice is likely to result in poor performance, poor staff relations and a missed opportunity to benefit from the different attributes and potential of the staff employed.

Discrimination may be a result of individual prejudice or have cultural or structural causes. Prejudice is a pre-conceived judgement that one group of people, or one person, is better or worse than others without any basis of knowledge or evidence.

False beliefs may be widely held and deeply ingrained; they are not easily changed, even in response to evidence to their contrary (Thompson and Thompson, 2008). If the false belief is not successfully challenged, it may be accepted as a fact and this may invoke an emotional response, which may be dislike or dismissal of the person or individuals associated with the belief.

Discriminatory, unfair behaviour often follows – inequitable treatment, exclusion, dismissal, becoming the butt of humour, being ridiculed or deliberately being marginalised are common outcomes. Threats and violence are extreme forms of discriminatory behaviour. Importantly, in the workplace much discriminatory behaviour may be covert and dressed up in the form of humour. Perpetrators may justify and trivialise their actions with statements such as 'It's just a bit of fun', 'She has no sense of humour', or 'He's so sensitive'. This trivialisation may make the behaviour difficult to address as individuals or staff may not want to be seen to be making a fuss or unable to take a joke. This requires a clear policy that is carried forward into practice, stating that singling out an individual's characteristics and using these to ridicule or humiliate them is completely unacceptable.

As a manager you need to ensure that you are well-versed in the effects of discrimination and understand how to tackle this in order to meet the needs of individuals in your care and workforce.

You should also be aware of the effects of oppression. This is the main outcome of an inappropriate use of power. Oppression as a result of discriminatory practice results in significant harm. It may manifest itself in the victim as a loss of confidence or undermine their self-belief and self-esteem. It can cause stress, anxiety or depression, all of which impact work performance and subsequent work opportunities. If the individual is unable to successfully challenge the oppression, there is a risk that the prejudicial belief or disabling structure takes on the significance of 'fact'. This then leads to the oppressed person responding defensively by avoiding situations and people that discriminate against them by trying to keep a low profile, leading to a negative cycle of oppression and defensive behaviour. If nobody challenges this, the perpetrators continue and the victim learns strategies to cope. However, this is clearly unfair.

Impact of inclusion

So far, much of the discussion has been focused on the impact of discrimination and strategies to redress unfairness. While this is clearly important, anti-discriminatory approaches are focused on the negative acceptance that discrimination is a fact of life and that energy should be spent on mitigating the effects. Inclusion, however, takes a more positive approach. A philosophy of inclusion is concerned with how things should and could be. Energies are spent on becoming better members of a community, by creating new visions for the community. The emphasis for inclusion is not on justifying reasons why someone should be included and developing policies and procedures to support this; inclusion starts from an assumption that everyone has equal rights and opportunities and that these should differ only when there is an appropriate reason to do so.

Supporting others

The first step in supporting others to challenge discrimination and exclusion is to accept that these exist and to acknowledge that discrimination is a significant factor in inhibiting equality. As managers it is necessary to communicate to staff that discrimination is fundamentally wrong and that it cannot be tolerated within an organisation. You should also be quick to challenge any sort of discriminatory behaviour in order to send out a strong message of zero tolerance. However, challenging discrimination is not easy.

Few people are exempt from prejudice or exclusive practice. What is important is that individuals are open to recognising their prejudices and are committed to change. It takes practice and time, but promoting policies that set out expectations of behaviour to others and that remind staff of disciplinary sanctions should they breach the policy will help. However, while it might be possible to get staff to comply with policies, that is only part of the picture. Policies alone do not change hearts and minds. The risk is that if only compliance is achieved, when not observed the behaviour will revert back to that which perpetuated inequality. For many people, understanding the consequences and impact of their actions will cause a change in behaviour and will encourage others to change, but you cannot assume this will be universal and managers must be vigilant.

We are all products of our culture, our experiences and our education. Discrimination and exclusion may not be intentional but may be the result of the belief that everyone experiences life in the same way. If we have never consciously experienced discrimination, we may not see it when it happens to others. One often needs to be able to relate to another person's experience in order to appreciate the injustice that is felt by others. It is not possible to be somebody else, but it is possible to ask them how it feels and to try to imagine what that must be like. Sometimes it is useful to assume the role of the impartial observer, setting aside emotion and experience and asking whether something is right or not.

Encourage reflection

It is imperative that you reflect critically on yourself and your values, attitudes and behaviours towards others. Where do these come from? Are they consistent with the values that one would choose to have? Reflective practice is an excellent vehicle for critical self-reflection and as a manager you need to encourage your staff to complete this task on a regular basis. By reviewing practice in this way, you can help staff to feel supported in their efforts to change practice. They will also feel empowered to challenge bad practice.

The simplest reflective model asks the participant to engage in three critical reflections:

- A detailed interrogation of the issue or situation.
- Why is this so or why did it happen?
- What does this mean?

Gibbs' (1988) model of reflection (Figure 34) is particularly useful in reflecting on values because it requires the reflector to consider and evaluate the morality of their thoughts and feelings.

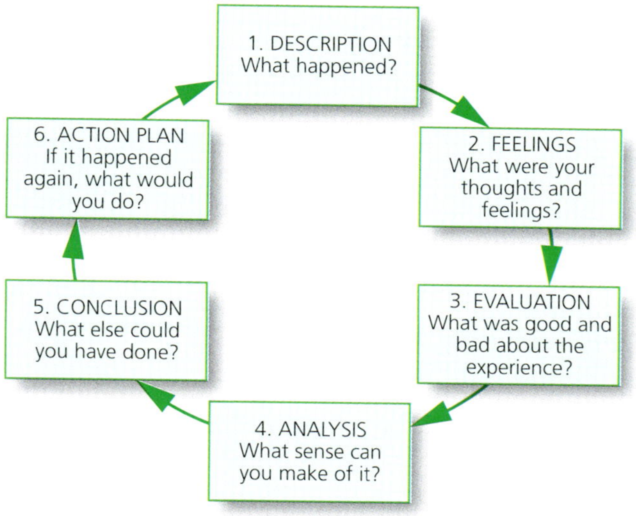

Figure 34 Gibbs' Model of Reflection

Model good practice

Discriminatory behaviour is often hidden, even from ourselves, and unless we take the time to reflect, be sensitive, question and change our responses to others, and evaluate the impact of our behaviours, individuals in our care will continue to be treated unjustly.

Managers must model good practice. You must be someone who positively challenges discrimination and supports others to do this. This requires you to be conscious of your own behaviour and to lead by example.

Dealing with discriminatory behaviour in staff and supporting others

Promoting equality and inclusion as positive concepts that are everybody's responsibility helps others to challenge discrimination when they encounter it. However, the way that you as manager respond could determine whether the individual is willing to do this again in any future situation. Importantly, any challenge should be taken seriously, and time must be given to listen to what the individual believes is occurring. You must investigate the situation impartially, trying to gain as much evidence as possible in order to ensure that you have the whole picture before you make any decisions. This includes talking to everyone involved, or to someone who has witnessed the potentially discriminatory behaviour, and taking statements.

Confidentiality should be maintained as these issues are often very sensitive. If the discrimination is found to be a reality, it is important to put in place an action plan to improve the situation and to provide managerial support to those affected. If discrimination has been proven, sanctions should be applied appropriately and proportionally. One purpose of investigating issues of concern is to resolve the particular situation, learn from it and, where possible, implement strategies to prevent something similar happening in the future. Where possible, actions should primarily be focused on enhancing and improving practice rather than on retribution or vengeance. Having clear processes that support individuals to raise concerns responsibly provides protection for those who wish to challenge discrimination and for those who may be under investigation.

Challenging discrimination and exclusion through training and development opportunities

One step in eliminating prejudice is to redefine beliefs and attitudes in the light of new information. You can do this through staff induction processes and in supervision and appraisal, where you may be able to challenge attitudes that come to light. The next step is to change behaviour in the light of that information, and also to challenge others who articulate similar prejudices. Training and development opportunities, staff appraisal and supervision can all be used as opportunities for achieving positive outcomes with respect to challenging discrimination.

None of these steps is easy, but challenging others can have a significant impact on breaking down discrimination and prejudice. Often prejudice is not only an individual issue but represents views that might be more widely held within a group or specific context. When a strong, widespread belief is apparent, challenging it is difficult and individuals who try to do so may fear ridicule, victimisation or reprisals if they stand up against the prevailing beliefs and practices. In an organisation, it is important that everyone is aware that prejudice and discriminatory practice cannot be tolerated. Individuals who become aware of such practice must be supported and protected to speak out.

Thompson (2011) points out that significant structural barriers exist that discriminate negatively on individuals. For example, there may be an unfair unwritten policy and agreement that women in their 20s and 30s are not employed in managerial posts because of the potential for them to leave or take maternity leave. Alternatively, the organisation that fails to provide accessible facilities for those in wheelchairs is discriminatory and in breach of the law. Staff should be aware of such circumstances and feel confident in speaking out against them.

Reflect on it

2.7 Labels and assumptions

Using an incident analysis model of reflection, reflect on thoughts, feelings and behaviours from a situation where you may have labelled, or have been tempted to label, someone, or made assumptions about their capabilities or trustworthiness, or when you felt anxious or threatened by someone you did not know.

Reflect on what caused you to respond in the way that you did. Was your response reasonable? Could you have behaved differently? What risks would there have been if you had behaved differently? Can you think of strategies to prompt you to behave differently in the future?

Reflect on it

2.7 Challenging discrimination and exclusion

Imagine yourself in a world in which you are seen as an inferior being. You have similar capabilities to others and yet these are dismissed because your characteristics mark you out as being of lesser value. You are constantly overlooked, marginalised and given the worst and dirtiest jobs to do. You do not have access to the developmental opportunities afforded to others. You are good humouredly ridiculed for the amusement of others. If anything goes wrong, it is assumed that you are responsible.

What sanctions do you think are appropriate to improve the situation and bring about a more equal environment? What are the risks, if any, of imposing sanctions? How could you support others in a similar situation to challenge discrimination and exclusion?

Management of complaints/service compliments and involvement and feedback from those in receipt of care and support

Creating a culture of discussion and tolerance is important in developing an open-minded community and in preventing abusive practice. You can ensure that your staff are acting in non-discriminatory ways by handling complaints and compliments in the organisation well. By involving individuals and their families in evaluating care you are also able to see how the process is working.

Many organisations are constrained by the premises and resources available to them in developing completely fair facilities. However, this is not an excuse for doing nothing. The expectation is that reasonable adjustments must be made and while these adjustments may not be perfect, they must be fit for purpose. Failure to address such issues may oppress certain groups in society simply because they cannot access a building or a service, thus undermining confidence and self-esteem.

Evidence opportunity

2.7 Support others to challenge discrimination and exclusion

Show your assessor evidence of how you lead and foster an environment where any discrimination or exclusion is actively challenged and addressed, for example through:

- ✔ training and development opportunities
- ✔ staff induction/supervision and/or appraisal
- ✔ management of complaints/service compliments
- ✔ involvement and feedback from those in receipt of care and support.

Research it

2.7 Support others to challenge discrimination and exclusion

Carry out a small-scale research study in your own setting which looks at diversity, equality and inclusion. Identify the strengths and limitations within your area of practice and make recommendations for improvement.

Legislation

Legislation	Key points
Equality Act 2010	Identifies that if a health or social care organisation provides goods, facilities, services or functions to the public then it must make sure that it does so within the requirements of the law.
Human Rights Act 1998	Outlines the basic human rights and principles of equality. It has five main principles: fairness, respect, equality, dignity and autonomy. Supports individuals' rights to dignity and respect and to be treated fairly when accessing care or support services.
Care Act 2014	Underpins all work with vulnerable adults ensuring that adults give consent for support that is tailored to them and has been chosen by them. Ensures that information and services for the provision of care and support are fair and clear to everyone involved.
Mental Capacity Act 2005	This act informs individuals about what they can do to plan and ensure that someone else can make decisions for them if they ever lack capacity to do so for themselves.
Special Educational Needs and Disability Act 2001	All education settings are required to make reasonable adjustments for people with disabilities so that they can be offered the same opportunities and choices as people who do not have disabilities.
Children and Families Act 2014 and the Special Educational Needs and Disabilities (SEND) Code of Practice 2014	Introduced legislation regarding adoption and family justice.

References

Care Quality Commission (2020) 'CQC publishes second part of independent review into its regulation of Whorlton Hall'. www.cqc.org.uk/news/stories/cqc-publishes-second-part-independent-review-its-regulation-whorlton-hall

Department of Health (2012) 'Transforming care: A national response to Winterbourne View Hospital. Department of Health Review: Final Report'. https://assets.publishing.service.gov.uk/government/uploads/system/uploads/attachment_data/file/213215/final-report.pdf

Gibbs, G. (1998) *Learning by Doing: A guide to teaching and learning methods*. Oxford: Oxford Further Education Unit.

Francis, R (2013) *Report of the Mid Staffordshire NHS Foundation Trust Public Inquiry*. London: TSO. https://assets.publishing.service.gov.uk/government/uploads/system/uploads/attachment_data/file/279124/0947.pdf

Mullins, L. (2009) *Management and Organisational Behaviour*. Harlow: Prentice Hall.

Thompson, N. (2011) *Promoting Equality: Working with diversity and difference*. Basingstoke: Palgrave Macmillan.

Thompson, N. and Thompson, S. (2008) *The Critically Reflective Practitioner*. London: Macmillan Education.

West Sussex Adult Safeguarding Board (WSASB) (2014) 'Orchid View Serious Case Review'. www.westsussex.gov.uk/media/5168/orchid-view-scr-final-report.pdf

Useful resources and further reading

Social Care Institute for Excellence (2020) 'Involvement and inclusion promoting dignity in care'. www.scie.org.uk/dignity/care/involvement

Unit 518

Leading and managing health and safety in adult care

GLH 30

About this unit

The purpose of this unit is to introduce you to health and safety in adult care and to enable you to understand the legislative requirements and how to manage risk. You will gain an understanding about how you can support and educate all work colleagues in health and safety guidance and procedures within the service/setting and will examine what your responsibilities are in leading teams to ensure that health and safety is prioritised.

Learning outcomes

By the end of this unit, you will:

1. Understand health and safety requirements in adult care.
2. Be able to lead the implementation of health and safety requirements in adult care.
3. Understand effective risk management.
4. Be able to lead the implementation of policies, procedures and practices to effectively manage risk.

Getting started

Before you study the unit, think about the following:

- What do you understand by the term 'risk management'?
- How much do you know about wider aspects of risk, danger and harm and how these may relate to your service?
- How do you support and educate colleagues to follow health and safety guidance and procedures within the service/setting?
- Why is it crucial that you understand your responsibilities in leading teams to ensure that health and safety is prioritised?
- Are there any risks that are particular to your service/setting?

LO1 Understand health and safety requirements in adult care

AC 1.1 Explain the current legislative framework for health and safety in adult care

Here, you will be required to explain how health and safety policies and procedures are reviewed and updated, including relevant legal and national regulations.

As a manager and leader in adult social care, your knowledge of the law and how it is translated into practice through policy and implemented by your staff must underpin your practice. Undoubtedly, you will already have a good working practice in the legal aspects of care work, but it is wise to revisit this from time to time.

In your role as manager you must offer strong induction activities and training for staff. Staff need to understand their roles and responsibilities with regard to health and safety record keeping and reporting and the importance of complying with policies, procedures and practice. Any breaches must be dealt with effectively and quickly to avoid unsafe practice. By monitoring compliance, ensuring that checks/audits take place and that risk assessments are updated you will be practising safely with respect to this part of your management role.

Relevant legal and national regulations

Under the Health and Social Care Act 2012 (and mentioned in the Care Act 2014), the Care Quality Commission (CQC) is the lead inspection and enforcement body for safety, quality of treatment and care matters involving individuals who receive a health or adult social care service from a provider registered with the CQC.

For individuals who receive a health or care service from a provider not registered with the CQC, local authorities are the lead inspection and enforcement bodies for health and safety matters.

When an incident occurs, the body that investigates will depend on the nature of the incident. For example, if an individual is seriously injured or dies after being physically restrained by staff, the police will become involved and the commissioning agency and CQC will investigate. If an employee suffers an accident at work, such as an injury caused by manual handling, then the Health and Safety Executive (HSE) and the local authority may investigate.

All the laws will be enshrined in the policies and procedures you are required to follow in your workplace.

As a manager, you must ensure that your staff understand the importance of practicing in accordance with policy, as failure to do so will have significant consequences for the individual, the staff member and the setting.

Health and safety means ensuring that people are safe and come to no harm in the workplace. This will inform policies, such as Control of Substances Hazardous to Health (COSHH), infection control, safe handling of medicine, moving and handling and fire safety. The HSE is the regulator or official supervisory body for the health, safety and welfare of people in work settings in the UK.

Health and Safety at Work Act 1974

The Health and Safety at Work Act 1974 (HASAWA), although drafted over 40 years ago, remains the main piece of UK health and safety legislation. See Unit 501 AC1.1 for more information on this Act.

Management of Health and Safety at Work Regulations 1999

These Regulations further highlight and detail in greater depth what employers are required to do to manage health and safety under the terms of HASAWA, but the main requirement is the need to carry out a risk assessment. Employers with five or more employees need to record significant findings of a risk assessment.

Safety Representatives and Safety Committees Regulations 1977

These Regulations make it a legal requirement for employers to consult with any nominated safety representatives in their workplaces. Safety representatives have legal rights and are recognised by trade unions. They represent everyone in the workplace on all matters of health and safety and can help to reduce the likelihood of accidents and ill health. They raise health and safety complaints and issues with management and can investigate hazards and accidents/incidents. To help them carry out the safety representative role, they can obtain information and facilities from employers and inspectors.

Other regulations to be followed

Table 7 outlines some examples of responsibilities. These are just examples and your job specification or agreed ways of working will offer more information. It will be up to you and your setting to be aware of your full duties and responsibilities with regard to legislation.

Table 7 Legislation, purpose, practice and examples of your responsibilities.

Legislation	Purpose	Practice: examples of your responsibilities
Care Act 2014	The Act aims to improve people's independence and wellbeing.	Local authorities must provide or arrange services that help prevent people developing needs for care and support, or delay people deteriorating so that they would need ongoing care and support. The responsibilities of the manager include ensuring that staff are operating fully in line with the Care Act through the policies developed in house and that they are trained accordingly.
Health and Safety (First Aid) Regulations 1981	To ensure that everybody has access to immediate first aid care in the workplace.	To maintain first aid training of designated first aiders and to supply resources for first aid.
Mental Health Act 1983	The MHA allows compulsory action to be taken, where necessary, to ensure that people with mental health disorders get the care and treatment they need for their own health or safety or for the protection of other people.	Staff need to be aware of the rights and choices individuals have under this act.
Mental Capacity Act 2005	The Act provides a legal framework for acting and making decisions on behalf of adults who lack capacity to make particular decisions for themselves.	To ensure that staff are fully informed of issues such as informed consent and legal application. This should be clearly stated in job descriptions and contracts of work.
Electricity at Work Regulations 1989	To minimise the risk due to electricity in the workplace.	To maintain upkeep and ensure that regular safety checks are made. As a manager, you will be required to keep records of regular testing that is undertaken.
Food Safety Act 1990	Sets out offences relating to sale of food, including serving food unfit for human consumption and food containing foreign bodies.	Ensure that any hazards are identified and controlled. Ensure that good personal hygiene procedures are upheld.
Food Safety and Hygiene (England) Regulations 2013	These Regulations lay down standards relating to the control and management of steps critical to food safety, cleanliness of equipment and premises, temperature control relating to food preparation, storage and serving, food handling practice including personal hygiene of food handlers and disposal of waste.	Staff who handle food are required to undertake training and food hygiene courses. As a manager, you need to ensure compliance with this.
Food Information Regulations 2014 (FIR)	Includes guidance on general food labelling, allergens, ingredients listing, best before and use by dates.	All staff must be trained in checking for any allergens contained in the food served in the setting. Staff need to be aware of the contents of the food that is served in order to comply with individuals' choices.
Manual Handling Operations Regulations 1992 (MHOR)	To reduce the risk of injury in manual handling.	A risk assessment for manual handling and moving must be in place and monitored. You must ensure that staff are trained in moving and handling protocols.
Lifting Operations and Lifting Equipment Regulations 1998 (LOLER)	Businesses and organisations whose employees use lifting equipment are subject to these Regulations, which place duties on organisations that own or operate lifting equipment to ensure that any lifting operation must be planned by a competent person, supervised and carried out safely. The equipment must also be maintained regularly, with records being kept of all examinations and defects reported. Note that some changes to rules and procedures have been made now the UK has left the EU.	Staff are required to undergo manual handling training to include use of lifting equipment on an annual basis. As their manager, you will be required to ensure that staff are compliant with the training and the use of the equipment.

Legislation	Purpose	Practice: examples of your responsibilities
Workplace (Health, Safety and Welfare) Regulations 1992	To minimise risks due to working conditions in the workplace.	Ensure that standards for heating, lighting, sanitation and building upkeep are maintained.
Personal Protective Equipment at Work Regulations 1992	To minimise the risk of cross-infection in the workplace.	To ensure that staff are aware of infection control procedures and are trained in dealing with potential cross-infection. To supply work wear and personal protective equipment (PPE). As a manager, your role is to ensure that staff comply with infection control procedures. There should be regular spot checks as well as annual training to ensure that infection risk is kept to a minimum.
Reporting on Injuries, Diseases and Dangerous Occurrences Regulations 1995 (RIDDOR)	Ensure that procedures are in place for the reporting of injury and illness to the HSE or local authority where appropriate.	Maintain the policy in the workplace and ensure that accident forms and reports are in place.
Provision and Use of Work Equipment Regulations 1998 (PUWER)	Risks due to the use of equipment must be minimised.	Train staff in the use of equipment and ensure that equipment is maintained and safe to use. This links with the LOLER regulations.
Data Protection Act 1998	Ensure that personal information is kept private and safe.	Check policy on confidentiality and arrange to undertake regular risk assessments.
Data Protection Act 2018	Replaces the Data Protection Act 1998.	See Unit 503 for more information on this Act.
Management of Health and Safety at Work Regulations 1999 (MHSWR) Amended 2003 and 2006	These Regulations were introduced to reinforce the Health and Safety Act 1974 and outline what employers must do to manage health and safety. It applies to every work activity and places duties on both employers and employees to maintain a safe and healthy workplace. The 2003 amendment allowed claims to be brought against employees by third parties who were affected by their work activity, e.g. members of the public. The 2006 amendment changed the civil liability provisions in the Regulations so as to exclude the right of third parties to take legal action against employees for contraventions of their duties under these Regulations.	Carry out risk assessments to minimise any risks to safety with respect to fire and safe handling of substances hazardous to health. Fire safety training is an annual process and you as the manager need to ensure that staff are up to date with the training.
Control of Substances Hazardous to Health Regulations 2002 (COSHH)	Minimise the risk from the use of substances that may be hazardous to health.	Carry out risk assessments and ensure that staff are trained in use of hazardous substances.
Regulatory Reform (Fire Safety) 2005	Minimise fire hazards.	Regular checks of fire safety procedures in the workplace.
Corporate Manslaughter and Homicide Act 2007	If a death occurs in suspicious circumstances, then an organisation may be convicted of negligence.	Ensure that staff are aware of duty of care and are following policy.
Health and Social Care Act 2012	Highlighted significant measures to modernise and integrate health and social care.	The changes that were introduced in 2012 mean that practitioners need to understand the reforms and how these may impact them and the individuals using their service. As a manager, you need to be aware of the changes and be able to direct staff to better understanding.

Legislation	Purpose	Practice: examples of your responsibilities
Health and Care Act 2022	Introduced new legislative measures that make it easier for health and care organisations to provide and deliver joined-up care for people who require multiple health and social care services.	The purpose of the Act is to establish in law collaboration and partnership-working to integrate services for individuals. As a care manager you will be required to lead the implementation of change, with more emphasis on integrating care, to enable improvements in population health and individuals' experience, particularly for those individuals living with multiple conditions.
Human Medicines Regulations 2012	These Regulations set out a regime for the authorisation of medicinal products for human use; for the manufacture, import, distribution, sale and supply of those products; and for their labelling and advertising.	Ensure that a medicines policy reflects the law and staff are continually trained and updated in this role. You are responsible for ensuring that medication is safely stored and administered. There are different policies operating in different settings and agency staff may need to be made aware of this. For example, controlled drugs differ. In some settings Oramorph is not classed as a controlled drug and is stored in the usual drug trolley. This will make a difference to who can administer the drug and how it is administered.
Equality Act 2010	This Act brings together over 116 separate pieces of legislation into one single act that provides a legal framework to protect the rights of individuals and advance equality of opportunity for all. The main pieces of legislation that have merged are: • Equal Pay Act 1970 • Sex Discrimination Act 1975 • Race Relations Act 1976 • Disability Discrimination Act 1995 • Employment Equality (Religion or Belief) Regulations 2003 • Employment Equality (Sexual Orientation) Regulations 2003 • Employment Equality (Age) Regulations 2006 • Equality Act 2006, Part 2 • Equality Act (Sexual Orientation) Regulations 2007	To ensure that policies and procedures reflect the Act and staff are aware of duties of care with respect to equality and diversity. This also relates to safeguarding as you will need to ensure that the individuals in your setting are treated fairly and given safe treatment regardless of any differences.
Health and Safety Information for Employees Regulations 1989	These set out the general duties that employers have towards employees and members of the public, and employees have to themselves and to each other.	Ensure that staff are aware of the arrangements for implementing the health and safety measures identified by a risk assessment. Be aware of emergency procedures. Have clear information and training. Be aware of the need to work together with other employers in the workplace. Undertake HASAWA risk assessment to manage health and safety risk in the workplace.

Research it

1.1 Legislation, policies and procedures

Look at the legislation listed in Table 7 and choose three. How does your chosen legislation affect policies and procedures in your setting, and your practice and responsibilities within the setting?

Evidence opportunity

1.1 Reviewing health and safety policies and procedures to reflect current legal, national and local requirements

Explain the current legislative framework for health and safety in adult care.

AC 1.2 Outline current key sources of information and guidance for health and safety management in the workplace

Here, you will be required to outline key sources of information that guide health and safety in the workplace and use the information to guide practice in your setting.

Britain's national regulator for workplace health and safety is the Health and Safety Executive (HSE). They publish guidance on health and safety issues and Approved Codes of Practice. Following their guidance is not compulsory but it is advised. For more information, go to their website.

The UK Health Security Agency and Office for Health Improvement and Disparities replaced Public Health England in October 2021. These two bodies are now the main source of public health information. For the latest information, go to their websites.

The Management of Health and Safety at Work Regulations 1999 set out how employers are required to manage health and safety under the terms of HASAWA. The Working Time Regulations 1998 also include relevant issues for health and safety regarding the number of hours that can be worked.

The Chartered Institute of Personnel and Development (CIPD) also provide information on health and safety in the workplace.

> **Research it**
>
> **1.2 Health and safety at work**
>
> Visit the CIPD website and look at the factsheet 'Health and safety at work' (CIPD, 2022). Read the section 'UK employers' health and safety obligations' and make a checklist of the areas your setting needs to address.

LO2 Be able to lead the implementation of health and safety requirements in adult care

AC 2.1 Explain the processes which ensure that health and safety requirements are met

Here, you are required to explain the legislation, guidance and specific information related to health and safety in the workplace.

Processes internal to the organisation

The implementation of health and safety requirements in adult care requires managers to ensure that policies and procedures are in place to keep the workforce and the individuals using the service safe.

Safeguarding

Care providers must provide a safe environment for individuals and a health and safety incident may overlap safeguarding protocols. For example, if an individual is harmed in an incident where manual handling equipment was faulty or they were scalded in a hot bath, while these are both reportable under the HSE guidance, there is also a safeguarding issue to be answered. In this case, the HSE will further investigate the incident and include the local safeguarding team. As a manager, you will need to know about the policies and procedures for safeguarding and ensure that staff are taught and trained in these.

Staff training and development

Not only is the need to train staff in health and safety a legal requirement for all employers, it is also part of the Care Certificate and is regulated by the CQC. Although settings may differ in the care they offer, health and safety training is mandatory and some certifications require updating annually.

Person-centred care

Person-centred care means ensuring that individuals are at the centre of all the care they receive and that the care given is based on their needs, wishes and preferences. You must ensure that any care given protects not only the physical state of the person but also their mental and emotional state. Each individual must be given respect and treated ethically and with dignity. Again, as a manager, you will need to ensure that your staff are aware of how they can apply a person-centred approach when they care for individuals.

Safety

People who require support in their own homes, outreach provision or care setting are vulnerable and so steps to reduce risks to their safety and address any environmental issues that may pose dangers to them and others must be taken.

Risk management practices, leadership and management practice

One of your responsibilities as a manager is to ensure the health and safety of your workplace so you must control the risks to those who use services, their carers and families, as well as staff. By giving thought to what might cause harm to people and conducting risk assessments, you can ensure that you are taking reasonable steps to prevent harm. You are required to carry out risk assessments in and for your setting by law.

Compliance with the Safety Representative and Safety Committee Regulations 1977 and the Health and Safety Consultations with Employees Regulations 1996 is part of the employer's role. As a manager, you need to ensure that everyone in your team understands that they are responsible for their own safety and also that of anybody with whom they interact in the workplace, and that staff are aware of their responsibilities when it comes to compliance with the legal aspects of health and safety.

Future practice

It is important to keep up to date with changes to the legislation surrounding health and safety, which is why annual updates must form part of your training schedule.

In order to demonstrate good practice as a manager, you can also do the following:

- **Make health and safety and safeguarding part of the agenda**: Health and safety and safeguarding should be a regular agenda item for your team meetings. In this way, staff can be updated on training opportunities, risk assessments and their outcomes, and general safety in the workplace issues. A poster giving details of the staff who are designated safety officers and first aiders is useful since it displays relevant information for staff and visitors to the area.
- **Be a good role model**: By demonstrating good practice in a consistent manner, you will inspire others to follow your lead. For example, by taking part in regular training updates for health and safety and manual handling with the staff, you will be sending positive messages with respect to good practice.
- **Be aware of your responsibility to staff and others**: You need to ensure that visitors to the site are aware of the systems in place for fire safety, infection control and COSHH. You might also want to include information about promoting positive behaviour.

As a manager, it is important that you monitor that staff are complying with the policies and procedures the setting has in place with respect to health, safety and risk management. Care setting failures have shown that although these policies may have been in place, lack of staff compliance led to poor performance and quality of care suffered.

External to the organisation

Potential future pandemics

External influences on the safety of staff and individuals include the changes to guidelines and practice with respect to infection control, particularly following the COVID-19 pandemic. With COVID-19 remaining an ongoing public health issue, the HSE website provides further guidance for workplaces.

To help countries better prepare for future pandemics, the WHO launched a new initiative to provide guidance on planning a response to respiratory pathogens, such as influenza or coronaviruses.

The new 'Preparedness and Resilience for Emerging Threats Initiative (PRET)', published in April 2023, provides tools and approaches for shared learning and collective action, which were established during the COVID-19 pandemic and other recent public health emergencies. For more information, see WHO (2023).

While there is no longer a requirement to consider COVID-19 in risk assessments or to have specific measures in place, employers are required to protect staff who will come into contact with the virus due to their work activity. Settings are expected to comply with the Workplace (Health, Safety and Welfare) Regulations 1992 for welfare facilities and the provision of sufficient ventilation in workplaces.

Under the terms of Control of Substances Hazardous to Health Regulations 2002, employers must protect care staff who come into contact with COVID-19 due to their work activity and, in these cases, employers must still do a risk assessment and implement control measures.

The Reporting of Injuries, Diseases and Dangerous Occurrences Regulations 1995 also include guidance on the circumstances under which you must report a health and safety incident.

Evidence opportunity

2.1 Ensuring health and safety requirements are met

Provide a written account explaining the internal and external processes that ensure that health and safety requirements are met in the workplace in respect of the topics discussed in this section.

Reflect on it

2.1 Applying policies and procedures

How do you apply health and safety policies and procedures in your own workplace in respect of the following areas? Go through each of the headings in turn and justify how they are used.

- Safeguarding: For example, look at incidents where an accident has been reported, then determine how it impacted safeguarding. What was done about it and how might it have been prevented?
- Staff training and development: For example, look at your staff training plans and evaluate how they might be improved. What is good about the training on offer and what gaps might need to be filled?
- Person-centred care: For example, determine how staff perceive person-centred care and demonstrate that individuals using the service are safe. What might be improved?
- Safety: For example, look critically at the accidents that are reported in your setting, then determine how you might make the place safer. What needs to be introduced to ensure that these accidents do not reoccur?
- Risk management practices: For example, look at the last risk assessment that was carried out. Was it useful? How might you improve it?
- Leadership and management practice: For example, how are you ensuring that staff comply with health and safety legislation and, as a manager, what have you put into place to check and audit this practice?
- Future practice: For example, what plans are in place to ensure that you have a safe environment for the future?

Adult social care that is delivered away from a base must be flexible. Domiciliary and outreach workers should meet regularly to plan how to ensure the health and safety of themselves and individuals in the setting. Good practice, with respect to health and safety, should be shared to encourage improved working practices.

AC 2.2 Support others to comply with relevant organisational health and safety practices, policies, procedures

Here, you will be required to demonstrate how health and safety information is disseminated to all colleagues, including any agency staff and non-care staff.

Health and safety training is an annual event, with all staff requiring updates. As their manager, it is important to establish that staff can access the training and also that you are recording that activity. Staff who are working in domiciliary or outreach settings should have regular updates provided through newsletters or staff meetings to ensure that they are made aware of health and safety legislation and the support that is available to them. People who attend a setting, such as agency staff or visitors, must be made aware of health and safety via posters on display. A mini introduction session could also be undertaken with them. You may also wish to ensure that they are trained and check their credentials when they arrive at the setting. Visitors, family and other adult care professionals must also be made aware of health and safety requirements.

Evidence opportunity

2.2 Supporting all team members to understand and be able to apply the policies and procedures

Explain to your assessor how health and safety information is disseminated to all colleagues, including agency staff and non-care staff. Discuss with them how you ensure that all staff are aware of the policies in place with respect to health and safety. How do you support all team members to understand and be able to apply the policies and procedures in their day-to-day work?

AC 2.3 Enable team members to access training to meet health and safety requirements

Here, you will be required to show how health and safety training is provided to all colleagues.

The HSE specifies that everyone who is employed in your setting needs to be trained in how to work safely and without risks to health. It may be that a simple annual update is required, with staff renewing their manual handling and COSHH training. New staff will require basic induction training in working safely, first aid, fire drills and evacuation. Whatever is required, clear instructions and information must be made available to all who enter the site.

If you are an outreach worker or a community carer, there are certain exceptions. HASAWA does not apply to activities such as 'domestic services', which are carried out in private households, but personal care provided within someone's own home will need to be considered on a case-by-case basis. For example, if you work for a local authority care provider or an employment agency, then HASAWA may apply.

Also, if complex care is being carried out, or you have been specially trained and are dealing with people with challenging behaviour, HASAWA is likely to apply. You may be offered basic health and safety training, but not require COSHH.

Some staff may also like to undertake further training, such as that provided by the National Examination Board in Occupational Safety and Health (NEBOSH), for example the National General Certificate in Occupational Health and Safety. The course covers legal, financial and moral reasons for managing health and safety as well as covering UK legislation and how to identify and manage hazards and risks in the workplace. For more information, see NEBOSH (n.d.).

> **Evidence opportunity**
>
> **2.3 Leading health and safety at work**
>
> Download a copy of 'Leading health and safety at work: Actions for directors, board members, business owners and organisations of all sizes' from the HSE website (HSE, 2013).
>
> How will you enable team members to access training to meet health and safety requirements and what training will be appropriate for your staff?

AC 2.4 Monitor compliance with safe working practices

Here, you will show how you ensure that safe working practices are maintained in the workplace.

Monitoring and reporting on health and safety incidents are crucial parts of a health and safety culture. As a manager you need sight of routine reports relating to health and safety. Looking at the documentation for accident reporting as well as general observations within the workplace of how staff manage health and safety in their daily routines will also be useful.

Information such as staff progress on training programmes and incident data such as accident reports and sickness absence rates are useful sources for monitoring progress in health and safety.

You can also make audits of the effectiveness of new procedures and work processes or any major health and safety failures.

Records of workplace health and safety data will give you much needed information on the organisation's performance against others in the sector.

> **Evidence opportunity**
>
> **2.4 Monitoring practices within the setting**
>
> Collect recent monitoring reports, accident reports and training plans and determine whether they meet safe working practices.

AC 2.5 Provide appropriate intervention if procedures are not adhered to

Here, you will demonstrate how breaches of health and safety policies are dealt with within the setting.

A breach of health and safety laws may result in fines or even a court case. You must therefore make sure that staff are fully trained and aware of their role in maintaining workplace safety.

A breach of health and safety is an incident that infringes the terms of the Health and Safety at Work Act. Staff who fail to undertake manual handling operations correctly or who do not adhere to actions required under the Personal Protective Equipment at Work Regulations may be putting themselves and the setting at risk.

In such cases, managers have a duty of care to uphold the law and staff who are not acting in accordance with legislation might face disciplinary action. Legal action can also be taken against a setting if there has been a failure to enforce good health and safety practice.

If a breach is reported to the commissioning agency or CQC, an investigation will be put in place to establish the facts. Once the investigation is complete, the course of action will depend on the following:

- the severity of the incident
- the level of risk involved
- whether it could have been prevented
- what measures were already in place.

The investigator may give improvement or prohibition notices, which give the setting time to address the issue. While prosecution may be avoided, a fine may still be issued. A severe breach, however, is likely to lead to criminal proceedings.

AC 2.6 Evaluate health and safety working practices, policies and procedures making improvements where required

Here, you will evaluate the setting's health and safety policies and assess potential improvements.

Evidence opportunity

2.5 and 2.6 Review health and safety policies

Undertake a thorough review of the health and safety policies in your setting and determine their strengths and weaknesses. How will you ensure that improvement can be made in the workplace to avoid breaches of policy and legislation? What are appropriate interventions if procedures are not adhered to?

AC 2.7 Complete records and reports on health and safety according to legislative and organisational requirements

Here, you will need to show that you can ensure that your service maintains health and care records in line with legislation and organisational requirements and review the need for further improvement(s).

The importance of good record keeping and report making cannot be underestimated. Should an incident occur with an individual using your service, you may be required to attend a commissioning agency review or a CQC hearing and report on the incident. Reports need to be written as soon after an incident as possible so that the details are accurate.

Records can be used in court as evidence of compliance with policies and procedures. Unfortunately, we live in a highly litigious society and so, in order to protect yourself when you are being held accountable for the care you give, you need to be aware of how important records are. If a complaint is made against you, it would be difficult to prove otherwise if you hold inadequate records. If negligence or a breach of health and safety is suspected in any care setting, any records and statements pertaining to the case will be seized and scrutinised.

If your records are less than accurate, you may find yourself in a difficult situation. All records must be accurate, ordered, up to date and stored safely and securely.

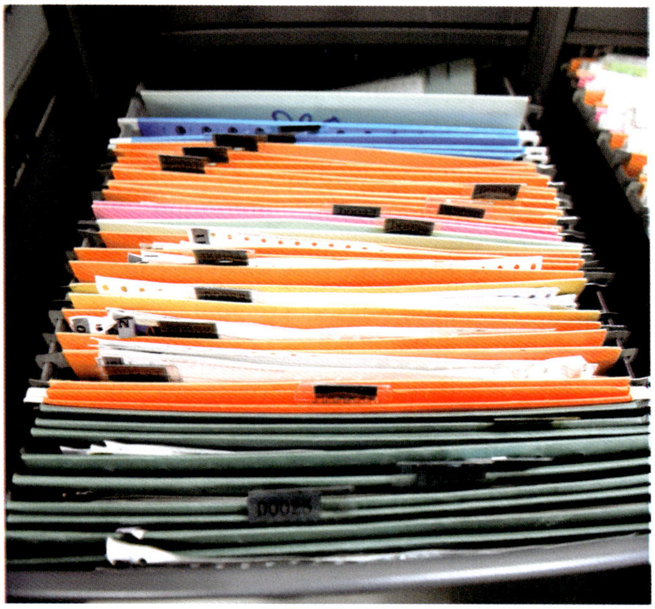

▲ **Figure 35** Good record keeping is vital in a social care setting

Compliance with the Data Protection Act 2018

The Data Protection Act 2018 is the UK's implementation of the General Data Protection Regulation and controls how personal information is used by organisations, businesses and the government.

It is a legal requirement to protect any data you may have on the individuals using your service and on staff, and to maintain it in a confidential way. Any unsuitable use of such information or any breach of confidentiality needs to be dealt with promptly and must be reported to you, the manager. The security of information is a safeguard for vulnerable individuals and any breach of that security can be detrimental to them.

The Health and Social Care Act 2008 (Regulated Activities) Regulations 2014: Regulation 17 states that 'providers must securely maintain accurate, complete and detailed records in respect of each person using the service and records relating to the employment of staff and the overall management of the regulated activity' (CQC, 2022).

You will be familiar with accident records and may have had to complete these from time to time. Although an incident may seem minor or trivial at the time, if you are involved in a legal case in the future, you need to be able to return to the accident records to remind you of what was actually done at the time.

Records therefore:

- provide an account of the care given
- give a record of continuous care (in the case of nursing and medical records)

- provide a source of reference for care
- provide an audit and quality assurance trail
- are a legal requirement
- give evidence of compliance with health and safety guidelines and law.

Additionally, anything that is of a serious nature, such as a reportable disease, serious injury or death, must be reported under RIDDOR.

Your responsibility with respect to record keeping is clear. You need to make records on the individuals using your service, but the way in which you use and store that information is paramount. You must handle all information effectively and be aware of the need to maintain its confidentiality. The following checklist may be useful to ensure that you and your staff are aware of good record keeping.

- Have I written legibly?
- Have I included information in chronological order?
- Have I included dates and times in the record, and are they accurately recorded?
- Have I included the individual's signs and symptoms? (Perhaps also recording how the individual is feeling.)
- Did I carry out a risk assessment?
- Have I included names of other people involved, such as visitors, and recorded information about them accurately?
- Have I written in a professional manner?
- Have I recorded things clearly? Are abbreviations clarified?
- Have I signed the forms/records?
- Have I completed the records in time, without delay?

Evidence opportunity

2.7 Health and safety records

Supply evidence to show how you complete records and reports on health and safety according to legislative and organisational requirements.

LO3 Understand effective risk management

AC 3.1 Describe what is meant by risk management

Here, you will describe your setting's risk assessment policies.

Risk management involves identifying potential risks and taking steps to minimise or avoid them altogether. Your policies should identify how you undertake risk assessment in your area and how you intend to manage risks that arise.

Unfortunately, attempting to manage risks can make you risk averse and you may have staff who constantly err on the side of caution and fail to enable individuals to undertake activities that are considered to be a safety risk. This sort of professional risk aversion will undoubtedly lead to a lack of choice and a loss of control and independence for the individuals using the service, which will in turn have an adverse effect on care and is potentially bad practice. Staff, then, need to be supported in carrying out a risk assessment that they feel confident about. Balancing the risk against its benefits and the rights of an individual can significantly improve a person's quality of life.

You will need to show that you can work with individuals, their family members and your colleagues to adopt a positive approach to risk assessment.

Evidence opportunity

3.1 Review risk management

Describe what is meant by risk management.

AC 3.2 Describe potential risks in own adult setting/service

Here, you will describe the potential risks within your setting.

Some of the most common risks in care settings are:

- moving and positioning – responsible for a significant proportion of accidents
- medication errors
- slips/trips
- verbal aggression, threats or physical violence
- food, due to allergies or choking
- food preparation, including burns and cuts
- infection control and prevention, including COVID-19.

Other common risks include:

- scalding and burning, for example from heating apparatus or bathing
- electrical, asbestos, fire and other premises-based risks that affect everyone
- Legionella – this bacteria can cause a pneumonia-type condition and is caught by breathing in tiny droplets of water containing bacteria; hospitals, hotels and offices are susceptible to contaminated water supplies

- staffing levels – low staffing levels will inevitably lead to some care practices being missed or not carried out well; safety demands that the ratio of staff to individuals according to the setting is upheld.

In domiciliary settings hazards may include some of the above, so a lone worker policy needs to be in place to protect the worker.

Evidence opportunity

3.2 Describe potential risks in setting

Describe your responsibilities to assess and manage risk.

Research it

3.2 Evaluate potential risks

The following table may apply to many settings. Complete it according to your setting, showing the actions you would take.

Risk	Evidence of this occurring (provide a report)	Action taken to prevent (show policy and procedure)
Moving and handling		
Medication error		
Slips and trips		
Behaviour management		
Food risks		
Infection prevention		
Staffing levels		

AC 3.3 Describe own responsibilities to assess and manage risk

Here, you will describe your policies and procedures in managing risk within the setting.

Risk management practice involves developing strategies that prevent negative events occurring and minimising harm. It also now includes ensuring that infection prevention and control is part of the risk management. You must ensure that your own practice is sound and this will require you to evaluate that practice and to establish that a risk management plan which documents identifiable risks in the setting, together with responses to these, is made available to staff.

Reflect on it

3.3 Implementing health and safety risk management

Think about how you implement health and safety risk management at work and what you might do to improve your own practice.

How has your management of infection control changed as a result of COVID-19?

AC 3.4 Explain methods and tools available to inform and undertake risk management activities

Here, you will explain the methods of managing risk and undertaking risk assessments.

Risk management requires a process for controlling health and safety risks caused by hazards in the workplace.

Steps to manage risk

1 Identify hazards

What in your workplace has the potential to cause harm? Consider the work being carried out and the equipment in use. Think about the chemicals and substances that are being used. Have you seen any unsafe work practices? What about the general state of repair of the setting or even the hazards that might apply due to danger from other people?

Look at accident and sickness records so you can begin to build a picture of less obvious hazards.

For each hazard, think about the harm that might come to your team, visitors or members of the public.

2 Assess the risks

Once you have a list of identified hazards, you can assess the likelihood of each of them occurring. You might think about who could be harmed or what the benefit of taking the risk is likely to be for the individual. Think about how and what you are doing to control the risks and about further action that might be needed, who needs to carry out that action and by when.

3 Control the risks

Reflect on what you are already doing to reduce the risk and determine whether you can remove the hazard altogether. If this is not possible, how do you intend to control the risks so that harm is unlikely?

It might simply be a case of replacing equipment, re-organising work or identifying the measures needed to work safely. If personal protective equipment is needed then this is a control that must be put in place.

It is not possible to eliminate all risks, but you must do everything 'reasonably practicable' to protect others from harm.

4 Record your findings

If your setting has five or more staff, you are required to record any significant findings. This means identifying the hazards, who might be harmed by them and what has been done to control the risks.

5 Review the controls

Finally, review these steps and the controls you have put in place to make sure they are working. It might be that they are no longer effective or there have been changes in the workplace and new risks have emerged. Staff may also highlight problems which need to be addressed.

Evidence opportunity

3.4 Risk management activities

Explain what methods and tools are available to you to inform and undertake risk management activities.

Research it

3.4 Risk assessment template

The HSE produce a risk assessment template. Download a template and complete it for your setting, then share with staff (HSE, n.d. a).

LO4 Be able to lead the implementation of policies, procedures and practices to effectively manage risk

AC 4.1 Develop policies, procedures and practices to identify, assess and manage risk

Here, you will show how you develop the setting's risk assessment policies and share them with colleagues.

The policies and processes of the setting must be developed, implemented and adhered to, to ensure that a positive approach to risk is developed and managed well.

Some settings may view policies and processes relating to risk management as documents to be read then forgotten. This is short sighted as policies provide valuable insight into what needs to be monitored and taken into consideration in the assessment of risk.

This makes for a safer environment and, as the manager, you need to ensure that staff are not simply ticking boxes when it comes to complying with the risk assessment policy.

Reflect on it

4.1 Risk management policies

Collect the policies relating to risk management together in a file. Use them at a team meeting to encourage staff to update their knowledge.

AC 4.2 Support team members to understand risk management and adhere to guidance which promotes safe practices

Here, you will demonstrate how as a manager you support your team in undertaking risk assessment and following best practice guidance.

Understand risk management

Care workers are duty bound to adopt a positive approach to risk assessment that balances individual choice with the duty of care to protect. Managing risks is a process that identifies the factors that could prevent care workers from providing safe, efficient care and staff need to be aware of and understand this.

If you believe that the safety of individuals using your service may be compromised in any way, you need to identify and report your concerns to ensure that safety controls can be put in place. You can do this by helping individuals to weigh up the potential benefits of a course of action against the harms of exercising it and also to look at alternative actions. Individuals, their family members and others involved in their care can all be part of the process to assess risk.

In assessing the seriousness of risk, you may want to address the following aspects in your workplace:

- factors that increase exposure to risk, e.g. environmental, social, financial, communication and recognition of abuse
- the support available to minimise risk
- the nature, extent and length of time of the risk
- the impact the risk may have on the individual and on others.

In addition to the above, you are bound by law as stated in Section 3(1) of the Health and Safety at Work Act 1974:

> *It shall be the duty of every employer to conduct his undertaking in such a way as to ensure, so far as is reasonably practicable, that persons not in his employment who may be affected thereby are not thereby exposed to risks to their health or safety.*

Adhere to guidance which promotes safe practices

The main reason for health and safety legislation is to protect people at work and those who are affected by work activities, so it is imperative that your setting's policies reflect these and that staff are fully aware of their responsibilities. Laws exist so that everyone in society knows which behaviours are acceptable and which are not. Health and safety is everybody's responsibility and your staff must be compliant in order to keep themselves and others safe.

> **Evidence opportunity**
>
> **4.2 Demonstrate how risk can be minimised**
>
> At your next team meeting provide evidence of how you support team members to:
>
> **a.** understand risk management
>
> **b.** adhere to guidance which promotes safe practices.

AC 4.3 Work with others to identify and assess risks

Here, you will show how you can work with colleagues in assessing risks.

Risks change, just as the care of an individual may change, and therefore they need to be reviewed on a regular basis, just as you would review a care/support plan. Although you may think of risk in terms of danger or injury, risk taking can have positive benefits for individuals' wellbeing. Balance must therefore be exercised in meeting the desires of people to undertake activities that require thought and planning to minimise risk.

Conflict may occur when families disagree with the individual as to their choice of activity. They may be risk averse, so the care staff can help them to understand how the decision has been arrived at. Showing families that decisions have been made based on clear reasoning regarding legislation, policies and procedures will help.

Safeguarding the individual receiving care is paramount and, in handling decisions about risk, information should be shared in accordance with the setting's protocols.

Developing a simple approach to identify, assess and manage risk will enable staff and individuals to seek clarification if they are unsure about what to do if complaints or concerns are raised.

For more on positive risk taking, see Unit 515 LO6.

AC 4.4 Work with others to manage risks to minimise their impact

Here, you will show how working as a team can help to minimise risks for individuals within the setting.

To help staff to assess and manage risk, you need to look at what is involved in the proposed course of action and identify the potential benefits and harm that could result. For example, an individual with a learning disability may express a wish to go on holiday with a friend. While the friend may be able to support them during the day, the support needed at night could be an issue. In determining the risk here, the potential benefits of the individual staying at home must be weighed against the benefits of the holiday and the individual's greater independence. Plans must be developed that reflect the positive wishes and priorities of the individual and resources made available to achieve the best outcomes for them while at the same time managing the risk and minimising potential harm.

> **Evidence opportunity**
>
> **4.3 and 4.4 Demonstrate positive approaches to risk assessments**
>
> Collect evidence that demonstrates how you work with staff, individuals, family members and colleagues to adopt a positive approach to risk assessment.

AC 4.5 Analyse the effectiveness of health and safety processes

Here, you will analyse your setting's health and safety policies.

Evidence opportunity

4.5 Analyse the effectiveness of risk assessment practice and health and safety in your setting

Provide an account of your own practice to show how you promote a balanced approach to risk taking for your own setting. Think about how you have helped individuals, staff and others such as family members to carry out risk assessments that support a positive risk-taking approach. How did you help them to understand the balance between risk and rights? Say how this practice has improved the care in your area. Determine how you might help an employee to understand the balance between risk and rights.

How might you change your risk assessment policy in the light of what you have learned?

AC 4.6 Evaluate existing processes and recommend changes where necessary

Here, you will evaluate your setting's policies and look for possible areas of improvement.

Risk management involves analysing risk and then developing policies to ensure that risks are minimised. A health and safety management plan will be successful if risks are properly identified and staff are trained to manage risks.

The risk management process involves four basic steps:

1. Identify and analyse the risks.
2. Prioritise the risk as to its harm and benefits.
3. Implement an action.
4. Monitor and determine practice changes if needed.

Risk from whatever source can cause uncertainty in any setting and staff may require supervision to help them to manage it confidently. You could start to consider ways that staff can supervise their peers so that the principles of risk become embedded in daily practice.

Compliance with respect to legislation will require you as the manager to ensure that policies and processes are up to date and reflect current safe practice. Failure to do so is breaking the law.

Legislation

See Table 7 for a list of relevant legislation in this area.

Evidence opportunity

4.6 Evaluate existing processes and recommend changes where necessary

Provide a report that shows how your setting is actively following policies and procedures and evaluate their effectiveness in respect of risk and management practices.

Make some recommendations for change where necessary.

References

Care Quality Commission (2022) 'Regulation 17: Good governance'. www.cqc.org.uk/guidance-providers/regulations-enforcement/regulation-17-good-governance

CIPD (2022) 'Health and safety at work'. www.cipd.org/uk/knowledge/factsheets/health-safety-factsheet/

Health and Safety Executive (2013) 'Leading health and safety at work: Actions for directors, board members, business owners and organisations of all sizes'. www.hse.gov.uk/pubns/indg417.pdf

Health and Safety Executive (n.d. a) 'Managing risks and risk assessment at work'. www.hse.gov.uk/simple-health-safety/risk/risk-assessment-template-and-examples.htm

NEBOSH (n.d.) 'National General Certificate in Occupational Health and Safety'. www.nebosh.org.uk/qualifications/national-general-certificate/

World Health Organisation (2023) 'Preparedness and Resilience for Emerging Threats (PRET)'. www.who.int/initiatives/preparedness-and-resilience-for-emerging-threats

Useful resources and further reading

Health and Safety Executive. www.hse.gov.uk

Health and Safety Executive (n.d. b) 'Sensible risk assessment in care settings'. www.hse.gov.uk/healthservices/sensible-risk-assessment-care-settings.htm

Office for Health Improvement and Disparities. www.gov.uk/government/organisations/office-for-health-improvement-and-disparities

Skills for Care (n.d.) 'GO Online: Inspection toolkit – managing risk'. www.skillsforcare.org.uk/Support-for-leaders-and-managers/Good-and-outstanding-care/inspect/Topic-examples.aspx?kloe=safe&topic=managing-risk&services=

UK Health Security Agency. www.gov.uk/government/organisations/uk-health-security-agency

Unit 519

Continuous development for leaders and managers in adult care

GLH 15

About this unit

In your role, you will need to know how you can most effectively manage yourself and your own behaviour, as well as manage others. In this unit, you will consider different strategies that you can use and that you can identify through self-reflection and reflective practice.

You will explore the importance of self-awareness and how you can manage your personal and professional behaviour in your role, as well as your professional development needs and how they affect the work you do. You will also learn about workload management.

Learning outcomes

By the end of this unit you will:

1. Be able to demonstrate commitment to own development.
2. Be able to demonstrate commitment to self-awareness.
3. Be able to manage own workload.

Getting started

Before you study the unit, think about the following:

- How do your belief systems and experiences affect your current work practice as a manager?
- How do your professional actions reflect a high standard of personal integrity?
- What is meant by work–life balance and how is this achieved? How do you achieve this?
- What opportunities for professional development are there to support your role?

LO1 Be able to demonstrate commitment to own development

AC 1.1 Evaluate own knowledge and performance using standards and benchmarks

Here, you will be required to evaluate your own professional skills, knowledge and behaviours against standards and benchmarks, feedback from others and organisational appraisal.

Standards and benchmarks

People working in the care sector are subject to a range of professional codes, expectations and standards of performance set by external organisations. All staff need to demonstrate that they are working to these standards. The requirement for professional development is reinforced in the following:

- legislation, for example the Data Protection Act 2018 and the Mental Capacity Act 2005
- minimum/essential standards that refer to the quality and safety of care and identify the experiences individuals are expected to have as a result of the care they receive
- CQC fundamental standards of quality and safety that must be met by care providers.

These documents articulate the standards that the public can expect from those delivering care. All codes and standards of practice make explicit reference to the need for those providing care to work within their levels of knowledge and experience and to address any knowledge deficits.

Evaluating your own knowledge and performance

Each individual is accountable for their professional development and you may be required to identify to your managers, to your profession and/or to a legal authority or commissioning agency how you have maintained this. You need to be able to evaluate and examine your practice knowledge so that you can identify any gaps and areas for development. It is essential that you can provide evidence of your knowledge and skills and how you have maintained these. As a manager and leader of others, it is your responsibility to ensure that you are appropriately equipped to effectively fulfil your role. This requires you to assess your own capabilities against your job description to ensure that you have the skills that are necessary to do your job well.

As well as identifying the standards of care to be achieved, codes of practice articulate the manner in which care should be delivered. All recipients of care should expect to receive competent care. An organisation that strives for excellence will also ensure that attention is paid to the value base of care provision, which facilitates good and excellent practice as opposed to merely competent or safe practice.

Evaluating your own performance requires you to examine your practice showing that your knowledge and skills are based on sound learning and that you always work within the standards required. You need to show that you are a lifelong learner and continually update your practice.

Feedback from others

360-degree feedback is a system by which employees receive feedback from the people who work with them. These can be other managers, stakeholders and peers. By asking others about your performance you can gather valuable insight into how others see your professional skills and behaviour. This can then help you to evaluate how you are developing in your role and identify any gaps in your learning. Remember that feedback does not have to be anonymous. It can be an open and honest discussion with staff members, where you ask for their thoughts on your performance. Remember to take feedback and criticism in a constructive manner, and not be offended by it. You should use it to improve your performance and practice, and not let it affect your performance or self-esteem negatively.

Reflect on it

1.1 Reflecting on your own role

Think about how much you have learned as a result of this course and your role. Look back to the start of the course and reflect upon how you have made changes to your management style as a result of what you have learned.

Organisational appraisal

In larger organisations you can expect to undergo an organisational appraisal in which information is gathered and the performance of the setting is assessed.

An organisational appraisal helps the management team to check how effective the organisation is by checking:

- whether policy and procedure are being complied with

- the effectiveness of leaders and staff
- how well resources are being used
- how well monitoring systems are working.

Even in a smaller setting you can still undertake checks of policy and procedure and determine how effective you are in your role in monitoring the systems and the resources. This process means that your skills, knowledge and behaviour within the organisation will come under scrutiny but you will gain valuable experience of how well you understand the organisation and where you may require development.

Evidence opportunity

1.1 Standards and benchmarks

Undertake a professional discussion with your assessor in which you evaluate your own professional skills, knowledge and behaviours against standards and benchmarks, feedback from others and organisational appraisal.

You might, for example, like to make a list of the codes and standards that govern your role.

When did you last review and reflect on your work against these standards?

How is your work influenced by these codes and standards?

Research it

1.1 360-degree feedback

Conduct a 360-degree feedback exercise to assess your professional skills, knowledge and experience.

AC 1.2 Prioritise own professional development needs and aspirations

Here, you will be required to select and prioritise your own goals and targets.

Identifying learning needs

Once you understand how you prefer to learn, you can identify areas for improvement and how this can be achieved. This can amount to nothing more than a wish list, so time spent reflecting on these wishes will help you to prioritise your development needs and these can then be shown as objectives. It is important that objectives are prioritised and committed to paper in the form of a plan and that timescales for completion and available resources are identified.

Developing a formal plan serves a number of purposes. It enables you to:

- structure and prioritise your learning and development
- set short- and long-term goals (using the SMART model)
- address those things that you must do, such as update your knowledge and skills
- devise more creative and personalised goals.

Remember, your short-term goals may or may not contribute to the longer-term ones. Writing your objectives in a plan gives them weight and structure and you are more likely to act on them, especially if the plan is shared with another person such as a line manager, who may commit to supporting it.

Use of tools

You might undertake what is known as a SWOT analysis. This acronym stands for Strengths, Weaknesses, Opportunities and Threats. Use it to look at these four key areas about yourself and to ask yourself questions. For example:

Strengths

- What are you good at in life and in the workplace?
- Which part of your job do you do well and why?
- What are the values and attitudes that you live by and that help you?
- What do others see you as an expert in?
- How do others value you?
- What qualifications do you have and could you make more use of them?

Weaknesses

- What areas of your job do you least enjoy?
- What makes you stressed?
- What would others say your weaknesses are?
- Are there skills you wish you had?

Opportunities

- What new skills are needed in your job role that you could learn?
- Do you have any skills that could be used to improve your performance that you currently do not use?
- What would you like to develop in your job role over the next year or so?
- What opportunities for promotion are currently presenting?

Threats

- During appraisal, have you been made aware of anything your manager is concerned about in respect of your performance? (In smaller settings you may simply have a one-to-one with the owner or your line manager but you can still gain feedback about how you are performing in your role).
- Is your job role changing and can you handle that change? (In smaller settings you may simply have a one-to-one with the owner or your line manager but you can still gain feedback about how you are performing in your role).
- What makes it harder for you to perform at work?
- Do you need to update your knowledge or technical expertise in order to continue to do your job?

Setting SMART targets with realistic short- and long-term goals

Setting SMART targets will help you to identify what it is you want to achieve, how you will do it, how you will know you have done it, and the specific timescale in which it will happen.

The SMART targets can be prioritised into the crucial activities you need to accomplish and those that can be left for later.

Setting timescales and managing interruptions

Timescales and deadlines must be set and then met and any interruptions to your plans should be dealt with flexibly. For example, potential interruptions such as illness, additional workload and personal issues will need to be addressed in your planning. Deadlines need to be realistic and attainable and milestones put in place, where needed, in order to meet those deadlines.

Managing multi-tasking

Multi-tasking is the ability to manage your time well and to focus on each task equally. You will need to decide how best to use your time effectively. You may also need to determine whether multi-tasking is the right thing to do in certain situations, or whether you can delegate tasks to others.

> **Evidence opportunity**
>
> **1.2 Prioritising your own development goals and targets**
>
> Show that you can select and prioritise your own goals and targets. You might discuss this with your assessor or prepare a presentation for them. You could, for example, undertake a SWOT analysis and use this tool to prioritise your goals and targets.

> **Research it**
>
> **1.2 SWOT and SMART**
>
> Compare the SMART model with a SWOT analysis What are the differences? Provide a written account.

AC 1.3 Implement plans to meet own professional development needs and aspirations

Here, you will be required to implement, establish and reflect on a personal and professional development plan.

When prioritising your objectives, think about how much you want to do something. Before embarking on development activities, you should be clear about what you are prepared to invest in achieving the goals that you set. This may include decisions about any personal motivations and the time you are prepared to make available, which is likely to be in addition to anything an employer will provide. You must be realistic about resources and, in particular, the financial burdens and who will be responsible for them. It is also important to acknowledge the potential impact that education and development can have on those around you, both at home and at work. This can be as a result of support that others must provide or the change that may occur in you as a result of the development. You must be realistic about these factors, but that does not mean you should not also have aspirations and set an ambitious plan.

A successful professional development plan will:

- clearly specify how the objectives will be achieved
- identify the timeframes and milestones against which progress can be measured
- suggest criteria against which the activity can be evaluated.

Personal goals for staff should be part of an organisation's goals. Although there may be barriers to developing staff, plans must be put in place to overcome those barriers and these plans need to be reviewed and changed if necessary. It is a requirement of the CQC standard on staffing that settings have suitably qualified, competent and experienced staff who are given the 'support, training and supervision' they need to do their job.

Clarify aims to ensure that the plan is designed to improve the effectiveness and impact of practice

In developing goals for the success of the setting, you must establish a plan that will have a positive impact on practice. There must be clarity about what it is you are trying to achieve and how you are going to do this.

Identify areas for improvement and development of skills

The plans should highlight the areas that need to be improved in the first instance and the skills that will be required of staff to achieve those goals. For example, you may feel that you need to improve your grasp of resource management recording and you notice that Microsoft Excel spreadsheets are a good way of doing this. You recognise that your lack of skills in the use of Excel currently limits your use of spreadsheets, so you will need to seek some help with this.

Establish SMART objectives that are time bound

The SMART targets that are set should have deadlines applied to them to ensure that the development is kept to target and accomplished. Without this, the plan is likely to fail.

A business case may need to be developed in order to ensure that any support required to meet the targets is costed and resources and finances are available to support the objectives.

Improve the effectiveness and impact of your practice

By undertaking a professional development plan you can be sure that you will be developing your skills and keeping up with changing trends in your role. Additionally, you can enhance your position in the job field and perhaps move on to higher roles within or external to your organisation.

It is important to identify how and with whom the plan will be reviewed, so set a date and a named person at the outset.

Evidence opportunity

1.3 Use personal and professional development planning

Have a discussion with your assessor about how you implement, establish and reflect on a personal and professional development plan. Address the areas discussed in this section.

If you have not developed a professional development plan, you might like to use a template similar to the one below. Ensure that you write objectives that can be measured and evaluated. Clearly show the evidence that will demonstrate whether or not you have achieved your objectives.

Overall learning development need	**What specifically do you need to know/learn?**			
Objectives	**Date for achievement**	**How will you achieve your objective?**	**Support required**	**Evidence and outcomes**
What specific end or steps do you have in mind? You must include a measurable verb in each objective statement in this column, e.g. 'Pass an accredited first-aid course.'	When will you assess progress? When will you have achieved your objective, e.g. the date of a training course?	How will you demonstrate that you have met the objective, e.g. attend a first aid course?	Human? Financial? Time? Learning resources?	What evidence will you have to confirm your achievement, e.g. a certificate of competence?
Avoiding barriers and blockers	What positive steps can you take to avoid barriers?			
Objective 1 Example: Develop IT skills to enable effective forward planning and publication of staff rotas for off-duty cover.	September this year.	Complete a course on how to use Microsoft Excel.	Either day release to attend the course or time to undertake online training.	Publication of all off-duty rotas using computerised support packages. Staff cover will be effective and planned and produced four weeks in advance.
What positive steps can you take to avoid barriers and blockers? Identify the need and the potential and actual benefits for the organisation. Research and present different methods of achieving the goal, with pros and cons identified. Discuss with and gain commitment from line manager through a signed agreement or financial support to enable attendance/completion of the course. Report progress.				

AC 1.4 Identify opportunities to support own professional development taking account of own learning style

Here, you will be required to research different methods of learning that will assist you in your personal development.

There are a number of sources of support to enable your learning and development. You may choose formal support such as training courses or supervision and appraisals. Informal support can be gained through mentoring and peer support opportunities within and outside the organisation. You might also access self-led and directed learning opportunities via the internet.

However you decide to undertake development, it is useful to understand how you like to learn. Individuals learn in different ways, and you should think about your preferred learning style so that, where possible, you can select an appropriate learning activity.

Think about different learning activities you have participated in. Do you like discussion and working with others? Do you prefer tutor guidance? Do you like exploring and learning on your own? Are computer programs a style of learning that you enjoy? If you enjoy the process of learning, you are more likely to stick with it, particularly if it is over a period of time. Your understanding of what development activities suit your learning style means you are likely to get more from your learning.

Having identified your strengths, deficits, training needs and ideas for service enhancements, it is important that these are transformed into tangible actions that can be articulated as objectives. Objectives are statements that describe what the end point of an activity will be. Objectives should be written with the SMART acronym in mind – that is, they should be Specific, Measurable, Achievable, Relevant and Time bound. When writing your objectives you should have the end in mind before you start. Think of it as a journey – it is not often that you set out on a journey not knowing where you want to end up. Your plan must be able to deliver what you set out to do and you must evaluate how successful you have been. Having information on which you can base your plan should secure the best chance of success.

Honey and Mumford (1992) developed a questionnaire that enables participants to distinguish between four ways of learning:

- Activists prefer to work intuitively, be flexible and spontaneous, generate new ideas and try things out. They like to learn from problem solving, discussion, group work and experience.
- Reflectors like to watch/listen and reflect, gathering data and taking time to consider options and alternatives. They like lectures, project work and information research.
- Theorists prefer to go through things thoroughly and logically, step by step. They like guidelines and prefer to learn from books, problem solving and discussion.
- Pragmatists learn by 'trying things out'. They are practical and realistic, and like work-based learning and practical application in real settings.

There may be a dominant style that fits your way of learning, but it's equally possible that more than one method is appropriate for you.

Barbe et al. (1979) identified the VARK (Visual, Auditory, Reading, Kinaesthetic) model of learning styles, which suggests that we learn better depending upon our most dominant sense. For example, a visually dominant person will learn better by seeing pictures, graphs and diagrams, whereas those who favour the auditory sense will prefer to listen and hear from others. They may learn better by listening to auditory books or lectures. The kinaesthetic learner is one who prefers to do things and have a more hands-on approach to learning, preferring to experience things and to undertake experiments.

Research it

1.4 Learning styles

Undertake some research on the VARK learning style and try to ascertain what your preference is.

Learning will be easier if you can be matched with your preferred style. Although this cannot always be fully accommodated, knowing your own style will help you to plan appropriately.

Evidence opportunity

1.4 Establish your own learning style

Think about your preferred learning style. What developmental opportunities are available to you? Research courses that might be a good fit for you.

AC 1.5 Create opportunities for others to provide feedback on own performance across all aspects of role

Here, you will ask your colleagues for feedback on your performance using a number of different possible methods.

As a manager of a team, teaching and encouraging staff to be self-reflective is important. It is also a crucial tool to use for your own wellbeing and self-awareness. Reflection can be a powerful tool. It can be used to improve practice by supporting you to question your routine work as you carry it out. In doing so, you can measure your behaviour against your values and those of the organisation to ensure that they are consistent. Alternatively, reflection may encourage you to try a new approach to an activity and evaluate its success. Reflective practice provides an opportunity for all practitioners to check their own standards of work and enhance practice.

360-degree reflection

360-degree reflection is similar to the 360-degree feedback cycle referred to in AC1.1 and seeks the views of others in the setting and also externally. Once you have gathered information from a range of individuals, both those in positions of authority over you and those over whom you have authority, you can use this to reflect on your behaviours and performance. You should gather information from people who will be honest and can be trusted to feed back responsibly and constructively. It is important that you do not only ask your friends – they are more likely to tell you what you want to hear rather than what you need to hear. To gain the most from the activity, you need to know how different people experience you and your actions. This can be empowering and being self-aware leads to growth, both personally and professionally. Getting all-round 360-degree feedback may provide you with insight about the following:

- a façade – information that suggests that you are better or worse at something than you think you are
- a blind spot – information that you did not know about yourself
- a suggestion about something that you could easily do that would make a positive difference
- an opportunity to stop doing something.

360-feedback is usually built around a questionnaire as this helps the individual to control the areas on which they want feedback. The criteria for writing questions for 360-feedback reflect general principles of performance appraisal systems and criteria, and include the following points:

- Questions should be relevant to the recipient's job.
- Each question should be concise, use plain English and omit qualifiers, such as 'when appropriate' and 'as necessary'. Vague and complex questions rarely produce clear feedback.
- Each question should relate to a clearly defined competency or function to avoid muddled feedback. It must be specific.
- Questions should set clear and appropriate standards. For example, 'makes decisions' is a poor criterion as the decisions made could be unclear, late or wrong. A better statement might be 'makes timely and effective decisions'.
- Open questions provide the opportunity to add comments in support of the answers to the rated questions and, as such, can be particularly helpful. The recipient is able to look for frequently used words or phrases and for common themes. When wording such questions, it is important to use clear language, for example 'What does the recipient do well?' and 'What does the recipient need to improve?'

Source: Adapted from CIPD (2022)

Additionally, you can gain feedback via other sources at your disposal such as appraisals, supervision and performance reviews. Appraisals are an opportunity for the employee and manager to get together to reflect and discuss their achievements over the past year, the aim of which is to have a shared view of the performance of the employee at the end of the meeting. Supervision is an ongoing process in which the manager oversees, supports and develops the knowledge and skills of the employee. By using a variety of methods, you are able to gain much-needed information about a person and enable them to develop their self-awareness.

The systems in the care setting to obtain feedback via surveys and customer satisfaction forms enable the carers, family and friends of those accessing care and support services to actively praise or make a complaint. They are useful for staff to gauge their performance and change it if necessary.

Reflect on it

1.5 Seek feedback on own leadership style

Seek feedback from staff regarding your leadership style. Ask them to anonymously complete sticky notes with suggestions for something you should stop, something you should start and something you should continue to do. For example:

Stop: Writing emails and talk to us.

Start: Taking your breaks!

Continue: Giving clear instructions.

Place the completed sticky notes on a poster and address each one in turn.

AC 1.6 Evaluate how own practice has been improved

Here, you will evaluate your own personal development.

Improved through implementation of a professional development plan

Now you have constructed a personal development plan and developed short- and long-term goals to guide your decisions about your career, you can use the plan to help you achieve your goals. The step-by-step process of self-assessment means you can examine your current job to see how it relates to the career goals identified in your plan. Once you have a clear idea about the skills you currently have, your next step is to identify areas in which you can improve and any skills gaps you need to address to reach your goals.

Improved through reflection on feedback from others

Reflective practice is a tool that can be used by practitioners individually to enhance their practice. It can also be used as a management tool, enabling managers to guide and support staff to reflect on key elements of their role and their performance. Prompts such as 'You did that really well. What was it that made that such a successful activity?' are useful. This approach develops individuals' self-esteem, confidence and a questioning and critical approach to their work. Reflection provides an ideal vehicle for learning that can be shared within the wider team. Teams can reflect as a group, particularly if they are keen to examine or change an aspect of practice that they have in common, and can share their learning with others.

Inevitably, when you reflect, no matter how candid you try to be, it is difficult to see the world from anything other than your own perspective. Reflection may require you to seek opinions and information from others in order to validate your reflections and to help you to see whether change is required. While information gained in this way can feel threatening, if managed and used sensitively 360-degree feedback can be illuminating and can challenge and refocus your perceptions of reality.

Improved through learning from achievements and adverse events

Adverse events or critical incidents occur in practice from time to time and you may need to react to an event that poses a risk to either yourself, your staff or the individuals using your service.

A critical incident is an event out of the range of normal experience and is often sudden and unexpected. It is an event that makes a contribution either positively or negatively to an activity or phenomenon. A critical incident may be a positive experience or a negative one, but an adverse event is always negative. Such events cause us to stop and think about the event afterwards and to review which behaviours were helpful or unhelpful in the situation.

In care, for example, a critical incident might be a medication error, or an individual testing positive for COVID-19. These events might be labelled as 'critical incidents' because they start a chain of events that need to be acted upon. Staff should be encouraged to reflect on what has happened as it challenges them to look at their practice and to consider what they might do differently next time.

Reflect on it

1.6 Evaluate how own practice has improved

Using the sticky note activity from the previous AC, evaluate how your own practice has improved and how you might work on areas that require improvement.

LO2 Be able to demonstrate commitment to self-awareness

AC 2.1 Use feedback from others to proactively increase own self-awareness

Here, you will review the feedback you have received and use this to assist your personal development.

Self-awareness is a characteristic of emotional intelligence and is about focusing on ourselves and becoming aware of how our actions, thoughts and emotions align with our internal standards and values. For example, a person who is highly self-aware is objective and can manage their emotions and align their behaviour well. It is a tool for self-control.

Change is inevitable in adult care work and sometimes you may find this difficult. However, a positive approach to the required changes will make the transition to new ways of working easier and more likely to be accepted by the staff you work with. If you view feedback as a way in which you can develop and grow, you will receive it in good grace, accept it openly and learn from it. Although negative feedback can sometimes be difficult to hear, if given in the right way it can have a positive impact upon the receiver, if they are willing to accept it as a learning experience.

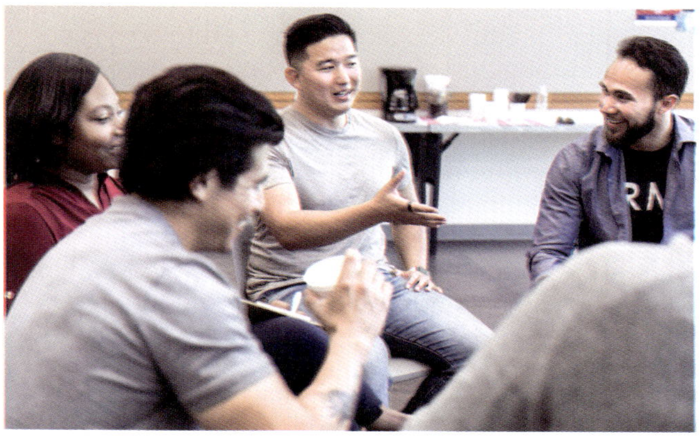

▲ **Figure 36** How does feedback from others help you to improve your performance?

Evidence opportunity

2.1 Responding to feedback

Reflect on how you respond to feedback from a range of sources, including a positive attitude towards change and a willingness to review your own behaviours and attitudes. Provide a written account or explain this to your assessor.

You might like to provide a reflective account demonstrating how you show willingness to review your own behaviours and attitudes to change. Think about how you react to both positive and negative feedback.

How do you respond to feedback from those senior to you? How do you respond to feedback from those you manage? How do you respond to feedback from individuals in your setting and their families? How do your reactions differ based on the people who give the feedback?

How do you ensure that you learn from the feedback you are given and maintain a positive attitude towards change?

AC 2.2 Reflect on own skills, values and behaviours to increase self-awareness and professional development

Here, you will reflect on your approach and use this analysis for your own personal development.

Reflective practice models were covered in Unit 505. Here you will review Gibbs' six stages to reflective practice (Gibbs, 1988), which uses structured questions to prompt reflection in a logical way. It is a good way to start reflection and these questions can be used to focus on incident analysis. To remind yourself of Gibbs' model, refer to Unit 505 AC1.10 now.

Using Gibbs' model can help you to structure a report of an incident. We often write descriptively, confusing evaluation and analysis, and this leads to repetition. By using the stages shown in Gibbs' reflective cycle, you can address each part of the report in a clear and constructive way.

Evidence opportunity

2.2 Reflecting on own skills

Using Gibbs' reflective cycle, reflect on your own skills, values and behaviours. How does this activity improve your self-awareness and professional development?

AC 2.3 Analyse how own values, belief systems and experiences impact own work practices

Here, you will analyse your own beliefs and look at how these affect your performance and personal development.

Your values and beliefs describe what you believe to be important and, as such, will influence the decisions you make in your life, work and behaviour. Sometimes, our values and beliefs support our decisions but on occasion they can cause conflict, and this may distress us. For example, if you are good at managing your time and value meeting deadlines, you may feel conflicted if you are too busy at work to maintain this.

Environmental factors

Where you are born and where you live may have some effect on the way your beliefs and values are formed. A child born in an overcrowded and deprived environment may be more prone to illness; their education may suffer as a result and this may shape the way in which they view their world and the choices they have in life. Your upbringing and the area and family environment in which you lived will have taught you the values and belief systems that you have brought to the way in which you work. You will also have been shaped by various experiences as you have grown up.

Family/family relationships

The way in which we are introduced into the world by our family and our upbringing, together with the experiences we have had in life through education and work, all help to formulate our personal system of values and beliefs. We learn through our parents and through observation of what is happening around us about what we feel is 'good'. We are taught how to behave in a manner that is polite and acceptable to others in our family and in wider society. This will carry into our working lives and, as a manager, you are likely to work alongside people who have very different values to you. Your role in this respect is to ensure that you promote values of respect, tolerance and democracy to ensure that you embed such values into the social care culture.

Social interactions including peers

As we grow older, the different social influences and interactions increase, and our friends and peers may become more important to us. As you learn, meet new people and experience new things, you could find some of your personal values are challenged and they may change to incorporate new thinking. In a social care setting, challenges can affect not only care workers but also the people who use the service and, in your role as manager, you need to ensure that you respect or even disagree with the challenges that present themselves. For example, some people are divided on political issues and this may affect the way in which they view certain groups in society.

Culture and religion

Parents or caregivers in the early years and family culture help to influence beliefs, and this includes adopting a religion or certain cultural practices. Being exposed at a young age to a religious upbringing or traditions will affect personal beliefs, and exposure to a culture helps to shape personal values.

The culture in which we are brought up also teaches us to value different things. For example, some cultures teach respect for the environment, which can directly influence personal beliefs about how we use natural resources. Some religions teach that modern medicine is to be avoided. Your culture and religion will influence the way in which you work and, as a manager, you need to be aware of the differences of others and be tolerant of these.

Social media

The internet, Facebook, Twitter, Instagram and other forms of media are useful additions to the way in which you gain information. However, a rising concern has been the use of social media to target vulnerable individuals with the intention of radicalising them – persuading them to adopt extreme political, social or religious views. Additionally, social media can expose people to 'fake news', where news stories supported by little evidence, or often completely made up, are presented as fact. Violence is also a major part of what people may be seeing on social media and this can influence behaviour and change attitudes. As a manager in an adult care setting, it is important that you do not let any of your personal views that may have been influenced by social media affect your interactions with the people you provide support to and work with. In addition, you must be acutely aware of how your staff are engaging with social media and ensure that they are not displaying unacceptable views or posting comments that may be considered inflammatory or damaging to others.

Education, professional career and working environments/situations

In 2014, the government introduced guidance on 'Promoting fundamental British values through SMSC' (spiritual, moral, social and cultural development), which aims to promote respect for British law and democracy, and mutual respect and tolerance for those from different beliefs and faiths and individual liberty (GOV.UK, 2014). It aims to ensure that young people in schools and colleges are exposed to the beliefs of others and to different attitudes and values, which then offers them wider choices and solutions. This sort of socialisation continues in the workplace, with employers in local authorities, healthcare, education and the justice system now bound to deliver the 'Prevent' strategy to employees, which is the government response to terrorism and radicalisation (GOV.UK, 2021).

Such exposure to different points of view, values and beliefs can help you to analyse your own values and belief systems and to understand how they affect working practices and the way we live our lives. Your role will be to ensure that you are embedding British values into staff training and the ethos of the setting.

Reflect on it

2.3 How your values and beliefs have developed and/or changed through your working practices

Think about a personal value you hold and try to trace it back to your very first experience of it. How did you acquire it?

What values and beliefs have changed as a result of your work and the exposure you have had to training? For example, think about something you have learned through the course of your work, which has made you question something you may have grown up believing. Alternatively, list some examples of personal values you hold about the following:

- environment
- family/family relationships
- social interactions including your peers
- culture
- religion
- media
- education
- professional career and working environments/situations.

Think back to the first time in your life that you were aware of them and how your values and beliefs have developed and/or changed through your working practices.

What changes have you made to your beliefs as a result of the work you now do?

Write a reflective account.

How your values and beliefs have developed and/or changed through working practices

Perhaps you believe that 'what will be will be' and you are subject to whatever fate brings you. Some universally accepted values highlight honesty and respect for others. It is possible that within your family you may have been brought up in a religion and, therefore, hold certain views about how you should live your life. Some people hold beliefs that certain groups of people are not to be trusted and these beliefs or stereotypes can affect them in their work. Decisions about others are made at an unconscious level and because of biases and stereotypes we may treat people in the workplace in different and less positive ways. We may find we prefer some people to others and unconsciously deal with them in a different manner. This can lead to poor decision making and behaving differently to some groups. Many organisations are now challenging this and are training their staff in 'unconscious bias', which addresses the negative attitudes we have towards others but which we fail to realise at a conscious level.

By questioning our beliefs through education we can develop self-awareness, and this can lead to changes in attitudes and bias. Indeed, as you have grown and lived through many new experiences, you may have started to question particular views and values and changed your outlook. By paying more attention to how you feel about something, or by reflecting on experiences and being truthful to yourself about how you feel, you can start to become more self-aware. This process can then help you to choose your own values rather than merely reflecting those of others and those you learned in childhood.

You may experience this sort of process within your career as a care worker. Having your values and beliefs challenged is not always a comfortable process, but it can be very liberating. For example, if you have always held the belief that certain groups of people cannot be trusted, a challenge to that belief can be quite uncomfortable. This might lead you to either dismiss the challenge and continue with your former belief or you may challenge it yourself. You can do this by analysing what caused you to believe this in the first place and where and how you learned it. You may also ask yourself if it is valid or whether there has been a time when this belief was not true. You may even find that you have a close friend who is part of this particular group!

The answers you come up with will help you to see that the belief is not as strong as you thought it was and you can then start to change it, or it may be that your belief is strengthened.

Evidence opportunity

2.3 Values, belief systems and experiences affecting working practice

Analyse your own values and belief systems in relation to the bullet points in the Reflect on it for AC2.3.

How have they affected your working practices and how have they been shaped by various life experiences? Provide a written account detailing your response.

AC 2.4 Analyse how own emotions affect own behaviour and impact others

Here, you will analyse how your feelings affect your own work and the work of others in the setting.

Self-awareness is the knowledge you have of yourself, while social awareness refers to the empathy and concern you have for other people's feelings, for example being able to acknowledge that people under threat in an organisation may show aggression and anger. Decisions affecting people's jobs may have to be made, and the manager who sees only the task in hand is failing to acknowledge the effect this is having on those at risk and those who have to continue to work in such a climate of change.

> **Research it**
>
> **2.4 Goleman's theories**
>
> Daniel Goleman is famous for his theories about emotional intelligence and this links to self-awareness (Goleman, 1995). You looked at Goleman's theories in Unit 500 AC1.2. Do some research into Goleman's work on self-awareness and write a short account to show how it can help you to become more self-aware.

How your emotions affect your behaviour and the behaviour of others

What sort of mood are you in today? Have you come to work feeling happy, sad, angry or frustrated? How do you think the way you feel will affect how you work and behave?

The way you feel and the emotions you have will affect the decisions you make and, as a manager working with staff and vulnerable people who can sometimes be challenging, you need to be aware of how your emotions affect your work. For example, think about how you feel when you are having a difficult conversation with a member of staff or you are required to address a problem with a visitor. This might make you feel anxious and it is helpful to recognise this. Do you let the anxiety get the better of you so that in future you try to avoid the situation? The emotions that you are feeling at this time and the anxiety this brings are worth investigating and you should reflect on how you are feeling. By analysing how your emotions affect your behaviour and the behaviour of others, you will develop self-awareness. For example, is the anxiety a reaction to the person or to your own feelings and emotions? Perhaps you fear failure in this situation? Perhaps it is not the person causing the anxiety but the situation you are in.

Difficult conversations with colleagues, other professionals, individuals, their families and carers

At some point in your working life, you will have difficult conversations with people and this can be a challenge. Perhaps you find it hard to talk to people who do not share your values and beliefs. These might include colleagues, individuals you provide care and support to, other professionals such as GPs or doctors, and the families and carers of individuals. For example, if you value diversity and are highly tolerant of people's beliefs and religious views, it may be quite difficult to talk to someone who does not. This can sometimes make situations uncomfortable but as a manager you will need to overcome this and manage the emotions you experience in a professional and respectful way.

Dealing with difficult situations

The things you value and believe are sometimes tested when you are working in difficult circumstances. For example, in a busy environment, where resources are low and demand on your service is high, you may find you are unable to give the care that individuals require and this may go against your beliefs about social care and the rights of individuals. The current crisis with staffing deficiencies in social care clearly shows how difficult situations at work affect staff in many ways. In such high-pressure environments, emotions can run high and this can affect the behaviour of staff as well as the behaviour of those in receipt of care and support, other professionals and family/carers.

Managing positive and negative emotions

What is a positive or a negative emotion? If you feel happiness, joy, love and contentment, you are showing positive emotions, and this affects the way in which you relate to others and the way you carry out your work. Not only do you feel good, but the people around you are likely to feel the same. Negative emotions, on the other hand, like sadness, anger or being self-critical and fearful, can be difficult, even painful at times, and when brought into the workplace they can have a negative effect on those around you. Being aware of the impact that emotions can have and managing them so that they do not impact you and others negatively is therefore important.

> **Reflect on it**
>
> **2.4 What is self-awareness?**
>
> Can Goleman's theory help us to manage others in a more effective manner? Think about what you know about yourself and the qualities and strengths you possess. Reflect also upon your limitations. How can this knowledge help you to grow as a person and as a manager?

Research it

2.4 Difficult work situations

Do some research around some of the issues affecting adult care currently, and some of the difficult work situations that may arise as a result.

You and your staff are likely to experience stress at times, especially during pressured situations. It is important to be aware of the staff you manage and how they are experiencing their workloads. For example, people behave differently and approach tasks in different ways. For some, a project they have to complete will trigger anxiety. They will be on edge until they have finished the task. For others, the stress may become apparent as the deadline approaches, but this may also have the effect of motivating them to get on with the task. Recognising how emotions affect your staff will be a real help in your decision making.

Reflect on it

2.4 The effects of emotions

Think about an emotion that crops up in situations at work, such as anxiety or anger, and write a short reflective piece about how it affects your behaviour.

Evidence opportunity

2.4 How your emotions affect your own behaviour and behaviour of others

Analyse how your emotions affect your behaviour and the behaviour of others in respect of:

- ✔ your leadership and management role and style
- ✔ dealing with difficult situations when working with colleagues, those in receipt of care and support, other professionals and family/carers
- ✔ managing positive and negative emotions within yourself and others.

Have a professional discussion with your assessor to analyse how your own emotions affect your behaviour and the behaviour of others in respect of the topics discussed in this section. You might like to record or document your discussion.

To analyse, you will need to ask questions about the emotions you are experiencing, how they affect you, and how this compares to how others experience these emotions.

LO3 Be able to manage own workload

AC 3.1 Use strategies and tools

Here, you will demonstrate different strategies for managing your workload.

Plan and identify priorities for work

Managing your workload effectively will improve your performance and enhance your work–life balance. It will also influence your team to adopt similar practices and hopefully reduce the risk of burnout and stress. With daily challenges, deadlines to meet and daily tasks that require completion, sometimes you can feel overwhelmed by what you need to achieve, but there are tools that can help. It is vital to make a plan and to take some time to view what needs to be done. You also need to ascertain what resources are at your disposal to make the most of staff time and their talents. Some of the daily tasks can then be allocated and delegated to others. A useful tool to use for this is the Covey matrix, developed by Stephen Covey in 1989. This identifies which tasks are important and urgent, and therefore should be prioritised, and which are not, and so may be left. For a reminder of the Covey matrix, see Unit 509 LO2.

The matrix helps you to divide work activities into management and leadership responsibilities and individual and/or service demands. Your day may be busy and feel quite overwhelming at times, but taking a step back and looking carefully at the tasks you are currently doing and prioritising them into important and unimportant may reveal that you are using valuable time to deal with tasks that are not increasing productivity but rather hindering it. For example, when staffing levels are low it is tempting to try to resolve this by helping staff with their work. This is counterproductive as it takes you away from your own work and not only could that be detrimental to your wellbeing, but it also fails to provide a long-term solution to the demands of your setting.

As a manager you need to work in a way that protects your wellbeing. You should prioritise the work you do to ensure that you meet the operational plans of the organisation as well as the general management of the day-to-day business at ground level. Good time management is the key to success, along with the ability to prioritise your workload. A balanced approach will ensure that you are also mindful of your own wellbeing in what can be a very stressful profession.

Having a mentor is a useful resource as they will understand the pressures of the role and can work with you, providing support when needed. In addition, training can help you to develop skills that you may require.

Research it

3.1 The Covey matrix

Undertake a time management analysis using the Covey matrix.

- In Quadrant 1 (top left) write down all the important, urgent items that you need to deal with immediately. A lot of people work solely in this area, but this is not a good place to be. By addressing this you reduce your risk of burnout.
- In Quadrant 2 (top right) write down the important but non-urgent items that do not require your immediate attention but still need to be planned. This is a good place to be because here you have the time to spend on important tasks.
- In Quadrant 3 (bottom left) highlight unimportant but urgent items that can be minimised or eliminated.
- In Quadrant 4 (bottom right) write down the unimportant and non-urgent items or the things that should be minimised or eliminated as these are the true time wasters.

Examples to help you are given below.

Important/urgent e.g. responding to the needs of an individual in your care	Important/non-urgent e.g. responding to interruptions from people knocking on your door
Unimportant/urgent e.g. arranging a staff meeting	Unimportant/non-urgent e.g. surfing the net or Facebook

Reflect on it

3.1 Time management

Having completed the time management exercise, you will be in a better position to see just how much time you really have.

Make notes about how time saved can be used towards better management of individuals in the workplace and the service demands of the organisation.

Revise plans when priorities change

One of the challenges of managing an adult care provision is that circumstances change rapidly. The needs of the individuals using the service are ever changing, and you may also be subject to unexpected situations arising from stakeholders and other services. For example, if an emergency arises with an individual, redeployment of staff may be required, placing demands on the setting. Staff may be required to escort individuals to other settings, leaving staffing short on your site, or domiciliary care staff and outreach workers may have traffic issues on the way to an urgent meeting with an individual in their care. These types of occurrences invariably increase demands upon staff.

As the manager, you need to be flexible and manage change in a calm and efficient manner. Plans may need to be adjusted and staff may need to be redeployed to accommodate changes.

Every day you are faced with challenges ranging from staff sickness to major incidents and everything in between. How you deal with unexpected demands upon your time is a useful measurement of how successful you are as a manager. Some managers are immediately stressed by any change; others do not deal well with staff who phone in sick. You may have been fortunate to work with managers who seem to be unfazed by emergencies and deal with them efficiently and with calm and ease. Which sort of manager do you aspire to be and how will you attain this?

Staff sickness demands that a manager responds by reallocating tasks, responsibilities and workload and perhaps liaising with agencies to access temporary staff. If the staff sickness is likely to be long term, you may need to have a contingency plan in place to assess your options and to understand what your responsibilities are with respect to handling the member of staff who is off sick.

Revise plans to take account of changing circumstances

You will need to show your assessor how you adjust your work to take into account changes in operational circumstances, like the ones discussed in this section. You could also request a witness testimony if this is agreed by your assessor and the individuals you approach.

Case study

Changing plans, revising circumstances

You come into work and have two staff off sick, a complaint from a relative about the care of their son who has autism and a deadline to meet on a report, which has proved very challenging to fulfil. How will you plan your day?

Provide a written account detailing your response to the above scenario. Then explain how you revise plans to take account of changing circumstances, including:

- staff absence and sickness
- needs and challenges presented by individuals in receipt of care and support
- unscheduled and unexpected demands from others – internal and external.

Access support mechanisms when workload is difficult to manage

An efficient business is a successful one and whether it is a large organisation or a small, family-run one every part of the organisation should recognise how it contributes to the overall success. It requires that every employee recognises their part in working together to reach the ultimate mission statement of the business. For example, in a large organisation employees need to be aware that strategic objectives are linked to departmental and team objectives and that their part in meeting team objectives is crucial to success. Organisations therefore need to take time to implement processes that reinforce this. When your workload becomes difficult to manage, staff need to be approached for help.

If you are working in a small setting you will still be working to objectives and will likely be made aware of the mission statement of the setting and its vision.

Work culture refers to the beliefs and attitudes of the employees and the ideologies and principles of the organisation. For example, the work culture may be one in which employees follow the rules and regulations and adhere to the existing guidelines and, as a result, are satisfied employees who respect each other and are valued by the employer. They will then be happy to support you when necessary.

Support can also be sought from your line manager. Regular updates about what is happening in the setting will keep higher management informed of any additional resources you might need to do your job.

Workforce planning

Workforce planning is about addressing two basic premises in terms of the workforce: how many staff and what sort of staff you need. You will need to understand the skills each team member has and ensure that during each period of duty the right people with the right skills are in place to deliver the care required. When putting together a workforce development plan, you should:

- identify the skills mix needed to deliver the sort of service you provide
- arrange any staff training needed to meet the needs of the individuals using your service
- look carefully at the working practices and the responsibilities of each staff member
- look at costs of staff and determine how these can be optimised.

Workforce planning is not only about your current provision; you need to consider future changes to the type or number of individuals coming to your setting so that your plan can highlight gaps to be filled.

You will require support from your own manager, particularly if you are currently experiencing a shortfall in staff. Support for partners and stakeholders may be sought and new ways of working in partnership might be part of your workforce plan for the future. For more on developing a workforce development plan, see Unit 503 AC1.2 and AC1.3.

Research it

3.1 Skills for care

The Skills for Care website provides guidance on 'Operational workforce planning', which describes how effective workforce planning can ensure that your setting is delivering personalised, safe and good quality services to individuals (Skills for Care, n.d.).

Make notes on the guidance and conduct checks against your own setting. How can you make improvements to your setting?

Evidence opportunity

3.1 Strategies and tools to identify priorities for work

Develop a workforce development plan for your setting. Start by giving evidence of the strategies and tools you use to identify the operational management priorities when setting priorities and goals for your teams.

AC 3.2 Use digital technology to enhance own and others' efficiency

Here, you will be required to demonstrate the application of different types of technology, which can enhance your efficiency at work and work plans.

Email

Email has certainly transformed business. Messages are fast and can be sent at any time of the day, and as long as you have access to a digital device, such as a laptop or a phone, you are able to send and receive email anywhere. Large files can be sent inexpensively and to multiple recipients, cutting out postage costs.

The disadvantages, however, are that emails can leave you open to viruses and spam, which can result in security issues and time wasting. Installing anti-virus and malware software is essential to ensure that your systems are not easily open to hacking. You and your staff should also use email efficiently and this might, for example, mean only checking emails at certain times of the day.

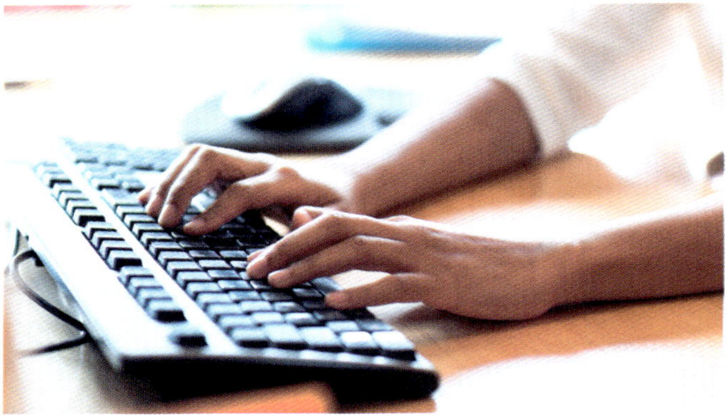

▲ **Figure 37** How do you promote efficiency in your staff by using digital technology?

Electronic reporting systems and specialist software for care plans/auditing

In care work, the use of electronic reporting systems, specialist software for logging observations and e-learning software has changed the way in which staff operate. There is also a wealth of auditing software that can be used to perform health and safety assessments and quality assurance tests.

It is now possible to inform other services of an individual's status simply by logging their current observations, results and status into a handheld device, which can then be accessed via a similar device in a setting. A disadvantage is that handheld devices can malfunction. Also, internet or broadband speed can cause delays.

e-learning software

A good example of an e-learning platform is Smart Screen, which provides high-quality online teaching and learning support. Aptem is another resource tool providing video, audio and text for students on diplomas in management and apprenticeships, such as those offered by Corndel. See their websites for further details.

One of the advantages of using e-learning software is that it can be accessed at various locations, which means you can undertake a course from your own home. Some courses are self-explanatory and are offered without tutor support, so you do not have to pay for someone to teach the course. A disadvantage is that sometimes the internet is unreliable and broadband access can be slow in some areas. It can be frustrating when access is unavailable.

Social media systems

Social media can be an effective way to engage and motivate staff if you use it appropriately. One advantage is that private groups can be set up on social media platforms to discuss topics on adult care in the news or to debate best practice. Social media can also be used to organise social gatherings.

The disadvantages are that not all staff may want to be part of such groups or may not be able to access the sites for various reasons. Also, there is a danger that confidential matters about individuals in your setting will be discussed in such groups. This is not the forum for such discussions.

Electronic conferencing

Electronic conferencing, such as Teams, Facetime, Google Meet and Zoom, enables you to speak face to face with people in different locations. The biggest advantages of electronic conferencing are that it enables meetings to take place without the need to travel and, during the COVID-19 pandemic, it became a powerful resource for keeping teams in touch with each other while working remotely. However, the disadvantages are that sometimes the internet cannot be relied upon to work when needed and some people may not have access to the software or be comfortable using it.

Research it

3.2 Specialist software

Research some of the specialist software that is available for care/support plans and auditing in adult care settings. You might, for example, wish to explore VitalPAC.

Evidence opportunity

3.2 Digital technology

Demonstrate the application of different types of technology that can enhance your efficiency at work and your work plans. Examples may include the ones discussed in this section. Provide a written account.

You might like to look at the headings in this section and compile a list of how these different types of technology have improved your ways of working. In each case, say which systems you use and how they have enhanced your work.

AC 3.3 Facilitate the development of team members to enable effective delegation

Here, you will be required to show how delegating is part of effective team management.

Delegation means giving a task to another member of staff to complete on your behalf. For example, you may delegate the task of compiling the work rota to another care worker, enabling you to do other things, which may be a more effective use of your time. You will need to use your judgement to ensure that you pick the right people to delegate tasks to; it must be someone who has the skills and knowledge to complete the task safely and effectively. It may be that you need to give them clear instructions, or even training if this is a bigger task. You must also ensure that the person you have delegated the task to has agreed to accept the task and supervise them if needed. As the manager, you are accountable for delegating the activity and must undertake to oversee the member of staff carrying out the task.

Delegation is a good way to empower employees, making them more motivated if they have been given tasks that managers would normally do. However, you should also be aware that it can have the opposite effect if they are being given mundane tasks to carry out that simply add to their workload rather than enhance their role.

Stretch and challenge

3.3 Delegating responsibilities to others

Show how delegation is part of your effective team management. You might like to demonstrate how you develop staff skills in order to make delegation possible in the future, and how you monitor the delegation process.

AC 3.4 Reflect on impact on own wellbeing when planning and responding to organisation priorities

Here, you will reflect on your own wellbeing and how this can be affected by your work.

Workplace culture can support or hinder your own and your staff's wellbeing. A culture that supports you to improve yourself in terms of career opportunities and encourages you to have a healthy work–life balance is one that will be successful. Organisational priorities and the ever-changing dynamic of care work will always be a challenge but it should never be to the detriment of your own or your team's health. Feeling stressed about deadlines or completing tasks is likely to lead to burnout and sickness. Limiting the amount of overtime you do and turning email notifications off when you are off duty is a good start. Make sure you take time to have a break and to eat. Taking holidays and switching off completely will also help. The staff will be led by your example so start to reinforce the idea of wellbeing and develop habits to show that this needs to come first.

Reflect on it

3.4 Organisational priorities and their impact on own wellbeing

What impact on your own wellbeing have you noticed when planning and responding to organisational priorities? What one thing can you change to improve your wellbeing?

Legislation

Legislation	Key points
Mental Health Act 1983, 2007 Mental Capacity Act 2005	While legislation relevant to mental health and capacity is not wholly relevant here, you should be aware of the issues around mental health and wellbeing for yourself, your staff, individuals in your setting and others you work with.

References

Barbe, W.B., Swassing, R.H. and Milone, M.N. (1979) *Teaching Through Modality Strengths: Concepts and practices*. Columbus, OH: Zaner-Bloser.

Chartered Institute of Personnel and Development (2022) 'Performance reviews: Understand the basics of performance reviews and how the process adds value to the organisation'. www.cipd.co.uk/knowledge/fundamentals/people/performance/appraisals-factsheet#gref

Covey, S. (1989) *The 7 Habits of Highly Effective People*. New York: Simon & Schuster.

Gibbs, G. (1988) *Learning by Doing: A guide to teaching and learning methods*. Oxford: Oxford Further Education Unit.

Goleman, D. (1995) *Emotional Intelligence*. New York: Bantam Books.

GOV.UK (2014) 'Promoting fundamental British values through SMSC'. www.gov.uk/government/publications/promoting-fundamental-british-values-through-smsc

GOV.UK (2021) 'Prevent duty guidance'. www.gov.uk/government/publications/prevent-duty-guidance

Honey, P. and Mumford, A. (1992) *Learning Styles Questionnaire*, Peter Honey Publications Ltd.

Skills for Care (n.d.) 'Operational workforce planning'. www.skillsforcare.org.uk/Support-for-leaders-and-managers/Workforce-commissioning-planning/Operational-workforce-planning.aspx

Useful resources and further reading

American Psychological Association (n.d.) 'Resilience'. www.apa.org/topics/resilience

Aptem. www.aptem.co.uk

Corndel Management College. www.corndel.com

GOV.UK (2016) 'Care Act 2014 factsheets'. www.gov.uk/government/publications/care-act-2014-part-1-factsheets/care-act-factsheets

Institute for Public Policy Research (2021) 'Revealed: NHS and care integration postcode lottery leading to unequal access to treatment and support'. www.ippr.org/news-and-media/press-releases/revealed-nhs-and-care-integration-postcode-lottery-leading-to-unequal-access-to-treatment-and-support

Psychology Today (n.d.), 'Resilience'. www.psychologytoday.com/basics/resilience

Social Care Institute for Excellence (2006) 'Workforce development'. www.scie.org.uk/workforce/Peoplemanagement/leadership/workforcedev/index.asp

Unit 520

Personal wellbeing for leaders and managers in adult care services

GLH 15

About this unit

Personal wellbeing is an important aspect of an organisation's culture and it is expected that employees are cared for in the workplace. While some organisations only comply with the basics, such as providing drinking water, sufficient toilet facilities, ventilation and heating, others recognise the importance of attracting and maintaining staff so are opting to provide benefits such as a subscription to a local gym, a cycle to work scheme, flexible working and childcare subsidies. As a manager, you will need to consider your role with regard to your own health and wellbeing and to ensure that your setting is a healthy place to work. In this unit you will also look at how to manage stress and anxiety.

Learning outcomes

By the end of this unit you will:

1 Understand own wellbeing.
2 Understand the importance of maintaining and improving own wellbeing.
3 Know how to maintain and improve own wellbeing.
4 Know how to manage own stress and anxiety.

Getting started

Before you study the unit, think about the following:

- What is the impact on personal wellbeing of undertaking a leadership and management role?
- What are the responsibilities of self, and the effects of not managing own wellbeing on others?
- What is the relation of resilience to stress and anxiety?

LO1 Understand own wellbeing

AC 1.1 Explain what is meant by personal wellbeing, self-care and resilience

Here, you will explain what is meant by wellbeing, learn about the factors that influence health and wellbeing and be able to recognise deterioration.

Personal wellbeing

Wellbeing is a subjective concept and is therefore personal. It can be affected by environmental factors or events experienced recently as well as many years ago. Personal wellbeing is about how we feel about ourselves and the quality of the relationships we have with others and is also our sense of purpose in the world. Our psychological needs are part of what makes us human and the emotions we experience, both positive and negative, matter to how we feel about ourselves and how happy we are.

The Office for National Statistics defines wellbeing using ten broad dimensions in its 'Measuring National Wellbeing Programme' (ONS, 2019). These are:

- personal wellbeing
- our relationships
- health
- what we do
- where we live
- personal finance
- economy
- education and skills
- governance
- environment.

Personal wellbeing is about how satisfied we are with our lives, and whether what we do in life is worthwhile. It is about how we experience happiness and anxiety and how that affects us.

Self-care

The World Health Organization's (WHO) definition of self-care is:

> *the ability of individuals, families and communities to promote health, prevent disease, maintain health, and cope with illness and disability with or without the support of a health worker.*

Source: WHO (n.d.)

Self-care is about making sound decisions based on knowledge to empower us to look after our own health and wellbeing. It involves making healthy lifestyle choices and avoiding unhealthy habits. It means being responsible in our use of prescription and non-prescription medicines and monitoring ourselves for signs of stress and anxiety, seeking help if necessary.

Resilience

The American Psychological Association defines resilience as 'the process and the outcome of successfully adapting to difficult or challenging life experiences' (APA, 2022). Resilience is the ability to adjust and demonstrate flexibility when faced with difficult situations and emotions. Everyone experiences stress and emotional suffering. When you are resilient you are more able to deal with the difficult issues and bounce back more quickly. Individuals who lack resilience may be overwhelmed and then seek out unhealthy coping mechanisms, such as alcohol or drugs. Resilient people look at their strengths and other support systems and use them to help them deal with challenges.

Care and support statutory guidance produced by the Department of Health and Social Care (GOV.UK, 2022) defines wellbeing as a broad concept. Although it was specifically designed for individuals using care services, you can still identify with the concepts it outlines and apply them to your own experience. Wellbeing relates to the following areas:

- personal dignity (including treatment with respect)
- physical and mental health and emotional wellbeing
- protection from abuse and neglect
- control by the individual over day-to-day life (including care and support)
- participation in work, education, training or recreation
- social and economic wellbeing, which means being actively engaged with life and with other people and having a positive standard of living based primarily on financial security
- domestic, family relationships and personal issues
- suitability of living accommodation
- the individual's contribution to society.

Caring for your own wellbeing requires you to be able to measure your state of wellbeing. When things are not going well, you may start to experience stress, worry and anxiety. Your psychological wellbeing becomes compromised and this will inevitably lead to a reduction in your quality of life. This can lead to depression and its subsequent effects on physical wellbeing and health.

Reflect on it

1.1 Resilience

Think about a person you consider to be resilient and another who lacks this quality.

How do they each react to a setback in life?

What effects do you think these reactions have on them?

AC 1.2 Describe factors that positively and negatively influence own wellbeing

Here, you will describe the lifestyle factors that may affect your own wellbeing.

A number of factors can affect your wellbeing. The NHS sets out five steps to mental wellbeing:

1. Connect with other people and build good relationships to help provide a sense of belonging and self-worth.
2. Be physically active, which will help to raise self-esteem.
3. Learn new skills to boost self-confidence and help build a sense of purpose.
4. Give to others. Research has shown that acts of giving and kindness can help improve mental wellbeing as they create positive feelings, a sense of reward and help you to connect with others.
5. Pay attention to the present moment and practice being mindful. This can positively change the way you feel about life and build resilience and is simply the practice of paying attention to the present moment and reflecting on your thoughts and feelings.

Source: Adapted from NHS (2022a)

In the period 2016–18, the Office for National Statistics (ONS) reported that in the UK 2.3 million people said their life satisfaction was low and 10.4 million were experiencing high anxiety. People with poor personal wellbeing are likely to be experiencing at least one of the following characteristics or circumstances:

- being in bad or very bad health
- unable to work due to long-term illness or disability
- being middle-aged and/or single, separated, widowed or divorced, which may lead to isolation and loneliness
- living in rented accommodation
- having little or no education.

Source: Adapted from What Works Wellbeing (n.d.)

Your genetic makeup, life experiences, upbringing and where you live all affect your health and wellbeing, both negatively or positively. Understanding how you think and respond to the situations you face can make it easier to ask for support when you need it.

Reflect on it

1.2 Factors influencing own health

Think about your own lifestyle and list the positive and negative factors influencing your health. What can you change?

AC 1.3 Describe indicators of own wellbeing

AC 1.4 Describe indicators that own wellbeing may be deteriorating

Here, you will describe your own wellbeing.

Reflect on it

1.3 and **1.4** Review own wellbeing

The ONS asks four personal wellbeing questions in its survey. People are asked to respond to the questions on a scale from 0 to 10, where 0 is 'not at all' and 10 is 'completely'. You can view the questions in 'Table 1: Four measures of personal well-being' at ONS (2018).

Answer the questions honestly then analyse your results. Do they suggest that your wellbeing is deteriorating or improving? Which areas of your wellbeing are most at risk and require intervention?

Evidence opportunity

1.3 and **1.4** Review own wellbeing

Describe how you feel when you are particularly well and describe the triggers or indicators that show that your wellbeing is deteriorating.

LO2 Understand the importance of maintaining and improving own wellbeing

AC 2.1 Analyse how own wellbeing impacts role and behaviour

Here, you will analyse how your wellbeing impacts areas of your work and others.

The Department of Health publication 'Wellbeing: Why it matters to health policy' (Department of Health, 2014) explains how wellbeing positively affects people's lives. Although the article is referring to health behaviours and illness it can still be applied to adult social care.

1. **Adds years to life**: Research shows that happy people live longer: subjective (or personal) wellbeing directly asks what people think and feel about their own wellbeing, to ascertain their life satisfaction, level of positive emotions and whether they feel their life has meaning. According to Diener and Chan (2011), high levels of subjective wellbeing contribute to better health and increased life expectancy compared with those with low levels of subjective wellbeing.
2. **Improves recovery from illness**: High levels of subjective wellbeing can protect an individual from developing illnesses. For example, individuals who experience positive emotions show greater resistance to developing the common cold. Additionally, people who had a tendency to experience negative emotions reported more unverified health complaints and more symptoms of other conditions (Cohen et al., 2003).
3. **Is associated with health behaviours in adults**: People with high wellbeing are more likely to eat healthily, undertake physical activity and are less likely to smoke. Smoking, excessive alcohol consumption and obesity are all to linked to a reduced wellbeing and health status.
4. **Is associated with broader positive outcomes**: Employment, crime, relationships and education all have an effect on wellbeing. Being unemployed reduces life satisfaction while being married improves it. Social isolation negatively impacts wellbeing. People who have spent less time in education have also been found to have higher levels of depression and anxiety, while those with higher levels of qualifications and who have continued formal and informal learning tend to have greater subjective wellbeing (ONS, 2012).
5. **Influences the wellbeing and mental health of those close to us**: Happiness spreads through social networks and if we are in close contact with happy people, we become happier as a result (Fowler and Christakis, 2008).
6. **Affects how care sector staff and providers work**: 'Where patients rate the care they receive as "bad", staff also feel their wellbeing is low due to the demands of their job and the risk of burnout. However, where patients rate their care as "good", staff feel much more supported, in a good team and with high job satisfaction' (Maben et al., 2012).
7. **Has implications for care practices and services**: The experience of illness and the services people receive is connected to how well and how quickly they recover. According to Thin (2010), giving individuals choice and ensuring that the care environment is attractive can positively affect their recovery and longevity.

Source: Adapted from Department of Health (2014)

Evidence opportunity

2.1 Analyse factors that impact own wellbeing

How does your wellbeing impact your behaviour and your role?

Analyse the effect this has on the way in which you do your job.

What changes will you make to improve your own wellbeing?

AC 2.2 Explain how own wellbeing impacts others

Here, you will explain the effects of any decline in your wellbeing on your colleagues and others.

Consider for a moment working in an environment where everybody is happy and content. Your team and the individuals, their families and visitors all display a good mood. You may also be in a good mood. Research supports the notion that happiness can be contagious – we can catch it from others and pass it on!

The Framingham Heart Study was a 20-year study by Fowler and Christakis (2008) that evaluated whether happiness can spread from person to person and whether niches of happiness form within social networks. Their findings showed that groups of happy and unhappy people were seen in the network, but that people's happiness can extend up to three degrees of separation, meaning that people who are surrounded by many happy people are more likely to become happy in the future. There was also the suggestion that clusters of happiness result from the spread of happiness. The conclusions showed that a person's happiness is affected by the happiness of the people to whom they are connected.

Our brains have a complex neural system and contain mirror neurons, which are responsible for us feeling empathy. Mirror neurons are brain cells that respond when we perform an action and also when we witness someone else perform the same action. For example, we may feel sympathy if we see somebody in pain, or we may feel excitement when we see a goal scored in a football match. Watching an action and performing an action could elicit the same feelings in people.

We experience the feelings of others inside ourselves so, for example, when we smile, others invariably do so as well. If we laugh, we find others joining in. Our good feelings can spread to others.

Your wellbeing can have a positive effect on others and helps you to bond and build better relationships. It can positively help you and your loved ones to have better health and will result in fewer conflicts.

Everyone has off days, but if you are often experiencing negative emotions then you should seek support rather than trying to repress them. Taking care of yourself and improving your wellbeing will affect those around you in a positive way. By practicing gratitude, mindfulness and compassion you may find that those around you also cope better with their own problems.

Mindfulness is a way of engaging with and paying attention to the present moment, using techniques such as meditation and breathing.

If we practice mindfulness, we become more aware of our thoughts, feelings and bodily sensations. If, for example, you are feeling overwhelmed, mindfulness can help you to feel calmer. A good exercise is to pay attention and take the time to experience your environment with all of your senses: touch, sound, sight, smell and taste. If you feel anxious, a useful exercise related to this is to think about five things you can see, four things you can touch, three things you can hear, two things you can smell and one thing you can taste in that moment. Practising this can reduce anxiety and calm the mind.

Evidence opportunity

2.2 How own wellbeing impacts others

How does your wellbeing, or lack thereof, affect those with whom you live and work. Describe how those around you are affected by your good days and your bad days.

AC 2.3 Describe challenges to own wellbeing

Here, you will describe the challenges to your own wellbeing and review your work–life balance.

One particular area for leaders to address is their work–life balance. Time is always an issue and you might find that the harder you work, the more the work piles up. Take a step back and think about how you can address this area of your life.

Reflect on it

2.3 Anxiety and stress

Think about the anxiety and stress in your life. Does it stop you from making decisions as you spend time listening to all options and opinions before taking action? If you are busy are you too tired to go to activities after work? Make some notes.

LO3 Know how to maintain and improve own wellbeing

AC 3.1 Explain why it is important to maintain and improve own wellbeing

Here, you will explain how to improve and maintain your own wellbeing.

We all know that a healthy diet and exercise are essential for our health and that having a good work–life balance is important. Yet we often ignore these things. So why is it important that we maintain our wellbeing?

Mental, physical and social wellbeing are interlinked. Good mental health is needed for a healthy lifestyle, good physical health and the ability to recover from illness. There are also social benefits of positive mental health including improved educational attainment, economic productivity, better relationships, social cohesion and overall quality of life.

Your wellbeing benefits you and others around you. Before you can promote a healthy lifestyle to your staff and the individuals using your service, you may need to make changes to how you live.

The NHS and Mind websites offer guidance about how your mental and physical wellbeing can be improved and maintained. For more information, go to the Mind website and NHS (2022).

AC 3.2 Identify a range of wellbeing support offers available to self and how to access them

Here, you will identify a range of support and how to access it.

The daily stresses of a busy workload and the inevitable lack of time to do essential work impacts the time you can spend on yourself. This can lead you to miss breaks at work, skip lunch and perhaps leave work late, all of which mean you are too exhausted to participate in the things you know will improve your lifestyle. It is important to take time to find ways to self-support your wellbeing and to look at ways you can improve the time you have available for yourself. If you require additional help to improve your wellbeing then your GP can suggest support groups or other ways in which you can get help.

Your setting may also subscribe to an employee assistance programme (EAP) should you require help with wellbeing.

Reflect on it

3.1 and 3.2 Improving own wellbeing

Take a few moments to think about the last week at work. How many breaks did you manage to take or lunches where you were not sitting at your desk? What exercise did you do? Who did you spend time with outside work?

Now think about time. You probably feel you don't have enough! There are 168 hours in a week. If you sleep for 8 hours a night that leaves 112 hours. If you work on average 40 hours a week that leaves 72 hours in the week after sleep and work have been taken into account. What are you doing in that time? Can you try to find time to do at least one of the following to improve your wellbeing?

- Arrange to meet a friend outside work.
- Spend part of your day with your family and take time to have a meal together.
- Switch off your phone for the evening and spend your free time doing something other than looking at social media.
- Undertake some exercise. Walking and running are free! Couch to 5K is a great way to start your regime. See NHS (2020).
- Learning a new skill can improve your self-esteem. Perhaps you could try out some new recipes or undertake a DIY project. There are also many free online courses where you can learn a language or develop a new skill.
- Undertake to help others. Research shows that acts of giving and kindness improve mental wellbeing by creating positive feelings and fostering a sense of purpose. Bake a cake for the team or think of a way that will show how you value them.
- During a busy day, undertake a reflective mindfulness activity.

AC 3.3 Explain strategies that maintain and improve own wellbeing

Here, you will explain strategies to maintain work–life balance and improve your own wellbeing.

We often prioritise work activity over wellbeing but it is important to develop strategies to help maintain wellbeing and to recognise when our wellbeing is deteriorating. One strategy you might use is the Covey matrix (Covey, 2004), which helps to identify which tasks are important and urgent as opposed to those which are important and non-urgent and may be left. Look at Unit 509 LO2 and Unit 519 AC3.1 for more on the Covey matrix.

Evidence opportunity

3.3 Wellbeing strategies

Explain strategies that you use to maintain and improve your own wellbeing.

Reflect on it

3.3 Using a Covey matrix

Using a Covey matrix, identify how you can make more time for your wellbeing. What might you now consign to the 'important and non-urgent' box which may have been previously placed in the 'important and urgent' box? Is there a lifestyle change you can think of?

A good work–life balance means that you can switch off from work when you go home and not allow work to intrude upon your home life. You need to set boundaries so that you work within the relevant timeframes, and do not spend time working at home, such as answering work emails. This could involve making sure you leave work on time and avoiding staying late. As a manager, you might feel that you are in a senior role and need to take work home with you. This might be something that you need to do at times, but you should not make a habit of it. If work demands are starting to impact your home life and leisure time then you are at risk of developing stress. There may be training that you can attend which can help with time management and working smartly.

Reflect on it

3.3 Planning strategies to maintain own wellbeing

How do you plan to meet your work priorities while maintaining your wellbeing?

Explain to your assessor or demonstrate to them how you do this. You could also write down how you are able to do this.

AC 3.4 Describe how to access support if needing professional therapeutic help to maintain own wellbeing

Here, you will describe the potential sources of support for your wellbeing.

If you feel that your wellbeing is being negatively affected to such an extent that it is causing you concern, then you may need to seek professional help. Symptoms of mental ill health, such as anxiety or depression, will affect the way you function in your daily life, so additional support can make a real difference to your mental health and wellbeing.

Start by speaking to your GP who can then work with you to find the right treatment. There are also local mental health support groups that can provide support when you require it. You could also contact a mental health professional such as a counsellor, therapist or psychologist. Do not underestimate the power of simply talking to a trusted friend or colleague, too.

Stretch and challenge

3.4 Provide details of local therapists and counsellors

Compile a list of local therapists and counsellors who you might be able to access should you require it.

LO4 Know how to manage own stress and anxiety

AC 4.1 Define what is meant by 'stress' and 'anxiety'

Here, you will be able to define stress and anxiety.

When the demands of work and life become too much, you may become stressed, which in turn can bring about anxiety. It is useful to know how you behave in times of stress and what makes you feel overwhelmed so that you can develop strategies to help you deal with it.

Other signs include showing irritation and anger towards others. You should be able to recognise these types of behaviours in yourself and find ways to overcome the stress in order to avoid serious health issues. You may find you are working too hard to maintain good health and this should encourage you to take a step back from work to try to achieve a good work–life balance. It is important to include yourself in any plans you make to help your staff to achieve a good work–life balance.

Relationship between pressure, anxiety and stress

When we feel under pressure, we often use the term 'stress' to describe it. Feeling unable to cope with the demands being put on us can lead to feelings of anxiety. This may well affect our work and can have an impact upon the people we work and live with. It might also affect the individuals we are caring for.

No matter how stressed you feel, it is inappropriate to take this out on those you care for. A care worker under stress and pressured to work more quickly may leave out parts of care that are essential for the wellbeing of others.

Psychological stress includes symptoms of anxiety and tension, and there may be a tendency for the sufferer to worry about things over which they have no control.

People who are irritable and distracted may also be unable to concentrate. The mind–body connection means that once these psychological symptoms are in place, physical symptoms of stress soon emerge and these can include difficulty in sleeping, loss of appetite or a tendency to overeat, tiredness, and aches and pains.

Stress affects us all in different ways and is a normal reaction when we are under pressure. It is often caused by something we think is harmful or poses a danger or threat to us. In such situations, when we are overwhelmed, tense or emotional, our body will react with the 'fight or flight' mechanism. Raised heart and breathing rates signify to us that our body is preparing to meet the challenge and is recognised biologically and psychologically. On a positive note, it is telling us that our body is working well to help us. This helps us to guard ourselves or fight and the body begins to secrete adrenaline to help us to do this. This can be harmful if the body remains in this state for long periods of time, however.

As a manager, you'll need to understand the causes of stress so that you are able to manage this in yourself. Work-related stress is not something that magically disappears when you return home and its continual presence can affect health and wellbeing and become chronic. This can lead to time off to deal with health issues such as high blood pressure, sleep problems and even heart disease and depression.

When dealing with the first signs of stress, it is a good idea to be aware of your stressors. Identify any situations at work that seem to create the most stress for you and analyse how you respond. For example, do you lose your temper, or find some other distraction to alleviate the feelings?

By looking at your diet and exercise regimes you can start to develop healthy responses to alleviating stress. Set boundaries with respect to how often you check work emails and make work phone calls when at home. Finding ways to switch off from work is important and taking time to relax is also helpful. Finally, you should seek support from work colleagues or your line manager and perhaps have discussions with a counsellor for additional help.

Reflect on it

4.1 Stress and anxiety

What is your definition of stress and anxiety? What do you spend time worrying about? What things cause your pulse rate to rise? Does this lead to anxiety and stress?

Take some time to think about how this affects your body, both mentally and physically, then make a determined effort to recognise the stressors and deal with them.

AC 4.2 Identify indicators of stress and anxiety in oneself

Here, you will identify the indicators of stress and anxiety.

Signs and symptoms of stress

Signs and symptoms of prolonged stress may include the following:

- problems with thought processes and only seeing the negative in life
- memory and concentration issues
- constant anxiety and worry
- irritability
- mood swings
- depression and isolation
- unexplained aches and pains
- upset digestive tract causing diarrhoea or constipation, nausea, dizziness
- chest pain, rapid heartbeat
- loss of sex drive/libido
- frequent infections
- poor sleeping habits
- using alcohol, cigarettes or drugs to relax
- low energy
- insomnia.

Only you can say how your own stress manifests itself and you need to be aware of the symptoms. Stress has a tendency to slowly accumulate so you are unaware of it happening until it is too late, and you suddenly feel overwhelmed. If you are aware of the signs and symptoms you can ensure that you are able to implement strategies to manage stress and maintain your own wellbeing and that of the people you support.

Reflect on it

4.2 Identifying symptoms of stress

Identify how stress in your life manifests itself.

What symptoms do you have? Once you recognise these symptoms for what they are, there is a tendency for them to lose their power.

AC 4.3 Describe factors that can trigger stress and anxiety in oneself

Here, you will describe your own possible sources of stress and anxiety.

Stress comes about as a response to many situations and can be triggered as a result of external stressors such as managing difficult situations and people, as well as the pressures associated with the day-to-day running of a department. Internal stressors come about as the result of the emotions and thoughts that sometimes cause you to feel uneasy.

External pressures come from the workplace itself and situations that develop daily with the individuals within the setting. They may be mundane issues, such as the duty rota or people calling in sick or even equipment not working, but they can all lead to pressure. These sources of stress are quite common and being aware of how they affect you and what situations may trigger them is the first line of defence in handling them. For example, if you find giving presentations to senior management or having difficult conversations with people in your team cause you anxiety, take some time to understand how you are feeling and develop ways that will help you manage the situations.

Stress triggers

These are stimuli that cause a stress response in you. They can come from external events or internal thoughts. For example, any major life change, even positive ones, such as promotion at work or moving house, or negative ones, such as illness or divorce, can trigger feelings of anxiety. At work, you may feel overburdened by an ever-increasing workload, or endless emails and urgent deadlines. Your internal thoughts may also trigger stress. Your beliefs, attitudes and even your fears come into play here. A fear of failure, for example, may cause stress to develop when you feel uncertain about what is happening around you, and may make you feel like you are losing control.

It is important to be aware of what triggers your stress levels and how they then affect your mind and body, so that you can better deal with stress. You may, for example, feel your heart rate increase slightly when there are work pressures or your workload has increased. If you are aware of these changes, then you can start to think about strategies to overcome them. You might, for example, take some time out and go for a walk.

Research it

4.3 Dealing with stress

Go to the NHS website and look at the section on stress and, in particular, the section 'Things you can try to help with stress' (NHS, 2022b). How might you use some of these suggestions to deal with your triggers?

AC 4.4 Explain how stress and anxiety may affect own reactions and behaviours towards others

Here, you will explain the effect that your stress may have on colleagues and others.

If a specific situation triggered stress in the past, you may experience a similar response if you encounter the situation again. For example, when things get pressured at work you might start to behave differently towards the staff. Maybe the pressure makes you become less amiable and more demanding. It might also mean you begin to give out orders, which is not your usual style. It is possible that the last time you had this sort of pressure you were concerned that you would not meet targets or be able to give a good standard of care, which may put the safety of individuals using your service at risk. Being faced with a similar situation now means you experience similar feelings and you may behave out of character again. This can affect how others view you and you may worry that you will lose credibility.

This type of behaviour has been shaped by a previous experience, which can be physical or emotional. This leads to a physical reaction, which repeats again and again when a similar situation occurs unless the pattern is interrupted. By understanding this you have the opportunity to change it by choosing another way to behave. You can start to think about alternative behaviours and make a conscious decision not to behave in this way. For example, you can start to analyse why the situation is troubling you and reframe it in your mind. Perhaps you are afraid of looking foolish or not coping. By looking at the situation from a different angle you may start to change the way you react.

Evidence opportunity

4.4 Impact of stress on own behaviour

Explain how stress and anxiety affect your behaviour towards others. Does your team know when you are stressed because of the behaviour you show?

AC 4.5 Explain how stress and anxiety may affect own health

Here you will explain the physical effects of stress on the body.

Stress symptoms affect us both physically and mentally. A common ailment, such as a cold or feeling sick or dizzy, may be put down to a virus but stress may be the cause. Being able to recognise common stress symptoms can help you to manage them (see AC4.2). Stress that is simply allowed to continue may lead to health problems such as high blood pressure, heart disease, obesity and diabetes.

Your behaviour can also be affected by stress symptoms. For example, having a headache may be due to anxiety and this can lead to either over or undereating.

A stomach upset could be due to sadness or depression but could mean that you don't take as much exercise as you should. Muscle or joint pains may occur, which could also stop you from doing exercise, and you might start to rely on sugary snacks, alcohol or smoking to help you manage stress.

Stress and anxiety have been shown to have long-term effects on the body and mind. Anxiety has been linked to chronic illnesses, such as gastrointestinal and digestive disorders and heart disease (Harvard, 2008).

In an article about Generalized Anxiety Disorder (GAD), The Mayo Clinic (2017) cited other symptoms such as worsening headaches, migraines, sleep issues and the increase of depressive states. Continued anxiety and stress can cause long-term issues if not treated.

Research it

4.5 Symptoms of stress

Go to the NHS website and look at the section on stress and, in particular, the sections on 'Physical symptoms', 'Mental symptoms' and 'Changes in behaviour' (NHS, 2022b). Do you recognise any of these symptoms in yourself? If so, how will you deal with them?

AC 4.6 Analyse strategies for managing own stress and anxiety

Here, you will analyse possible strategies for managing your own stress and anxiety.

Resilience

Having good emotional health gives you the ability to cope with difficult situations and maintain a positive outlook. In traumatic circumstances you can remain focused and flexible and able to deal with adversity. This is commonly known as resilience – the ability to recognise emotions and express them appropriately while diverting depression, anxiety or other negative moods. Another factor in managing anxiety and stress is being part of a network of people that you can rely on for support and encouragement.

The notion of resilience is often used to describe an individual's ability to recover from difficult or stressful situations. While it appears to be a quality that some people possess in abundance and others lack, emotional resilience is a trait that involves actions, thoughts and behaviours that can be learned and developed by anybody.

A resilient person is generally positive, optimistic and aware of their emotions. If they fail at a task they can bounce back quickly and use the failure as feedback to do better next time.

Some effective ways to cope with stress include exercise, which helps to release endorphins and sparks positive feelings, helping others, and ensuring that you put measures in place to establish a good work–life balance.

When we are stressed or anxious we may think that smoking or alcohol will help, but this is not the case. These can make matters worse in the long term, so you should find a different way to tackle the cause of your stress. Working long hours may leave you feeling exhausted, but connecting with friends and family in social situations can help mitigate stress. Try to meet up with a friend and do not rely on social media for your connections.

Key techniques for managing stress include building your emotional strength and being in control of the situation. We cannot control everything that happens, so rather than worrying about things you cannot change, focus on what you can do instead and try to accept what you cannot control.

We discussed earlier how using mindfulness exercises and paying attention to the present moment can help you to positively change how you are feeling. If your anxiety causes you to panic then a calming breathing exercise may help. This can be accomplished standing, sitting or lying down, whatever is comfortable for you at that time. Let your breath flow deep down into your belly and try breathing in through your nose and out through your mouth. Start to breathe in gently and regularly, then count steadily from 1 to 5. Let your breath flow out gently, counting from 1 to 5 again. This type of regular breathing is calming to the mind and body.

Wellbeing and work–life balance

Taking action and making small changes to your life to increase resilience will improve mental wellbeing. You may know people who always seem able to display positivity in adversity and who are able to carry on despite difficult times. It is possible that you will also be aware of people who become very stressed when faced with challenges and who believe they cannot cope.

The fact is, we all experience hard times and painful situations. Disappointments, loss and change are part of everybody's lives, and they cause stress and anxiety even in the healthiest individuals. An individual who has good mental and emotional health will be able to cope with this anxiety and they do this by seeing the setback for what it is and by maintaining their emotional balance in dealing with it. Is this something you can teach yourself and encourage others to adopt?

Evidence opportunity

4.6 Identify and manage your stress indicators

Review some of the strategies you have learned for dealing with stress and anxiety. Analyse the strategies that work for you. What is the most useful way in which you manage your anxiety and stress?

AC 4.7 Describe how to access a range of support offers for managing own stress and anxiety

Here, you will describe ways of getting support for managing your stress and anxiety.

As a manager, it is crucial that you understand how to manage the demands of your own work and develop an appropriate work–life balance. You may also be concerned about the stress levels of others, but you must not neglect your own wellbeing needs. Think of the safety talk that is always given before a flight. Passengers are told to put on their oxygen mask first before helping others and this analogy can be applied to wellbeing too.

Ensure that you have stress management strategies for yourself in place. You can start by managing your time effectively. Seek support from colleagues if you feel overwhelmed by the work you have to do. Maybe you can delegate a task to give yourself some space. Working smarter not harder is an expression you may have heard before. Prioritising your workload and putting aside things that are not urgent is not a sign of failure. Ensure that you take breaks. You may be used to sitting at your desk for coffee and tea breaks and even for lunch. A more disciplined effort to step away from your desk and perhaps take a short walk will be useful for managing stress. Other areas of support may come from external sources, such as support groups or self-help apps and websites. There might be local groups near you to support people with anxiety. Your employer may also offer an Employer Assistance programme and you could contact these agencies for counselling. Do not underestimate the power of buddying up with a colleague or connecting with somebody at work as a mentor.

Reflect on it

4.7 Managing stress and work–life balance

Describe the range of support you have for managing your own stress and anxiety and how you can access it.

Reflect on it

4.7 Stress

Evaluate the psychological and physiological effects of work-related stress. Think about each of the areas discussed in this section and what your role as the manager is.

You might think about the psychological effects of stress that you notice in your staff. How does their anxiety affect their behaviour? How do you help them to manage this and what are the advantages and disadvantages of the strategies you suggest for them? How do they help?

References

American Psychological Association (2022) 'Resilience'. www.apa.org/topics/resilience

Cohen, S., Doyle, W.J., Turner, R.B, Alper, C.M. and Skoner, D.P. (2003) 'Emotional style and susceptibility to the common cold'. *Psychosomatic Medicine*, 65, 652–57.

Covey, S. (2004) *The 7 Habits of Highly Effective People*. New York: Simon & Schuster.

Department of Health (2014) 'Wellbeing: Why it matters to health policy'. https://assets.publishing.service.gov.uk/government/uploads/system/uploads/attachment_data/file/277566/Narrative__January_2014_.pdf

Diener, E. and Chan, M.Y. (2011) 'Happy people live longer: Subjective wellbeing contributes to health and longevity'. *Applied Psychology: Health and Wellbeing*, 3(1), 1–43.

Fowler, J.H. and Christakis, N.A. (2008) 'Dynamic spread of happiness in a large social network: Longitudinal analysis over 20 years in the Framlingham Heart Study'. *British Medical Journal*, 337, a2338. https://doi.org/10.1136/bmj.a2338

GOV.UK (2022) 'Care and support statutory guidance'. www.gov.uk/government/publications/care-act-statutory-guidance/care-and-support-statutory-guidance

Harvard (2008) 'What to do about social anxiety disorder'. www.health.harvard.edu/newsletter_article/What_to_do_about_social_anxiety_disorder

Maben, J., Peccei, R., Adams, M., Robert, G., Richardson, A., Murrells, T. and Morrow, E. (2012) *Exploring the relationship between patients' experiences of care and the influence of staff motivation, affect and wellbeing*, National Institute for Health Research Service Delivery and Organisation Programme.

Mayo Clinic, The (2017) 'Generalized anxiety disorder'. www.mayoclinic.org/diseases-conditions/generalized-anxiety-disorder/symptoms-causes/syc-20360803

NHS (2020) 'Get running with Couch to 5K'. www.nhs.uk/live-well/exercise/running-and-aerobic-exercises/get-running-with-couch-to-5k/

NHS (2022a) '5 steps to mental wellbeing'. www.nhs.uk/mental-health/self-help/guides-tools-and-activities/five-steps-to-mental-wellbeing/

NHS (2022b) 'Stress'. www.nhs.uk/mental-health/feelings-symptoms-behaviours/feelings-and-symptoms/stress/

Office for National Statistics (2012) 'Measuring national well-being, education and skills'. https://webarchive.nationalarchives.gov.uk/ukgwa/20160105160709/http://www.ons.gov.uk/ons/dcp171766_268091.pdf

Office for National Statistics (2018) 'Surveys using our four personal well-being questions'. www.ons.gov.uk/peoplepopulationandcommunity/wellbeing/methodologies/surveysusingthe4officefornationalstatisticspersonalwellbeingquestions

Office for National Statistics (2019) 'Measures of national well-being dashboard'. www.ons.gov.uk/peoplepopulationandcommunity/wellbeing/articles/measuresofnationalwellbeingdashboard/2018-04-25

Raleigh, V.S., Hussey, D., Seccombe, I. and Qi, R. (2009) 'Do associations between staff and inpatient feedback have the potential for improving patient experience? An analysis of surveys in NHS acute trusts in England'. *Quality and Safety in Health Care*, 18(5), 347–54.

Thin, N. (2010) *Social Happiness – Theory into Policy and Practice*. Bristol: The Policy Press.

What Works Wellbeing (n.d.) 'What affects our wellbeing?' https://whatworkswellbeing.org/about-wellbeing/what-affects-wellbeing/

World Health Organization (n.d.) 'Self-care interventions for health'. www.who.int/health-topics/self-care#tab=tab_1

Useful resources and further reading

De Neve, Diener, Tay and Xuereb (2013) 'The objective benefits of Subjective Wellbeing' in Helliwell, J., Layard, R. and Sachs, J. (eds.) *World Happiness Report 2013*. New York: UN Sustainable Development Solutions Network. https://ssrn.com/abstract=2306651

Kiecolt-Glaser, Marucha, Malarkey, Mercado & Glaser (1995). 'Slowing of wound healing by psychological stress'. *The Lancet*, 346, 1194–96. www.thelancet.com/pdfs/journals/lancet/PIIS0140-6736(95)92899-5.pdf

Mind. www.mind.org.uk/

Glossary

6Cs: These are the values that underpin social care – care, compassion, commitment, communication, courage and competence.

Accountable: Taking responsibility and being liable or answerable for something.

Action orientation: A type of leadership in which practical action is taken to deal with a problem or situation.

Active listening: A way of listening and responding to improve understanding. It involves skill in questioning, clarifying, summarising, reflecting, paying attention to body language, offering encouraging verbal cues and refraining from judgement.

Active participation: In this context, this refers to enabling individuals to be included in their care and to be able to voice how they wish to live their life and obtain their own care.

Advance directive: Also known as a living will, this is a legal document that specifies what actions should be taken for a person if they cannot make decisions for themselves because of illness or incapacity.

Advocate: An individual who acts for or on behalf of another, particularly if the person lacks capacity in some way or simply requires help to speak out.

Agreed ways of working: Procedures and policies that workers in an organisation are required to follow.

Appraisal: A process where employees and line managers discuss their performance, developmental needs and the support they need in their role. It is used to provide evidence and evaluation of recent performance and focus on future goals, opportunities and resources. Sometimes referred to as performance appraisal.

Authoritarian/autocratic: Having total authority and control over decision making; keeping everything under close scrutiny.

Care Quality Commission (CQC): The independent regulator and lead inspection and enforcement body for all social care services in England.

Change management: A systematic approach to dealing with the transition or transformation of an organisation's goals, processes or technologies. The purpose of change management is to implement strategies for effecting change, controlling change and helping people to adapt to change.

Collaboration: The practice of care professionals working in partnership with individuals and members of the public to improve health outcomes.

Consent: To give permission for something to happen. It may be verbal, written or implied but always needs to be obtained.

Contingency theories: A theory that suggests there is no single best style of leadership; the leader's effectiveness will depend on the situation.

Continuing professional development (CPD): The planned process of improving and increasing capabilities of staff. It is an ongoing process and includes training and education activities to ensure that staff remain fit to practise.

Continuous quality improvement: Continual actions to improve the outcomes for individuals and to develop the workforce.

Co-production: Working in partnership and sharing power between people who require care and support. It includes carers, families and citizens.

Critical incident: An unintended event that occurs when an individual in care is involved in something that results in a consequence to them; for example, a fall.

Democratic/participative: Sharing type of leadership in which employees' participation in the decision making is favoured.

Disclosure: Making new or secret information known.

Discrimination: Treating people unfairly or unlawfully because they have a disability, or are of a different race, gender or age, for example.

Diversity: In this context, means equal respect for people who are from different backgrounds.

Diversity champions: People in your organisation who drive inclusion and diversity objectives and make sure they are achieved. Champions are responsible for supporting and developing the equality, diversity and inclusion agenda.

Duty of Candour: Requires providers to be open and transparent with individuals about their care and treatment. If treatment goes wrong, the care provider must inform the individual about the incident, provide support and offer an apology.

Emotional intelligence: Being aware of and having the ability to control your emotions in order to manage interpersonal relationships empathetically (i.e. thinking about and understanding how others are feeling and seeing things from their point of view).

Empathy: Being able to understand and share the feelings of another person or having the ability to experience another person's condition from their perspective.

Empowerment: Giving someone authority.

Equality: Treating individuals or groups of individuals fairly and equally irrespective of race, gender, disability, religion or belief, sexual orientation and age.

Evidence-based practice: Refers to using information from high-quality research and applying it within practice to make informed decisions about an individual's care.

Experiential learning: The process of learning through experience.

Feedback: An open two-way communication between two or more parties.

Golden thread: A description of how an organisation's goals, vision and values link together to inform its processes.

Governance procedures: Monitoring actions, practices and policies which guide the decisions of organisations and their stakeholders.

Harassment: Unwanted behaviour towards another person that is designed to intimidate or degrade.

Imposter syndrome: Feelings of doubt that a person might experience about their abilities, which can lead them to feel like a fraud or assume that their success is due to luck rather than talent. People suffering from imposter syndrome often feel that they are underqualified or lacking in ability to do their job properly.

Inclusion: Exhibiting positive behaviour to ensure that all people have an opportunity to be included and not excluded because of their individual characteristics.

Inclusion health groups: People who are socially excluded and who often have overlapping risk factors, such as poverty, violence and complex trauma. They include people who experience homelessness, drug and alcohol dependence, vulnerable migrants, Gypsy, Roma and Traveller communities, sex workers, people in contact with the justice system and victims of modern slavery.

Interlinked work: Work that is connected and has similar objectives.

Key performance indicator (KPI): A way to measure performance over time for a specific objective or target. KPIs state what must be achieved and when and can be used to assess and manage performance.

Laissez faire: Leadership style that favours leaving things to take their own course, without interference.

Lasting Power of Attorney (LPA): A legal document that allows anybody over the age of 18 to appoint one or more people to support the decision-making process should the individual become unable to do so. The person must have the mental capacity to undertake this step.

LGBTQIA+: Stands for lesbian, gay, bisexual, transgender, queer/questioning, intersex, asexual and other terms (such as non-binary and pansexual).

Liberty Protection Safeguards (LPS): Introduced in the Mental Capacity (Amendment) Act 2019, these will provide protection for people aged 16 and over who lack the capacity to give consent to arrangements for their care or treatment and who need to be deprived of their liberty in order for that care or treatment to be given. They will replace the DoLS and provide a less bureaucratic system.

Line reports: Members of staff who report to you.

Microaggressions: Subtle and indirect statements or incidences of discrimination against a particular group.

Multidisciplinary groups: Groups of people with different specialist skills. For example, the group may have people with medical and care expertise and others with specialist knowledge of housing and other services.

Multidisciplinary team (MDT): One in which care professionals from a range of disciplines and organisations work together to deliver streamlined care to individuals.

Objective measures: Examine the factors that affect someone's life; they include measures of education, employment, health, housing, income and environmental quality, which can be used to monitor how people feel and function.

Objective wellbeing: This is based on material, quantitative indicators and is measured by what people have in society. Educational opportunity, housing and the built environment in which a person lives, being part of a community and having enough money are all indicators of objective wellbeing.

Obligation: An action or restraint from action that a person is morally or legally bound to owe to (an)other(s).

Ordinary Power of Attorney (OPA): A temporary arrangement that allows a person to nominate an attorney to undertake financial decisions while they are temporarily incapacitated.

Outcomes-focused care: An outcomes-based approach is similar to person-centred care in that people should be at the centre of their own care and support planning. By identifying what is important to their lives, and ensuring that the person's independence and quality of life is maximised, everyone involved in the support works together, actively listening to the person without judgement. This differs from the task-based approach, which concentrated on meeting task targets. This was previously common but is gradually being replaced.

Partnership working: The use of inclusive and mutually beneficial relationships in care work that improve the quality and experience of care. It refers to the relationships between individuals, their carers, service providers and care professionals.

Perception awareness: The ability to recognise how and what we are communicating to others through our non-verbal communication.

Person-centred practice: A way of working that recognises the complexity and unique nature of individuals and places them at the centre of the care given, respecting their needs, preferences and knowledge.

Policy: A plan or principle of action proposed by an organisation, also known as a guideline or code.

Policy drivers: Documents, research, laws and information that can lead to change in practice and drive forward new procedures and ways of working.

Positive risk taking: Identifying the potential risks and then developing plans and actions that reflect the potential benefits and harm of exercising one course of action over another. It is a way of seeing the risk in a positive way that enhances the quality of life for an individual.

Prejudice: An unreasonable, preconceived judgement or opinion that is not based on knowledge, evidence or experience.

Presenteeism: Being at work for more hours than is required, or when ill, because of insecurity about one's job.

Procedures: These state how policies will be carried out or actioned in a setting.

Protocol: A set of rules that explains the correct procedure to be followed in a situation.

Psychological safety: The 'absence of interpersonal fear' or the ability to speak out at work without fear of reprisal.

Qualitative data: Collected through interviews and observations, this type of information is descriptive and will try to find a meaning in certain phenomena.

Quantitative data: Data that is numerical in nature. It will answer questions such as 'how much' or 'how many'.

Reflective practice: The act of stopping and thinking about what you are doing in practice and analysing the decisions you make in the light of theory and the things you have learned. By doing this you are more able to relate theory to practice, helping you to generate new knowledge and ideas.

Regulation: A rule or order that is underpinned by law. In care settings, apart from those concerned with health and safety care, regulations with respect to health protection and control of disease are also available.

Risk management: Forecasting potential risks and taking steps to minimise or avoid them altogether. Your policies should identify how you undertake risk assessment in your area and how you intend to manage risks that arise.

Safeguarding: The CQC defines this as 'protecting people's health, wellbeing and human rights, and enabling them to live free from harm, abuse and neglect. It is fundamental to high-quality health and social care'.

Safeguarding Adults Reviews: Previously known as serious case reviews, these take place after a person is seriously injured or dies, particularly if abuse or neglect is thought to have been a causative factor. It looks at what might be learned from the occurrence in order to help prevent similar incidents from happening in the future.

Self-awareness: The ability to notice the self and to be able to recognise our behaviour and personality.

Serious case review: This takes place after a person who should be safeguarded is seriously injured or dies, particularly if abuse or neglect is thought to have been a causative factor. It looks at what can be learned from the situation to help prevent similar incidents in the future. Serious case reviews are now known as Safeguarding Adults Reviews (SARs).

Service delivery teams: Teams within multidisciplinary groups such as the primary care team, social care team, hospital, housing and other services used within your own setting.

SMART: Targets that are specific, measurable, achievable, realistic/relevant and time bound.

Social care providers: Care providers who operate on one or more sites; these settings vary and can range from individuals' homes to specialised care settings to hospitals.

Socialisation: The process through which we are taught the norms, customs, roles, values and beliefs of our society. We are socialised first into our own families and communities and this is termed primary socialisation. Secondary socialisation occurs when we enter the education system or have contact with religion and the media.

Stigma: This implies that a characteristic held by some people or groups deviates from social expectations. For example, some people will not admit to being depressed because of the stigma of mental illness in society.

Subjective measures: Measure what people say about how they are feeling. Standardised daily self-reports on symptoms and feelings can be used to measure how individuals are feeling at any given time.

Subjective wellbeing: This relates to how an individual feels and how satisfied with life they are. Levels of subjective wellbeing are influenced by internal factors, such as personality and outlook on life but also external factors, such as the society in which an individual lives. Also referred to as personal wellbeing.

Systems leadership: How the best resources from other settings and disciplines can be used to bring about improvement and beneficial change across partnership systems in other organisations. The style of leadership is characterised by a belief that leadership is the responsibility of teams, rather than individuals, and is collaborative in nature.

Training needs analysis: Determines the current knowledge, skills and abilities of all staff and identifies the gaps that might need to be filled to strengthen the organisation. It is the process of identifying training needs to improve staff job performance.

Unconscious bias: Holding unfavourable or unreasonable beliefs and views about other people that are outside our conscious awareness and control.

Voluntary sector providers: These are part of charitable trusts or groups who simply volunteer services to support social care services.

Warning notice: This is issued when the quality of care falls below what is legally required. A section 29 warning notice for all types of regulated provider is issued in writing when there has been regulation breach. A warning notice will state the relevant regulation that has been breached or the section of the Act or condition that is not being complied with and what further action will be taken and in what timescale if compliance is not met.

Whistle blowing: Making a disclosure or revealing information that is in the public interest.

Workforce planning: Allocating staff with the necessary skills to a task when they are needed in order to deliver organisational objectives.

Work–life balance: Giving equal priority to the demands of work and the demands of our personal life.

Index

D

E

F

G

H

I

K

L

M

N

O

P